RADIOGRAPHY PREP

EDITION

10

D.A. Saia, MA, RT(R)(M)
Radiography Educator and Consultant
Adjunct Professor, Manhattanville College
Purchase, New York

McGraw Hill

New York   Chicago   San Francisco   Athens   London   Madrid   Mexico City
Milan   New Delhi   Singapore   Sydney   Toronto

Radiography PREP, Program Review and Exam Preparation, Tenth Edition

1 2 3 4 5 6 7 8 9 LWI 28 27 26 25 24 23

ISBN: 978-1-264-69253-8
MHID: 1-264-69253-6

Notice

Medicine is an ever-changing science. As new research and clinical experience broaden our knowledge, changes in treatment and drug therapy are required. The author and the publisher of this work have checked with sources believed to be reliable in their efforts to provide information that is complete and generally in accord with the standards accepted at the time of publication. However, in view of the possibility of human error or changes in medical sciences, neither the author nor the publisher nor any other party who has been involved in the preparation or publication of this work warrants that the information contained herein is in every respect accurate or complete, and they disclaim all responsibility for any errors or omissions or for the results obtained from use of the information contained in this work. Readers are encouraged to confirm the information contained herein with other sources. For example and in particular, readers are advised to check the product information sheet included in the package of each drug they plan to administer to be certain that the information contained in this work is accurate and that changes have not been made in the recommended dose or in the contraindications for administration. This recommendation is of particular importance in connection with new or infrequently used drugs.

This book was set in Minion Pro by Graphic World, Inc.
The editors were Dana Thimons and Christina M. Thomas.
The production supervisor was Richard Ruzycka.
Project management was provided by Graphic World, Inc.

Library of Congress Cataloging-in-Publication Data

Names: Saia, D. A. (Dorothy A.), author.
Title: Radiography PREP : program review and exam prep / D.A. Saia.
Description: Edition 10. | New York : McGraw Hill LLC, [2024] | Includes bibliographical references and index. | Summary: "Hailed by Doody's Review Service as "the gold standard among instructors and students," Radiography PREP delivers a concise summary of the entire radiography curriculum in a readable narrative. Written by an experienced program director, this is a true "must read" for certification or recertification. Readers will find more than 900 ARRT-style review questions with detailed answer explanations for correct and incorrect answers, a practice exam, hundreds of illustrations and radiographic images, and powerful learning aids such as summary boxes and a glossary"— Provided by publisher.
Identifiers: LCCN 2023015406 (print) | LCCN 2023015407 (ebook) | ISBN 9781264692538 (paperback) | ISBN 1264692536 (paperback) | ISBN 9781264693054 (ebook)
Subjects: MESH: Radiography | Technology, Radiologic | Examination Questions
Classification: LCC RC78.15 (print) | LCC RC78.15 (ebook) | NLM WN 18.2 | DDC 616.07/572—dc23/eng/20230510
LC record available at https://lccn.loc.gov/2023015406
LC ebook record available at https://lccn.loc.gov/2023015407

McGraw Hill books are available at special quantity discounts to use as premiums and sales promotions, or for use in corporate training programs. To contact a representative, please visit the Contact Us pages at www.mhprofessional.com.

Dedication
Spiritus Sancti gratia, illuminet sensus et corda nostra.

CONTRIBUTORS

Thai Chan-Grullon, MS, RT(R)(CT)(M)(ARRT)
Program Director and Clinical Assistant Professor
Radiologic Technology
Manhattanville College
Purchase, New York

Jayme A. Scheckler, MS, RT(R)(ARRT)
Adjunct Professor
Radiologic Technology
Manhattanville College
Purchase, New York

Gregory Torsiello, MS, RT(R)(CT)(ARRT)
Assistant Director and Assistant Professor
Radiologic Sciences
St. John's University
Queens, New York

REVIEWERS

Daniel Fink, MBA, RT(R)(CT)
Radiography Program Director
Division Director of Allied Health
Galveston College
Galveston, Texas

Idamae Jenkins, MA, RT(R)
Clinical Coordinator, Radiologic Technology
Radiologic Sciences & Imaging Program
Kettering College
Kettering, Ohio

Olive Peart, MS, RT(R)(M)
Radiologic Technology Program Chair
Fortis College
Landover, Maryland

CONTENTS

Preface .... *xi*

Acknowledgments .... *xiii*

Master Bibliography .... *xv*

I. PATIENT CARE 1

1. Ethical and Legal Aspects 3
   Chapter Review Questions *13*

2. Interpersonal Communication 17
   Chapter Review Questions *26*

3. Ergonomics, Monitoring, and Medical Emergencies............. 29
   Chapter Review Questions *49*

4. Infection Prevention and Control 53
   Chapter Review Questions *66*

5. Pharmacology 69
   Chapter Review Questions *83*

II. PROCEDURES 87

6. General Procedural Considerations 89
   Chapter Review Questions *102*

7. Anatomy, Positioning, and Pathology 105
   Chapter Review Questions *234*

III. SAFETY 247

8. Radiation Physics and Radiobiology 249
   Chapter Review Questions *270*

9. Patient Protection 273
   Chapter Review Questions *290*

10. Personnel Protection 293
    Chapter Review Questions *304*

11. Radiation Exposure and Monitoring 307
    Chapter Review Questions *319*

IV. IMAGE PRODUCTION 321

12. Image Acquisition and Technical Evaluation.................... 323
    Chapter Review Questions *357*
    Chapter Review Questions *376*

13. Equipment Operation and Quality Assurance 381
    Chapter Review Questions *399*
    Chapter Review Questions *418*
    Chapter Review Questions *432*
    Chapter Review Questions *442*
    Chapter Review Questions *461*

Chapter Review Questions..*475*

Chapter Review Questions..*490*

Chapter Review Questions..*502*

V. PRACTICE TEST **505**

14. Practice Test **507**

Index..*561*

This 10th edition of *Radiography PREP* is intended to be useful throughout all phases of radiography education. This text is designed to be useful for regular coursework, helping the student to extract fundamental key concepts from reading assignments and class notes. Its use will make study and test preparation easier and more productive.

Radiography PREP is also useful for students preparing for their American Registry of Radiologic Technologists (ARRT®) certification examination. It helps students direct their study efforts toward examination-related material and includes registry-type multiple-choice questions designed to help them practice test taking and critical thinking skills they will need for the ARRT radiography examination—and for their professional careers.

The ARRT's Content Specifications for the Examination in Radiography list the examination's four content categories and provide a detailed list of the topics addressed in each category. *Radiography PREP* is divided into four parts reflecting each of the four examination content categories. Part content reflects changes to the ARRT Content Specifications approved by the ARRT board in January 2021 and implemented in January 2022. The Safety and Image Production sections have each been divided into two separate sections for more focused study. Some basic introductory CT material is also included—an area becoming increasingly important for the entry-level radiographer. As this field continues to grow, there is increasing need to include its fundamentals in the radiography curriculum. Particularly important is updated and expanded content in digital imaging. Obsolete content on radiographic film and intensifying screens have been deleted. SI units are used exclusively, with occasional equivalent traditional unit of measure provided for reference. Thus, study becomes even more directed and focused on examination-related material.

A *series* of tools is available for effective coursework study followed by preparation for the certification test. *Radiography PREP* is recommended for use with regular coursework. Used with its companion book, *Lange Q&A Radiography Examination, Radiography PREP*, provides a thorough preparation for the certification examination administered by the ARRT. Finally, certification examination preparation can be extended to include the computerized testing, RadReview, offered at the website https://www.radreviewmhe.com.

KEY FEATURES AND USE

- More than 400 ***illustrations and images*** appeal to the visual learner as well as the verbal learner. The essence of radiography is visual, and the graphics and radiographic images given in *Radiography PREP* visually express the written words. This new edition is now in full color.

- The numerous ***summary boxes*** serve to call the student's attention to the most important facts in a particular section. Students can use summary boxes as an overview of key information.

- ***Inside covers*** list a number of formulae, radiation protection facts, conversion factors, body surface landmarks, digital imaging facts, acronyms and abbreviations, radiation quality factors, and minimum filtration requirements. A "last-minute cheat sheet" is provided for some things that students often forget because they may not use them on a regular basis.

- The ***final review sections*** allow students to assess chapter material in two ways. The first review section, ***Comprehension Check,*** requires short essay answers; exact page references follow each question, providing answers in chapter material. The second section, ***Chapter Review Questions***, consists of registry-type multiple-choice questions followed by detailed explanations. To make the most of their study efforts, students are encouraged to review in that order: Comprehension Check first, followed by the multiple-choice questions.

- Chapter 13 (Equipment Operation and Quality Assurance) in Part IV, includes a section on Computed Tomography. As this field continues to grow, there is increasing emphasis on at least fundamental concepts in the radiography curriculum.

- Part V is Practice Test; a simulation of the actual certification examination with questions designed to test your problem-solving skills and your ability to integrate facts that fit the situation. The questions are designed to provide focus and direction for your review, thus helping you do your very best on your certification examination.

Following completion of the Chapter Review Questions and the Practice Test, the student is ready for final self-evaluation by answering even more "registry-type" questions in the companion text, *Lange Q&A Radiography Examination*, 12th Edition, and supplemental study at the RadReview's website https://www.radreviewmhe.com.

ACKNOWLEDGMENTS

I am grateful to those who have generously contributed their insight and expertise to this project. Foremost among those are my teachers and colleagues who have contributed to my knowledge over the years and the many students on whom I have had the privilege of sharpening my knowledge and skills.

This 10th edition of *Radiography PREP* has been enhanced by the participation of three contributors; Thai Chan-Grullon, Greg Torsiello, and Jayme Scheckler have provided valuable updates and contributions. Working with these educators has been a rewarding experience for me, and their participation is greatly appreciated. An outstanding group of reviewers was recruited for this edition of *Radiography PREP*. Daniel Fink, Idamae Jenkins, and Olive Peart are invaluable resources to the health care and the radiologic imaging communities. They reviewed the manuscript and offered suggestions to improve style and remove ambiguities and inaccuracies. Their participation in this project is deeply appreciated.

Review, updates, and supplemental information about venipuncture in Chapter 5 were graciously provided by Clinton Vass, RT(R)(CT).

Richard M. Kovatch, RT(R) generously supplied equipment photographs.

It has been a pleasure to once again work with several of the product providers in our Radiology Imaging community. A huge measure of gratitude goes to Rob Fabrizio, Gregg Cretella, and Douglas Young of FUJIFILM Healthcare Americas Corp. They responded to endless emails and questions, and provided many valuable illustrations for this text.

Carol Locke at Shielding International was so helpful obtaining color images and expediting permission for their use.

Tiffani Frey and Dana Banks of Landauer as well as Dan Wold and Lena Hansson of RaySafe, a division of Fluke Electronics Corporation, were all incredibly helpful and patient in providing figures and obtaining permission for this edition.

Melanie Fayta, Joe Sorci, and Dan Galanti of TIDI Products, LLC, graciously provided color images and permission to use their images.

Much appreciation goes to Laura Jensen of Mirion Technologies Inc., for obtaining updated photos of their product and permission for their use in this text.

The professional staff of McGraw Hill have again supported and guided me through this project. Much appreciation is extended to Bob Boehringer, Dana Thimons, Lior Raz-Farley, Christina Thomas, Rachel Norton, and Richard Ruzycka. Their confidence and support are truly appreciated. A note of gratitude to Jason McAlexander of MPS North America LLC, who once again shared his art expertise. Sunil Kumar of GW Tech was the Production Manager for this project. This project could not have been completed without his patience and his help keeping me organized. Thank you, Sunil!

I also extend my appreciation to Conrad P. Ehrlich, MD, for granting permission to use several radiologic images. The CT section in Chapter 13 could not have been accomplished without the help of several individuals; I am grateful to Sarah Bull, MS, DABR; Angie Dohan, RT(R); Conrad Ehrlich, MD; Paula Hill, RT(R)(CT)(CV)(M); Doug Schueler, RT(R)(CT); and Teresa Whiteside, BA, RT(R)(BD)(CT)(CBDT).

The preparation of previous editions was always made easier by the loving encouragement and support of my late husband, Tony. Happy memories endure, and the work of this edition is performed in loving memory of him.

Adler AM, Carlton RR, Stewart K. *Introduction to Radiologic and Imaging Sciences and Patient Care.* 8th ed. St. Louis, MO: Saunders Elsevier; 2023.

ARRT Standards of Ethics. https://assets-us-01.kc-usercontent.com/406ac8c6-58e8-00b3-e3c1-0c312965deb2/6bf7867c-b0fa-4773-ae18-2ebd78023931/arrt-standards-of-ethics.pdf Published September 1, 2022

ASRT Practice Standards. https://www.asrt.org/main/standards-and-regulations/professional-practice/practice-standards-online

Bushong SC. *Radiologic Science for Technologists.* 12th ed. St. Louis, MO: Mosby; 2021.

Carlton RR, Adler AM, Balac V. *Principles of Radiographic Imaging.* 6th ed. Albany, NY: Delmar; 2020.

Carroll QB. *Radiography in the Digital Age.* 3rd ed. Springfield, IL: Charles C Thomas; 2018.

Carter C, Vealé B. *Digital Radiography and PACS.* 3rd ed. St. Louis, MO: Mosby Elsevier; 2019.

Dutton AG, Ryan TA. *Torres' Patient Care in Imaging Technology.* 9th ed. Philadelphia, PA: Lippincott; 2019.

Ehrlich RA, Coakes DM. *Patient Care in Radiography.* 10th ed. St. Louis, MO: Mosby; 2021.

Lampignano JP, Kendrick LE. *Bontrager's Textbook of Radiographic Positioning and Related Anatomy.* 10th ed. St. Louis, MO: Mosby Elsevier; 2021.

Long BW, Rollins JH, Smith BJ. *Merrill's Atlas of Radiographic Positioning and Procedures.* Vols 1-3. 14th ed. St. Louis, MO: Mosby; 2019.

Mills WR. e relation of bodily habitus to visceral form, tonus, and motility. *Am J Roentgenol.* 1917;4:155–169.

NCRP Report No. 184. *Medical Radiation Exposure of Patients in the United States.* NCRP; 2019

NCRP Report No. 102. *Medical x-ray, Electron Beam and Gamma-Ray Protection for Energies up to 50 MeV* (Equipment Design, Performance and Use). NCRP; 1989.

NCRP Report No. 116. *Recommendations on Limits for Exposure to Ionizing Radiation.* NCRP; 1987.

NCRP Report No. 160. *Ionizing Radiation Exposure of the Population of the United States.* NCRP; 2009.

NCRP Report No. 99. *Quality Assurance for Diagnostic Imaging.* NCRP; 1990.

Peart O. *Lange Radiographic Positioning Flashcards.* New York, NY: McGraw-Hill; 2014.

Peart O. *Mammography and Breast Imaging PREP.* 3rd ed New York, NY: McGraw-Hill; 2022.

Saia DA. *Radiography PREP.* 9th ed. New York, NY: McGraw-Hill; 2018.

Saladin KS. *Anatomy and Physiology: e Unity of Form and Function.* 7th ed. New York, NY: McGraw-Hill; 2015.

Seeram E, Brennan PC. *Radiation Protection in Diagnostic X-ray Imaging.* Burlington, MA: Jones and Bartlett Learning; 2017.

Seeram E. *Digital Radiography: An Introduction.* Clifton Park, NY: Delmar Cengage Learning; 2011.

Selman J. *The Fundamentals of Imaging Physics and Radiobiology.* 9th ed. Springfield, IL: Charles C Thomas; 2000.

Statkiewicz-Sherer MA, Visconti PJ, Ritenour ER, Haynes KW. *Radiation Protection in Medical Radiography.* 9th ed. St. Louis, MO: Mosby; 2022.

Takahiro KAWAMURA*, Satoshi NAITO*, Kayo OKANO* and Masahiko YAMADA*. *Improvement in Image Quality and Workflow of X-ray Examinations Using a New Image Processing Method, Virtual Grid Technology.*

White Victor. *Selman's The Fundamentals of Imaging Physics and Radiobiology.* 10th ed. Springfield, IL: Charles C Thomas; 2020.

*Imaging Technology Center, Research & Development Management Headquarters, FUJIFILM Corporation

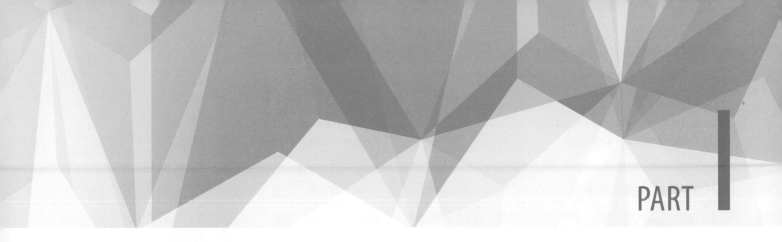

PART I

Patient Care

CHAPTER 1
Ethical and Legal Aspects
Patients' Rights
  Patient Confidentiality
  Informed Consent
  Patients' Bill of Rights/Patient Care Partnership
Legal Issues
  X-ray Examination Requests
  Law/Medicolegal Issues
Standards of Ethics
  ARRT Standards of Ethics
  Honor Code

CHAPTER 2
Interpersonal Communication
Communication Skills
Types of Communication
Communication With Patients
  Patient Identification
  Verbal/Written and Nonverbal Communication
  Patient Education
  Examination Instructions
Communication Challenges
  Impediments
  Medical Terminology
  Strategies to Improve Communication

CHAPTER 3
Ergonomics, Monitoring, and Medical Emergencies
Physical Assistance and Transfer
  Body Mechanics
  Ergonomic Transfer Devices
  Patient Safety and Transfer Considerations

Patient Support Equipment
  Oxygen
  Suction
  Tubes and Catheters
Patient Monitoring and Documentation
  Assessment
  Physical Signs
  Vital Signs
  Documentation
Medical Emergencies
  Allergic Reactions
  Latex
  Anaphylactic Responses
  Renal Function
Other Medical Emergencies
  Vomiting
  Fractures
  Spinal Injuries
  Epistaxis
  Postural Hypotension
  Vertigo
  Syncope
  Convulsion
  Seizure
  Unconsciousness
  Acute Abdomen
  Shock
  Respiratory Failure
  Cardiopulmonary Arrest
  Stroke

CHAPTER 4
Infection Prevention and Control

Terminology and Basic Concepts
    Microorganisms
    Pathogens
    Medical and Surgical Asepsis
    Hand Hygiene
    Personal Care
    Chain of Infection
CDC Standard Precautions
    Infection Prevention and Control: Basic Guidelines
    Health Care–Associated Infections
    Transmission-Based Precautions

CHAPTER 5
Pharmacology

Patient History
Administration
    Routes of Administration
    Equipment
    Venipuncture
Contrast Media
    Patient History
    Purpose
    Types and Properties of Agents
    Scheduling and Preparation Considerations
    Contraindications and Patient Education
Reactions and Complications
    Local Effects
    Systemic Effects
    Laboratory Values and Medications
    Documentation

Ethical and Legal Aspects

OBJECTIVES

At the conclusion of this chapter, the student will be able to:

- Discuss the ethics relative to behavior and values, and their relationship to the health care professions.
- Identify the acronym HIPAA and discuss that legislation's impact on patient information.
- Identify the purpose of an Advance Health Care Directive and its impact on patient autonomy and decision-making.
- Discuss the radiographer's responsibilities regarding patient examination requests.
- Describe examples of potential professional negligence.
- List the parts of the ARRT® Standards of Ethics.
- Identify where guidelines for the radiographer's professional conduct can be found.

Ethics refers to a set of principles of *right and wrong behavior*, a system of *values* that guides conduct in relationships among people in accordance with expected patterns of behavior. Ethical conduct is particularly important in the health care professions. The effects of our actions and/or behavior can harm others, put them at risk for harm, or violate their rights.

> ### Ethical Behavior
>
> - The effects of our actions and/or behavior can harm others, put them at risk for harm, or violate their rights.

PATIENTS' RIGHTS

Patient Confidentiality

Most institutions now have computerized, paperless systems (known as hospital information systems or HIS) to accomplish information transmittal; these systems must ensure *confidentiality* in compliance with Health Insurance Portability and Accountability Act (HIPAA) of 1996 regulations. A health care professional generally has access to a computerized system only via a personal password, thus helping ensure confidentiality of patient information. All medical records and other individually identifiable health information—whether electronic, on paper, or oral—are covered by HIPAA legislation and by subsequent Department of Health and Human Services (HHS) rules that took effect in April 2001.

All health care practitioners must recognize that their patients comprise a community of people belonging to different religions, races, and economic backgrounds, and that each patient must be afforded their best efforts. Every patient should be treated with consideration of his or her worth and dignity. Patients must be provided *confidentiality* and *privacy*. They have the right to be informed, to make *informed consent*, and to refuse treatment.

Informed Consent

Patient *consent* could be verbal, informed, or implied. For example, if a patient arrives for emergency treatment alone and is unconscious, implied consent is assumed. A patient's previously granted or implied consent can be withdrawn at any time. Informed patient consent is required before any examination that involves greater than the usual risk, for example, invasive vascular examinations requiring the use of injected iodinated contrast agents. Adequate informed consent includes associated risks of the procedure and any alternative treatments. For lower risk procedures, the consent given on admission to the hospital is generally sufficient.

It is imperative that the radiographer takes adequate time to thoroughly *explain* the procedure or examination to the patient. An informed patient is a more cooperative patient, and a better examination is more likely to result. Patients should be clear about what is expected of them and what to expect from the radiographer. This must be considered the *standard of care* for each patient, to fulfill not only legal mandates but also professional and humanistic obligations.

Patients' Bill of Rights/Patient Care Partnership

The American Hospital Association's (AHA's) Management Advisory presented a *Patients' Bill of Rights* that was first adopted by the AHA in 1973, then revised and approved by the AHA Board of Trustees in October 1992. The 1992 Patients' Bill of Rights detailed 12 specific areas of patients' rights and the health care professional's ethical (and often, legal) responsibility to adhere to these rights. The Patients' Bill of Rights is summarized as *the right to*

1. considerate and respectful care
2. be informed completely and understandably
3. make decisions about plan of care/refuse treatment
4. have an advance directive (e.g., a living will, health care proxy) describing the extent of care desired
5. privacy
6. confidentiality
7. review his or her records (access to his or her health care information)
8. request appropriate and medically indicated care and services

---

Conditions for Valid Patient Consent

- The patient must be of legal age.
- The patient must be of sound mind.
- The patient must give consent freely.
- The patient must be adequately informed about the procedure about to take place.

9. know about institutional business relationships that could influence treatment and care

10. be informed about, consent to, or decline participation in proposed research studies

11. continuity of care

12. be informed about hospital policies and procedures relating to patient care, treatment, and responsibilities

The AHA replaced the Patients' Bill of Rights with *The Patient Care Partnership—Understanding Expectations, Rights, and Responsibilities.* Their plain-language brochure includes the essentials of the Bill of Rights and reviews what patients can/should expect during a hospital stay.

The Patient Care Partnership statement addresses *high-quality hospital care*—combining skill, compassion, and respect and the right to know the identity of caregivers, whether they are students, residents, or other trainees. It includes *a clean and safe environment*, free from neglect and abuse, and information about anything unexpected that occurred during the hospital stay. The Patient Care Partnership identifies *involvement in your care;* it elaborates on patient discussion/understanding of their condition and treatment choices with their physician, the patient's responsibility to provide complete and correct information to the caregiver and understanding who should make decisions for the patient if the patient cannot make those decisions (including "living will" or "advance directive").

The Patient Care Partnership statement also identifies *protection of your privacy*—describing the ways in which patient information is safeguarded. It also describes *help when leaving the hospital*—availability of and/or instruction regarding follow-up care. Finally, the Patient Care Partnership statement addresses *help with your billing claims*—including filing claims with insurance companies, providing patient physicians with required documentation, answering patient questions, and assisting those without health coverage.

The above-mentioned patient rights can be exercised on the patient's behalf by a *designated surrogate or proxy* decision maker if the patient lacks the decision-making capacity, is legally incompetent, or is a minor. Many people believe that potential legal and ethical issues can be avoided by creating an *Advance Health Care Directive* or *Living Will.* Because all individuals have the right to make decisions regarding their own health care, this legal document preserves that right in the event an individual is unable to make those decisions. An Advance Health Care Directive, or Living Will, names the individual authorized to make all health care decisions and can include specifics regarding *DNR* (do not resuscitate), *DNI* (do not intubate), and/or other end-of-life decisions.

The Patient Care Partnership

What to expect during your hospital stay:

1. High-quality hospital care
2. A clean and safe environment
3. Involvement in your care
4. Protection of your privacy
5. Help when leaving the hospital
6. Help with your billing claims

Source: The American Hospital Association.

Advance Health Care Directive/Living Will

- Preserves a person's right to make decisions regarding his or her own health care
- Names the individual authorized to make all health care decisions for them
- Can include specifics regarding DNR, DNI, and other end-of-life decisions

---

LEGAL ISSUES

It is essential that radiographers, like other health care professionals, should be familiar with their *Practice Standards* published by the American Society of Radiologic Technologists (ASRT). The Standards provide a *legal role definition* and identify Clinical, Quality, and Professional Standards of practice—each Standard has its own rationale and identifies general and specific criteria related to that Standard. The student radiographer can access the individual Standards, their rationale, and criteria on the ASRT website.

X-ray Examination Requests

X-ray examinations must be requested by authorized individuals, typically by a physician, a physician assistant, or nurse practitioner. Request forms for radiologic examinations must be carefully reviewed by the radiographer prior to commencement of the examination. Many hospitals and radiology departments have specific rules about exactly what kind of information must appear on the requisition.

An all-important first step is careful and accurate patient identification and verification. Patient identification, and correctly matching the patient with the intended examination, is a routine activity in the health care environment. The health care worker has primary responsibility for checking/verifying patient identity. Most facilities require verification using *at least two patient identifiers*. Rigorous observance of "timeout" processes prior to procedures can avoid costly events, including those involving patient identification.

It is important that the radiographer obtains a short but adequate pertinent patient *history* or reason the examination has been requested. Because patients are rarely examined or interviewed by the radiologist, observations and information obtained by the radiographer can be a significant help in making an accurate diagnosis. The radiographer must be certain to obtain all clinical information in a manner and environment that ensures patient privacy.

The requisition is usually printed with the patient's personal information (name, address, age, admitting physician's name, and the patient's hospital identification number). When examining a patient who is admitted to the hospital, the requisition should also include the patient's mode of travel to the radiology department or other imaging facility (e.g., wheelchair or stretcher), the type of examination to be performed, pertinent diagnostic information, and any infection control or isolation information. The radiographer, having access to confidential patient information, must be mindful of compliance with HIPAA regulations.

The radiographer must be certain to understand and, if necessary, clarify the information provided, for example, any abbreviations used and any vague terms such as *leg* or *arm* (femur vs. tibia, humerus vs. forearm). The radiographer must also be alert to note and clarify conflicting information, for example, a request for a left ankle examination when the patient complains of, or has obvious injury to, the right ankle. The radiographer should also ascertain that clinical indicators match the requested examination. Computerized systems or department policy may require that there be appropriate and accurate diagnostic information accompanying every request for diagnostic procedure. Documentation is essential if any changes are made to the initial order, for example, if any medical event occurred that requires modification of the originally requested procedure.

Law/Medicolegal Issues

The four primary *sources of law* are the Constitution of the United States, statutory law, regulations and judgments of administrative bureaus, and court decisions.

The *Constitution* expresses the categorical laws of the country. Its impact with respect to health care and health care professionals lies, in part, in its assurance of the *right to privacy*. The right to privacy indicates that the patient's modesty and dignity will be respected. It also refers to the health care professional's obligation to respect the confidentiality of privileged information. Communication of privileged information to anyone but the appropriate health care professionals is inexcusable.

Statutory law refers to laws enacted by congressional, state, or local legislative bodies. The enforcement of statutory laws is frequently delegated to administrative bureaus such as the Board of Health, the Food and Drug Administration, and the Internal Revenue Service. It is the responsibility of these agencies to enact *rules and regulations* that will serve to implement the statutory law.

Court decisions involve the interpretation of *statutes* and various regulations in decisions involving individuals. For example, the decision of an administrative bureau can be appealed, and the court would decide if the agency acted appropriately and correctly. Court decisions are called *common law*.

There are two basic kinds of law—*public law* and *private (civil) law*. *Public* laws are those that regulate the relationship between individuals and government. *Private*, or civil, laws include laws that regulate the relationships among people. *Litigation* involving a radiographer's professional practice is most likely to involve the latter.

A *private (civil) injustice, injury, or misconduct is a tort*, and the injured party may seek reparation for damage incurred. Torts are described as either *intentional* or *negligent/unintentional*.

Examples of *intentional* (misconduct) torts include false imprisonment, *assault* and *battery*, defamation, and invasion of privacy. *False imprisonment* is the illegal restriction of an individual's freedom. Holding a person against his or her will or using unauthorized *restraint* can constitute false imprisonment. Various types of *immobilization* devices (e.g., carefully placed positioning aid such as a sponge or sandbag) can be used, with consent, to effectively reduce motion from involuntary muscular tremors resulting from anxiety or pain.

Assault is to threaten harm; *battery* is the carrying out of the threat. A patient might feel sufficiently intimidated to claim assault by a radiographer who threatens to repeat a difficult examination if the patient does not try harder to cooperate. A radiographer who performs an examination on a patient without his or her consent, or after the patient has refused the examination, can be guilty of *battery*. A charge of battery may also be made against a radiographer who treats a patient roughly or who performs an examination on the *wrong* patient.

The assessment of *duty* (what *should* have been done) is determined by the professional standard of care (that level of expertise generally possessed by reputable members of the profession). The determination

---

Tort

- A private/civil injustice
- Reparation can be sought
- Is either intentional or unintentional

For Negligent Tort Liability, Four Elements Must Be Present

- Duty (what should have been done)
- Breach (deviation from duty)
- Injury sustained
- Cause (as a result of breach)

Negligence

- Medical *malpractice* lawsuits are principally initiated on the basis of the *negligence* theory of liability.

Legal Doctrines

- *Res ipsa loquitur*—"the thing speaks for itself"
- *Respondeat superior*—"let the master answer"

---

of whether the standard of care was met is usually made by determining what another reputable practitioner would have done in the same situation. Medical *malpractice* lawsuits are principally initiated on the basis of the *negligence* theory of liability, that is, failure to use reasonably prudent care.

Examples of *negligent/unintentional* torts include imaging the wrong patient, radiographing the opposite limb, and causing injury to a patient as a result of a fall when left unattended on an x-ray table in a radiographic room, or on a stretcher without side rails or safety belt.

A radiographer who discloses confidential information to unauthorized individuals can be found guilty of invasion of privacy. If disclosure of the information is detrimental to the patient (e.g., causing ridicule or loss of job), the radiographer can be accused of *defamation*. *Spoken* defamation is *slander*; *written* defamation is *libel*.

The term *malpractice* is usually used with reference to *negligence*. Three areas of frequent litigation in radiology involve patient falls and positioning injuries, pregnancy, and errors or delays in *diagnosis*.

Patient falls and positioning injuries. Examples: A sedated patient left unattended in the radiographic room falls from the x-ray table; a patient with a spinal injury is moved from the stretcher to the x-ray table, resulting in irreversible damage to the spinal cord.

Pregnancy. Example: The radiographer fails to inquire about a possible pregnancy before performing a radiologic examination. Sometime later, the patient contacts the health care facility, expressing concern about her fetus.

Errors or delays in diagnosis. Example: The patient undergoes an x-ray examination in the emergency department and is sent home. The radiologist interprets the images and fails to notify the emergency department physician of the findings. The physician gets a written report 2 days later. Meanwhile, the patient suffers permanent damage from an untreated condition.

If patient injury results from misperformance of a duty in the routine scope of practice of the radiographer, most courts will apply *res ipsa loquitur*, that is, "the thing speaks for itself." If the patient is injured obviously as a result of the radiographer's/caregiver's actions, it becomes the radiographer's/caregiver's burden to *disprove* negligence. Examples of this include imaging the wrong patient/incorrect limb, surgical removal of a healthy organ or limb, and leaving a sponge or clamp in a patient's body during surgery. Additional examples can include manipulation of, or changes made in, electronic data—for example, cropping or masking an electronic x-ray image of a larger area to make it look like a collimated smaller area; not only does patient tissue receive unnecessary exposure but also potentially useful information can be eliminated via cropping/masking. Other examples can include modification of exposure indicator (EI) values, processing algorithms, and manipulation of brightness and/or contrast values. In many instances, the hospital and/or radiologist will also be held responsible according to *respondeat superior*, or "let the master answer." The "master," or employer, can be held liable for wrongful acts of the "servant," or employee, in causing injury during employed activities.

STANDARDS OF ETHICS

The mission of the American Registry of Radiologic Technologists (ARRT®) is to promote high standards of patient care by recognizing qualified individuals in medical imaging, interventional procedures, and radiation therapy. As every radiography student knows, the ARRT develops and administers examinations that assess the knowledge and skills underlying the intelligent performance of the tasks typically required by professional practice in the modality. In addition, the ARRT adopts and upholds:

- standards for educational preparation for entry into the profession
- standards of professional behavior consistent with the level of responsibility required by professional practice

Practitioners of the profession of radiologic technology, like other health care professionals, have an ethical responsibility to adhere to the principles of professional conduct and to provide the best services possible to the patients entrusted to their care. These principles are detailed in the ARRT two-part *Standards of Ethics*, which includes the Preamble, the Code of Ethics (Part A), the Rules of Ethics (Part B), and the Administrative Procedures. The 10-part *Code* of Ethics is *aspirational*; the 22 *Rules* of Ethics are *enforceable,* and any violation can result in sanction/injunction. The Rules of Ethics elaborate on fraudulent or deceptive practices, subversion, unprofessional conduct, scope of practice, fitness to practice, management of patient records, violations of state and/or federal laws or regulations, and duty to report. The complete ARRT Standards of Ethics was last revised and published on September 1, 2022, and can be found on the ARRT website.

> **ARRT Standards of Ethics Comprises**
>
> - Preamble
> - Statement of Purpose
> - Code of Ethics (aspirational)
> - Rules of Ethics (enforceable)
> - Administrative Procedures

ARRT Standards of Ethics

A critical component of ARRT governing documents with which students and ARRT-certified technologists must be familiar with is the ARRT Standards of Ethics. Situations can occur that make us wonder what is the "right" thing to do—circumstances that require us to make ethical decisions. The Standards of Ethics provides guidelines for making these very important decisions; the decision we make could impact our entire professional career.

The ARRT Ethics Committee provides peer review of cases to ensure adherence to standards of professional behavior. Radiographers, like all health care providers, must have the moral character required to practice in the health care professions. If their actions demonstrate that moral character is lacking, those individuals can be sanctioned. The sanction can be in the form of a reprimand, a suspension of registration, revocation of registration, ineligibility for certification, or other sanctions deemed appropriate by the Ethics Committee. The student should carefully study the ARRT Rules of Ethics.

For example, if you become aware that one of your coworkers is in violation of one of the Rules of Ethics, what should you do? Your professional obligation is to report your knowledge to your supervisor and then to the ARRT (according to Rule #21, *you* are in violation if you fail to report to the ARRT); *and* you must report to the State if your State has the licensing authority.

The radiographer must remember that failure to disclose a conviction is a violation of Ethical Rules #1 and #19 and involves falsification of ARRT information. The ARRT can become aware of an unreported conviction as part of an employment background check. This could actually result in a more serious sanction than the original offense!

The radiographer needs to be familiar with the ARRT Standards of Ethics, as these provide very important information and answers to tough questions that can be encountered during the radiographer's professional practice.

Honor Code

The word *honor* implies an effective regard for the standards of one's profession, a refusal to lie or deceive, an uprightness of character or action, a trustworthiness, and incorruptibility (being incapable of falling short in a trust or responsibility). Other words used to describe these qualities are *honesty*, *integrity*, and *probity*.

Certainly, these are the qualities required of students and health care professionals. This honor/integrity can only be achieved in an environment where intellectual honesty and personal integrity are highly valued, and where the responsibility for communicating and maintaining these standards is widely shared.

All candidates for primary, postprimary, and continuing pathway ARRT certification must meet ethical/honor code requirements. The ARRT Rules of Ethics indicate that felonies, misdemeanors, and various criminal procedures must be reported. Any primary pathway candidate may use the pre-application process to determine his or her ethical eligibility *before* enrolling in a radiography program or any time *during* the program. Many educational programs have a specific Honor Code to which students are required to adhere.

If a student has been suspended or dismissed/expelled from a/any radiography program, that incident must be indicated on the ARRT application and submitted with a detailed explanation, with accompanying documentation.

A student radiographer having any question regarding a violation reportable on his or her ARRT examination application should contact the ARRT Ethics Requirements Department.

A radiographer (or student radiographer) convicted of a misdemeanor or felony must report that to the ARRT. The Ethics Committee will conduct a peer review of the case and make a determination regarding possible *sanction*. One important consideration will be whether the actions were job related and could present a risk to the welfare of the patient.

Summary

- Patient consent can be verbal, written, or implied; a valid patient consent includes four conditions.

- Hospital information systems must ensure confidentiality in compliance with Health Insurance Portability and Accountability Act (HIPAA) of 1996 regulations.

- The AHA Patient's Bill of Rights details 12 specific areas of patient rights that the health care professional is obligated to respect.

- The AHA's six-part Patient Care Partnership has replaced the Patients' Bill of Rights.

- An Advance Health Care Directive, or Living Will, names the individual authorized to make all health care decisions and can include specifics regarding DNR, DNI, and/or other end-of-life decisions.

- The radiographer has the primary responsibility for verification of patient identity prior to a radiologic examination; most facilities require checking at least two patient identifiers.

- The ASRT Practice Standards identify the level of knowledge and skill required of a professional radiographer.

- Radiologic examinations must be requested by a qualified professional (MD, PA, etc.).

- The radiographer should examine the requisition carefully before bringing the patient to the radiographic room.

- Most health care facilities require that examination requests include pertinent diagnostic information and any infection control or isolation information.

- A civil injustice is a *tort*; a tort can be intentional or negligent.

- Negligence litigation in radiology most frequently involves injuries from falls, positioning injuries, pregnancy, and errors or delays in diagnosis.

- The ARRT Standards of Ethics consists of the Preamble, the Statement of Purpose, the Code of Ethics, the Rules of Ethics, and the Administrative Procedures.

- The Code of Ethics details guidelines for the radiographer's professional conduct and is *aspirational*. The Rules of Ethics are mandatory and enforceable.

- All candidates for primary pathway/continuing ARRT certification must meet the ethical/honor code requirements.

COMPREHENSION CHECK

Congratulations! You have completed this chapter. If you are able to answer the following group of comprehensive questions, you can feel confident that you have mastered this section. You are then ready to go on to the "registry-type" multiple-choice questions that follow.

For greatest success, do not go to the multiple-choice questions without first completing the following short-answer questions.

1. What does the term *ethics* refer to? How/why is ethical behavior important in the health care professions (p. 3)?

2. What are the two parts of the ARRT Standards of Ethics? Which part is mandatory and enforceable (p. 12)?

3. How can Honor Code violations impact a candidate for an ARRT examination (p. 10)?

4. Discuss the AHA Patient Care Partnership with respect to legal considerations pertinent to radiography (p. 5).

5. Describe an Advance Health Care Directive and possible elements that it might address. What is its purpose (p. 5)?

6. Discuss the purpose of the ASRT Practice Standards for the radiographer (p. 5, 6).

7. List the conditions necessary for valid consent (p. 4).

8. Discuss public versus private (civil) law (p. 7).

9. Differentiate between assault and battery; slander and libel (p. 7).

10. Give examples of intentional and unintentional torts (p. 7, 8).

11. List the four elements of a negligent tort (p. 7, 8).

12. On the basis of which theory of liability are medical malpractice lawsuits are principally initiated (p. 8)?

13. Identify the areas of litigation that most frequently involve radiology (p. 8).

14. List the patient information usually found on examination request forms (p. 6).

15. What does the acronym HIPAA refer to (p. 3)?

16. Describe the impact of the 1996 HIPAA regulations on radiologic patient care considerations (p. 3, 4).

17. Identify the types of clarification that may be required before beginning the x-ray examination (p. 6).

18. Review the ARRT Rules of Ethics and give an example of how one or more of these could impact a radiography student (p. 9, 10).

19. Discuss the differences between restraint and immobilization (p. 7).

20. Give examples of positioning aids and describe their use (p. 7).

21. List various patient verification processes that can be used by the radiographer. (p. 8).

22. List various patient verification processes required of the radiographer (p. 6).

CHAPTER REVIEW QUESTIONS

1. The ASRT document that defines the radiographer's role is the

    (A) Standards of Ethics

    (B) Practice Standards

    (C) Standard of Care

    (D) Legal Standards

2. Occurrences that can keep a radiography student from meeting ARRT certification requirements include

    1. being suspended from a radiography program

    2. being dismissed/expelled from a radiography program

    3. falling more than one course in his or her radiography program

    (A) 1 only

    (B) 2 only

    (C) 1 and 2 only

    (D) 1, 2, and 3

3. Violations of the ARRT Rules of Ethics include

    1. accepting responsibility to perform a function outside the scope of practice

    2. failure to obtain pertinent information for the radiologist

    3. failure to share newly acquired knowledge with peers

    (A) 1 only

    (B) 1 and 2 only

    (C) 1 and 3 only

    (D) 1, 2, and 3

4. Which organization has the authority to impose professional sanction on a radiographer?

    (A) ARRT

    (B) ASRT

    (C) JRCERT

    (D) TJC

5. A radiographer who discloses confidential information to unauthorized individuals may be found liable for

    (A) assault

    (B) battery

    (C) intimidation

    (D) defamation

6. The Patient Care Partnership includes

    1. the right to refuse treatment

    2. the right to confidentiality

    3. the right to possess one's medical records

    (A) 1 only

    (B) 1 and 2 only

    (C) 1 and 3 only

    (D) 1, 2, and 3

7. A radiographer who performs an x-ray examination on a patient without the patient's consent, or after the patient has refused the examination, may be liable for

    (A) assault

    (B) battery

    (C) slander

    (D) libel

8. An individual's legal document identifying his or her specific wishes regarding medical care to be provided in the event that he or she is unable to make or communicate decisions is called

    1. Advance Health Care Directive

    2. informed consent

    3. last will and testament

    (A) 1 only

    (B) 1 and 2 only

    (C) 2 and 3 only

    (D) 1, 2, and 3

9. The legislation that guarantees confidentiality of all patient information is

    (A) HSS

    (B) HIPAA

    (C) HIPPA

    (D) MQSA

10. If a patient lacks decision-making capacity, his or her rights can be exercised on his or her behalf by

    1. designated surrogate

    2. designated proxy

    3. no one

    (A) 1 only

    (B) 2 only

    (C) 1 and 2 only

    (D) 3 only

Answers and Explanations

1. (B) Radiographers should be familiar with the *Practice Standards* published by the American Society of Radiologic Technologists (ASRT). The Standards provide a legal role definition and identify Clinical, Quality, and Professional Standards of practice—each Standard has its own rationale and identifies general and specific criteria related to that Standard. The student radiographer can access the individual standards, their rationale, and criteria on the ASRT website.

The American Registry of Radiologic Technologists (ARRT) establishes principles of *professional conduct* to ensure the best services possible to patients entrusted to our care. These principles are detailed in the ARRT two-part *Standards of Ethics*, which includes the Code of Ethics and the Rules of Ethics. The 10-part *Code* of Ethics is aspirational; the 22 *Rules* of Ethics are enforceable, and their violation can result in professional sanction.

2. (C) Honor/integrity can only be achieved in an environment where intellectual honesty and personal integrity are highly valued, and where the responsibility for communicating and maintaining these standards is widely shared. To meet ARRT certification requirements, candidates for the ARRT examination must answer the question "Have you ever been suspended, dismissed, or expelled from an educational program that you attended in order to meet ARRT certification requirements?" in addition to reading and signing the "Written Consent under FERPA," allowing the ARRT to obtain specific parts of their educational records concerning violations to an honor code. If the applicant answers "yes" to that question, he or she must include an explanation and documentation of the situation with the completed application for certification. If the applicant has any doubts, he or she should contact the ARRT Ethics Requirements Department at (651) 687-0048, ext. 8580.

3. (A) Accepting responsibility to perform a function outside the scope of practice is a violation of Ethical *Rule* #7, which states that it is a violation to "delegate or accept delegation of a radiologic technology function or any other prescribed health care function when the delegation or acceptance could reasonably be expected to create an unnecessary danger to a patient's life, health, or safety. Actual injury to a patient need not be established under this clause." So, accepting a responsibility outside the scope of practice is a violation of an ARRT *rule*. However, choices 2 and 3 are in violation of the *aspirational Code* of Ethics.

4. (A) The ARRT establishes principles of professional conduct to ensure the best services possible to patients entrusted to our care. These principles are detailed in the ARRT two-part *Standards of Ethics*, which includes the Code of Ethics and the Rules of Ethics. The 10-part *Code* of Ethics is aspirational; the 23 *Rules* of Ethics are enforceable, and their violation can result in professional sanction. The ARRT Ethics Committee provides peer review of cases (misdemeanor, felony, etc.) to ensure adherence to standards of professional behavior and possession of the moral character required to practice in the health care professions. If the violator's actions demonstrate that moral character is lacking, that individual can be sanctioned—that is, reprimanded, suspended, revoked, ineligible for certification, and so on—or other sanctions deemed appropriate by the Ethics Committee.

5. (D) A radiographer who discloses confidential information to unauthorized individuals may be found guilty of *invasion of privacy or defamation*. A radiographer whose disclosure of confidential information is in some way detrimental to the patient may be accused of defamation. Spoken defamation is *slander;* written defamation is *libel. Assault* is to threaten harm; *battery* is to carry out the threat.

6. (B) The AHA's Patient Care Partnership identifies six important Rights/Expectations during a hospital stay. These include the right to refuse treatment (to the extent allowed by law), the right to confidentiality of records and communication, and the right to continuing care. Other patient rights identified are the right to informed consent, privacy, respectful care, *access* to personal medical records, refusal to participate in research projects, and an explanation of one's hospital bill.

7. (B) *Assault* is to threaten harm; *battery* is to carry out the threat. A patient may feel sufficiently intimidated to claim assault by a radiographer who threatens to repeat a difficult examination if the patient does not try to cooperate better. A radiographer who performs an examination on a patient without the patient's consent or after the patient has refused the examination may be liable for battery. A charge of battery may also be made against a radiographer who treats a patient roughly or who performs an examination on the wrong patient. A radiographer who discloses confidential information to unauthorized individuals may be found liable for *invasion of privacy* or *defamation*. A radiographer whose disclosure of confidential information is in some way detrimental to the patient may be accused of defamation. Spoken defamation is *slander;* written defamation is *libel*.

8. (A) Many people believe that potential legal and ethical issues can be avoided by creating an *Advance Health Care Directive*. Because all individuals have the right to make decisions regarding their own health care, this legal document preserves that right in the event an individual is unable to make or communicate those decisions. An Advance Health Care Directive lists the individual's specific wishes, names the individual authorized to make health care decisions, and can include specifics regarding *DNR* (do not resuscitate), *DNI* (do not intubate), and/or other end-of-life decisions.

9. (B) Most institutions now have computerized, paperless systems for patient information transmittal (hospital information system [HIS]); these systems must ensure confidentiality in compliance with Health Insurance Portability and Accountability Act (HIPAA) of 1996 regulations. A health care professional generally has access to a computerized system only via a personal password, thus helping ensure confidentiality of patient information. All medical records and other individually identifiable health information—electronic, on paper, or oral—are covered by HIPAA legislation and by subsequent Department of Health and Human Services (HHS) rules that took effect in April 2001.

10. (C) Patients' rights can be exercised on the patient's behalf by a *designated surrogate or proxy* decision maker if the patient lacks decision-making capacity, is legally incompetent, or is a minor. Many people believe that potential legal and ethical issues can be avoided by creating an Advance Health Care Directive or Living Will. Because all individuals have the right to make decisions regarding their own health care, this legal document preserves that right in the event an individual is unable to make those decisions. An Advance Health Care Directive, or Living Will, names the individual authorized to make all health care decisions and can include a living will, giving specifics regarding *DNR* (do not resuscitate), *DNI* (do not intubate), and/or other end-of-life decisions.

Interpersonal Communication

OBJECTIVES

At the conclusion of this chapter, the student will be able to:

- Identify the types of communication and cite examples of each.
- Discuss the importance of effective communication skills in medical imaging.
- List various challenges to effective communication and discuss tools and strategies available to meet these challenges.
- Discuss techniques to reduce patient anxiety in various age-specific groups.
- Discuss the radiographer's responsibility related to patient education.

COMMUNICATION SKILLS

Radiographers interact with many individuals every workday. Their *communication* with patients, families, and other professionals must be with care, accuracy, clarity, and sensitivity. The importance of effective and professional communication skills cannot be overstressed. Interaction between the patient and the radiographer can leave the patient with a lasting impression of his or her health care experience. Interaction between the radiographer and other health professionals can impact the delivery and efficiency of health care.

TYPES OF COMMUNICATION

Of course, communication refers to not only the spoken word (i.e., *verbal* communication) but also unspoken/*nonverbal* communication. *Facial expression* can convey care and reassurance or impatience and disapproval. Pursed lips, pointed fingers, frowns, and hands on hips all indicate disapproval. Similarly, a radiographer's *touch* can convey his or her commitment to considerate care, or it can convey a rough, uncaring, and hurried attitude. Making *eye contact* while speaking is generally considered polite and respectful in the United States, whereas it can be considered just the opposite in other cultures (e.g., Asian, East Indian, Native American). Our *appearance* gives an impression about how we feel about our work and our patients; it is very much a part of communication, and we should strive for a professional appearance/image.

COMMUNICATION WITH PATIENTS

Patient Identification

Effective patient communication begins with establishing trust and rapport. The radiographer/student introduces himself or herself to the patient and then follows with verification of the patient *identity*. Care must be taken when making the initial patient identification. Patient identification, and correct matching of the patient with the intended examination, is a routine activity in the health care environment. The health care worker has primary responsibility for checking/verifying the patient identity. Most facilities require checking *at least two patient identifiers*. Rigorous observance of "timeout" processes (verification of correct procedure, patient, and site, according to The Joint Commission and other accrediting agencies such as HFAP [Healthcare Facilities Accreditation Program] and ACHC [Accreditation Commission for Health Care]) prior to procedures can avoid costly events, including those involving patient identification.

If the radiographer calls out a name into a rather full waiting room or asks a patient whether he is Mr so-and-so, an anxious patient might readily respond in the affirmative without actually having heard his or her name being called. The radiographer must check the patient's wristband *and* ask the patient for a second verification, such as his or her birth date. If the patient has no wristband, definite identification must be documented by having the patient state his or her full name and date of birth.

Effective communication with a patient should also begin with a review of relevant patient *history*, often including ascertainment of the patient's current medication(s). The acquisition of pertinent clinical history from the patient is one of the most valuable contributions to the diagnostic process. Because the diagnostic radiologist rarely has the opportunity to speak with the patient, this is a crucial responsibility of the radiographer. For instance, to report that the patient indicates most pain at his or her medial malleolus is far more valuable than simply saying that his or her leg hurts. Review of the patient information *before* bringing the patient to the radiographic department also enables the radiographer to have the x-ray room prepared, with all equipment and accessories readily available. *However*, it is exceedingly important to respect patient privacy and HIPAA (Health Insurance Portability and Accountability Act) regulations. Ensure to interview the patient in a manner/place that your conversation cannot be overheard by individuals not involved with that patient's examination.

Verbal/Written and Nonverbal Communication

Scenario #1: Consider the *nonverbal* messages communicated to a patient brought into a disorderly examination room or by a radiographer's sloppy, poorly groomed appearance. What about the grim-faced

---

Effective Communication Begins With

- Verifying patient identity
- Establishing trust and rapport

Patient Identification/Verification

- Most facilities require checking at least two patient identifiers

professional who hurries the patient along to the radiographic room, gives rapid-fire instructions to the patient while searching for missing markers and other accessories, tosses the patient onto the x-ray table, and finally dismisses the patient with a curt "you can go now"?

The disorderly x-ray room and sloppy appearance of the radiographer indicate disrespect for the patient and a negative feeling about oneself and one's profession. That impression is further cemented by lack of preparedness, as well as an apathetic and generally uncaring attitude toward the patient.

Scenario #2: Consider another patient, greeted by a smiling professional who introduces himself or herself and brings the patient to a neat and orderly radiographic room where everything is in readiness for the procedure. This radiographer explains the procedure, listens to what the patient has to say, and carefully answers the patient's questions. At the end of the examination, the patient is escorted back to the waiting area and clear instructions are given for any required postprocedural care.

Which scenario provides the patient with a more comfortable, anxiety-free examination? Which patient leaves the hospital or clinic environment with a more favorable impression of his or her health care experience? Which patient is likely to return to that facility for any additional required diagnostic studies? Which experience would *you* prefer for yourself or a loved one?

The volume of the radiographer's *voice* and the rate of speech are also important factors to consider in effective communication. The radiographer should face the patient and make *eye contact* during communication. Loud, rapid speech and/or movement are unpleasant to most people and particularly uncomfortable for the sick and/or the elderly patient. A conscious effort should be made to use a well-modulated tone and to maintain a calm demeanor. Patients with even minor hearing loss will greatly benefit when the speaker faces him or her. If the patient and/or radiographer is wearing a mask, care must be taken to ensure comprehension.

X-ray examinations may be requested by an appropriately qualified individual—usually a physician, physician assistant, or other licensed provider. Written and/or verbal instructions and requests received by the radiographer must be clearly understood. Request forms for radiologic examinations should be carefully reviewed by the radiographer prior to commencement of the examination. If the radiographer has any question about the examination to be performed, or receives conflicting/questionable information from the patient, it is his or her duty to *clarify all information and documentation before proceeding.* Many hospitals and radiology departments have specific rules about exactly what kind(s) of information is required to be included on requisition forms.

Patient Education

It is imperative that the radiographer takes adequate time to thoroughly explain the procedure or examination to the patient. In addition, there are times when the radiographer must inquire whether proper diet and/or

---

Verbal Communication Is *Impacted* By

- Tone and rate of speech
- Eye contact
- Vocabulary

Examples of Nonverbal Communication

- Personal appearance
- Appearance of work area
- Facial expression
- Touch
- Eye contact
- Other body language

other preparation instructions have been followed prior to the examination. The radiographer requires the cooperation of the patient throughout the course of the examination; therefore, providing a thorough *explanation* will alleviate patient anxieties and permit full cooperation. The radiographer is responsible for verification of the patient consent, when applicable, for certain examinations/procedures.

The radiographer must use good listening skills, that is, looking at the patient and listening carefully without interruption. Patient anxiety can be relieved by explaining procedures and answering questions in a simple, clear, and direct manner, avoiding the use of elaborate medical terminology or abbreviations.

Effective communication skills require the use of layman's terms, and an explanation should be given for any technical terms used. The patients should be clear about what will be expected of them and what they may expect from the radiographer.

The patients often have questions about other scheduled diagnostic imaging procedures, such as mammography, computed tomography (CT), magnetic resonance (MR) imaging, sonography, or nuclear medicine studies. They often inquire about the length of an examination, as well as ask other questions relating to safety of or contraindications for an examination. The diagnostic radiographer must be well informed and able to effectively respond to questions relating to all types of examinations. If the radiographer is unsure about how to answer a patient's concerns, he or she must know where to get the proper information. Patient concerns are often related to diet restrictions or other preparation that may be required for CT or sonography, concerns, or contraindications for some examinations such as MR imaging, and positioning techniques such as compression used in mammography. The radiographer should also be able to help the patient obtain information about these and other services he or she might require, for example, social services, rehabilitation, and spiritual counseling.

Examination Instructions

Radiologic examinations using contrast media usually require preexamination and/or postexamination patient instructions. The radiographer must be able to provide the patient with accurate instructions, ascertain that the patient is properly prepared, and provide clear postexamination/discharge instructions.

To alleviate the anxiety associated with diagnostic imaging examinations and procedures, the patients could be encouraged to repeat explanations or instructions (to the radiographer) to be certain that they understood; some may have an additional question or two they must ask to clarify their thoughts. The radiographer's patience and understanding at these times are greatly appreciated by the anxious patient or relative.

The radiographer should also be able to respond to rudimentary questions the patient may have regarding radiation dose and/or other imaging procedures, for example, CT, MR imaging, sonography, and mammography, for which he or she may be scheduled.

COMMUNICATION CHALLENGES

Impediments

Gaining the patient's confidence and trust through effective communication is an essential part of the radiographic examination. Some patients present challenges that require a greater use of the radiographer's communication skills—patients who are seriously ill or injured; traumatized patients; patients with vision, hearing, speech, or cognitive impairments; situations requiring wearing of masks or other protective apparel; infants and children; non–English-speaking patients; elderly and infirm people; people with physical, emotional, or cognitive disabilities; people who abuse alcohol and drugs; the families of patients—radiographers must adapt their communication skills to meet the needs of all individuals.

Radiographers, like other health care professionals, can often care for patients experiencing loss or grief. This can be loss of a treasured possession, physical mobility, social status, or a loved one. The patients with terminal conditions or illnesses sometimes face anticipatory grief. When caring for a patient dealing with grief, the health care professional may understandably experience strong emotion. It is important for the professional to understand his or her own attitude concerning loss and grief. Studying and understanding the grieving process phases can help the health care professional provide empathetic and supportive care.

The grieving process varies with everyone. The length and order of these phases can depend on several factors including cultural, religious, and ethnic factors. Dr Elisabeth Kübler-Ross was one of the first to recognize this and summarized the process, though noting that it can vary considerably with each individual. She summarized the grieving process phases as follows:

Phase 1: *Denial* is a defense mechanism, which helps the individual to begin to adapt to this truth.

Phase 2: *Anger* is expressed when experiencing frustration, helplessness, and seeming injustice.

Phase 3: *Bargaining* behavior is exhibited as being a "good" patient, very tolerant and uncomplaining.

Phase 4: *Depression* is experienced as the patient begins to accept impending loss and mourn for past life. The patient is quiet and withdrawn.

Phase 5: *Acceptance* is expressed by loss of interest in everything except the support of the loved ones/caregivers close at hand and his or her immediate surroundings. The patient begins to disengage from life.

Diversity of culture is often thought of as ethnic diversity—a difference in nationality. But cultural groups include religious groups, age groups, racial groups, socioeconomic groups, geographic groups, groups of people with disabilities, generational groups, gender groups and sexual preference groups.

Misunderstandings between cultures can occur because of seemingly innocuous circumstances—such as standing too close while speaking to another, looking directly into someone's eyes, or the use of certain gestures.

Cultural Groups Include

- Religious groups
- Age groups
- Racial groups
- Socioeconomic groups
- Groups with disabilities
- Gender groups
- Sexual preference groups
- Geographic groups

Gestures have different meanings in different countries. In the United States and Europe, the "thumbs-up" gesture has a positive implication. However, it is considered rude in Australia and obscene in the Middle East. Other examples of potentially misunderstood gestures include the following: If you compliment a Mexican child, you must touch that child's head, whereas in Asia, it is not acceptable to touch the head of a child; in the Philippines, it is rude to beckon with the index finger.

Furthermore, there are significant cultural differences regarding "personal space." In the United States, people are comfortable speaking approximately 18 inches apart; in the Middle East, people stand much closer together to speak, whereas in England, people stand further apart when speaking.

Ethnocentrism is the belief that one's own cultural ways are superior to any other way. Ethnocentrism can be found in all cultures and is the most significant barrier to good intercultural communication. It is essential that we have an awareness of our own ethnocentrism.

Medical Terminology

Although many individuals nowadays are knowledgeable health care consumers, we cannot assume that all patients understand the medical terminology or technical jargon of radiologic procedures. Using language that is not comprehensible to the patients can make them feel intimidated and give them unnecessary anxiety.

Patient anxiety can be relieved by explaining procedures and answering questions in a simple, clear, and direct manner—avoiding the use of elaborate medical terminology. Let the patients know that you are there for them—not simply to perform the x-ray examination but to help them understand and to be as comfortable as possible.

Strategies to Improve Communication

Many patients are anxious about their illness/condition and are unfamiliar with the procedure they are about to undergo. Communication difficulties can be simply and significantly resolved through explanation. Because *anxious* patients require more time to think and to move, a radiographer who takes the time to explain the procedure and the unfamiliar terminology, and answer the patient's questions will be long remembered and appreciated by that patient.

Elderly patients, for example, are uncomfortable being pushed or hurried about. They appreciate the radiographer who is compassionate enough to take the extra few minutes necessary for comfort. Some patients with dementia are easily confused; it is best to address them by their full name and to keep instructions simple and direct. The elderly patients deserve the same courteous, dignified care as all other patients. Many people nowadays enjoy longer and quite active lives. Consequently, the term *elderly* is likely to be defined differently by different people. Many textbooks describe old/elderly as older than 80 years, but even that varies with the individual. *Ageism* is discrimination against aged persons.

Another special population that should be considered carefully in the imaging department comprises infants and children. Communication and care challenges can be quite different with *children*, depending on their age; they must be provided with a safe environment and never left unattended.

Infant (birth to 1 year) care includes minimizing separation anxiety by keeping the infant and the parent(s) together, keeping a familiar object or two (toy, blanket) with the infant, and limiting the number of staff present in the x-ray room.

Toddlers (1–2 years) should be spoken to at the eye level; the radiographer should be cheerful and unhurried. Talking to the child cheerfully and having a playful manner can significantly reduce his or her anxiety and help him or her to be more cooperative.

Preschoolers (3–5 years) benefit from simple explanations of what you will be doing and how they can help you. Be honest with *school-aged children* (6–12 years), explain what you will be doing, and let them help whenever possible.

Adolescents (13–18 years) require privacy and modesty. Establish rapport by striking up conversation about hobbies or other interests.

Young adults are described as 19–45 years old. These years, especially early on, are usually a time of gaining greater independence. Later, the demands of career, marriage, and children are of the greatest importance. It is a time of beginning to recognize one's own vulnerability more clearly. The young adult depends on a calm, competent professional to ease his or her apprehensions.

The *middle adult* is described as 46–64 years old and the *older adult* as 65–79 years old. As baby boomers age, the older adult groups are increasing in number. During this time, common issues that can arise deal with vision, hearing, bone mass, muscle tone, weight gain, and diet restrictions.

Older adults and the elderly frequently exhibit increased pain threshold, breakdown of skin, and atrophy of fat pads and sweat glands. Many changes occur as our bodies age. Although muscle is replaced with fat, the amount of subcutaneous fat is decreased and the skin atrophies. Therefore, a geriatric patient requires *extra gentle treatment*. A mattress pad should always be placed on the radiographic table to help prevent *skin injury* or abrasions. If a tape is required, the paper tape should be used instead of the adhesive tape. Geriatric patients are also more sensitive to *hypothermia* because of the breakdown of the sweat glands and always should be kept covered both to preserve modesty and to provide extra warmth. *Loss of sensation* in the skin increases pain tolerance, so the geriatric patient may not be aware of excessive stress on bony prominences such as the elbow, wrist, coccyx, and ankles. These individuals are often concerned about loss of autonomy. The radiographer can help by keeping them involved with their examination and allowing them to make any possible choices.

Communication difficulties can arise with non–English-speaking patients. Most hospitals and large clinics have a list of resources such as people, automated systems, LanguageLine, special dual-headset phones, or similar accommodations to assist with interpretation when there is a language barrier. A certified interpreter is most helpful because he or she translates exactly what has been said—rather than a family member or friend who might edit or try to explain what he or she *thinks* is implied. People whose second language is English occasionally lose their ability to communicate in that second language during times of

---

Age-Specific Care

- Infant: birth to 1 year
- Toddler: 1–2 years
- Preschooler: 3–5 years
- School-aged: 6–12 years
- Adolescent: 13–18 years
- Young adult: 19–45 years
- Middle adult: 46–64 years
- Older adult: 65–79 years
- Elderly: older than 80 years

trauma, illness, or stress. Volume, speed, and tone of voice may also be determined by culture. In addition, expressions/figures of speech such as "a piece of cake" or "home free" may not be understood by these patients or their families.

Summary

- The radiographer has primary responsibility for verifying the patient identity prior to the radiologic examination.
- The radiographer should examine the requisition carefully before bringing the patient to the radiographic department.
- Patients must be identified by checking their wristbands and requesting a second identifier verification such as birth date.
- Most health care facilities require that examination requests include pertinent diagnostic information, mode of transport, and any infection control or isolation information.
- *Verbal* communication involves the tone and rate of speech, as well as what is being said. It involves personalization and respect.
- *Nonverbal* communication involves facial expression, touch, eye contact, professional appearance, orderliness of the radiographic department, and the preparation and efficiency of the radiographer.
- The radiographer must clarify any unclear or contradictory information or documentation before proceeding with the examination.
- A thorough explanation of procedures reduces the patient's anxiety, increases cooperation, and results in a better examination.
- The radiographer must be able to provide accurate *preexamination* and *aftercare* information and ably address the patient's questions about other imaging studies.
- Patients should receive explanations in a simple, clear, and direct manner, without the use of elaborate medical terminology.
- Communication challenges can arise with many patients, for example, the seriously ill, traumatized patients; patients with impaired senses or cognition; children; non–English-speaking patients; elderly; substance abusers; and patients' families.

COMPREHENSION CHECK

Congratulations! You have completed your review of this chapter. If you are able to answer the following group of comprehensive questions, you can feel confident that you have mastered this section. You are then ready to go on to the "registry-type" questions that follow. For greatest success, do not go to the multiple-choice questions without first completing the following short-answer questions:

1. Explain the importance of reviewing the examination request and other patient information before bringing the patient to the radiographic department (p. 18).

2. Discuss the best way(s) to ensure correct identification of a patient (p. 18).

3. Explain the importance of obtaining patient history (p. 18).

4. Discuss the importance of explaining the procedure to the patient (p. 19, 20, 22).

5. Discuss five ways through which the radiographer communicates *verbal* messages to the patient (p. 17, 18, 19).

6. List five ways through which the radiographer communicates *nonverbal* messages to the patient (p. 17, 18, 19).

7. Discuss some qualities of verbal communication likely to evoke a *positive* response from the patient; qualities likely to evoke a *negative* response (p. 18, 19).

8. Explain the value of making as many preparations as possible before bringing the patient to the radiographic department/room (p. 18, 19, 20).

9. List the five phases of the grieving process as identified by Dr Kübler-Ross and discuss how their order and length might vary (p. 21).

10. Discuss five patient-related challenges that might require special communication efforts by the radiographer (p. 23, 24).

11. List five benefits of effective communication skills (p. 20, 22).

12. Discuss potential sources/causes of cultural misunderstanding (p. 21, 22, 23).

13. List various age groups and discuss appropriate age-specific care for each group (p. 23).

14. Discuss typical responsibilities of the radiographer regarding patient education (p. 19, 20).

CHAPTER REVIEW QUESTIONS

1. Which of the following communicate(s) messages to the patient?
   1. Facial expression
   2. Eye contact
   3. Personal appearance
   (A) 1 only
   (B) 1 and 2 only
   (C) 3 only
   (D) 1, 2, and 3

2. Examples of nonverbal communication include
   1. appearance
   2. eye contact
   3. touch
   (A) 1 only
   (B) 1 and 2 only
   (C) 2 and 3 only
   (D) 1, 2, and 3

3. Successful, effective communication includes proficiency in the following skills:
   1. writing
   2. speech
   3. observation
   (A) 1 only
   (B) 1 and 2 only
   (C) 2 and 3 only
   (D) 1, 2, and 3

4. Which of the following should be the first step in performing a radiographic examination?
   (A) Obtaining clinical history
   (B) Providing appropriate patient assistance
   (C) Verifying patient identity
   (D) Using appropriate infection control

5. All of the following are useful resources for non–English-speaking patients, *except*
   (A) automated language lines
   (B) special dual-headset phones
   (C) a certified interpreter
   (D) a family member or friend

6. A patient, aged 55 years, is most accurately described as
   (A) young adult
   (B) middle adult
   (C) older adult
   (D) elderly

7. Increased pain threshold, breakdown of skin, and atrophy of fat pads and sweat glands are all important considerations when working with which of the following groups of patients?
   (A) Infants
   (B) Children
   (C) Adolescents
   (D) Geriatric patients

8. A radiographer should recognize that geriatric patients often have undergone physical changes that include loss of
   1. muscle mass
   2. bone calcium
   3. mental alertness
   (A) 1 only
   (B) 1 and 2 only
   (C) 1 and 3 only
   (D) 1, 2, and 3

9. The belief that one's own cultural ways are superior to any other is termed
   (A) ethnology
   (B) ethnobiology
   (C) ethnocentrism
   (D) ethnography

10. Misunderstandings between cultures can happen as a result of
    1. looking directly into someone's eyes
    2. using certain gestures
    3. standing too close while speaking to another
    (A) 1 only
    (B) 1 and 2 only
    (C) 2 and 3 only
    (D) 1, 2, and 3

Answers and Explanations

1. (D) The interaction between a patient and a radiographer generally leaves a lasting impression on the patient's health care experience. Communication may be verbal or nonverbal. *Verbal communication* involves tone and rate of speech, as well as what is being said. It involves personalization and respect. *Nonverbal communication* involves facial expression, professional appearance, orderliness of radiographic department, and preparation and efficiency of the radiographer.

2. (D) The importance of effective and professional patient *communication* skills cannot be overemphasized; the interaction between the patient and the radiographer generally leaves the patient with a lasting impression of his or her health care experience. Of course, communication refers to not only the spoken word (i.e., *verbal* communication) but also unspoken/ *nonverbal* communication. *Facial expression* can convey care and reassurance or impatience and disapproval. Pursed lips, pointed fingers, frowns, and hands on hips all indicate disapproval. Similarly, a radiographer's *touch* can convey his or her commitment to considerate care, or it can convey a rough, uncaring, and hurried attitude. Making *eye contact* while speaking is generally considered polite and respectful in the United States, whereas it can be considered just the opposite in other cultures (e.g., Asian, East Indian, Native American). Our *appearance* gives an impression of how we feel about our work and our patients; it is very much a part of communication, and we should strive for a professional appearance/image.

3. (D) Communication can be achieved in many forms; those forms can be verbal or nonverbal. Effective and professional patient communication skills are essential; the interaction between the patient and the radiographer generally leaves the patient with a lasting impression of his or her health care experience. The radiographer's communication skills must include a proficiency in *observational* skills, *listening* skills, *speaking* skills, and *writing* skills.

4. (C) Although each of these steps is part of a complete radiologic examination, an all-important first step is careful and accurate patient identification. Patient identification, and correctly matching the patient with the intended examination, is a routine activity in the health care environment. The health care worker has primary responsibility for checking/verifying the patient identity. Most facilities require checking *at least two patient identifiers*. Rigorous observance of "timeout" processes prior to procedures can avoid costly events, including those involving patient identification.

5. (D) Communication difficulties can arise with non–English-speaking patients. Most hospitals and large clinics have a list of resources such as people, automated systems, LanguageLine, special dual-headset phones, or similar accommodations to assist with interpretation when there is a language barrier. A certified interpreter is most helpful because he or she translates exactly what has been said, rather than a family member or friend who might edit or try to explain what he or she *thinks* is implied. People whose second language is English occasionally lose their ability to communicate in that second language during times of trauma, illness, or stress. Volume, speed, and tone of voice may also be determined by culture. In addition, expressions/figures of speech such as "a piece of cake" or "home free" may not be understood by these patients or their families.

6. (B) Young adults are described as 19–45 years old. These years, especially early on, are usually a time of gaining greater independence. Later, the demands of career, marriage, and children are of the greatest importance. It is a time of beginning to recognize one's own vulnerability more clearly. The young adult depends on a calm, competent professional to ease his or her apprehensions.

The *middle adult* is described as 46–64 years old and the *older adult* as 65–79 years old. As baby boomers age, the older adult groups are increasing in number.

7. (D) Increased pain threshold, breakdown of skin, and atrophy of fat pads and sweat glands are all important considerations when working with *geriatric patients*. Many changes occur as our bodies age. Although muscle is replaced with fat, the amount of subcutaneous fat is decreased and the skin atrophies. Therefore, a geriatric patient requires *extra gentle treatment*. A mattress pad should always be placed on the radiographic table to help prevent *skin injury* or abrasions. If a tape is required, the paper tape should be used instead of the adhesive tape. Geriatric patients are also more sensitive to *hypothermia* because of the breakdown of the sweat glands and always should be kept covered both to preserve modesty and to provide extra warmth. *Loss of sensation* in the skin increases pain tolerance, so the geriatric patient may not be aware of excessive stress on bony prominences such as the elbow, wrist, coccyx, and ankles.

8. (B) *Gerontology* is the study of the elderly. *Geriatrics* deals with the care of the elderly. Although bone demineralization and loss of muscle mass occur to a greater or lesser degree in most elderly individuals, the radiographer must not assume that all geriatric patients are hard of hearing, clumsy, or not mentally alert. Nowadays, many elderly people remain very active, staying mentally and physically agile well into their "golden years." The radiographer must keep this in mind as he or she provides age-specific care to the geriatric patients.

9. (C) *Ethnocentrism* is the belief that one's personal experience and perception of the world are superior to the experiences and perceptions of others, that is, the belief that one's own cultural ways are superior to any other. Ethnocentrism can be found in all cultures and is the most significant barrier to good intercultural communication. *Ethnology* is the comparative study of various cultures. *Ethnobiology* is the study of biological characteristics of various races. *Ethnography* is the study of a single society's culture.

10. (D) Misunderstandings between cultures can occur as a result of the use of gestures, which have different meanings in different countries. In the United States and Europe, the "thumbs-up" gesture has a positive implication. However, it is considered rude in Australia and obscene in the Middle East. Other examples of potentially misunderstood gestures include the following: If you compliment a Mexican child, you must touch the head, whereas in Asia, it is not acceptable to touch the head of a child; in the Philippines, it is rude to beckon with the index finger; furthermore, in the United States, people are comfortable speaking approximately 18 inches apart, whereas in the Middle East, people stand much closer together when they talk; in England, people stand further apart.

Ergonomics, Monitoring, and Medical Emergencies

OBJECTIVES

At the conclusion of this chapter, the student will be able to:

- List rules of body mechanics appropriate for the radiographer.
- Compare transfer methods for wheelchair-/stretcher-bound patient transport.
- Provide examples of objective and subjective patient information.
- Identify the use of various tubes and central lines.
- Identify the vital signs and their norms.
- Discuss the factors and conditions that can affect vital sign norms.
- Explain the use of various oxygen delivery systems.
- Define the terms related to allergic reactions.
- Discuss the importance of being alert to any change in patient condition.
- List various potential medical emergencies and identify the radiographer's role in each.
- Define the infection prevention and control terminologies.
- Discuss the role of personal hygiene in preventing the spread of infection.

PHYSICAL ASSISTANCE AND TRANSFER

Body Mechanics

Radiographers work with many patients whose capacities for *ambulation* vary greatly. Outpatients are usually *ambulatory*, that is, able to walk and not confined to bed. Ambulatory inpatients generally travel by wheelchair, whereas patients confined to bed must travel by stretcher. For the safety of the patient and the radiographer, it is essential that the radiographer uses proper techniques and *body mechanics/physical ergonomics* when transferring the patients, whether they are inpatients or outpatients. Modes of patient transportation include ambulation, wheelchair, and stretcher.

Not all patients need, or want, well-intentioned assistance. Many prefer to manage on their own. The radiographer should recognize this

---

Other Rules of Good Body Mechanics/Ergonomics

1. When carrying an object, hold it close to the body.
2. The back should be kept straight; avoid twisting.
3. When lifting an object, bend the knees and use the leg and abdominal muscles to lift (rather than the back muscles).
4. Whenever possible, push or roll heavy objects (rather than lifting or pulling).

but be ever alert and watchful should the patient need assistance. Other patients find it reassuring and feel an added sense of security with an attentive radiographer. The professional radiographer develops a sense of awareness of each patient's needs and concerns.

To transfer the patient with maximum safety, the radiographer must correctly use certain concepts of body mechanics. First, *a broad base of support* lends greater stability; therefore, the radiographer should stand with feet approximately 12 inches apart and with one foot slightly forward. Second, stability is achieved when the body's *center of gravity* (center of the pelvis) is positioned over its base of support. For example, leaning away from the central axis of the body makes the body more vulnerable to losing balance; if the feet are close together, balance is even more difficult to maintain.

Even the ambulatory outpatient might be somewhat unsteady, so a ready, supporting hand at the elbow can be very helpful. The radiographer should keep a watchful eye on the patient and assist him or her as needed.

Ergonomic Transfer Devices

The *patient transfer board* is also known as a *smooth mover* or *patient shifter*. It is a thin, smooth, polyethylene board with an antistatic surface and hand grips on the surrounding edges. Its function is to bridge the gap between two surfaces to enable the safe transference of a patient from one surface to another (i.e., from a stretcher to an examination table). To use the transfer board, the recumbent patient is rolled to one side and the board is slipped halfway under the patient's body, under the drawsheet. The board covers the space between the stretcher and the x-ray table. The patient is rolled back into the supine position. With the patient's arms folded safely across his or her chest, two people grip the drawsheet and slide the patient smoothly and safely across the board. The board is radiolucent and may be removed or kept under the patient during the x-ray examination.

The *gait belt*, or *transfer belt*, can be used for transferring a patient from the bed to the wheelchair and vice versa or in general assistance when mobility or weakness might be an issue. A gait belt is usually approximately 2–4 inches (5–10 cm) wide and made of canvas or nylon with a buckle at one end. The belt is placed around the patient's waist, over clothing, with buckle in front. The belt is securely buckled; it should be snug but with enough room for the radiographer's fingers under it. The radiographer supports the patient with his or her fingers under the belt. Gait belts are useful in helping the patient to stand and walk from one location to another. Gait belts must never be used over incisions, stitches, tubes, or lines, and never on a pregnant patient.

A *Hoyer* patient lift, or a *sling lift*, is a portable patient lift operated by electric, hydraulic, or battery power. There is a sling-type surface that slides under the patient's body to secure and transfer him or her between bed/chair/wheelchair/toilet.

Patient Safety and Transfer Considerations

Health care practitioners have the responsibility to ensure patient safety and comfort while the patient is in their care. The radiographer should make a mental note of what the patient has in his or her possession when he or she enters the department, such as glasses or a purse. Patient belongings should be properly secured according to institution or department policy. The radiographer must be certain that the radiographic department is hazard-free, that all equipment and accessories are used properly and safely, and that the patient is as comfortable as possible.

When moving a patient to or from the wheelchair or stretcher, he or she should always be assisted or, at least, given careful attention. The x-ray tube must be *moved away* from the x-ray table, the x-ray table lowered, or a footstool must be in place to assist the patient from the table, and the radiographer must be there to guide or assist the patient safely to the correct dressing room.

If an injured patient requires assistance with dressing and undressing, it is important to remember that clothing should be *removed* from the *uninjured* side first, in comparison to being *placed* on the *injured* side first.

Special consideration must be given to each patient according to his or her condition. Elderly and very thin patients, and those who will be required to lie on the x-ray table for a lengthy period, benefit greatly from a foam pad between them and the x-ray table. Lumbar strain is relieved by a pillow or positioning sponge placed under the knees. An extra pillow for the head or cushioning under the heels or ischial tuberosities can make a big difference in patient care. Special care and attention should be given to the skin of the elderly patients because it bruises and bleeds easily.

Patients who are sedated, senile, in shock, or under the influence of alcohol or drugs must never be left unattended. Patients should never be left alone on the x-ray table because they may be active, disoriented, and, occasionally, combative. Indeed, many radiology departments have rules stating that *no* patient may *ever* be left unattended in the radiographic department.

Patients with IV *infusions* in place require additional attention. The IV bag should be 18–24 inches above the level of the vein. The infusion site should be checked periodically for any signs of tissue infiltration. Swelling around the needle site generally indicates that the needle or catheter is no longer in the vein and that the medication is infiltrating the surrounding tissues. The radiographer should turn off the IV tube and notify the physician or nurse.

Difficulty in communication can be encountered with a patient having a *tracheostomy* tube in place. These individuals are often anxious because they cannot communicate verbally, and they are fearful of choking because they cannot remove the secretions that accumulate in their throats. They require careful attention. The nurse should be available to suction secretions if the patient starts to breathe noisily or with difficulty. The radiographer can relieve much patient anxiety by careful explanation of the examination. The patient can be provided with a pencil and pad to communicate any questions or concerns. Other patients that can benefit from this technique are those with chest tubes and other drains, catheters, and orthopedic devices.

Just as health care practitioners provide safety and comfort to the patients, they must ensure their own safety by practicing good physical ergonomics/body mechanics, infection control, and standard precautions.

Safety/Comfort Guidelines

- Secure the patient's belongings
- Ensure hazard-free environment to avoid unnecessary/painful movement
- Use the equipment properly
- Remove clothing first from the uninjured side
- Place clothing first on the injured side

Should an accident ever occur, and a patient or a health care practitioner be injured, no matter how small or insignificant the injury seems, it must be reported to the supervisor and an incident report completed. The risk management team, or similar group, requires all such information for legal *documentation* and as a means of identifying and resolving potential hazards.

Summary

- Modes of patient transportation include ambulation, wheelchair, and stretcher.
- Patient and radiographer safety requires the use of proper and safe ergonomics/body mechanics.
- Wheelchairs and stretchers must be locked, and wheelchair footrests positioned out of the way prior to the patient transfer.
- One person should be responsible for the safe transport of IV lines, catheters, and other tubes.
- Patient transfer between the radiographic table and the stretcher should involve pulling, not pushing; safe patient handling devices include the transfer board, gait belt, and Hoyer lift.
- The knees should be bent when lifting heavy objects; use leg and abdominal muscles instead of the back muscles.
- Heavy objects should be carried close to the body; the back should be kept straight, and twisting motions should be avoided.
- Heavy objects (e.g., mobile x-ray unit) should be pushed or rolled (instead of pulled or lifted) whenever possible.
- Patient belongings should be properly secured according to the policy while the patient is in the radiographer's care.
- The radiographer must be always alert to patient safety and comfort; patients should not be left unattended in the radiographic department.
- Should an accident occur involving the patient and/or the radiographer, accurate documentation should be completed regardless of how minor the incident is.

PATIENT SUPPORT EQUIPMENT

Oxygen

One of the most basic physiologic needs of human beings is an adequate supply of oxygen. Oxygen is taken into the body and supplied to the blood to be delivered to all body tissues. Any tissue(s) lacking in, or devoid of, an adequate blood supply can suffer permanent damage or can die. Diminished oxygen supply (*hypoxia*) can result from an airway obstructed by *aspirated* material, laryngeal edema as a result of *anaphylaxis*, or a pathologic process such as *emphysema*. Oxygen supplementation may be required in cases of severe anemia, pneumonia, pulmonary edema, and shock. Other conditions often requiring oxygen therapy are chronic obstructive pulmonary disease (COPD), pneumonia, severe asthma, and cystic fibrosis.

The radiographer must be knowledgeable enough to recognize symptoms and respond appropriately. The proper response to respiratory distress might be to perform the *Heimlich maneuver,* to summon the code team, or to check the flow of oxygen already in place.

Symptoms of inadequate oxygen supply include *dyspnea, cyanosis, diaphoresis,* and distention of the veins of the neck. A patient who experiences any of these symptoms will be very anxious and must not be left unattended. The radiographer must *call* for help, assist the patient to a sitting or semi-*Fowler position* (the recumbent position makes breathing more difficult), and have oxygen and emergency drugs available.

In areas that patients will occupy for extended periods (e.g., patient department, operating room, emergency department, and radiology department), oxygen is available through wall outlets at a pressure of 60–80 psi (pounds per square inch) equipped with an easily adjustable flowmeter to regulate the administration of oxygen. It is important to administer *humidified* oxygen to avoid drying and irritation of the respiratory mucosa. In other areas, oxygen will be available in tanks, with one valve to regulate its flow and another to indicate the amount of oxygen remaining in the tank.

Methods of Delivery. There are various devices available to deliver oxygen to patients. Their use is determined by the amount of oxygen and its concentration required by the patient. Oxygen is typically delivered at 24%–45% concentration at a rate of 1–6 L/min. Oxygen delivery is frequently classified as *low* or *high flow.* Patients with COPD require low-flow therapy. High-flow systems provide more accurate control of concentration and rate. Excessive or inappropriate high-flow delivery can result in apnea (temporary cessation of breathing).

The *nasal cannula* is the most frequently used device to supplement the oxygen in room air; its short prongs extend approximately 1 cm into the nares. The nasal cannula, also called *nasal prongs,* is a low-flow small-percentage oxygen device used for the patients experiencing mild hypoxia. It is convenient and fairly comfortable for the patient, although it can be somewhat easily dislodged, for example, during sleep.

There are various types of oxygen *masks* available for delivery of oxygen. The *simple face mask* (low flow) is best suited for short-term oxygen therapy. With extended use, the plastic becomes warm and sticky. Communication is difficult, the mask is easily displaced, and it must be removed at mealtime.

The *Venturi mask* mixes oxygen with room air and can deliver higher, carefully controlled, concentration to select patients with COPD, emphysema, and other lung conditions that cause difficulty breathing.

The *partial rebreathing mask* (low flow) and *nonrebreathing mask* (low flow) deliver more precise concentrations of oxygen to the patient who needs high-concentration oxygen but does not require breathing assistance. Examples include patients who are suffering from trauma, carbon dioxide poisoning, and smoke inhalation.

Mechanical ventilators (high flow) are most frequently encountered in a hospital critical care unit and are used when a patient is unable to breath on his or her own. Patients on ventilators have an artificial airway such as intubation or tracheostomy in place, whereas the ventilator controls the respiratory rate and volume.

Special considerations: Although oxygen is not a flammable substance, it does *support combustion* (i.e., materials burn more readily in its presence), so care must be taken to avoid spark or flame where oxygen is in use. No one should ever smoke in an area where oxygen is in use. Oxygen canisters must be kept away from flame. The use of petroleum-based lotion/cream should be avoided because petroleum is a highly flammable mixture of hydrocarbons; rather, water-based products should be used.

Suction

The use of a *suction* device is occasionally required to maintain a patient's airway by *aspirating* secretions, blood, or other fluids. Suctioning may be indicated when the patient is unconscious, when secretions have high volume or viscosity, when coughing is ineffective, or when the individual is otherwise unable to clear his or her airway. Suction is available either from a wall outlet, similar to oxygen, or as a mobile apparatus. It is unlikely that the radiographer would be required to suction the tracheobronchial tree, but he or she might be needed to assist with the procedure. Suction tubing must have a disposable catheter attached to its end for collection of airway secretions. It is essential to use the correct diameter catheter; too large a diameter can result in airway occlusion, leading to hypoxia and/or atelectasis when suction is applied. The radiographer should be familiar with the location of suction equipment and replacement of disposable catheters.

Tubes and Catheters

Following thoracotomy or other thoracic surgery, a *chest tube* may be put in place for the purpose of treating pneumothorax or hemothorax (removing air and/or fluid from the pleural space). The *chest drainage system* usually has three compartments: suction control chamber; collection chamber; and water seal chamber, which prevents atmospheric air from entering the chest cavity. The drainage system must always be kept below the level of the patient's chest.

Radiographers might encounter chest drainage systems when performing mobile radiographic examinations on postsurgical patients. The radiographer must be careful not to disturb chest tubes during patient or equipment manipulation and must immediately report any sudden change in the patient's condition and/or patient's complaint of chest pain or discomfort.

Gastrointestinal (GI) tubes can be *nasogastric* (NG), *nasointestinal* (NI), or *nasoenteric* (NE), and are often simply called NG tubes. NG tubes, such as the Dobhoff tube, are used as feeding tubes for patients whose condition prevents normal swallowing. NI/NE *tubes* can be used following digestive tract surgery to remove gastric fluids and/or air (decompression, e.g., Levin and Salem Sump tubes). NG and NI/NE tubes may be single or double *lumen* and can sometimes be temporarily disconnected for radiographic examinations.

The *single*-lumen NG or NI/NE tube can be clamped, but the *double*-lumen tube must *never* be clamped. If clamped, the walls of the double-lumen tube could adhere permanently. Instead, the tip of a syringe is inserted into the lumen and the syringe, and the tube then pinned (open side up) to the patient's gown. Care must be taken not to disturb the placement of the GI tube. Examples of single-lumen NE tubes are the Cantor and Harris tubes; the Miller–Abbott tube is a double-lumen NE tube. The Sengstaken–Blakemore tube is a triple-lumen tube with a gastric balloon, an esophageal balloon, and a gastric suction port; it is often used in the treatment of bleeding esophageal varices.

There are several specialized tubes/catheters used to provide regular or continual access to the *circulatory* system for long-term care requirements such as dialysis, blood transfusion, drug therapy such as chemotherapy, and parenteral nutrition. They can also be used for laboratory blood draws and for monitoring central venous pressure. These are called *central venous catheters* (CVCs or *central lines*). Examples of these central lines include the Port-A-Cath, the Hickman, the Raaf, and the peripherally inserted central catheter (PICC). For x-ray verification of position placement, they usually have a radiopaque distal tip. The distal tip should be located in the superior or inferior vena cava near the right atrium. During mobile radiography of the chest for tube placement, it is often necessary to *move the radiopaque external wires out of the way* as much as possible to avoid artifacts that can interfere with the accurate diagnosis.

Classification	Purpose	Example
Short-term, external/ nontunneled	Administer medications, draw blood, monitor RA BP	PICC, CVC
Long-term, external/ nontunneled	Administer medications, draw blood	PICC
Long-term, tunneled	Parenteral nutrition, dialysis	Hickman, Raaf
Long-term implanted venous access	Chemotherapy, blood transfusion	Port-A-Cath

Urinary catheterization may be used postsurgically either to assist in the healing of tissues or to assist an incontinent patient in the elimination of urine. It is essential that equipment used for the catheterization procedure is sterile and that subsequent care is given to the catheterized patient to prevent infection because *urinary tract infections* (UTIs) *account for the greatest number of nosocomial* (health care–acquired) *infections.* Urinary catheters are made of plastic, rubber, polyvinylchloride (PVC), and silicone. The type selected is dependent on how long it is expected to remain in the bladder. Plastic and rubber catheters are generally used for short-term use, whereas PVC or silicone catheters can be in place for up to 3 months. The urine collection container must be *kept below the level of the bladder;* backflow of urine into the bladder can lead to infection. When transporting or transferring the catheterized patient, care must be taken that the catheter does not become entangled or dislodged.

Summary

- Oxygen is usually available through wall outlets with adjustable flowmeters or in tanks with a flow-regulating valve and an indicator showing the quantity of oxygen left in the tank.

- Oxygen can be administered via nasal cannula, masks, or mechanical ventilators; oxygen supports combustion, so it must be used away from flame.

- Suction devices are used to aspirate secretions; suction is available from wall outlets or portable suction mechanisms.

- Chest tubes function to remove fluids or air from the thoracic cavity.

- NG and NI/NE tubes assist in the removal of gastric secretions or air and/or are used for the administration of water-soluble contrast material.

- GI tubes can be single or double lumen and can be used for diagnostic and/or therapeutic purposes.

- To prevent UTIs, urinary collection containers must be kept below the level of the bladder, and catheterization procedures must be sterile.

- Continual access tubes are used for long-term care requirements.

PATIENT MONITORING AND DOCUMENTATION

Assessment

The radiographer must *assess* a patient's condition before bringing the patient to the radiographic department and during the diagnostic examination. A good place to begin with is a review of the patient's chart. Other useful information includes the admitting diagnosis and recent nurses' notes including information about the patient's degree of ambulation, any preparation for the x-ray procedure and how it was tolerated, notes regarding laboratory tests, and possible need to save patient urine.

As the radiographer obtains a brief pertinent clinical history, he or she also assesses the patient's condition by *observing* and *listening*. To provide safe and effective care, the radiographer must be able to assess the severity of a traumatized patient's injury, the patient's degree of motor control, and the need for support equipment or radiographic accessories. Can the patient move or be moved from the stretcher? Can the anatomic part be imaged adequately and with less pain on the stretcher or in the wheelchair? Will the use of sponges and/or sandbags result in a more comfortable, safer, and better imaged examination? Routine and continuous monitoring of the patient's condition is essential so that any change in condition can be addressed *before* it becomes a medical emergency.

Physical Signs

When the patient is first approached, and as the diagnostic examination progresses, the radiographer should be alert to the patient's appearance and condition, and any subsequent changes in them. These are often called *objective* signs. It is important to notice the color, temperature, and moistness of the patient's skin. Paleness frequently indicates weakness; the *diaphoretic* patient has pale, cool skin. The *febrile* patient usually exhibits hot, dry skin. "Sweaty" palms may indicate *anxiety*. A patient who becomes *cyanotic* (bluish lips, mucous membranes, or nail beds) needs oxygen and requires immediate medical attention.

It is important that the radiographer be aware of the patient's gross and fine *motor control* to avoid patient injury. Gross/general motor control refers to basic body movement and locomotion such as walking or waving one's arm. Fine motor control involves the coordination of bones, muscles, and nerves to produce smaller and more precise movements/tasks such as zipping a zipper or grasping and writing with a pencil. Conditions of the brain, spinal cord, nerves, muscles, and bony articulations (e.g., in Parkinson's disease) impair fine motor control.

Subjective signs are those perceived by the patient—how he or she feels, what is the level of his or her pain, and so on. Subjective information can be just as valuable as objective information, and the radiographer's listening skills can have a great deal to do with the patient's lasting impression of his or her health care experience.

Vital Signs

Vital signs can provide crucial information about an individual's state of health. The radiographer employed in an office environment often finds vital signs measurement part of his or her routine duties. If a medical emergency arises in the hospital radiology area, the radiographer may be required to assist by obtaining the patient's vital signs. Although checking vital signs is not a routine function, the radiographer should be proficient and confident if and when the need arises. Practicing the skills associated with taking vital signs during "slow" periods can benefit the patient during an emergency, and those on whom you practice will learn their baseline signs—which provides valuable information for everyone.

Obtaining *vital signs* involves the measurement of *body temperature, pulse rate, respiratory rate,* and *arterial blood pressure.*

Body temperature varies with the time of day and site of measurement. It can be measured via a thermometer in the mouth, rectum, axilla, bladder, heart chamber, external auditory canal, or temporal artery. Elevated body temperature, or *fever,* often signifies infection. Symptoms of fever include general malaise, increased pulse and respiratory rates, flushed skin that is hot and dry to the touch, and occasional chills. Patients who experience very high, prolonged fevers can suffer irreparable brain damage.

Normal body temperature varies from person to person depending on several factors, including age. A normal *adult* body temperature taken orally is 98.6°F (37°C). Rectal temperature is generally 0.5°F–1.0°F

Vital Signs

- Body temperature
- Pulse rate
- Respiratory rate
- Arterial blood pressure

Normal Body Temperatures

Adult	
Oral	98.6°F
Rectal	99.1°F–99.6°F
Axillary	97.6°F–98.1°F
Infants to children aged 4 years	97.9°F–100.4°F (rectal)
Children aged 5–13 years	97.8°F–98.6°F

higher, whereas axillary temperature is usually 0.5°F–1.0°F lower. A variation of 0.5°F–1.0°F is generally considered within normal limits. Body temperature is usually lowest in the early morning and highest at night. Infants and children have a wider range of body temperature (rectal: 97.9°F–100.4°F) than adults; the elderly patients have lower body temperatures than others. Infants and children up to 4 years of age have normal (tympanic) body temperatures between 96.4°F and 100.4°F. *Children* aged 5–13 years have a normal body temperature range of 97.8°F–98.6°F.

Body areas with superficial arteries are best suited for determination of a patient's pulse rate. The *seven most readily palpated pulse points* are the radial, carotid, brachial, femoral, popliteal, temporal, and dorsalis pedis pulses. Of these, the radial pulse is the most frequently used pulse. The apical pulse, at the apex of the heart, may be readily evaluated with the use of a stethoscope. The pulse rate should be counted for 30 s and multiplied by 2. Attention should be given to pulse regularity and volume.

Pulse rate depends on the person's age, sex, body exertion and position, and general state of health. Children and the elderly individuals have higher pulse rates. Pulse rate increases in the standing position, after exertion, and with certain conditions such as fever, organic heart disease, *shock,* and alcohol and drug use. Certain variations in the regularity and strength of the pulse are characteristic of various maladies. Pulse rates vary between men and women, and among adults, children, and infants; athletes often have lower pulse rates.

The act of *respiration* serves to deliver oxygen to all the body cells and rid the body of carbon dioxide. The radiographer must be able to recognize abnormalities or changes in the patient respiration. The general term used to describe difficulty breathing is *dyspnea.* Symptoms of inadequate oxygen supply include retracted intercostal spaces, cyanosis, diaphoresis, and neck vein distention; sitting and semi-Fowler positions are helpful for patients with dyspnea. More specific terms used to describe abnormal respirations include *uneven, spasmodic, strident* (shrill, grating sound), *stertorous* (labored, e.g., snoring), *tachypneic* (abnormally rapid breathing), *orthopneic* (difficulty breathing while recumbent), and *oligopneic* (abnormally shallow, slow).

Respirations should be counted after counting the pulse rate while still holding the patient's wrist. Respiratory action may become more deliberate and less natural in the patient who is aware that his or her respirations are being counted. Respirations should be counted for at least 30 s; 15-s counting multiplied by 4 can result in a fairly large error. The normal *adult* respiratory rate is 12–18 breaths/min. The respiratory rate of young *children* is somewhat higher, up to 30 breaths/min. Although the radiographer is counting respirations, he or she should also be assessing the respiratory pattern (even, uneven) and depth (normal, shallow, deep).

Blood pressure measures the degree of force applied to arterial walls as the heart pumps blood throughout the body. It is measured by using a mercury-based manometer and read in millimeters of mercury

Common Pulse Points

Artery	Location
Radial	Wrist; at the base of the thumb
Carotid	Neck; just lateral to the midline
Temporal	In front of the upper ear
Femoral	Inguinal region; groin
Popliteal	Posterior knee
Brachial	Medial to bicep tendon near antecubital fossa
Dorsalis pedis	Dorsum of foot between the 1st and 2nd toes

Normal (Resting) Pulse Rates (Beats/min)

Men	68–75
Women	72–80
Children	70–100
Infants	100–160

(mm Hg). As with other vital signs, the measurement is made with the patient in the sitting position and having rested for approximately 5 min prior to measurement.

Blood pressure among individuals varies with age, sex, fatigue, mental or physical stress, disease, and trauma. The blood pressure within vessels is highest during ventricular *systole* (contraction) and lowest during *diastole* (relaxation). Blood pressure measurements are recorded with the systolic pressure on top and the diastolic pressure on the bottom, as in 100/80 (read "one hundred over eighty"). Normal adult systolic pressure ranges between 90 and 120 mm Hg; the normal diastolic range is between 60 and 79 mm Hg. Prehypertension is present when blood pressure measurements are between 120 and 140 mm Hg systolic and/or between 80 and 90 mm Hg diastolic. Blood pressure consistently above 140/90 mm Hg is considered hypertension. Left undiagnosed and untreated, hypertension can lead to renal, cardiac, or brain damage. Hypotension is characterized by a systolic pressure of less than 90 mm Hg. Hypotension is seen in individuals with a decreased blood volume as a result of hemorrhage, infection, fever, and anemia. *Orthostatic* hypotension occurs in some individuals when they rise quickly from a recumbent position.

Blood pressure is measured by using a *sphygmomanometer* and a stethoscope. The patient may be recumbent or seated with the arm supported. The cuff of the sphygmomanometer is wrapped snugly around the upper arm, with its lower edge just above the *antecubital fossa*. With the stethoscope earpieces in place, the brachial artery pulse is palpated in the antecubital fossa and the bell (diaphragm) of the stethoscope is placed over the brachial artery. The valve on the bulb pump is closed and the cuff is inflated *enough to collapse the brachial artery* (~180 mm Hg). The valve is then opened very slowly. The first sound heard is the systolic pressure; as the valve pressure is slowly released, the sound becomes louder and then suddenly gets softer—this is the diastolic pressure. After the blood pressure measurements are recorded, the stethoscope earpieces and bell should be cleaned.

Blood Pressure Can Be Affected By

- Cardiac output
- Blood volume
- Vascular resistance

Blood Pressure

- Measured by using a sphygmomanometer and a stethoscope
- Cuff inflation sufficient to collapse the brachial artery
- First sound heard is systolic pressure

Documentation

The *chart* of a hospitalized patient is a collection of information, records, and laboratory and imaging reports. Information includes the patient's condition, progress, medications, treatments, and so on.

Documentation required of the radiographer should be entered directly on the patient's examination *requisition,* or in the radiology computer system *notes*. Notes are made regarding pertinent patient history, illness, or injury.

Any incident, accident, or unusual occurrence that causes injury or potential injury/harm to the patient (or visitor, or staff) must be reported to a radiology supervisor and an incident report completed. This is very important for the hospital's risk management department— both for liability considerations and for possible procedural alterations to prevent future similar incidents.

Summary

- Patient condition may be assessed through chart information, observation, questioning, and vital signs.
- A patient's vital signs are temperature, pulse and respiration rates, and blood pressure.
- A normal adult oral body temperature is 98.6°F, axillary temperatures is 0.5°F–1°F lower, and rectal temperatures is 0.5°F–1°F higher.
- The *pulse* represents regular expansion and contraction of an artery as waves of blood travel through it.
- The arterial pulse points include radial, carotid, temporal, femoral, and popliteal.
- The normal adult pulse rate is 70–80 beats/min; pulse rates of infant and children are higher.
- The normal adult respiratory rate is 12–18 breaths/min, with children's respirations being higher (up to 30 breaths/min).
- Dyspnea refers to difficulty breathing; other terms are used to describe specific respiratory abnormalities.
- Symptoms of inadequate oxygen supply include dyspnea, cyanosis, diaphoresis, and neck vein distention; sitting and semi-Fowler positions are helpful for patients with dyspnea.
- Blood pressure is measured by using a sphygmomanometer and a stethoscope.
- The average normal adult systolic blood pressure is 90–120 mm Hg, and average normal adult diastolic blood pressure is 60–80 mm Hg; blood pressure varies with a person's age, sex, fatigue, mental or physical stress level, disease, and trauma.
- When reading blood pressure, systolic pressure (contraction) is the top number and diastolic pressure (relaxation) is the bottom number.

MEDICAL EMERGENCIES

Radiographers must be prepared to provide immediate attention and appropriate response to any serious and unexpected patient event. A number of potential medical emergencies and their appropriate responses are identified as follows.

Allergic Reactions

An *allergy* is an abnormal, acquired immune response to a substance (i.e., *allergen*) that would usually not trigger a reaction. An initial exposure to the allergen (i.e., *sensitization*) is required. Subsequent contact with the allergen then results in an *inflammatory response*. Examples of such responses include hay fever, urticaria, allergic rhinitis, eczema, and bronchial asthma. Allergens can be introduced into the body via contact, ingestion (e.g., food), inhalation (e.g., dust, pollen), or injection (e.g., medication, drugs). Allergic reactions of particular importance to the radiographer involve the use of *latex* products and *contrast media*.

Medications are administered to meet specific patient needs; medications can have harmless *side effects* in some individuals. If the side effect offsets the benefit, the medication might be discontinued. Medications can also have a *toxic effect*. Toxic effects can occur because of sensitivity, overdose, or poor metabolism. An *antidote* is used to treat a toxic effect.

Latex

Latex products are manufactured from a milky fluid derived from the rubber tree, and several chemicals are added to the fluid during the manufacture of commercial latex. Some proteins in latex can produce mild-to-severe allergic reactions. In addition, chemicals added during processing can cause skin rashes. When *powdered* latex gloves are worn, more latex proteins reach the skin. In addition, when gloves are changed, latex protein/powder particles get into the air, where they can be inhaled and come in contact with the body membranes. Studies have indicated that when unpowdered gloves are worn, there are extremely low levels of the allergy-producing proteins present. Health care professionals should help educate latex-sensitized persons about the latex content of common objects.

A wide variety of products contain latex: medical supplies, personal protective equipment, and many household items. The intermittent use of latex products generally causes no health problems. However, workers in the health care industry (physicians, technologists, nurses, dentists, etc.) are at risk for developing *latex allergy* because they use latex gloves frequently. Other workers with frequent glove use (hairdressers, housekeepers, food service workers, etc.) and those involved in the manufacture of latex products are also at risk.

Irritant Contact Dermatitis. The most common reaction to latex products is *irritant contact dermatitis*. It is characterized by the development of irritated, dry, itchy areas on the skin, usually the hands. Irritant contact dermatitis is a skin irritation resulting from the use of gloves and/or from exposure to other workplace products and chemicals. Irritant contact dermatitis can also be caused by repeated handwashing, incomplete drying, use of sanitizers, and exposure to glove powder. *Irritant contact dermatitis* is not defined as a true allergy.

Allergic Contact Dermatitis. Allergic contact dermatitis (*delayed hypersensitivity*) results from exposure to the chemicals added to latex during its manufacture. These chemicals can cause skin reactions such as those produced by poison ivy, in which the rash usually begins 24–48 hours following contact and can lead to oozing skin blisters and/or spread to areas away from the area of initial contact. Wearing latex gloves during episodes of hand dermatitis may increase skin exposure and the risk of developing latex allergy.

Latex Allergy. Latex allergy (*immediate hypersensitivity*) can be a much more serious reaction to latex. Certain proteins in latex can cause sensitization, and although the amount of exposure needed to cause this sensitization is unknown, even very low level exposure can trigger allergic reaction in some sensitized individuals.

Medical Equipment That Could Contain Latex

- Disposable gloves
- Tourniquets
- Blood pressure cuffs
- Stethoscopes
- Intravenous tubing
- Oral and nasal airways
- Enema tips
- Endotracheal tubes
- Syringes
- Electrode pads
- Catheters
- Wound drains
- Injection ports

Types of Reactions to Latex

- Irritant contact dermatitis
- Allergic contact dermatitis (delayed hypersensitivity)
- Latex allergy (immediate hypersensitivity)

Reactions usually begin within minutes of exposure to the latex but can occur hours later. *Mild* reactions involve skin redness, hives, or itching. *More severe* are respiratory reactions, for example, itchy eyes, runny nose, sneezing, difficulty breathing, and wheezing. A *life-threatening reaction* such as shock is rarely the first sign of latex allergy. Such reactions are similar to those seen in some persons with allergy after a bee sting.

Anaphylactic Responses

Potentially *life-threatening (anaphylactic) systemic responses* include respiratory failure, shock, and death within minutes. *Early* symptoms of an anaphylactic reaction include itching of the palms and soles, wheezing, constriction of the throat (possibly caused by laryngeal edema), *dyspnea, dysphagia, hypotension,* and *cardiopulmonary arrest.* The radiographer must maintain the patient's airway, summon the radiologist and/or nursing staff, and call a "code." The radiographer should then be prepared to stay with the patient and assist until the arrival of the code team.

Renal Function

With the use of iodinated contrast agents, there can be concern for increased renal damage in patients with acute kidney injury (AKI) and/or in patients with severe chronic kidney disease (as determined by estimated glomerular filtration rate [eGFR]). In addition, patients taking oral medication to control blood sugar, such as metformin (Glucophage), can be susceptible to kidney damage from the use of iodinated contrast agents. Current (February 2022) American College of Radiology (ACR) recommendations state that "Although the true risk of CI-AKI remains unknown, prophylaxis with intravenous normal saline is indicated for patients without contraindication (eg, heart failure) who have acute kidney injury (AKI) or an estimated glomerular filtration rate (eGFR) less than 30 mL/min/1.73 m^2 who are not undergoing maintenance dialysis. In individual high-risk circumstances, prophylaxis may be considered in patients with an eGFR of 30–44 mL/min/1.73 m^2 at the discretion of the ordering clinician."

https://www.acr.org/-/media/ACR/Files/Clinical-Resources/ACK-NKF-Consensus-Iodinated-Contrast.pdf

Summary

- An *allergy* is an abnormal, acquired immune response.
- Allergens can be introduced into the body via contact, ingestion, inhalation, or injection.
- Initial *sensitization* to the allergen is required, subsequent contact results in an *inflammatory response.*
- Proteins in *latex* can produce mild-to-severe allergic reactions; types of reactions to latex include irritant contact and delayed or immediate hypersensitivity.
- An *anaphylactic* reaction is a life-threatening systemic response that requires immediate attention by the code team.
- Patients with diabetes taking metformin should follow the ACR recommendations.

OTHER MEDICAL EMERGENCIES

The importance of radiographers' careful evaluation of their patients is never more obvious than when an emergency arises. An emergency is defined as *a sudden change in a patient's condition requiring immediate medical intervention.* Most patients arrive in the radiology department in a stable condition; a few arrive for diagnostic evaluation of a medical crisis. The radiographer must note the patient's condition on arrival and be alert to any subsequent sudden change in that condition. The value of continual review of the knowledge and skills required for emergencies cannot be overemphasized. Many of these emergencies can occur with little or no warning. Many can be life threatening if not dealt with immediately and correctly.

Vomiting

Patients with vomiting who are sitting or standing should be provided with a basin, tissues, and water for rinsing their mouths. It is essential that recumbent patients have their heads turned to the side to prevent choking from aspiration of vomitus. Patients who report feeling nauseous are often apprehensive and may get some relief by breathing slowly and deeply through their mouths.

Fractures

An *unsplinted* fracture must be moved with great care, with *areas proximal and distal to the fracture site adequately supported.* Any motion is very painful and can result in further injury to tissues surrounding the fracture. Muscle spasm can cause additional pain and can interfere with proper reduction of the fracture. A *splint* should never be removed from an extremity except by a physician or under the direct supervision of a physician. Some splinting devices are not radiolucent, and their removal may be required before the radiographic examination.

Rib fractures may be associated with lung trauma and sternum fractures with heart lacerations. Rib fractures can be very painful—the patient experiences pain just from breathing. *Pelvic* fractures are often associated with injuries to pelvic and abdominal viscera, and extreme care must be taken to avoid *hemorrhage.*

Spinal Injuries

Patients arriving for radiographic evaluation with possible spinal injuries must not be moved. The position of any sandbags or other supportive mechanisms must not be changed. A *horizontal (cross-table) lateral projection* should be evaluated by the physician first to determine the extent of injury and necessity for further radiographs. If the patient must be placed in a lateral position, the logrolling method is usually advised. *A physician must be present whenever the patient's position is changed.*

Epistaxis

A nosebleed (*epistaxis*) may be a result of any one of many causes including *hypertension*, dry nasal mucous membranes, sinusitis, or trauma. The patient should be sitting or in a Fowler position. The radiographer should place cold cloths over the patient's nose and back of the neck. Compressing the sides of the nose against the nasal septum for 6–8 min is also helpful. Continued hemorrhage should be brought to the attention of the physician because cautery or nasal packs might be required.

Postural Hypotension

Orthostatic, or postural, *hypotension* is a decrease in blood pressure that occurs on rising to the erect position. It can be severe enough to cause fainting in individuals who have been confined to bed for several days. The radiographer should assist patients slowly and be watchful for signs of weakness.

Vertigo

Objective vertigo is the sensation of having *objects* (or "the room") spinning around the person; *subjective vertigo* is the sensation that a *person* is spinning in space. It is usually associated with an inner-ear disturbance. Patients experiencing true vertigo (as opposed to dizziness or lightheadedness) are often very nauseous and must be protected from falls with the use of side rails and/or safety belts.

Syncope

A patient who reports feeling dizzy or faint is experiencing *syncope* and should be immediately assisted to a chair. Bending forward and placing the head between the knees will often help relieve the lightheadedness as blood flow to the brain increases. In more severe cases, a patient who cannot be assisted to a chair should be *lowered to a recumbent position*. Elevation of the lower legs or use of the Trendelenburg position is helpful. If the patient loses consciousness, the radiographer should make certain that the airway is open and that clothing, especially at the collar, is loose. Once the patient is recumbent, recovery is usually swift; however, a physician should be notified and the cause of *syncope* identified.

Convulsion

Involuntary muscular contractions and relaxations, often associated with epilepsy or other neurologic disorder, characterize a *convulsion*. *Febrile* convulsions are associated with fever, especially in children. During convulsion, no attempt must be made to restrain the patient's movements. The radiographer's responsibility is to keep the patients from injuring themselves. Tight clothing can be loosened, and objects that could harm the patient should be moved out of the way. The use of a padded tongue blade is no longer usually recommended; it can induce emesis or cause tooth breakage. Most convulsions are of short duration and self-limited. Medical intervention is often unnecessary; it is most important that the patient be protected from injury from objects lying close by.

The term *seizure* is often used interchangeably with the term *convulsion*. However, there are many different types of seizures. Some seizures have very mild symptoms, with little or none of the body movement that characterizes the convulsion.

Seizure

The type of *seizure* known as *petit mal* is so subtle that it goes unnoticed by the patient and the observer. It is characterized by brief loss of consciousness (10–30 s) and accompanied by eye or muscle fluttering. A *grand mal* seizure is characterized by loss of consciousness and falling, followed by generalized muscle spasms. The radiographer should remove any objects in the area that could harm the patient and loosen any tight clothing. The patient's head should be turned to the side to allow any secretions to flow from the mouth.

Unconsciousness

Unconsciousness is the state of being partially or completely unaware of external stimuli. This state occurs during normal sleep and can also occur in illness and trauma. Pathologic unconsciousness can be caused by a wide variety of conditions including insulin overdose, fainting, uremia, concussion, heat *stroke,* and intoxication. It is important to remember, as we image the unconscious patient, that the sense of hearing is believed to be the last sense that one loses. Imagine how comforting it can be to the unconscious patient to hear his or her caregiver(s) talking to him or her and explaining what is going on around him or her.

There are various levels of consciousness, and the condition of an acutely ill patient can rapidly deteriorate from being fully aware and responsive to diminished or inappropriate responsiveness to complete unresponsiveness. The unconscious patient must never be left unattended. The radiographer must be alert to changes in the patient's level of consciousness and notify the physician immediately of any deterioration.

Acute Abdomen

Patients arriving for radiographic evaluation with a diagnosis of "acute abdomen" are usually suffering from severe abdominal pain, nauseous and vomiting, and frequently close to being in shock. They are indeed very sick patients. The radiographer must perform the examination swiftly and efficiently and remain alert to any sudden changes in the patient condition.

Shock

Shock is a general term and is characterized by diminished peripheral blood flow and insufficient oxygen supply to body tissues. Shock can be caused by a number of conditions including allergic reaction, trauma, hemorrhage, myocardial infarction, and infection. A patient in shock is pale and may become cyanotic; the pulse is rapid and weak, breathing is shallow and rapid, and blood pressure drops sharply. The radiographer should keep the patient warm and flat, or in the Trendelenburg position, and be prepared to assist with emergency procedures.

Respiratory Failure

The inability of the lungs to perform ventilatory functions is respiratory distress and may be described as *acute* or *chronic.* Acute respiratory distress can be caused by impaired gas exchange processes (requiring positive-pressure ventilation) or airway obstruction (requiring the Heimlich maneuver). Chronic respiratory failure is a result of a disease process that impairs breathing such as emphysema, bronchitis, *asthma,* or cystic fibrosis.

The radiographer should be able to distinguish between respiratory arrest (absence of chest movement and breathing sounds) and cardiopulmonary arrest (absence of pulse and respiration with loss of consciousness) and be able to initiate lifesaving actions.

Cardiopulmonary Arrest

The *sudden cessation of productive ventilation and circulation* is called cardiopulmonary arrest. The radiographer should be trained in basic life support for health care providers. The American Heart Association uses the acronym CAB, representing circulation, airway, breathing, to help individuals remember cardiopulmonary resuscitation (CPR) step sequence. Compressions should be approximately 100–120/min. After approximately 30 compressions, airway should be established by using the head-tilt, chin-lift movement. If the victim is not breathing normally, the professional rescuer should begin mouth-to-mouth breathing. One cycle is considered to be 30 chest compressions, followed by two rescue breaths.

Many health care facilities require their employees to be certified in basic lifesaving skills. It is wise for radiographers (and the general public) to be familiar with skills such as the Heimlich maneuver (abdominal thrust) and CPR should the need arise.

Stroke

A *stroke,* or cerebrovascular accident (CVA), is an interference with blood supplied to the brain as a result of occlusion or rupture of a cerebral vessel. If the condition results from a partial vessel occlusion, the interference is usually mild and temporary and is called a *transient ischemic attack* (TIA). The patient may experience temporary blindness in one eye, *dysphasia* or *aphasia, hemiparesis* or hemiplegia, or anesthesia.

If the cerebral vessel is totally occluded or ruptures into the brain or subarachnoid space, a much more serious event has occurred. The patient frequently experiences sudden loss of consciousness and one-sided paralysis (*hemiparesis*), although the onset can be slower if the *occlusion* is caused by *thrombus* formation. Other symptoms include speech disturbances and cool, sweaty skin. The patients should have their head and shoulders elevated or be in the lateral recumbent position; an open airway must be maintained. Because a stroke can occur without warning at any time, the radiographer should be familiar with the signs of an impending stroke and be able to provide appropriate immediate care. The American Stroke Association developed the FAST acronym, which is an easy guide to help identify the signs of a stroke.

Summary

- It is essential that the radiographer be alert to *any* sudden changes in the patient condition; how well the radiographer recognizes and is prepared to meet the challenges of emergencies can have significant impact on the outcome of the emergency.

- F—Face drooping: One side of the face is numb/drooping; when the patient smiles, smile is uneven.
- A—Arm weakness: Weakness/numbness in one arm; when the patient raises both arms, one moves downward.
- S—Speech difficulty: The patient's speech suddenly slurred or difficult to understand/unintelligible; the patient may be unable to repeat a simple sentence.
- T—Time: If any of these symptoms is present, it is time to call 911. Make note of the time when the symptoms started.

COMPREHENSION CHECK

Congratulations! You have completed your review of this chapter. If you are able to answer the following group of comprehensive questions, you can feel confident that you have mastered this section. You are then ready to go on to the "registry-type" questions that follow. For greatest success, do not go to these multiple-choice questions without first completing the following short-answer questions:

1. Discuss the importance of careful and accurate patient assessment; what are the components of a good assessment (p. 38)?

2. Discuss some special needs that a patient undergoing tracheostomy might have (p. 31).

3. Discuss three modes of patient transport (p. 29, 30, 31).

4. Identify, with respect to physical ergonomics/body mechanics and patient transfer (p. 30, 31):

   A. position of the radiographer's feet (as a base of support)

   B. the body's center of gravity (vis-à-vis stability) and when moving heavy objects: push versus pull; use of knees, legs, and back; proximity of the object to the body

   C. three types of ergonomic transfer patient devices; discuss indications for use of each

   D. position of chair, footrests, and locks during wheelchair transfers

   E. position of locks, use of drawsheet and plastic mover, and push versus pull in stretcher transfer

   F. care of IV lines, catheters, oxygen, safety belts, and side rails

5. Discuss objective versus subjective signs; give examples of each (p. 37).

6. Identify the manner in which ambulatory patients should be directed onto and removed from the x-ray table (p. 30, 31).

7. Explain how clothing should be removed from a patient with unilateral injury (p. 31).

8. Identify techniques used to reduce discomfort of elderly and/or thin patients recumbent on the radiographic table (p. 31).

9. Discuss the types of patients likely to be at greater risk if left unattended on the radiographic table (p. 31).

10. Discuss the importance of being alert to the initial patient condition and any subsequent changes in his or her condition (p. 37).

11. Identify and describe the two types of motor control (p. 36, 37).

12. List the four vital signs, identify their adult norms, and list/identify equipment necessary for their assessment (p. 37, 38, 39).

13. What does the palpable pulse represent? What are some variables that can affect pulse rate? List common pulse points (p. 38).

14. Define the terms *diaphoretic, cyanotic, febrile, hypertension, systole, bradycardia,* and *hypoxia* (p. 32, 37, 39).

15. Identify the following with respect to body temperature (p. 37):

    A. normal adult, infant, and child temperatures

    B. the significance of fever, that is, what it usually indicates

    C. symptoms usually associated with fever

    D. difference between oral, rectal, and axillary temperatures

16. Identify the following with respect to pulse rate (p. 38, 39):

    A. the normal, average adult pulse rate for men and women

    B. normal and abnormal conditions under which pulse rate will vary/change

    C. the usual site of pulse determination; other possible sites/any special equipment needed

17. Identify the following with respect to respiration (p. 38):

    A. its function

    B. the ideal time to determine patient respiration rate; why?

    C. the normal, average adult respiratory rate

18. Identify the following with respect to blood pressure (p. 38, 39):

    A. equipment necessary

    B. position of the patient

    C. position of the cuff and the bell

    D. first and second sounds heard

    E. maximum norms for systolic and diastolic pressures

    F. prehypertensive and hypertensive pressures

19. Identify illnesses/conditions that might require supplemental oxygen (p. 32, 33).

20. What condition specifically requires a low-flow rate of oxygen (p. 33)?

21. List the subjective symptoms of inadequate oxygen; identify the body position frequently helpful for the patient with dyspnea (p. 33).

22. Describe four methods of oxygen delivery and identify when each might be indicated (p. 33).

23. Identify any hazards involved in the use of oxygen (p. 34).

24. Describe the circumstance(s) in which suction might be required; identify types of suction devices available (p. 31, 34, 35).

25. Explain the function of chest tubes and precautions that should be taken by the radiographer (p. 34).

26. Describe the function of NG and NI tubes and any precautions that should be taken by the radiographer (p. 34, 35).

27. Identify the classification and purpose of the PICC, Hickman, and Port-A-Cath lines (p. 35).

28. Describe the function of urinary catheters and any precautions that should be taken by the radiographer (p. 35).

29. List/name the three parts of a chest drainage system (p. 34).

30. Identify the level at which urinary collection containers should be kept (p. 35, 36).

31. Define *allergy;* discuss *sensitization* and *inflammatory* responses (p. 40, 41).

32. Distinguish between a *side effect* and a *toxic effect* (p. 41).

33. List the three types of latex reactions; discuss the effect *powder* can have on latex gloves (p. 41).

34. Discuss the difference between *delayed* and *immediate* hypersensitivity (p. 41).

35. Discuss the importance of observing initial patient condition and any subsequent changes (p. 34).

36. Describe precautions the radiographer should take when radiographing a patient with a *fracture* (p. 43).

37. Discuss precautions to be taken with patients having suspected *spinal injuries* (p. 43).

38. Describe first aid for *epistaxis* (p. 43, 44).

39. Distinguish between postural hypotension, vertigo, and syncope; discuss precautions taken and care given by the radiographer (p. 44).

40. Discuss any unique considerations that should be addressed when caring for an unconscious patient (p. 45).

41. Describe symptoms of *acute abdomen* and *shock;* indicate any precautions that should be taken by the radiographer (p. 45).

42. Discuss the difference between *convulsion* and *seizure.* Distinguish between grand mal and petit mal seizures; discuss care appropriate for a patient experiencing a grand mal seizure (p. 45, 46).

43. Distinguish between respiratory arrest and cardiopulmonary arrest; discuss appropriate responses by a radiographer (p. 46).

44. Describe stroke, including some symptoms, and discuss appropriate responses by a radiographer (p. 46, 47).

45. Define and discuss the importance of the acronym FAST (p. 47).

CHAPTER REVIEW QUESTIONS

1. Which of the following is/are symptom(s) of inadequate oxygen supply?

   1. Diaphoresis
   2. Cyanosis
   3. Retracted intercostal spaces

   (A) 1 only
   (B) 1 and 2 only
   (C) 2 and 3 only
   (D) 1, 2, and 3

2. A patient's feeling of spinning, or the room spinning around him or her, is called

   (A) orthostatic hypotension
   (B) epistaxis
   (C) vertigo
   (D) syncope

3. Types of NG/NI/NE tubes include

   1. Port-A-Cath
   2. Sengstaken–Blakemore
   3. Miller–Abbott

   (A) 1 only
   (B) 1 and 2 only
   (C) 2 and 3 only
   (D) 1, 2, and 3

4. A patient's IV container should be hung

   (A) 18–24 inches above the vein
   (B) 18–24 inches below the vein
   (C) 18–24 inches above the heart
   (D) 18–24 inches below the heart

5. All of the following are correct concepts of good physical ergonomics/body mechanics during patient lifting/moving, *except*

   (A) the radiographer should stand with feet approximately 12 inches apart and with one foot slightly forward
   (B) the body's center of gravity should be positioned over its base of support
   (C) the back should be kept straight; avoid twisting
   (D) when carrying a heavy object, hold it away from the body

6. Partial restriction of blood supplied to the brain as a result of a temporary or mild occlusion of a cerebral vessel is called

   (A) TIA
   (B) CVA
   (C) syncope
   (D) epistaxis

7. Blood pressure is measured in units of

   (A) millimeters of mercury (mm Hg)
   (B) beats per minute
   (C) degrees Fahrenheit (°F)
   (D) liters per minute (L/min)

8. Which blood vessels are best suited for determination of pulse rate?

   (A) Superficial arteries
   (B) Deep arteries
   (C) Superficial veins
   (D) Deep veins

9. Medical equipment that might contain latex include

   1. catheters
   2. endotracheal tubes
   3. syringes

   (A) 1 only
   (B) 1 and 2 only
   (C) 2 and 3 only
   (D) 1, 2, and 3

10. When a radiographer is obtaining a patient history, both subjective and objective data should be obtained. An example of *subjective* data is that

    (A) the patient appears to have a productive cough
    (B) the patient has a blood pressure of 130/95 mm Hg
    (C) the patient states that she experiences extreme pain in the upright position
    (D) the patient has a palpable mass in the right upper quadrant of the left breast

Answers and Explanations

1. (D) Oxygen is taken into the body and supplied to the blood to be delivered to all body tissues. Any tissue(s) lacking in or devoid of an adequate blood supply can suffer permanent damage or die. Oxygen may be required in cases of severe anemia, pneumonia, pulmonary edema, and shock. Symptoms of inadequate oxygen supply include *dyspnea, cyanosis, diaphoresis, retraction of intercostal spaces, dilated nostrils,* and distention of the veins of the neck. A patient who experiences any of these symptoms will be very anxious and must not be left unattended. The radiographer must call for help, assist the patient to a sitting or semi-Fowler position (the recumbent position makes breathing more difficult), and have oxygen and emergency drugs available.

2. (C) *Objective vertigo* is the sensation of having *objects* (or the room) spinning about the person; *subjective vertigo* is the sensation of the *person* spinning about. It is often associated with an inner-ear disturbance. Patients experiencing true vertigo (as opposed to dizziness or lightheadedness) are often very nauseous and must be protected from falls. A patient who reports feeling dizzy or faint (*syncope*) should be immediately assisted to a chair. Bending forward and placing the head between the knees will often help relieve the lightheadedness as blood flow to the brain increases. In more severe cases, *a patient who cannot be assisted to a chair should be lowered to a recumbent position.* Elevation of the lower legs, or use of the Trendelenburg position, is helpful. *Orthostatic, or postural, hypotension* is a decrease in blood pressure that occurs on rising to the erect position. It can be severe enough to cause fainting in individuals who have been confined to bed for several days. A nosebleed (epistaxis) may be a result of any one of many causes including hypertension, dry nasal mucous membranes, sinusitis, or trauma. The patient should be sitting or in a Fowler position. The radiographer should place cold cloths over the patient's nose and back of the neck.

3. (C) Gastrointestinal (GI) tubes can be *nasogastric* (NG), *nasointestinal* (NI), or *nasoenteric* (NE). NG tubes, such as the Dobhoff tube, are used as feeding tubes for patients whose condition prevents normal swallowing. NI/NE tubes can be used following digestive tract surgery to remove gastric fluids and/or air (decompression; e.g., Levin and Salem Sump tubes). NG and NI/NE tubes may be single or double *lumen* and can sometimes be temporarily disconnected for radiographic examinations.

The *single*-lumen NG or NI/NE tube can be clamped, but the *double*-lumen tube must *never* be clamped. If clamped, the walls of the double-lumen tube could adhere permanently. Instead, the tip of a syringe is inserted into the lumen and the syringe and the tube then pinned (open side up) to the patient's gown. Care must be taken not to disturb the placement of the GI tube. Examples of single-lumen NE tubes are the Cantor and Harris tubes; the Miller–Abbott tube is a double-lumen NE tube. The Sengstaken–Blakemore tube is a triple-lumen tube with a gastric balloon, an esophageal balloon, and a gastric suction port; it is often used in the treatment of bleeding esophageal varices.

4. (A) The IV container should be hung 18–24 inches *above the level of the vein*. If placed lower than the vein, solution will stop flowing and blood will return into the tubing. If hung too high, solution can run too fast. Occasionally, the position of the needle or catheter in the vein will affect the flow rate. If the bevel is adjacent to the vessel wall, flow may decrease or stop altogether. Often, just changing the position of the patient's arm will remedy the situation.

5. (D) Rules of good physical ergonomics/body mechanics include the following: When carrying a heavy object, hold it *close* to the body; the back should be kept straight; *avoid twisting* when lifting an object; bend the knees and *use leg and abdominal* muscles to lift (rather than the back muscles); and whenever possible, *push or roll* heavy objects (rather than lifting or pulling). To transfer the patient with maximum safety, the radiographer must correctly use certain concepts of physical ergonomics. First, *a broad base of support* lends greater stability; therefore, the radiographer should stand with his or her feet approximately 12 inches apart and with one foot slightly forward. Second, stability is achieved when the body's *center of gravity* (center of the pelvis) is positioned over its base of support. For example, leaning away from the central axis of the body makes the body more vulnerable to losing balance; if the feet are close together, balance is even more difficult to maintain.

6. (A) A *stroke*, or *cerebrovascular accident* (CVA), is an interference with blood supplied to the brain as a result of occlusion or rupture of a cerebral vessel. If the condition results from a *partial* vessel occlusion, the interference is usually *mild and temporary* and is called a *transient ischemic attack* (TIA). The patient may experience temporary blindness in one eye, dysphasia *or* aphasia, hemiparesis or hemiplegia, or anesthesia. *Syncope* is the feeling of lightheadedness, faintness, or dizziness. A patient should be immediately assisted to a chair. Bending forward and placing the head between the knees will often help relieve the lightheadedness as blood flow to the brain increases. A nosebleed (*epistaxis*) may be a result of any one of many causes, including hypertension, dry nasal mucous membranes, sinusitis, or trauma. The patient should be sitting or in a Fowler position. The radiographer should place cold cloths over the patient's nose and back of the neck.

7. (A) Blood pressure is measured in *millimeters of mercury* (mm Hg). Heart rate, or pulse, is measured in units of *beats per minute*. Temperature is measured in *degrees Fahrenheit* (°F). Oxygen delivery is measured in units of *liters per minute* (L/min). Table 3-1 outlines the normal ranges for vital signs in healthy adults.

TABLE 3-1. Normal Ranges for Vital Signs in Adults

Blood pressure	90–120/60–80 mm Hg
Pulse rate	60–80 beats/min
Temperature	97.7°F–99.5°F
Respiratory rate	12–20 breaths/min

8. (A) *Superficial arteries* are best suited for determination of pulse rate. The five most easily palpated pulse points are the radial, carotid, temporal, femoral, and popliteal pulses. The radial pulse is the most frequently used pulse. The apical pulse, at the apex of the heart, is the most accurate and can be determined with the use of a stethoscope.

9. (D) *Latex* products are manufactured from a milky fluid derived from the rubber tree, and several chemicals are added to the fluid during the manufacture of commercial latex. Some proteins in latex can produce mild-to-severe allergic reactions; chemicals added during processing can also cause skin rashes. A wide variety of products contain latex: medical supplies, personal protective equipment, and many household items. Medical equipment that could contain latex include disposable gloves, catheters, tourniquets, endotracheal tubes, syringes, enema tips, and stethoscopes. The intermittent use of latex products generally causes no health problems. However, workers in the health care industry are at risk for developing *latex allergy* if they use latex gloves frequently. Other workers at risk because of frequent latex glove use are hairdressers, housekeepers, food service workers, and so on, and those involved in the manufacture of latex products.

10. (C) Obtaining a complete and accurate history from the patient for the radiologist is an important aspect of a radiographer's job. Both subjective and objective data should be collected. *Objective* data include signs and symptoms that can be observed, such as a cough, a lump, or elevated blood pressure. *Subjective* data relate to what the patient feels and to what extent. A patient may experience pain, but is it mild or severe? Is it localized or general? Does the pain increase or decrease under different circumstances? A radiographer should explore this with the patient and document the information on the requisition for the radiologist.

Infection Prevention and Control

OBJECTIVES

At the conclusion of this chapter, the student will be able to:

- Discuss pathogens as causative and opportunistic agents.
- Discuss and distinguish between antisepsis, medical asepsis, disinfection, and surgical asepsis.
- Identify the most important precaution in the practice of aseptic technique and infection prevention.
- Identify the appropriate use of antiseptics, disinfectants, and germicides.
- Discuss the importance of the health care professional's personal care.
- Explain the cycle involved in transmitting infectious disease.
- Identify the three main modes of infection transmission and their transmission-based precautions.
- Discuss the radiographers' approach to dealing with neutropenic isolation/precautions.
- Discuss appropriate precautions for various hazardous materials.
- Identify the OSHA requirements for MSDSs for hazardous materials.

TERMINOLOGY AND BASIC CONCEPTS

Microorganisms

Living organisms too small to be seen with the naked eye are called *microorganisms*. Most microorganisms do not produce infection or disease; many reside harmlessly. Many are beneficial for our good health, for example, bacteria, protozoa, and fungi found on/in particular body areas. Specific permanent floras are found, for example, in the mouth, upper respiratory tract, and intestines; many of these microorganisms inhibit the growth of *pathogens* in their natural sites, but can cause infection if introduced into a site where they do not normally reside, or when introduced into an immunocompromised host.

Pathogens

Pathogens are causative agents—microorganisms capable of producing disease. Pathogens can cause infection or disease by destroying cells or tissues, or by secreting toxins. Pathogenic microorganisms can be transmitted from one host to another. Because hospitals are the places that treat and care for people with infection and disease, it stands to reason that health care practitioners must be particularly vigilant against transmission of pathogenic microorganisms. Pathogens termed *opportunistic* are usually harmless but can become harmful if introduced into a part of the body where they do not normally reside, or when introduced into an immunocompromised host. *Blood-borne* pathogens reside in blood and can be transmitted to an individual exposed to the blood or body fluids of the infected individual. Common blood-borne pathogens include hepatitis C virus (HCV), hepatitis B virus (HBV), and human immunodeficiency virus (HIV).

The prevention and control of infection must be a hospital-wide effort; each department is required to have its own infection prevention and control protocol, designed according to the risks unique to the services provided. Because radiography often involves exposure to sickness and disease, the radiographer must be aware of, and conscientiously practice, effective prevention and control measures to reduce the spread of infection.

Medical and Surgical Asepsis

Antisepsis is a practice that retards the growth of pathogenic microorganisms. The practice of *medical asepsis* reduces the likelihood of transferring pathogenic microorganisms (bacteria) to a vulnerable individual. The destruction of pathogens by using chemical materials is termed *disinfection*. Examples of disinfectants are hydrogen peroxide, chlorine, iodine, chlorhexidine, and formaldehyde. *Surgical asepsis* (*sterilization*) refers to the removal of all microorganisms *and* their spores (reproductive cells) and is practiced in the surgical suite. Health care practitioners must practice medical asepsis at all times.

Hand Hygiene

Ignaz Semmelweis was a Hungarian physician who is known as the "Father of Infection Control" and as the "Savior of Mothers." He believed that pathogens were transmitted via *direct contact* from the physician to the patient. While working in a maternity clinic in Vienna, in 1847, Dr Semmelweis began encouraging interns to cleanse their hands. The fatal puerperal fever (childbed fever) incidence was immediately reduced from 5%–30% to 1%–2%. However, the ideas of Semmelweis were ridiculed, and he was dismissed from the hospital. Nowadays we know that *the most important precaution in the practice of aseptic technique is proper handwashing*.

The radiographer's hands should be thoroughly washed with soap and warm running water, or by using an alcohol sanitizer, for at least 20 s before and after each patient examination. If the faucet cannot be operated with the knee, it should be opened and closed by using paper towels (to avoid contamination of, or by, the faucet). The radiographer's uniform should not touch the sink. The hands and forearms should always be kept lower than the elbows; care should be taken to wash all surfaces and between fingers. Hand lotions may be used to prevent hands from chapping because broken skin permits the entry of microorganisms.

Alcohol-based hand antiseptic sanitizers have been recommended as an alternative to handwashing with soap and water, except when there is visible soiling or after caring for a patient with *Clostridium difficile* (*C. difficile*) infection. Antiseptics, disinfectants, and germicides are substances used to kill pathogenic bacteria, and some of these products are used in handwashing substances. Disinfectants and germicides are often used for *hard surfaces*, whereas antiseptics are generally used for *tissue*. Disinfection of environmental services is essential to reduction in health care–associated infections (HAIs). High-touch surfaces such as call buttons, bed rails, over-the-bed tables, and other reusable equipment that can be moved between rooms can contribute to inadvertent infections in the absence of adequate disinfection.

Personal Care

A clean uniform should be worn daily because clothing becomes contaminated during patient care. Microorganisms can find safe harbor in jewelry, especially in rings with stones and other crevices, and many facilities do not permit health care workers to wear artificial nails, for they can harbor fungi and microbes. The Centers for Disease Control and Prevention (CDC) *Guideline for Hand Hygiene in Healthcare Settings* (*Morb Mortal Wkly Rep.* 2002;51(RR-16):1–44) states, "HCWs (Heath Care Workers) who wear artificial nails are more likely to harbor Gram-negative pathogens on their fingertips than are those who have natural nails, both before and after handwashing." The only jewelry a health care practitioner should wear is a wristwatch and simple wedding band. *Many microorganisms can remain infectious while awaiting transmission to another host.*

Sterile technique is used during invasive procedures, such as biopsies, and for the administration of contrast media via the *intravenous* (IV) (e.g., CT studies) and *intrathecal* (e.g., myelography) routes.

When radiography is required in the surgical suite, every precaution must be made to maintain the surgical asepsis required in surgical procedures. This requires proper dress, cleanliness of equipment, and restricted access to certain areas. One example of a restricted area is the "sterile corridor," the area between the draped patient and the instrument table. Only the surgeon and the instrument nurse occupy this area.

Chain of Infection

The CDC describes the chain of infection as follows.

Reservoir of Infection. The reservoir (source) of infection is any environment where pathogens can survive and reproduce, and ultimately pose a risk of transmission to a susceptible host. This environment must afford an appropriate temperature, moisture, and nutrients—all conditions found in the human body.

Chain of Infection

1. Reservoir of infection
2. Portal of exit
3. Modes of transmission
4. Portal of entry
5. Susceptible host

Examples of reservoirs of infection include a patient with active tuberculosis, a visitor with an upper respiratory infection, or a health care professional with conjunctivitis.

Some people, called "carriers," can appear healthy yet harbor infectious microorganisms. Carriers may unwittingly infect a susceptible host (patient or coworker). Probably the most famous example of an unwitting carrier was Mary Mallon (Typhoid Mary), a healthy Irish immigrant whose employment as a cook was traced back to 1900; the food she prepared was the *vehicle* that transported typhoid microorganisms. It was found that typhoid outbreaks had followed Mallon's employment from job to job. From 1900 to 1907, Mallon worked at seven places of employment in which 22 people had become ill with typhoid fever shortly after Mallon came to work for them. Once traced, Mallon did not understand how a healthy person could possibly spread disease. But Mallon was tried in court, subsequently ran from health officials, was recaptured, and forced to live in relative seclusion on an island off New York. Mary Mallon was the first healthy carrier of typhoid fever in the United States. An example of healthy carriers nowadays includes asymptomatic carriers of HIV.

Although we might think of the human body as the typical reservoir for infection, any environment that can provide appropriate temperature (warm), moisture (damp), and lack of cleanliness will provide welcome accommodations for pathogenic microorganisms. Animals, arthropods, plants, and soil are all potential reservoirs of infection.

Portal of Exit. A portal of exit from the reservoir can be any pathway by which pathogens are able to leave the reservoir. Examples of portals of exit include urine, feces, blood, respiratory droplets, and contaminated solutions.

Modes of Transmission. Transmission via *direct contact* occurs when the host is touched by an infected person and the infectious pathogenic organisms come in contact directly with susceptible tissue such as mucous membrane or broken skin. Diseases transmitted by direct contact include skin infections such as boils, and multidrug-resistant organisms (MDROs). Direct contact also includes *droplet* spread from a sneeze, cough, or even speaking. The droplets are relatively large and comprise a short-range (a few feet) aerosol effect.

Transmission via *indirect contact* involves the transportation of infectious pathogenic microorganisms via airborne/suspended particles, vehicles/inanimate objects, or vectors/animals.

The *airborne* mode of transmission involves suspended particles of wet droplets, dust, or fungus. Examples of diseases transmitted in this manner include the common cold, COVID-19, measles, mumps, influenza, chicken pox, tuberculosis, and anthrax. These are the infectious agents that have settled on a surface and then carried and circulated by an air current. These droplets are exceedingly small and can remain suspended in air for long periods of time and/or be blown over a great distance.

Vehicle transmission of infectious microorganisms occurs with contaminated food, water, blood, and fomites. A *fomite* is an object that has been in contact with an infectious organism; examples include the x-ray table, IV pole, contaminated positioning aids, bedding, and handkerchiefs.

Vector-borne transmission mode, as described by the CDC, can be either *mechanical* or *biologic*. These are the diseases carried by flies, mosquitoes, ticks, fleas, and others. Flies can transmit disease by their body hairs or via their appendages when they land on surfaces/food. This is mechanical transmission. However, ticks transmit disease via their saliva when biting the host; this is an example of biologic transmission.

Portal of Entry. The pathway by which infectious organisms gain entry to the body is termed the *portal of entry*. Potential portals of entry include breaks in the skin; the gastrointestinal tract; mucous membranes of eyes, nose, or mouth; the respiratory tract; and the urinary tract. Entry can be accomplished by ingestion, injection, and inhalation, and across mucous membrane; the placenta serves as a portal of entry between the mother and the fetus.

Susceptible Host. The most susceptible hosts include the sick, infirmed, immunocompromised, very young, elderly, poorly nourished, weak, or fatigued—all who have a diminished natural resistance to infection. Host susceptibility can also depend on immune and genetic factors. *HAIs,* also called *nosocomial* infections, are the infections acquired by *patients* (susceptible hosts) while they are in the hospital, unrelated to the condition for which the patients were hospitalized.

Hospital personnel can also be susceptible hosts. The most important precaution is proper hand hygiene. Hand lotions may be used; broken skin permits the entry of microorganisms. Antiseptics, disinfectants, and germicides are the substances used to retard growth of pathogenic bacteria or to kill pathogenic bacteria and are frequently used in hand-hygiene substances. Alcohol-based hand sanitizers have been recommended as an alternative to handwashing with soap and water and may be used as described earlier. Uniforms worn in patient areas should not be worn elsewhere; a clean uniform should be worn daily, and minimal jewelry should be worn. *Microorganisms can remain infectious while awaiting transmission to another host.*

Modes of Transmission

Direct
- Direct contact (with contaminated person or vegetation)
- Droplet spread (large droplets from sneeze, cough, etc.)

Indirect
- Airborne (suspended tiny particles of wet droplets, dust, etc.)
- Vehicle borne (contaminated food, water, blood, fomites)
- Vector borne (mechanical or biologic/flies, fleas, ticks, etc.)

Summary

- Most microorganisms do not produce infection or disease; many are harmless, and many are beneficial.
- Pathogenic microorganisms can cause an infection/a disease; pathogenic microorganisms can be transmitted from one host to another.
- Many microorganisms can remain infectious while awaiting transmission to another host.
- Antiseptics retard the growth of bacteria.
- Medical asepsis refers to the destruction of bacteria by using disinfectants/antiseptics.
- Disinfectants (germicides) are used in handwashing liquids to kill microorganisms.
- Surgical asepsis refers to the destruction of all microorganisms and their spores through sterilization.

- The practice of medical asepsis is always required, whereas surgical asepsis is required for invasive procedures.
- The single most important component of medical asepsis is proper and timely hand hygiene.
- A clean uniform must be worn daily; uniforms become contaminated and should not be worn elsewhere; pathogenic microorganisms thrive in jewelry crevices and chipped nail polish.
- The six factors in the chain of infection are the infectious organism, the reservoir of infection, the portal of exit, the means of transmission, the portal of entry, and the susceptible host.
- Transmission can occur via direct contact with infected person or vegetation.
- Transmission can occur as indirect contact via air, vehicle, or vector.

THE CDC STANDARD PRECAUTIONS

Infection Prevention and Control: Basic Guidelines

The CDC and the Hospital Infection Control Practices Advisory Committee have revised and simplified infection control guidelines for hospitals and other health care facilities. The various types of isolation techniques, disease-specific precautions, and varied terminology have been reviewed, revised, and updated. All of these considerations are now incorporated into *standard precautions* and *transmission-based precautions*.

Exposure to infectious microorganisms is a daily concern for health care professionals, especially with a possible risk of exposure to HIV/AIDS (acquired immunodeficiency syndrome) and *HBV* infections. HIV-infected individuals may be symptomless and go undiagnosed for 10 years or more, yet they are carriers of the infection and have the potential to spread the disease. *Epidemiologic* studies indicate that HIV infection can be transmitted only by intimate contact with blood or body fluids of an infected individual. This can occur through the sharing of contaminated needles, through sexual contact, from mother to baby at childbirth, and from transfusion of contaminated blood. Inanimate objects such as water fountains, telephone surfaces, or toilet seats *cannot* transmit HIV. *Hepatitis B* is another blood-borne infection that affects the liver. It is thought that more than 1 million people in the United States have chronic hepatitis B and, as such, can transmit the disease to others.

Because no symptoms may be evident in patients infected with particular diseases, such as HIV/AIDS, and hepatitis B, all patients must be treated as potential sources of infection from blood and other body fluids. The practices associated with this concept are called *standard precautions*. This rationale treats *all* body fluids and substances as infectious and serves to prevent the spread of microorganisms to other patients by the radiographer, as well as to protect the radiographer from contamination. Body fluids and substances that may be considered

---

Guidelines for Standard Precautions

The radiographer is now legally, as well as ethically, responsible for strict adherence to standard precaution principles identified in the following guidelines:

- Avoid cross-contamination of soiled (with body fluids) patient care linens/equipment.
- Clean reusable equipment properly before using on another patient; properly discard single-use items.
- Clean and disinfect environmental surfaces on a routine basis.
- Patients who can contaminate the environment should be placed in private rooms.
- Blood and body fluid spills should be carefully cleaned and disinfected by using a solution of 1 part bleach to 10 parts water.
- Used needles must not be separated from the syringe or resheathed and must be placed in designed puncture-proof containers.
- Prescribed procedures must be followed, and sufficient care and attention given to risky tasks to avoid needlesticks and other skin penetrations from cutting instruments (sharps).
- Emergency cardiopulmonary resuscitation (CPR) equipment must include resuscitation bags and mouthpieces.

infectious include blood, breast milk, vaginal secretions, amniotic fluid, semen, peritoneal fluid, synovial fluid, cerebrospinal fluid, feces, urine, secretions from the nasal and oral cavities, and secretions from the lacrimal and sweat glands.

It is essential, then, that the radiographer makes the practice of blood and body fluid precautions *standard;* that is, they must be practiced on all patients without exception. This involves the use of personal protective equipment (PPE), or barriers, such as gowns and masks as indicated, to provide a separation between the patient's blood and body fluids and the radiographer or other health care worker. Special precautions must also be taken with the *disposal* of biomedical waste, such as laboratory and pathology waste; all sharp objects; and liquid waste from suction, bladder catheters, chest tubes, and IV tubes, as well as drainage containers. The syringe with needle connected should be placed immediately into the sharps disposal container. Any contaminated materials such as dressings, gauze and tubing must be placed in biohazard waste disposal bags. Any uncontaminated (nonsharp) materials are placed in a standard trash container.

Biomedical waste is packaged in special, easily identifiable, impermeable, puncture-proof containers and removed from the premises by an approved biomedical waste hauler.

Health Care–Associated Infections

HAIs are the infections acquired by patients while they are in the hospital; these are also termed *nosocomial* infections. Many of these infections are acquired by patients whose resistance has been diminished by their illness and are unrelated to the condition for which the patients were hospitalized. Infection resulting from physician intervention is termed *iatrogenic.* The CDC estimates that from 5% to 15% of all hospital patients may acquire some type of HAI. Hospital personnel can also become infected (occupationally acquired infection).

It is somewhat surprising, yet understandable, that many infections can be acquired in the hospital: Surprising because hospitals are places where people go to regain their health, yet understandable because individuals weakened by illness or disease are more susceptible to infection than the healthy individuals. The most common HAI is the *urinary tract infection,* often related to the use of urinary catheters, which can allow passage of pathogens into the patient's body. Other types of HAIs include sepsis, wound infection, and respiratory tract infection.

Health care practitioners must exercise strict infection prevention and control precautions so that their *equipment* and/or technique will not be the source of HAI. *Contaminated* waste products, equipment such as emesis basins, tubing and catheters, soiled linen, and improperly sterilized equipment are all means by which microorganisms can travel. Not every patient will come in contact with these items; however, the health care professional is in constant contact with patients and is therefore a constant threat to spread infection. Microorganisms are most commonly spread by way of the hands; spread of infection can be effectively reduced by proper disposal of contaminated objects and proper hand hygiene before and after examining each patient. *Disinfectants, antiseptics,* and *germicides* are used in many hand-hygiene liquids.

Use of PPE

- PPE, or barriers, such as masks and/or gowns must be used as indicated.

- Shielding for the face and eyes must be in place whenever the possibility of blood or body fluid splashes may occur near the face.

- Plastic aprons or gowns must be worn whenever the possibility of blood or body fluid splashes may occur on the clothing.

- Gloves must be worn whenever there is a possibility of touching blood or body fluids, and whenever there is a possibility of handling equipment or touching surfaces contaminated with blood or body fluids.

- Hands must also be washed/sanitized before and after gloves are worn, patient contact, and between changing from contaminated gloves to a clean pair.

Transmission-Based Precautions

Health care professionals adhere to *standard precautions* in the care of all patients. Standard precautions are based on assessing risk, making use of common sense practices, and making use of PPE to protect the health care professional from infection and to prevent the spread of infection from one patient to another. These common sense practices include proper hand hygiene, correct use of PPE, correct handling/disinfection of equipment and environment, and proper laundry care.

The CDC identifies *transmission-based precautions* as the second tier of basic infection control and are to be used in addition to standard precautions for patients infected with known or suspected infections. These have been replaced by *transmission-based precautions: airborne, droplet,* and *contact* (Table 4-1). Under these guidelines, some conditions/diseases can fall into more than one category.

Airborne. *Airborne precaution* is implemented in patients suspected or known to be infected with the *tubercle bacillus (TB), chicken pox (varicella), measles (rubeola),* and *disseminated herpes zoste*r (shingles). Patients infected with *airborne diseases* require a *private, specially ventilated (negative-pressure) room* (Table 4-1). Airborne precaution requires the patient to wear a surgical string mask to avoid the spread of acid-fast bacilli (in bronchial secretions) or other pathogens during coughing, particularly if the patient must be transported. The health care staff must wear personal N95 respirators whenever they enter an airborne isolation room. This special mask requires periodic fit testing. Those who cannot be fitted for an N95 mask may need to wear a powered air-purifying respirator instead. The radiographer should wear gloves, but a gown is required only if flagrant contamination is likely.

Airborne Precautions

They are used to prevent airborne disease transmission in the health care setting.

- Airborne transmission occurs when small airborne droplet nuclei float through the air and travel distances, becoming a risk for inhalation.
- Patients are isolated in private rooms with special air handling and ventilation systems (negative-pressure rooms). If a private room is not available, patients are cohorted.
- Health care personnel must wear personal N95 respirators whenever they enter an airborne isolation room.
- Patient transport must be limited as much as possible; when patient transport is essential, the patient must wear a surgical string mask.

TABLE 4-1. Transmission-Based Precautions

Examples	Protection

Airborne
  TB
  Varicella
  Rubeola
	· Patient: wears a surgical string mask; private, negative-pressure room
	· Radiographer: wears an N95 particulate respirator mask if the patient is not able to wear a mask, gloves; gown for blatant contamination

Droplet
  Rubella
  Mumps
  Influenza
	· Patient: wears a surgical string mask; private room
	· Radiographer: gown and gloves as indicated; surgical string mask if the patient is not able to wear a mask, except for H1N1 influenza when an N95 particulate respirator mask would be worn

Contact
  Mumps }
  MDROs }
(antibiotic-resistant organisms such as MRSA and VRE)
	· Patient: private room; wears a mask if required by the facility
	· Radiographer: gloves and gown; mask for MRSA, if required by the facility

MRSA, methicillin-resistant *Staphylococcus aureus*; VRE, vancomycin-resistant enterococci.

Droplet. A private room is indicated for all patients on *droplet precaution*, that is, diseases transmitted via large droplets expelled from the patient while speaking, sneezing, or coughing. The patient must wear a mask. The pathogenic droplets can infect others when they come in contact with mouth or nasal mucosa or conjunctiva. *Rubella* (German measles), *mumps,* and *influenza* are among the diseases spread by droplet contact; a private room is required for the patient, and health care practitioners must wear a regular (string) mask to enter a droplet-precaution isolation room, except for H1N1 influenza, where an N95 particulate respirator mask may need to be worn instead, when involved in aerosol-generating procedures.

Contact. Any disease that spreads by direct or close (indirect) contact, such as methicillin-resistant *Staphylococcus aureus (MRSA)*, *C. difficile*, and some wound, skin, gastrointestinal, or respiratory infections require *contact precautions*. Contact-precaution procedures require a *private patient room* and the use of *gloves and a gown* for anyone coming in direct contact with the infected individual or the infected individual's environment. PPE is donned on entering the patient room, then properly discarded before exiting the room. Some facilities may require health care workers to wear a mask when caring for a patient with MRSA.

Patients in *contact isolation* occasionally must be transported to the radiology department for examination. When this is the case, the department should be notified first to prepare properly. The patient should wash his or her hands first if possible. The wheelchair or stretcher should first be covered with a clean sheet, followed by a second sheet or thin blanket to cover the patient. The radiographic room should be available and ready for the patient to be taken in directly. The x-ray table should be covered with a clean sheet before the patient is transferred to it. One radiographer (wearing gloves) must be responsible for patient positioning and the other for equipment controls and operation (to avoid contamination of equipment and possible transmission of disease to others via indirect contact or fomites).

After the examination is completed, the patient is transferred to the wheelchair or stretcher and transported back to his or her room. Any contaminated *linens* should be placed in an appropriate linen hamper and contaminated disposables such as tissues should be placed in a separate trash receptacle for disposal.

The radiographic table and other equipment should be cleaned with a disinfectant while wearing clean gloves (not the gloves worn to care for the patient). Hands should be carefully washed before applying gloves and after glove removal at the completion of the task.

Mobile radiography performed on patients on *contact isolation* generally requires special precautions and the teamwork of *two* radiographers. The first (or "dirty") radiographer dons a gown, gloves (gloves must cover gown cuffs), and a mask (if indicated), usually available outside, or just inside, the patient's room. The necessary image plates (IPs) must be placed in a plastic bag or pillowcase to protect them from contamination. The mobile x-ray unit is brought into the room, and all possible adjustments must be made and/or covers applied before the radiographer touches anything else.

Droplet Precautions

They are used to prevent contact with droplets expelled while speaking, sneezing, or coughing.

- Patients are isolated in private rooms.
- Patients must wear masks.
- Health care personnel must wear string masks while in patient rooms; an N95 mask is indicated in case of H1N1 influenza.

Diseases transmitted via droplet include influenza, mumps, and rubella.

Contact Precautions

They are used to prevent contact transmission of disease in the health care setting.

- Patients are isolated in private rooms or cohorted.
- Health care personnel must use gloves and gowns as indicated to prevent unprotected exposure.
- Hands must be disinfected before and after gloving.
- Patient transport should be limited as much as possible; when necessary, special precautions are taken.
- All x-ray imaging requires special precautions and a two-radiographer team.
- Equipment should be dedicated to a single patient or cohort, or equipment must be cleaned and disinfected between patients.

The equipment and IP are positioned, and the patient is adjusted properly. *At this point, the mobile x-ray unit must not be touched* until the radiographer disposes of the gloves he or she has on, cleanses his or her hands, and replaces the used gloves with a clean pair of gloves.

The exposure is then made; the covered IP is removed from behind/under the patient and brought to the door. The "dirty" radiographer slides the pillowcase or plastic cover away from the IP and the second member of the team (the "clean" radiographer) grasps the uncovered IP. Just inside the patient room door, the contaminated gloves should be removed properly, and then the gown ties untied and the gown removed by folding the gown forward (with the dirty surfaces touching) and pulling the sleeves inside out, rolling the gown into a ball with the clean side now on the outside of the rolled gown. The mask, if worn, may now be removed by untying strings and removing without touching the front surface of the mask.

The discarded garments must be placed in the container provided. The radiographer should then carefully wash/sanitize his or her hands, dry them with paper towels, and take care not to touch the faucets. After leaving the room, *the mobile unit must be thoroughly cleaned* with a disinfectant while wearing gloves and then hands carefully washed/sanitized after glove removal at the completion of this task.

It should be noted that these patients may feel ostracized and relegated to a kind of solitary confinement. The radiographer must remember that these patients have the same needs as other patients (indeed, perhaps greater needs) and be certain to treat them with dignity and care.

Patients Whose Immune Systems Are Compromised. The purpose of *neutropenic* (protective or reverse) *isolation* is to keep the susceptible patient whose immune system is compromised (immunosuppression) from becoming infected. Patients suffering from burns have lost their means of protection, their skin, and have increased susceptibility to bacterial invasion. Patients whose immune systems are compromised (e.g., transplant recipients, leukemia, chemotherapy) are unable to combat infection and are more susceptible to infection. These patients are treated with strict isolation technique, taking care to protect the *patient* from contamination.

The teamwork of two radiographers is also required for care of the patient with a compromised immune system, although the purpose and procedure are largely opposite to that of the other isolation categories. Preparation for cleanliness and hygiene starts *before* entering the patient room. The "clean" radiographer touches only the patient and that which comes in contact with the patient.

Hazardous Materials. Special precautions must be taken with the disposal of biomedical waste, such as laboratory and pathology waste; used bandages and dressings; discarded gloves; all sharp objects; and liquid waste from suction, bladder catheters, chest tubes, and IV tubes, as well as drainage containers.

Biomedical waste must be packaged in special, easily identifiable, impermeable bags and removed from the premises by an approved biomedical waste hauler.

Spills in the imaging department can pose a chemical hazard as well as the risk of injury from falls. The work area must be monitored for potential hazards and facilities management called to clean up as necessary.

Hazardous substances must be stored in a safe area as designated. Toxic chemicals must be clearly marked with the name of the substance and identified with a hazard warning. They must remain in their original container that lists the name and address of the manufacturer.

Imaging department personnel should know the location of contact information for the local poison control center.

The imaging department must have posted emergency instructions to be followed in case of accidental poisoning.

Contrast media and other drugs must be kept in a safe storage area with access restricted to radiographers trained in their use.

OSHA requires that all chemicals be properly labeled and that Material Safety Data Sheets (MSDSs) for all hazardous materials be on file and easily accessible to personnel. The MSDS for any chemical will indicate the required equipment and procedure for safe handling in the event a spill occurs. The radiographer can ensure the patient safety as follows:

- by limiting access to the area
- by evaluating the risks involved
- by ensuring access to required equipment and the expertise to clean the spill safely
- if lacking the necessary skill/equipment, by calling the supervisor and/or facilities management

> In case of accidental spill of hazardous substances, the first aid guidelines are as follows:
>
> - *Eye contact:* Flush eyes with water for 15 min or until irritation subsides; consult a physician.
> - *Skin contact*: Remove affected clothing; cleanse skin with gentle soap and water.
> - *Inhalation*: Remove from exposure area; if breathing has stopped, begin CPR; call emergency number and a physician.
> - *Ingestion*: Do not induce vomiting; call emergency number and poison control center.

Summary

- Because no symptoms may be evident in patients afflicted with certain communicable diseases, all patients must be treated as potential sources of infection from blood and other body fluids; this is the standard precautions concept.
- The practice of standard precautions and transmission-based precautions helps prevent spread of infection to the health care professional and to other patients.
- Infections acquired in hospitals are called health care–associated infections (HAIs) or nosocomial infections; the most common HAI is the urinary tract infection.
- The health care professional is legally and ethically responsible for adhering to standard precautions principles; these principles must be practiced on all patients at all times without exception.
- Biomedical waste (body substances and their containers) must be disposed of in carefully controlled circumstances.
- Transmission-based precautions include airborne, droplet, and contact.
- Airborne precaution requires that the patient wear a surgical string mask and be admitted to a private, specially ventilated, negative-pressure room. Examples include tubercle bacillus, varicella, rubeola, and disseminated herpes zoster.

- Droplet precaution and a private room are required for patients with rubella, mumps, and influenza and others spread by droplet contact. The patient must be masked.

- Contact precautions are required for methicillin-resistant *Staphylococcus aureus* (MRSA), *C. difficile,* and some wound, skin, gastrointestinal, or respiratory infections. It requires that the radiographer use a gown and gloves when in direct contact with the patient and, on occasion, a mask.

- Radiography of a patient with contact precaution requires the teamwork of two radiographers.

- Neutropenic isolation (also called protective or reverse isolation) is used to keep the susceptible patient from being infected.

- Special precautions are required for disposal of biomedical waste such as laboratory waste, used bandages, gloves, all sharps, and liquid drainage waste.

- Hazardous substances must be labeled; personnel must be aware of correct storage and handling of hazardous substances.

COMPREHENSION CHECK

Congratulations! You have completed your review of this chapter. If you are able to answer the following group of comprehensive questions, you can feel confident that you have mastered this section. You are then ready to go on to "registry-type" questions that follow. For greatest success, do not go to these multiple-choice questions without first completing the following short-answer questions:

1. List three disinfectant agents (p. 54).

2. Describe the correct method of handwashing, including *when* hands should be washed, opening/closing faucets, and position of hands and forearms (p. 54, 55).

3. Define *pathogen* and discuss types of pathogens (p. 54).

4. Describe the importance of the radiographer's personal care related to disease control (p. 55, 59).

5. Identify and differentiate between the three basic means of transmitting infectious microorganisms (p. 56).

6. List three means of indirect transmission of pathogenic microorganisms (p. 56, 57).

7. Identify the most common type of hospital-acquired infections (p. 59).

8. List five possible sources of HAI infection in the radiology department (p. 59).

9. Describe precautions used to prevent airborne disease transmission (p. 56).

10. Identify the means by which microorganisms are spread (p. 56).

11. What substances are added to handwashing liquids to kill microorganisms (p. 54, 55)?

12. Discuss the rationale of standard precautions (p. 58).

13. Discuss each of the following with respect to standard precautions (p. 58, 59):

    A. when should a face shield be used?

    B. when should appropriate PPE be used?

    C. when should hands be washed?

    D. when should gloves be used?

    E. how should body fluid and substance spills be cleaned?

    F. how should care of used needles be performed?

    G. what are the special devices available for CPR?

    H. on whom should standard precautions be practiced?

14. Differentiate between medical and surgical asepsis (p. 57).

15. Identify and explain the most important practice in good aseptic technique (p. 54, 55).

16. Discuss the function of uniforms worn by health care practitioners, and the hazards of jewelry and nail polish (p. 57).

17. List the three types of transmission-based precautions (p. 61).

18. Explain the precautionary measures taken in airborne precaution regarding apparel (and for whom) and patient room (p. 60).

19. List three communicable diseases spread by droplet contact, which require droplet precaution (p. 61).

20. Describe/demonstrate the method of performing mobile chest radiography on patients with contact precaution, to include the following (p. 61, 62):

    A. what is the number of persons needed?

    B. what is the required apparel for a radiographer?

    C. how should IPs be protected from contamination?

    D. why is an extra pair of gloves needed in the patient room?

    E. what is the role played by the second individual?

    F. how should protective clothing be removed?

    G. what are the steps required for care of the x-ray machine at completion of the examination?

21. Describe the proper method of transporting a contact-precaution patient to the radiology department (p. 61, 62).

22. Describe the purpose of protective isolation (p. 62).

23. Discuss any special needs the isolation patient may have (p. 62).

24. What is biomedical waste and how must it be cared for (p. 62)?

25. Discuss special precautions that are required for safe disposal of biomedical waste such as laboratory waste, used bandages, gloves, sharps, and liquid drainage waste. (p. 62, 63)

26. Discuss the content and purpose of MSDSs. (p. 63)

CHAPTER REVIEW QUESTIONS

1. Pathogens are
   1. always harmful
   2. sometimes harmful
   3. capable of producing disease
   (A) 1 only
   (B) 2 only
   (C) 1 and 3 only
   (D) 2 and 3 only

2. Diseases that can be transmitted by direct contact include
   1. skin infections
   2. MDROs
   3. malaria
   (A) 1 only
   (B) 1 and 2 only
   (C) 2 and 3 only
   (D) 1, 2, and 3

3. Protective, or reverse, isolation is indicated in the following conditions:
   1. transplant recipient
   2. chemotherapy recipient
   3. leukemia
   (A) 1 only
   (B) 1 and 2 only
   (C) 2 and 3 only
   (D) 1, 2, and 3

4. Which of the following is/are means of transmission of microorganisms?
   1. Vector
   2. Fomite
   3. Airborne
   (A) 1 only
   (B) 1 and 2 only
   (C) 3 only
   (D) 1, 2, and 3

5. What is the single most effective means of controlling the spread of infectious microorganisms?
   (A) Wearing gloves
   (B) Wearing masks
   (C) Handwashing
   (D) Sterilization

6. What is the name of the practice that serves to retard the growth of pathogenic bacteria?
   (A) Antisepsis
   (B) Bacteriogenesis
   (C) Sterilization
   (D) Disinfection

7. Which of the following diseases require(s) airborne precaution?
   1. TB
   2. Varicella
   3. Rubella
   (A) 1 only
   (B) 1 and 2 only
   (C) 3 only
   (D) 1, 2, and 3

8. The radiographer must perform the following procedure(s) before entering an isolation room with a mobile x-ray unit:
   1. wear a gown and a mask
   2. wear a gown, gloves, and possibly a mask
   3. disinfect the mobile x-ray unit
   (A) 1 only
   (B) 2 only
   (C) 1 and 3 only
   (D) 2 and 3 only

9. Lyme disease is a condition caused by bacteria carried by deer ticks. The tick bite may cause fever, fatigue, and other associated symptoms. This is an example of transmission of an infection by
   (A) droplet contact
   (B) the airborne route
   (C) a vector
   (D) a vehicle

10. Which of the following can be transmitted via infected blood?
    1. TB
    2. AIDS
    3. HBV
    (A) 1 only
    (B) 1 and 2 only
    (C) 2 and 3 only
    (D) 1, 2, and 3

Answers and Explanations

1. (D) *Pathogens* are causative agents—microorganisms capable of producing disease. Pathogens termed *opportunistic* are usually harmless but can become harmful if introduced into a part of the body where they do not normally reside, or when introduced into an immuno-compromised host. *Blood-borne* pathogens reside in blood and can be transmitted to an individual exposed to the blood or body fluids of the infected individual. Common blood-borne pathogens include hepatitis C virus (HCV), hepatitis B virus (HBV), and human immunodeficiency virus (HIV). Because radiography often involves exposure to sickness and disease, the radiographer must be aware of, and conscientiously practice, infection prevention and control measures.

2. (B) Infectious microorganisms can be transmitted from one patient to other patients or to health care workers, and from health care workers to patients. They are transmitted by means of either direct or indirect contact. *Direct contact* involves touch. Diseases transmitted by direct contact include skin infections, such as boils and multidrug-resistant organisms (MDROs).

Indirect contact involves transmission of microorganisms via airborne contamination, fomites, and vectors. Pathogenic microorganisms expelled from the respiratory tract through the mouth or nose can be carried as evaporated droplets through the air or on dust and settle on intermediate objects such as clothing, utensils, or food. Patients with respiratory tract infections and diseases transported to the radiology department, therefore, should wear a mask to prevent such transmission during a cough or sneeze; it is not necessary for the health care professional or transporter to wear a mask (as long as the patient does). Many such microorganisms can remain infectious while awaiting transmission to another host. A contaminated inanimate object such as a food utensil, doorknob, or intravenous (IV) pole is called a fomite. A vector is an insect or animal carrier of infectious organisms, such as a rabid animal (e.g., rabies; although the rabid animal is the vector, rabies is contracted by contact), a mosquito that carries malaria, or a tick that carries Lyme disease.

3. (D) *Protective, or reverse, isolation is used to keep the susceptible patient from becoming infected.* Burn patients who have lost their means of protection (their skin) have increased susceptibility to bacterial invasion. Protective isolation is particularly important in caring for immunodeficient patients such as those who have received chemotherapy, transplant recipients, and patients with leukemia. These patients are unable to combat infection and are more susceptible to infection. They are treated with strict isolation technique, that is, taking care to protect the *patient* from contamination.

4. (D) Microorganisms can be transmitted via *droplet, air,* and *contact (direct or indirect)*. Other sources of transmission are *vehicle* and *vector*. Pathogenic microorganisms expelled from the respiratory tract through the mouth or nose can be carried as evaporated droplets through the air or on dust and settle on clothing, utensils, or food. A contaminated inanimate object such as a pillowcase, x-ray table, or IV pole is called a *fomite*. A *vector* is an insect or animal carrier of infectious organisms, such as a rabid animal (rabies), a mosquito that carries malaria, or a tick that carries Lyme disease.

5. (C) Health care practitioners must exercise strict infection control precautions so that they or their equipment will not be the source of health care–associated infections (HAIs). Contaminated waste products, soiled linen, and improperly sterilized equipment are all means by which microorganisms can travel. Not every patient will come in contact with these items; however, the health care professional is in constant contact with patients and is therefore a constant threat to spread infection. *Microorganisms are most commonly spread by way of the hands; therefore, handwashing/sanitizing before and after examination of each patient is the most effective means of controlling the spread of microorganisms.* Disinfectants, antiseptics, and germicides are used in many handwashing liquids.

6. (A) *Antisepsis* retards the growth of pathogenic bacteria. Alcohol is an example of an antiseptic. *Medical asepsis* refers to the destruction of pathogenic microorganisms through the process of *disinfection*. Examples of disinfectants are hydrogen peroxide, chlorine, and boric acid. *Surgical asepsis (sterilization)* refers to the removal of all microorganisms and their spores (reproductive cells) and is practiced in the surgical suite. *Bacteriogenesis* refers to the formation of bacteria.

7. (B) *Airborne precaution* is implemented in patients suspected or known to be infected with the tubercle bacillus (TB), chicken pox (varicella), and measles (rubeola). Airborne precaution requires the patient to wear a surgical string mask to avoid the spread of acid-fast bacilli (in bronchial secretions) and other pathogens during coughing. If the patient is unable or unwilling to wear a mask, the radiographer must wear one. An N95 particulate respirator is the mask required for health care workers. The radiographer should wear gloves, but a gown is required only if flagrant contamination is likely. Patients with airborne precautions require a private, specially ventilated (negative-pressure) room (Table 4-1).

A private room is indicated for all patients on *droplet precaution*, that is, diseases transmitted via large droplets expelled from the patient while speaking, sneezing, or coughing. The pathogenic droplets can infect others when they come in contact with mouth or nasal mucosa or conjunctiva. Rubella (German measles), mumps, and influenza are among the diseases spread by *droplet* contact; a private room is required for the patient, and health care practitioners must wear a mask. An N95 particulate respirator mask may be required while a patient with H1N1 is receiving an aerosol-generating procedure.

8. (B) When performing bedside radiography in an isolation room, the radiographer should wear a gown, gloves, and sometimes a mask. The IPs are prepared for the examination by placing a pillowcase over them to protect them from contamination. Whenever possible, one person should manipulate the mobile unit and remain "clean," while the other handles the patient. The mobile unit should be cleaned with a disinfectant before *exiting* the patient's room.

9. (C) Lyme disease is a condition that results from transmission of an infection by a vector ("deer" tick). *Vectors* are insects and animals carrying disease. *Droplet contact* involves contact with secretions (from the nose, mouth) that travel via a sneeze or cough. *Airborne* route involves evaporated droplets in the air that transfer disease.

10. (C) Epidemiologic studies indicate that HIV/AIDS can be transmitted only by intimate contact with blood or body fluids of an infected individual. This can occur through the sharing of contaminated needles, through sexual contact, from mother to baby at childbirth, and from transfusion of contaminated blood. Inanimate objects cannot transmit HIV and AIDS. HBV is another blood-borne infection and affects the liver. It is thought that more than 1 million people in the United States have chronic hepatitis B and, as such, can transmit the disease to others. Acid-fast bacillus isolation is implemented in patients suspected or known to be infected with the TB. Acid-fast bacillus isolation requires that the patient wear a mask to avoid the spread of acid-fast bacilli (in bronchial secretions) during *coughing*.

Pharmacology

OBJECTIVES

At the conclusion of this chapter, the student will be able to:

- Discuss the value of complete and accurate patient assessment.
- Identify component parts of patient history.
- List the various routes of medication administration.
- Describe anatomy and procedural technique pertaining to venipuncture.
- Identify the types of contrast media; cite examples of their use and identify potential complications/contraindications.
- Discuss the difference between side effect and toxic effect.
- Describe the levels of contrast media untoward responses.

PATIENT HISTORY

The radiographer *assesses* a patient's condition before bringing the patient to the radiographic department and continues to be alert to the patient's condition and any changes as the examination proceeds. *Assessment* begins with a review of the patient's chart; useful components of patient history include admission diagnosis, current medications, nurses' notes, any allergy, degree of ambulation, preparation for the radiologic procedure and its effectiveness (e.g., premedication, effectiveness of cathartic/cleansing enemas), results of laboratory tests (e.g., creatinine, blood urea nitrogen [BUN], glomerular filtration rate [GFR]), any requirements for collecting the patient's urine, and so on. Some radiologic procedures, especially those using contrast media, may require appropriate scheduling, premedication, and attention paid to any potential contraindications. Scheduling, contrast media, medications, and potential contraindications are covered in this chapter. Patient shielding will be addressed in chapters on radiation safety.

The radiographer obtains a brief pertinent *clinical history* and assesses patient condition by *observing* and *listening*. Facts are gathered to obtain information useful in providing adequate care and accurate diagnosis. To provide safe and effectual care, the radiographer will *assess* the severity of any traumatic injury, degree of motor control, and any need for support equipment or radiographic accessories. Is the patient able to move? Has the patient been NPO (nothing by mouth)? Does the patient have any history of intolerance to contrast material? Has the patients' radiologic procedure been scheduled appropriately with other required imaging procedures? Are there any laboratory values or diagnoses that might contraindicate the use of contrast material (e.g., intestinal perforation, diabetes)?

The radiographer is always alert to patient appearance and condition. Awareness of gross and fine *motor control* is critical to avoid patient injury. Sudden changes in color, temperature, and moistness of the patients' skin should be noted. Paleness can indicate weakness; the *diaphoretic* patient has pale, cool skin; *fever* is frequently accompanied by hot, dry skin; "sweaty" palms might indicate *anxiety;* a patient who is *cyanotic* (bluish lips, mucous membranes, nail beds) needs oxygen and requires immediate attention. Chronic obstructive pulmonary disease (COPD) patients receive low flow rates of oxygen; acute exacerbations are managed with inhaled bronchodilators. High flow rates of oxygen are contraindicated for COPD patients because of the higher levels of carbon dioxide in the blood.

ADMINISTRATION

In cases requiring documented informed consent, the radiographer will take special care to ensure that all unanswered patient questions are addressed and that the required *documentation is verified and in place.*

Routes of Administration

Although radiographic contrast media are usually administered orally or intravenously, there are a number of *routes* and methods of drug administration. Drugs and medications may be administered either orally or parenterally. Parenteral administration refers to any route other than via the digestive tract and includes topical (i.e., applied to the surface), subcutaneous (i.e., beneath the skin), intradermal (i.e., within the dermis/skin), intramuscular (IM; i.e., within a muscle), intravenous (IV; i.e., within a vein), intrathecal (i.e., within the spinal canal), and inhalation (e.g., in asthma control) administration. Sublingual and buckle administrations are considered variations of topical method.

Equipment

Oral administration of contrast material is usually required for the upper gastrointestinal system, small bowel, and the lower gastrointestinal tract (large bowel). Barium sulfate suspension is generally used except in patients with suspected or known stomach or intestinal perforation; in that case water-soluble iodinated contrast material should be used instead of barium sulfate. Air is also often used as a negative contrast in double-contrast studies. Necessary equipment for these studies includes prepared barium sulfate suspension for drinking. Gas-producing crystals are often used in conjunction with barium to produce the desired double-contrast effect. An enema kit is required for barium enema (BE)

Methods of Administration

Enteral
- PO (by mouth), through digestive system

Parenteral
- Topical
- Subcutaneous
- Intradermal
- Intramuscular
- Intravenous
- Intrathecal
- Inhalation
- Sublingual (variation of topical)
- Buccal (variation of topical)

procedures. A colostomy catheter may be required for patients with an existing colostomy.

IV fluids and/or medications are administered to meet specific patient needs. Medications administered intravenously result in rapid patient response; medications are often delivered in this manner in emergency and critical situations. Patients who are dehydrated and require fluid and electrolyte replacement will have these (normal saline or D5W [a solution of 5% dextrose in water]) administered intravenously. *IV equipment* includes needles, syringes, fluids such as normal saline or D5W, IV catheters, heparin locks, IV poles, and infusion sets. Care must be taken to flush the IV line in advance of, and following, delivering medicines. This ensures the IV line remains clean and prevents blockages.

The inner diameter of a needle is identified as its *gauge.* As the gauge increases, the *bore* becomes smaller. Hence, a 23-gauge needle has a smaller diameter bore than an 18-gauge needle. Hypodermic needles are generally used for phlebotomy (blood samples), whereas butterflies and IV catheters are used more frequently for injections such as contrast media. If an *infusion* injection is required, an IV catheter is generally preferred. The *hub* of the hypodermic needle is attached to a syringe, whereas the hub of the butterfly tubing or IV catheter may be attached to a syringe or an IV container via an IV infusion set.

Venipuncture

Medication or contrast material is often mixed with normal saline or D5W. Some IV medications are given at intervals through an established heparin lock. A *heparin lock* consists of a venous catheter established for a certain length of time to make a vein available for medications that have to be administered at frequent intervals. This helps prevent the formation of scarred, sclerotic veins because of frequent injections at the same site. When repeated administrations of a medication are needed, an *IV catheter* is often used. This is a two-part device consisting of a solid (without a bore) needle and a flexible plastic catheter. After the needle is introduced into the vein, the catheter is advanced over the needle, secured with tape, and the needle removed.

The IV container should be hung 18–24 inches *above the level of the vein.* If it is placed lower than the vein, the solution will stop flowing and blood will return into the tubing. If it is hung too high, the solution can run too fast. Occasionally, the position of the needle or catheter in the vein will affect the flow rate. If the bevel is adjacent to the vessel wall, flow may decrease or stop altogether. Often, just changing the position of the patient's arm will remedy the situation.

Anatomy and Technique. The *antecubital* vein, located superficially on the anterior medial side of the elbow, is the most commonly used *venipuncture* site for contrast medium administration. It is not used for infusions that take longer than 1 h because of its location at the bend of the elbow (Fig. 5-1). The *cephalic* vein located superficially in the lateral aspect of the arm and forearm may also be used (Fig. 5-1A). The *basilic* vein, located on the dorsal surface of the medial side of the hand (Fig. 5-1B), is used when the antecubital vein is inaccessible.

Needles

- Gauge: identifies diameter of needle bore/lumen
- Larger gauge: smaller bore diameter
- Smaller gauge: larger bore diameter
- Hub: part of needle attached to syringe or IV tube

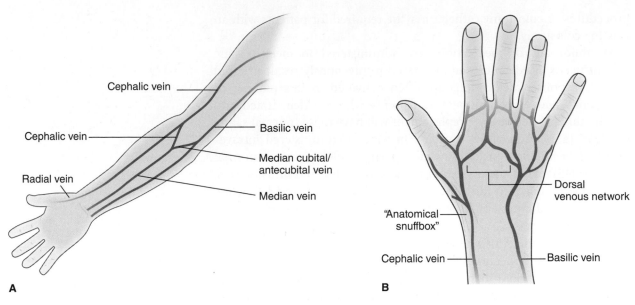

Figure 5-1. Veins commonly selected for venipuncture. **(A)** Anterior aspect, right forearm. **(B)** Posterior aspect, left hand.

A warm compress can be applied to the area of intended injection to increase the area of blood circulation and improve access to the intended vein. The needle is inserted into the vein at an acute angle of approximately *15°*; blood will flow back into the tubing when the needle is correctly positioned. Strict aseptic technique must be used for all IV injections.

Battery-powered peripheral "vein-finder" devices are available commercially. They use high-intensity LED lights to transilluminate the patient's subcutaneous tissue; in doing so, the device highlights the veins via their absorption (rather than reflection) of the light. These devices can be particularly useful for locating hard-to-find veins in obese adults, infants, and small children.

Summary

- Drugs and medications may be administered either orally or parenterally.
- *Parenteral* administration includes topical, oral, subcutaneous, intradermal, IM, IV, and intrathecal administration.
- Needle size is indicated by gauge; larger gauge means smaller needle bore.
- Butterfly sets or IV catheters are generally used for IV injection of a contrast medium.
- A heparin lock makes a vein accessible for medications administered at frequent intervals.
- IV solutions should be elevated 18–24 inches above the injection site.
- The median cubital/antecubital vein is the most commonly used venipuncture site for contrast medium administration.
- Injections can be subcutaneous, intravenous, or intramuscular.

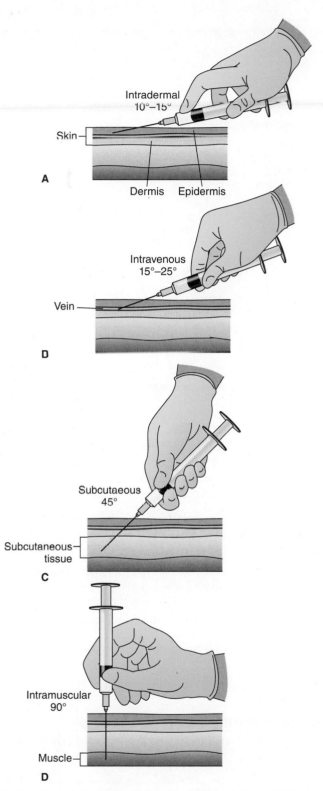

Injection Site	Needle Angle
Intradermal (Fig. 5-2A)	10°–15°
Intravenous (Fig. 5-2B)	15°–25°
Subcutaneous (Fig. 5-2C)	45°
Intramuscular (Fig. 5-2D)	90°

Figure 5-2. Needle position for injection sites: **(A)** Intradermal, **(B)** intravenous, **(C)** subcutaneous, and **(D)** intramuscular.

Steps for Venipuncture/Placement of Peripheral Intravenous Line

Assemble necessary materials:

- Tourniquet
- Antimicrobial agent to cleanse the site (70% alcohol or chlorhexidine gluconate swab)
- Needle (appropriate gauge)
- Gauze
- Saline syringe
- IV extension tubing
- Luer lock (leak-proof connector)
- Tegaderm dressing
- Tape
- Bandage

Confirm patient identity (two identifiers).

Review patient history (allergies, blood thinners, etc.).

Perform hand hygiene, wear protective gloves.

Place tourniquet proximal to where you will place the IV (above the vein).

Open and close fist to help to visualize vein (can also apply warm, moist compress over venipuncture site for several minutes to dilate the vein).

Select vein (visually or via palpation).

Clean the IV site for a minimum of 30 s, using circular motion. Let air-dry, do not blow on or fan the site (can cause contamination of area).

Using thumb of the nondominant hand, gently pull the skin below the IV site. This makes the skin taut and immobilizes the vein to prevent rolling.

Insert into vein using shallow angle (15°–30°) with bevel up.

When flashback seen (blood in the catheter chamber), advance catheter over stylet/needle until hub reaches skin and catheter is in the vein.

Apply pressure proximal to insertion site (to prevent blood from leaking out of the catheter); retract, remove, dispose of stylet/needle in appropriate bin.

Remove the tourniquet.

Attach IV extension tubing to the catheter.

Attach a luer lock connector to a saline syringe, ensuring to purge the air from the syringe. Connect the syringe to the IV extension tubing.

Draw back on the syringe to be certain there is blood return, then flush the catheter to ensure patency of the vessel. Significant pain or swelling indicates unsuccessful placement and should be removed.

Secure the catheter in place with Tegaderm dressing; tape extension tubing to the patient's arm.

If the catheter is to be indwelling, place a label on the Tegaderm with your initials and current time/date. Otherwise, remove the catheter and apply pressure with gauze and bandage.

CONTRAST MEDIA

Patient History

It is important for the radiographer to obtain a short but adequate patient history including reason(s) the examination has been requested. This history should be obtained in a manner and environment that ensures patient privacy. Because patients are rarely examined or interviewed by the radiologist, observations and information obtained by the radiographer can be a significant help in making an accurate diagnosis.

Purpose

The purpose of a contrast medium is to artificially increase subject contrast in body tissues and areas where there is little natural subject contrast. The abdominal viscera, for example, have very little subject contrast; that is, it is very difficult to identify specific organs or distinguish one organ from another. However, if a contrast agent is introduced into a particular organ such as the kidney or stomach, or into a vessel such as the aorta or one of its branches, we may more readily visualize these anatomic structures and/or evaluate physiologic activity.

Types and Properties of Agents

Contrast media or contrast agents can be described as either positive (radiopaque) or negative (radiolucent). Positive, or radiopaque, contrast agents have a higher atomic number than the surrounding soft tissue, resulting in a greater attenuation/absorption of x-ray photons, thereby increasing image contrast. Examples of positive contrast media are *iodinated agents* (both water based, and oil based) and *barium sulfate* suspensions. The inert characteristics of barium sulfate render it the *least toxic* contrast medium. On the other hand, iodinated contrast media have characteristics that increase their likelihood of producing *side effects* and *reactions*.

Negative, or radiolucent, contrast agents used are *air* and various *gases*. Because the atomic number of air is also quite different from that of soft tissue, high subject contrast is produced. Carbon dioxide is absorbed more rapidly by the body than by air.

In examinations, negative contrast is often used *with* positive contrast, which is termed *double-contrast studies*. The function of the positive agent is usually to *coat* various parts under study, whereas the air *fills* the space and permits visualization through the gaseous medium. Examinations that frequently use double-contrast technique are contrast enema (BE), upper GI (UGI) series, and arthrography.

Scheduling and Preparation Considerations

Multiple Examinations. When patients are scheduled for multiple x-ray examinations, each requiring the use of a contrast medium, the examinations must be scheduled in the correct sequence. For example, if a particular patient must be scheduled for a UGI or SB (small bowel) series, BE, and intravenous urogram (IVU), what sequence will permit optimal visualization of the required structures? Remember that it is important that residual barium does not overlie structures of interest. IVUs are rarely requested nowadays—being supplanted by other imaging methods—but should the examination be requested, the call-out box Sequencing Contrast Examinations indicates where it should be placed in the imaging sequences.

Examinations using a contrast medium that is excreted quickly and completely should be scheduled *first*. Therefore, if an IVU has been

---

Contrast Media

Positive (radiopaque)
- Barium sulfate
- Iodinated

Negative (radiolucent)
- Air
- Other gases

Sequencing Contrast Examinations

Sequence
- Sonography
- Radiologic imaging:
  - IVU*
  - Contrast enema
  - UGI
  - SBS

IVU examinations are infrequently performed, often replaced by other imaging methods.

requested, the IVU should be scheduled first. If the UGI or SB series were scheduled next, residual barium would be in the large bowel the next day, thus preventing adequate visualization of the large intestine. Therefore, the contrast enema/BE should be scheduled prior to the UGI/SBS; any residual barium is unlikely to interfere with the UGI/SBS, although a preliminary scout image of the abdomen should be seen first to be certain.

Patient Preparation. Patient preparation is somewhat different for each of these examinations. A patient scheduled for a *UGI or SB* series must be NPO after midnight. A contrast enema/BE (*lower GI*) requires that the large bowel be very clean prior to the administration of barium; this requires a low-residue diet 2–3 days before the procedure and only clear liquids 24 h prior, along with the administration of *cathartics* (laxatives) and cleansing enemas. Preparation for an *IVU* requires that the patient be NPO after midnight; some institutions also require that the large bowel be cleansed of gas and fecal material.

Aftercare for the contrast enema is very important. Patients are typically instructed to take milk of magnesia, increase their intake of fiber, drink plenty of water, expect changes in stool color until all barium is evacuated, and call their physician if they do not have a bowel movement within 24 h. Because water is removed from the barium sulfate suspension in the large bowel, it is essential to make patients understand the importance of these instructions to avoid barium impaction in the large bowel.

Contraindications and Patient Education

Radiopaque contrast media are most frequently used for radiographic procedures. *Barium sulfate* is one type of radiopaque contrast agent that is used to visualize the GI tract. Mixed with water, it forms a suspension that is usually administered orally for demonstration of the UGI tract (esophagus, stomach, and progression through the small intestine), and rectally for demonstration of the lower GI tract (large intestine).

Barium sulfate is *contraindicated* if a *perforation* is suspected somewhere along the course of the GI tract (e.g., a perforated diverticulum or gastric ulcer). Escape of barium sulfate into the peritoneal cavity can result in peritonitis. In these cases, a water-soluble, absorbable, iodinated contrast medium is generally used instead of barium. The water-soluble preparations are available as a ready-mixed liquid or as a powder requiring appropriate dilution with water. A patient with an NG tube can have the contrast medium administered through it for the purpose of locating and studying any site of obstruction. This procedure is called *enteroclysis.*

Barium preparations in the large bowel become thickened as a result of absorption of their fluid content, a process called *inspissation,* causing symptoms from mild constipation to bowel obstruction. Constipation can be a serious problem, particularly in the elderly, and fecal impaction or obstruction can result. It is essential that the radiographer provides clear instructions for follow-up aftercare, especially to outpatients. Patients are usually advised to expect light-colored stools for the next few days, to drink plenty of fluids, to increase their intake of fiber, and to take a mild laxative such as milk of magnesia following a barium study.

Patient Preparation

UGI/SBS

NPO after midnight

Contrast enema/BE

Low-residue diet 2–3 days before the procedure

Only clear liquids for 24 h

Cathartics, cleansing enemas

IVU

NPO after midnight, cleansing enemas, empty bladder before scout image

Iodinated contrast agents are another type of radiopaque contrast medium. These may be *oil based or water based.* Oil-based contrast media are rarely used nowadays, being replaced by water-soluble iodinated contrast media. Oil-based contrast media are not water soluble and not readily absorbed by the body; they remain in body tissues for a long period. Examinations that formerly used oil-based contrast agents are myelogram, lymphangiogram, sialogram, and bronchogram.

Water-based contrast media are either *ionic* or *nonionic.* These agents are principally used to delineate the urinary and vascular systems, and the GI tract when barium sulfate is contraindicated.

Ionic contrast media have a *higher osmolality,* that is, a greater number of particles in a given amount of solution. *Nonionic,* or *low-osmolality,* contrast agents are used especially with children, the elderly, patients with renal disease, patients with a history of *allergic* reaction to contrast media, or patients with multiple allergies. Side effects and allergic reactions are less likely and less severe with these media. Nonionic contrast agents are associated with less injection discomfort and a lower incidence of *nausea,* vomiting, and cardiovascular complications. Their only disadvantage is their cost, which is far greater than that of ionic contrast agents.

Iodinated contrast agents can become more *viscous* at normal room temperature, making injection more difficult. Warming the contrast to body temperature, in a special warming oven, reduces *viscosity,* permitting an easier and more comfortable injection.

REACTIONS AND COMPLICATIONS

Local Effects

The term *infiltration* refers to the diffusion of the injected material further into adjacent tissues. Extravasation is a local effect. The term *extravasation* refers to leakage of a medication or contrast medium from a vein rupture or inadvertent introduction into a tissue outside the vein. We often use these terms interchangeably in diagnostic imaging, although they are technically different. The needle should be removed and pressure applied to prevent formation of a *hematoma.* The recommended treatment is that the affected extremity be elevated above the heart and cold compresses applied topically. Extravasation of small amounts of contrast agent will cause some pain, minimal swelling, and localized erythema that rapidly decreases. Another potential local effect is *phlebitis.* If there is any skin blistering, increasing pain, and so on, the patient should be referred to the emergency department. If larger volumes of contrast are extravasated, extensive tissue and skin necrosis can occur.

Systemic Effects

Medications are administered to meet specific patient needs; medications can have harmless *side effects* in some individuals. If the side effect offsets the benefit, the medication might be discontinued. *Diabetic* patients taking insulin and scheduled for a UGI series are generally instructed to withhold their morning insulin and bring it with them to take following their examination. Should the patient take his or her

---

Qualities of Iodinated Contrast Agents That Contribute to Discomfort, Side Effects, and Reactions

Viscosity. More viscid (thick, sticky) agents are more difficult to inject and produce more heat and vessel irritation; the higher the concentration, the greater is the viscosity; viscosity also increases as room temperature decreases.

Toxicity. Potential toxicity is greater with higher concentration agents and ionic agents.

Miscibility. Contrast agents should be readily miscible (able to mix) with blood.

Osmolality. Low-osmolality agents have fewer particles in a given amount of solution and are less likely to provoke an allergic reaction.

insulin before the examination and remain NPO for a length of time, a reaction might occur because of a drop in blood sugar, especially if the examinations were delayed for any reason. UGI examinations on diabetic patients should be among the first examinations scheduled each day and priority should be given to these patients.

Medications can also have a *toxic effect.* Toxic systemic effects can occur because of sensitivity, overdose, or poor metabolism. An *antidote* is used to treat a toxic effect.

An *allergy* is an abnormal, acquired immune response to a substance (i.e., *allergen*) that would not usually trigger a reaction. An initial exposure to the allergen (i.e., *sensitization*) is required. Subsequent contact with the allergen then results in an *inflammatory response.* Examples of such responses include hay fever, urticaria, allergic rhinitis, eczema, and bronchial asthma. Allergens can be introduced into the body via contact, ingestion (e.g., food), inhalation (e.g., dust, pollen), or injection (e.g., medication, drugs). Allergic reactions of particular importance to the radiographer involve the use of *latex* products and *contrast media.*

Anaphylaxis is a life-threatening allergic reaction that affects millions of Americans every year and can be caused by a variety of allergens. *Anaphylaxis* can result from the body's sensitivity and allergic reaction to certain foods, insect venom, medications, anesthetics, and latex. The reaction can be the result of *ingestion, injection,* or *absorption* of the sensitizing agent.

Because iodinated contrast media are potentially toxic, the radiographer must be knowledgeable and alert to the possible adverse effects of their use (although the risk of a life-threatening reaction is relatively rare). Reactions to contrast media generally occur within 2–10 min following injection and can affect all body systems.

The body's response to the introduction of contrast material is the production of histamines, which brings about various symptoms. Symptoms of a *mild* systemic reaction include a flushed appearance, nausea, a metallic taste in the mouth, nasal congestion, a few hives (*urticaria*), and, occasionally, vomiting. Treatment of these minor symptoms generally consists of administration of either an *antihistamine* such as diphenhydramine (Benadryl), which blocks the action of the histamine and reduces the body's inflammatory response, or an epinephrine to raise the blood pressure and relax the bronchioles (see Table 5-1).

Potentially *life-threatening (anaphylactic) systemic responses* include respiratory failure, shock, and death within minutes. *Early* symptoms of an anaphylactic reaction include itching of the palms and soles, wheezing, constriction of the throat (possibly caused by laryngeal edema), *dyspnea, dysphagia, hypotension,* and *cardiopulmonary arrest.* The radiographer must maintain the patient's airway, summon the radiologist, and call a "code." The radiographer should then be prepared to stay with the patient and assist until the arrival of the code team.

Laboratory Values and Emergency Medications

BUN and *creatinine* values are indicators of renal function. The usual normal BUN range for adults is approximately 6–20 mg/dL; the normal creatinine range is 2.0 mg/dL. Elevated BUN and/or creatinine is indicative of potential renal damage resulting from the use of iodinated contrast medium.

Reactions Can Result From

- Ingestion
- Injection
- Absorption of the sensitizing agent

TABLE 5-1. Common Medications and Their Applications

Type	Effect	Example
Adrenergic	Vasopressor, stimulates sympathetic nervous system: increases BP, relaxes smooth muscle of respiratory system	Epinephrine (adrenaline)
Analgesic	Relieves pain	Aspirin, acetaminophen (Tylenol), codeine, meperidine (Demerol)
Antiarrhythmic	Relieves cardiac arrhythmia	Quinidine sulfate, lidocaine (Xylocaine)
Antibacterial	Stops growth of bacteria	Penicillin, tetracycline, erythromycin
Anticholinergic	Depresses parasympathetic system	Atropine, scopolamine, belladonna
Anticoagulant	Inhibits blood clotting; keeps IV lines and catheters free of clots	Heparin, warfarin
Anticonvulsant	Prevents/relieves convulsions	Carbamazepine (Tegretol) Phenytoin (Dilantin)
Antidepressant	Prevents/alleviates mental depression	Fluoxetine (Prozac) Paroxetine (Paxil) Sertraline (Zoloft) Nortriptyline (Pamelor, Aventyl)
Antihistamine	Relieves allergic symptoms	Diphenhydramine hydrochloride (Benadryl)
Antipyretic	Reduces fever	Aspirin, acetaminophen
Antitussive	Reduces coughing	Dextromethorphan (Romilar)
Barbiturate	Depresses CNS, decreases BP and respiration, and induces sleep	Phenobarbital sodium (Nembutal), secobarbital sodium (Seconal)
Cardiac stimulant	Increases cardiac output	Digitalis
Cathartic	Laxative, relieves constipation, prepares colon for diagnostic tests	Bisacodyl (Dulcolax), castor oil
Diuretic	Stimulates urine	Furosemide (Lasix)
Emetic	Stimulates vomiting	Activated charcoal, ipecac
Hypoglycemic	Lowers blood glucose	Insulin, chlorpropamide (Diabinese), metformin (Glucophage)
Narcotic (opioid)	Sedative/analgesic; potentially addictive	Morphine, codeine, meperidine (Demerol)
NSAID	Nonsteroidal pain relief	Aspirin (Bayer and others) Ibuprofen (Motrin and others) Naproxen (Aleve and others)
Stimulant	Stimulates the CNS	Caffeine, amphetamines
Tranquilizer	Reduces anxiety	Diazepam (Valium), alprazolam (Xanax)
Vasodilator	Relaxes and dilates blood vessels, decreases BP	Nitroglycerine, verapamil

Metformin (Glucophage) is an antidiabetic agent indicated for the treatment of type 2 diabetes mellitus.

With the use of iodinated contrast agents, there can be concern for increased renal damage in patients with acute kidney injury (AKI) and/or in patients with severe chronic kidney disease (as determined by estimated glomerular filtration rate [eGFR]). In addition, patients taking oral medication to control blood sugar, such as metformin (Glucophage), can be susceptible to kidney damage from the use of iodinated contrast agents. Current (February 2022) American College of Radiology (ACR) recommendations state, "Although the true risk of CI-AKI remains unknown, prophylaxis with intravenous normal saline is indicated for patients without contraindication (e.g., heart failure) who have acute kidney injury (AKI) or an estimated glomerular filtration rate (eGFR) less than 30 mL/min/1.73 m^2 who are not undergoing maintenance dialysis. In individual high-risk circumstances, prophylaxis may be considered in patients with an eGFR of 30–44 mL/min/1.73 m^2 at the discretion of the ordering clinician" (*https://www.acr.org/-/media/ACR/Files/Clinical-Resources/ACK-NKF-Consensus-Iodinated-Contrast.pdf*).

Medications that are used to treat hypertension include beta-adrenergic blockers and calcium channel blockers. Individuals taking beta-adrenergic blockers are at an increased risk for anaphylactic reactions. Individuals taking calcium channel blockers are at an increased risk for abrupt blood pressure decrease during cardiac catheterization.

The radiographer checks these laboratory values and medications before proceeding with the procedure and confirms with the radiologist whether the examination should proceed. If the radiologist has a question, he or she will have conversation with the referring physician to determine whether the examination should proceed.

Documentation

The *chart* of a hospitalized patient is a collection of information, records, and laboratory and imaging reports. Information includes the patient's condition, progress, medications, treatments, allergies, and so on. It is important that the radiographer is familiar with patient chart so as to check for laboratory values, medications, allergies, contraindications, and so on.

Documentation required of the radiographer should be entered directly on the patient's examination *requisition* and/or in the radiology computer system *notes*. Notes are made about pertinent patient history, or patient's illness or injury.

Any incident, accident, or unusual occurrence that causes injury or potential injury/harm to the patient (or visitor, or staff) must be reported to a radiology supervisor and an incident report completed. This is very important for the hospital's risk management department—for liability considerations and for possible procedural alterations to prevent future similar incidents.

Summary

- Patients must be appropriately prepared and scheduled for the contrast examination(s) for which they are scheduled.

- Artificial contrast media function to increase insufficient subject contrast; they can be positive (radiopaque) or negative (radiolucent).

- Positive contrast media include barium sulfate and iodinated (oil- or water-based) agents; negative and positive contrast agents are often used together in "double-contrast" studies.

- Qualities of iodinated contrast media that contribute to their risk include viscosity, toxicity, and miscibility.

- Water-soluble (absorbable) contrast agents are used in place of barium sulfate when visceral *perforation* is suspected.

- Patients require clear and complete postprocedural instructions, particularly following barium examinations.

- Allergens can be introduced into the body via contact, ingestion, inhalation, or injection. An *allergy* is an abnormal, acquired immune response.

- Initial *sensitization* to the allergen is required; subsequent contact results in an *inflammatory response.*

- *Extravasation* refers to leakage of a medication or contrast medium from a vein rupture or inadvertent introduction into a tissue outside the vein. *Infiltration* refers to diffusion of the injected material into adjacent tissues. Treatment includes removing the needle, applying pressure to prevent *hematoma* formation, and applying *a cold pack* to relieve pain and limit further infiltration.

- Nonionic iodinated contrast agents produce far less side effects than their ionic counterparts; nonionic contrast agents are more expensive.

- Reactions to ionic agents usually occur within 2–10 min following injection.

- Symptoms of a mild reaction include mild urticaria, flushing, nausea, nasal congestion, and metallic taste; an antihistamine is usually given to the patient.

- The radiographer must confirm that patients taking antidiabetic medication, beta-adrenergic blockers, or calcium channel blockers have had their laboratory values checked and approved by the radiologist and/or referring physician.

COMPREHENSION CHECK

Congratulations! You have completed your review of this chapter. If you are able to answer the following group of comprehensive questions, you can feel confident that you have mastered this section. You are then ready to go on to the "registry-type" questions that follow. For greatest success, do not go to these multiple-choice questions without first completing the following short-answer questions:

1. Discuss the importance of careful and accurate patient assessment. What are the components of a good assessment (p. 69, 70)?

2. Identify how a needle bore changes with increasing/decreasing gauge (p. 71).

3. Describe the function and uses of a heparin lock (p. 71).

4. Identify the correct needle angle for subcutaneous, intravenous, and intramuscular injections (p. 73).

5. Identify the height at which IV containers should be hung (p. 71).

6. Explain how contrast medium extravasation/infiltration should be treated (p. 77).

7. Identify the vein(s) commonly selected for venipuncture (p. 71, 72).

8. Define *allergy;* discuss *sensitization* and *inflammatory* response (p. 78).

9. Distinguish between *side effect* and *toxic effect* (p. 77, 78).

10. Discuss the importance of observing initial patient condition and any subsequent changes (p. 70).

11. Describe the difference between oral and parenteral drug administration; list five types of parenteral administration (p. 70).

12. Explain the purpose of artificial contrast media (p. 75).

13. Identify the two types of contrast media, describe their characteristics, and give examples of each (p. 75).

14. Explain the appropriate patient preparation for UGI/SBS, contrast enema/BE, and IVU (p. 75, 76).

15. Describe the *risks* associated with iodinated contrast media and identify the type of iodinated media associated with less risk (p. 78, 79, 80).

16. Describe three *qualities* of iodinated contrast media that contribute to the production of side effects (p. 77).

17. Explain how double-contrast examinations can serve to better demonstrate certain anatomic parts (p. 75).

18. Describe *contraindications* to the use of barium sulfate; identify the alternative contrast medium (p. 76).

19. Explain the importance of *aftercare* explanations, especially following barium examinations (p. 76).

20. Identify the correct sequence for scheduling radiologic contrast examinations. (p. 75)

21. Discuss orderly sequence of placement of peripheral intravenous line. (p. 74).

22. Identify the basic difference between ionic and nonionic contrast media and identify when use of nonionic agents is indicated (p. 77).

23. Describe symptoms a patient with a *mild* reaction to iodinated contrast media might experience and their usual treatment (p. 78).

24. Describe the symptoms of a possible *impending anaphylactic reaction* and the radiographer's responsibilities (p. 78).

25. Give examples of local versus systemic reactions (p. 77, 78).

26. Which medications have the potential for untoward physical reaction with iodinated contrast agents (p. 79)?

27. List components of a typical patient chart (p. 69).

28. List various equipment necessary for IV drug administration (p. 74).

CHAPTER REVIEW QUESTIONS

1. Equipment that might be needed for intravenous drug/contrast medium administration include(s)

   1. heparin lock
   2. needles
   3. infusion set

   (A) 1 only
   (B) 1 and 2 only
   (C) 2 and 3 only
   (D) 1, 2, and 3

2. Body reaction to a sensitizing agent can occur as a result of

   1. absorption
   2. injection
   3. ingestion

   (A) 1 only
   (B) 1 and 2 only
   (C) 2 and 3 only
   (D) 1, 2, and 3

3. Example(s) of negative contrast agents include

   1. air
   2. iodine
   3. barium sulfate

   (A) 1 only
   (B) 1 and 2 only
   (C) 2 and 3 only
   (D) 1, 2, and 3

4. Which of the following gauge needles has the smallest bore?

   (A) 12
   (B) 18
   (C) 20
   (D) 23

5. What should be the angle formed between the needle and the skin surface for an intravenous injection?

   (A) 15°
   (B) 45°
   (C) 60°
   (D) 90°

6. Parenteral administration of drugs may be performed

   1. intrathecally
   2. intravenously
   3. orally

   (A) 1 only
   (B) 1 and 2 only
   (C) 3 only
   (D) 1, 2, and 3

7. What is the most frequently used site for an intravenous injection of contrast agents?

   (A) Basilic vein
   (B) Cephalic vein
   (C) Antecubital vein
   (D) Femoral vein

8. Mild systemic reaction to intravenous contrast material include all of the following, *except*

   (A) nausea
   (B) metallic taste in mouth
   (C) wheezing
   (D) flushed appearance

9. Terms correctly associated with positive contrast agents include all the following, *except*

   (A) radiopaque
   (B) iodinated
   (C) high atomic number
   (D) carbon dioxide

10. The usual patient preparation for a UGI examination is

    (A) NPO 8 h before the examination
    (B) only light breakfast the morning of the examination
    (C) only clear fluids the morning of the examination
    (D) 2 ounces of castor oil and enemas until clear

Answers and Explanations

1. (D) IV fluids and/or medications are administered to meet specific patient needs. Medications administered intravenously result in rapid patient response; medications are often delivered in this manner in emergency and critical situations. Patients who are dehydrated and require fluid and electrolyte replacement will have these (normal saline or D5W) administered intravenously. *IV equipment* includes needles, syringes, fluids such as normal saline or D5W (a solution of 5% dextrose in water), IV catheters, heparin locks, IV poles, and infusion sets.

2. (D) Anaphylaxis is a life-threatening allergic reaction that affects millions of Americans every year and can be caused by a variety of allergens. It can result from the body's sensitivity and allergic reaction to certain foods, insect venom, medications, anesthetics, and latex. The reaction can be the result of *ingestion, injection,* or *absorption* of the sensitizing agent.

3. (A) *Negative, or radiolucent, contrast agents* used are *air* and various *gases*. Because the atomic number of air is also quite different from that of soft tissue, high subject contrast is produced. Carbon dioxide is absorbed more rapidly by the body than by air.

Negative contrast is often used *with* positive contrast in examinations termed *double-contrast studies*. The function of the positive agent is usually to *coat* the various parts under study, whereas the air *fills* the space and permits visualization through the gaseous medium. Examinations that frequently use double-contrast technique are BE, UGI series, and arthrography.

4. (D) The diameter of a needle is identified as its *gauge*. As the diameter of its *bore* decreases, the *gauge* increases. Hence, a 23-gauge needle has a smaller diameter bore than an 18-gauge needle. Hypodermic needles are generally used for phlebotomy (i.e., blood samples), whereas butterflies and IV catheters are used more frequently for injections such as contrast media. If an infusion injection is required, an IV catheter is generally preferred. The hub of the hypodermic needle is attached to a syringe, whereas the hub of the butterfly tubing or IV catheter may be attached to a syringe or an IV container via an IV infusion set.

5. (A) The antecubital vein is the most commonly used *venipuncture* site for contrast medium administration. The basilic vein, located on the dorsal surface of the hand, is used when the antecubital vein is inaccessible. The cephalic vein may also be used (see Fig. 5-1). The needle is inserted into the vein at a *15° angle;* blood will flow back into the tubing when the needle is correctly positioned. Strict aseptic technique must be used. The needle forms a 90° angle with the skin in intramuscular injections and a 45° angle in subcutaneous injections.

6. (B) Although radiographic contrast media are usually administered orally or intravenously, there are a number of routes or methods of drug administration. Drugs and medications may be administered either *orally* or *parenterally*. *Parenteral* administration refers to any route other than the digestive tract (orally) and includes *topical, subcutaneous, intradermal, intramuscular, intravenous,* and *intrathecal* administration.

7. (C) The *antecubital* vein is the most commonly used injection site for contrast medium administration. It is not used for infusions that take longer than 1 h because of its location at the bend of the elbow. The basilic vein, located on the dorsal surface of the hand, is used when the antecubital vein is inaccessible. The cephalic vein may also be used. Strict aseptic technique must be used for all intravenous injections.

8. (C) Any reaction to contrast media generally occurs within 2–10 min following injection and can affect all body systems. The body's response to the introduction of contrast material is the production of histamines, which brings about various symptoms. Symptoms of a *mild systemic* reaction include a flushed appearance, nausea, a metallic taste in the mouth, nasal congestion, a few hives (*urticaria*), and, occasionally, vomiting. Treatment of these minor symptoms generally consists of administration of either an *antihistamine* such as diphenhydramine (Benadryl), which blocks the action of the histamine and reduces the body's inflammatory response, or an epinephrine to raise the blood pressure and relax the bronchioles (see Table 5-1). Potentially *life-threatening/anaphylactic systemic responses* include respiratory failure, shock, and death within minutes. *Early* symptoms of an anaphylactic reaction include itching of the palms and soles, wheezing, constriction of the throat, *dyspnea, dysphagia, hypotension,* and *cardiopulmonary arrest.* The radiographer must maintain the patient's airway, summon the radiologist, and call a "code." The radiographer should then be prepared to stay with the patient and assist until the arrival of the code team.

9. (D) Contrast media or contrast agents can be described as either positive (radiopaque) or negative (radiolucent). Positive, or radiopaque, contrast agents have a higher atomic number than the surrounding soft tissue, resulting in a greater attenuation/absorption of x-ray photons, thereby increasing image contrast. Examples of positive contrast media are *iodinated agents* (both water based and oil based) and *barium sulfate* suspensions. The inert characteristics of barium sulfate render it the *least toxic* contrast medium. On the other hand, iodinated contrast media have characteristics that increase their likelihood of producing *side effects* and *reactions. Negative, or radiolucent, contrast agents* used are *air* and various *gases.* Carbon dioxide is absorbed more rapidly by the body than by air. Negative contrast is often used *with* positive contrast in examinations termed *double-contrast studies.* The function of the positive agent is usually to *coat* the various parts under study, whereas the air *fills* the space and permits visualization through the gaseous medium. Examinations that frequently use double-contrast technique are contrast enema (BE), upper GI (UGI), and arthrography.

10. (A) Patient preparation differs for various contrast examinations. To obtain a diagnostic examination of the stomach, it must first be empty. The usual *UGI* preparation is NPO (nothing by mouth) after midnight (approximately 8 h before the examination). Any material in the stomach can simulate the appearance of disease. An iodinated contrast agent, usually in the form of several pills, is taken by the patient the evening before a scheduled *GB* examination and only water is allowed the morning of the examination. The patient scheduled for a *BE* (lower GI) requires a large bowel that is very clean prior to the administration of barium; this requires the administration of cathartics (laxatives) and cleansing enemas. Preparation for an *IVU* requires that the patient be NPO after midnight; some institutions may require that the large bowel be cleansed of gas and fecal material. *Aftercare* for barium examinations is also very important. Patients are typically instructed to take milk of magnesia and to drink plenty of water. Because water is removed from the barium sulfate suspension in the large bowel, it is essential to make patients understand the importance of these instructions to avoid barium impaction in the large bowel.

PART II

Procedures

CHAPTER 6
General Procedural Considerations
Body Planes
Body Habitus
Surface Landmarks and Localization Points
Preliminary Steps and Procedural Guidelines
Immobilization and Respiration
Modified and Additional Projections

CHAPTER 7
Anatomy, Positioning, and Pathology
The Skeletal System
The Appendicular Skeleton
    Upper Limb and Shoulder Girdle
    Lower Limb and Pelvis

The Axial Skeleton
    Vertebral Column
    Thorax
    Head and Neck
Body Systems
    Respiratory System
    Biliary System
    Digestive System
    Urinary System
    Female Reproductive System
    Central Nervous System
    Circulatory System

General Procedural Considerations

OBJECTIVES

At the conclusion of this chapter, the student will be able to:

- Define anatomic/positioning terms.
- Identify the body planes.
- Discuss various procedural modifications the radiographer can use in nonroutine/emergency circumstances.
- Discuss how an understanding of patient body habitus and body surface landmarks impacts ease and accuracy of imaging procedures.
- Explain the concepts and steps involved in performing an accurate and efficient imaging procedure.

The development of positioning skills requires a thorough knowledge of normal *anatomy,* an awareness of *pathologic conditions* and their impact on positioning limitations, and selection of prudent *technical factors.*

A review of basic positioning principles and terminology is essential to an overview of radiographic procedures. Therefore, several tables and figures in this chapter summarize the fundamental principles of imaging procedures: *body planes* (see Fig. 6-2), *body habitus* (see Figs. 6-4 and 6-5), *four quadrants* and *nine regions* of the abdomen (see Fig. 6-6), *body surface landmarks* and *localization points* (see Fig. 6-7), and *standard terminology* (see Fig. 6-3). The student should be thoroughly acquainted with these before approaching the study of specific positioning skills.

It must be emphasized that a patient's condition often impacts his or her ability to move readily on the x-ray table or maintain positions for a longer period. Most of the descriptions of *positions of a part* in Chapter 7 can be readily used with patients not severely injured and patients without debilitating pathology; in many instances, suggested modifications for *traumatized* patients are included. One measure of a skilled radiographer is his or her ability to be cautious and resourceful when examining injured or debilitated patients having pathologic or traumatic conditions such as arthritis, bone fractures, metastatic bone disease, and gastrointestinal or respiratory distress, patients in shock, or victims of stroke.

The use of *body surface landmarks* and *localization points* (see Fig. 6-7) as external indicators of anatomic structures can increase the ease and accuracy of positioning.

Modifications that radiographers can make to aid in patient comfort and completion of a thorough, diagnostic examination include thoughtful placement of a cushioning sponge, the use of a horizontal beam (cross-table) for *lateral* projections instead of moving the patient (Fig. 6-1), and performing an examination in an *erect* position if the *recumbent* position is uncomfortable. The radiographer must also be aware of how various pathological processes can impact the need to alter technical factors.

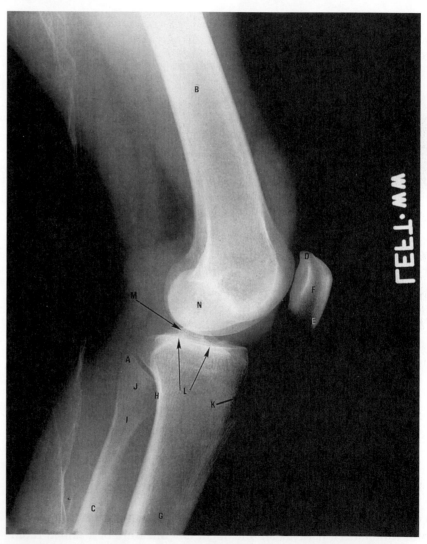

Figure 6-1. *Horizontal beam lateral* projection of the knee performed in the supine position on a patient with multiple injuries. A horizontal (cross-table) x-ray beam was used to reduce discomfort and risk of further injury. Observe the bedsheet artifact from the mattress pad beneath the patient. Use this radiograph to *review the skeletal anatomy* of the knee and correctly identify the lettered parts. A, styloid process of fibula; B, femur; C, fibula; D, patella—base; E, patella—apex; F, patella—body; G, tibia; H, proximal tibiofibular articulation; I, neck of fibula; J, head of fibula; K, tibial tuberosity; L, tibial plateau; M, intercondylar eminence; N, femoral condyle. (Photo contributor: Stamford Hospital, Department of Radiology.)

BODY PLANES

Body planes are illustrated in Figure 6-2. Positioning descriptions and methodology are described using these planes. The student radiographer must understand these body planes and their relationship to each other and that of the x-ray beam and the image receptor. The body planes are described as follows:

- Midsagittal or median sagittal plane (MSP): divides the body into left and right halves
- Sagittal plane: any plane parallel to the MSP
- Midcoronal plane (MCP): divides the body into anterior and posterior halves
- Coronal plane: any plane parallel to the MCP
- Transverse/horizontal plane: perpendicular to the MSP and MCP and divides the body axially into superior and inferior portions

BODY HABITUS

In 1916, R. Walter Mills presented an article at the American Roentgen Ray Society meeting in Chicago (published in *American Journal of Roentgenology,* April 1917) describing "The Relation of Bodily Habitus

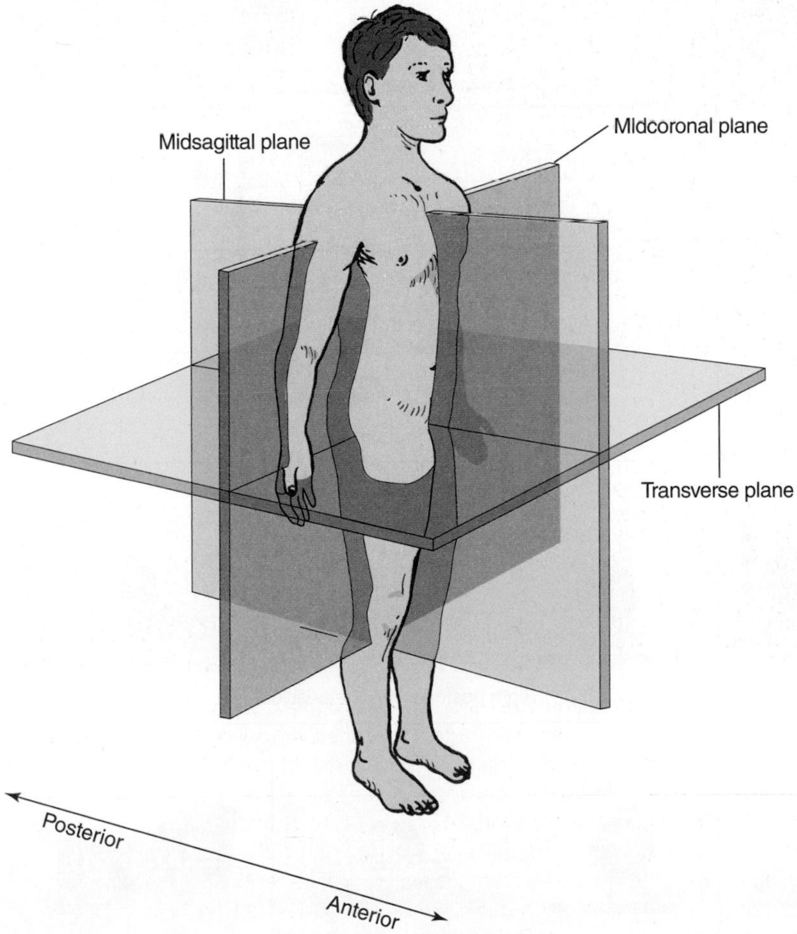

Anatomic/Positioning Terminology (Fig. 6-3)

The following terms are used to indicate anatomic direction:

Superior	Toward the upper part of the structure
Inferior	Toward the lower part of the structure
Anterior/ventral	Nearer to or at the front of the body
Posterior/dorsal	Nearer to or at the back of the body
Medial	Nearer the midline of the body
Lateral	Away from the midline of the body
Proximal	Nearer to the point of attachment
Distal	Farther from the point of attachment
Cephalad	Toward the head
Caudad	Toward the feet

Figure 6-2. Body planes.

Positioning Terminology

Radiographic position
Refers to body's physical position, e.g., recumbent, erect, prone, supine, Trendelenburg

Radiographic projection
Describes the path of the CR, e.g., PA (CR enters posteriorly, exits anteriorly)

Radiographic view
Describes the body part as seen by the IR, e.g., palmar view of the hand; infrequently used

General Terminology

1. Recumbent/lying down in any position
   * lying on back, face up = *supine*
   * lying on abdomen, face down = *prone*
   * supine, prone, or lateral, using horizontal CR = *decubitus*
2. Erect/upright/standing or sitting up
   * facing the IR = *anterior position*
   * with back toward IR = *posterior position*
3. Oblique position—erect or recumbent
   * *RAO/Right Anterior* Oblique: body rotated, with right anterior aspect nearest the IR
   * *LAO/Left Anterior Oblique:* body rotated, with left anterior aspect nearest the IR
   * *RPO/Right Posterior Oblique:* body rotated, with right posterior aspect nearest the IR
   * *LPO/Left Posterior Oblique:* body rotated, with left posterior aspect nearest the IR

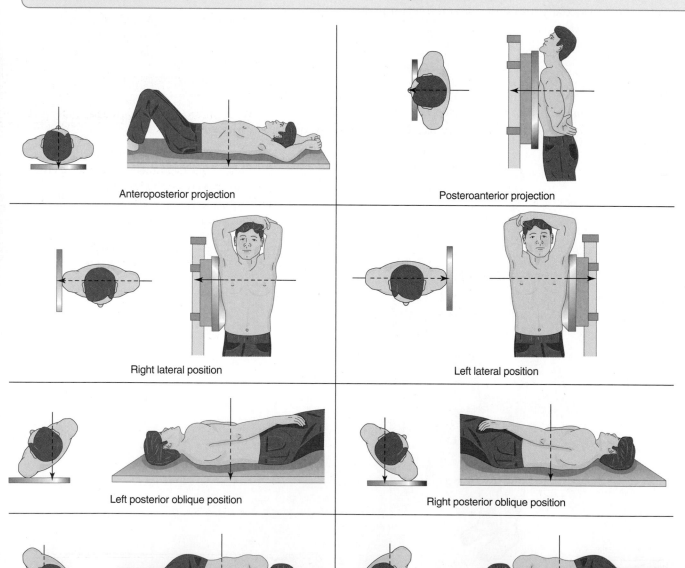

Anteroposterior projection

Posteroanterior projection

Right lateral position

Left lateral position

Left posterior oblique position

Right posterior oblique position

Left anterior oblique position

Right anterior oblique position

Figure 6-3. Standard terminology provides descriptions and interpretation of accepted radiologic positioning language.

to Visceral Form, Position, Tonus and Motility." In his article, he coined the terms *hypersthenic, sthenic, hyposthenic,* and *asthenic* to describe the various body types. He noted that most physicians came into the field prejudiced by their early anatomic teachings and had fixed conceptions, "which the revelations of the Roentgen ray ruthlessly outraged."

Patients come in all shapes and sizes. The term *body habitus* refers to the body's physical appearance. Variations in body habitus have a significant effect on the *shape, location,* and *position* of thoracic and abdominal organs and can affect their function and motility. Figure 6-4

Body Habitus: Types, Characteristics, and Prevalence

Hypersthenic and asthenic types characterize the *extremes* in body types:

Hypersthenic (5)

- Body large and heavy
- Bony framework thick, short, and wide
- Lungs and heart high
- Stomach transverse (Fig. 6-5A)
- Colon/large bowel peripheral
- Gallbladder high and lateral

Asthenic (10)

- Body slender and light
- Bony framework delicate
- Thorax long and narrow
- Stomach very low and long (fish hook) (Fig. 6-5B)
- Colon/large bowel low, medial, and redundant
- Gallbladder low and medial

Sthenic and hyposthenic types characterize the *more average* body types:

Sthenic (50)

- Build average and athletic
- Similar to hypersthenic but modified by elongation of the abdomen and thorax

Hyposthenic (35)

- Somewhat slighter, less robust
- Similar to asthenic, but stomach, intestines, and gallbladder situated higher in the abdomen

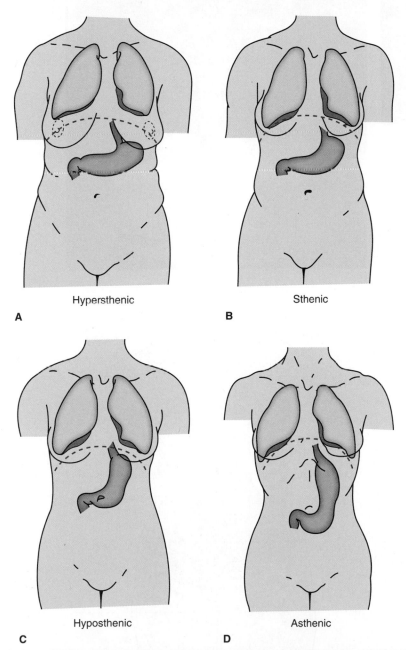

Hypersthenic

A

Sthenic

B

Hyposthenic

C

Asthenic

D

Figure 6-4. (A–D) The *position, shape,* and *motility* of various organs can differ greatly from one *body habitus* to another. Each of the body habitus types is shown, and the characteristic variations in shape and position of the diaphragm, lungs, and stomach are illustrated. The radiographer must consider these characteristic differences while performing radiographic examinations on individuals of various body habitus types.

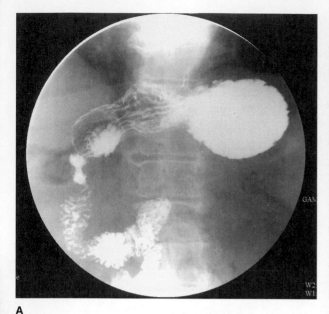

A

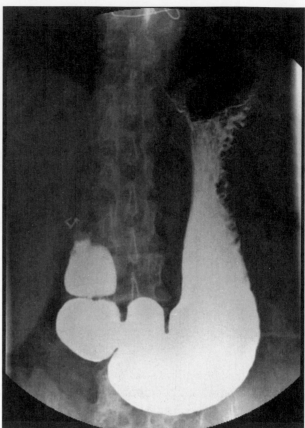

B

Figure 6-5. (A) Example of hypersthenic stomach. **(B)** Example of asthenic stomach. (Photo contributor: Stamford Hospital, Department of Radiology.)

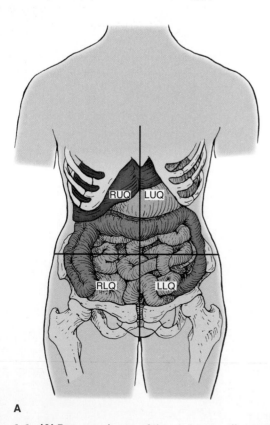

A

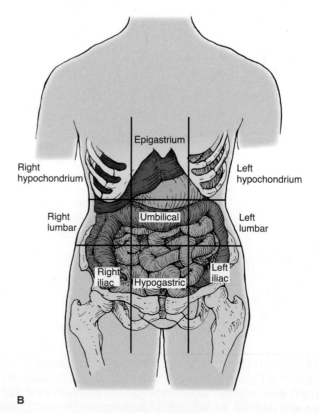

B

Figure 6-6. (A) Four quadrants of the abdomen, illustrating position of major organs. **(B)** Nine regions of the abdomen, illustrating position of major organs.

illustrates how greatly the position of the diaphragm, lungs, and stomach can differ among the various body habitus types. Radiographers should be knowledgeable about the variable characteristics of each habitus and how to use that knowledge when imaging patients of various body habitus types.

The *hypersthenic* habitus is the largest of the four types. This type is broad and heavy; the chest area is short with a high diaphragm. The viscera (stomach, large intestine, and gallbladder) are usually high and lateral.

The *sthenic* habitus is defined as an average athletic build. Compared with the hypersthenic habitus, it is characterized by a longer chest and abdomen, with viscera located more medially.

The *hyposthenic* habitus is a slighter version of the sthenic habitus—less athletic/strong.

The *asthenic* habitus is the smallest/slightest of the four types. This habitus can be frail-looking, slender, and slight. The chest is long, and the abdominal viscera are located quite low and medially.

SURFACE LANDMARKS AND LOCALIZATION POINTS

A number of surface anatomic points and particular vertebral levels are effectively used in radiographic positioning. These are illustrated in Figure 6-7A (anterior view) and Figure 6-7B (lateral view). The radiographer uses surface landmarks that are both bony prominences and

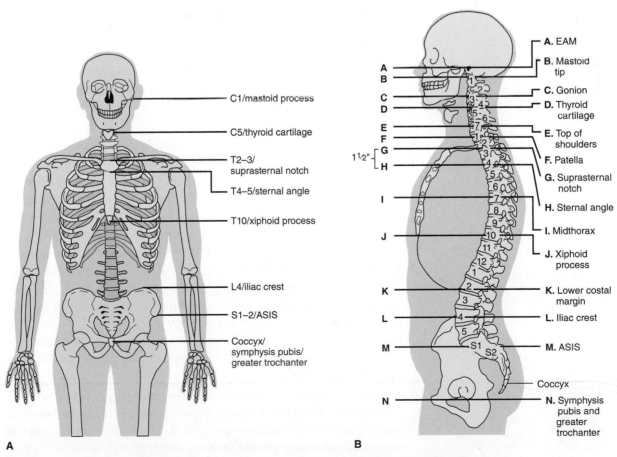

Figure 6-7. Body surface landmarks and localization points: **(A)** anterior view and **(B)** lateral view.

Vertebra(e)		Localization Point
Cervical region	C1	Mastoid process
	C5	Thyroid cartilage (Adam's apple)
	C7	Vertebra prominens
Thoracic region	T2–T3	Suprasternal (jugular) notch
	T4–T5	Sternal angle
	T7–T8	Inferior angle of scapula
	T9	Xiphoid (ensiform) process
	T10	Xiphoid process
Lumbar region	T12–L3	Kidneys
	L1	Transpyloric plane
	L3	Inferior costal margin
	L3–L4	Umbilicus
	L4	Iliac crest
Sacral and coccygeal regions	S1–S2	Anterosuperior iliac spine (ASIS)
	Coccyx	Symphysis pubis and greater trochanter

projections to identify anatomic structures and positional accuracy, and to locate internal structures/organs that are known to correspond to the bony prominences or vertebral levels. Accurate use of surface landmarks and localization points can effectively avoid the need for repeat images. Knowledge of these relationships improves accuracy of patient positioning and the central ray entry/exit points.

PRELIMINARY STEPS AND PROCEDURAL GUIDELINES

Providing skillful patient care in an *orderly* fashion is exceedingly important. Having the diagnostic room prepared with all necessary accessories available *before* bringing the patient in the room is the correct way to begin a diagnostic x-ray procedure.

The following are ordered steps and procedures that help ensure high-quality patient care and diagnostic radiographs:

1. Read the request carefully, noting the type of examination, condition of the patient, and mode of travel. (Make mental notes of any modifications or accessory equipment that may be required.)

2. Prepare the radiographic department. Be certain that the x-ray room is neat and orderly, with a clean x-ray table and a fresh pillowcase. All accessories needed for the examination should be in the x-ray room before bringing in the patient.

3. Identify the correct patient, quickly evaluating any special needs. *Introduce* yourself and establish rapport en route to the radiographic department, being careful not to discuss confidential issues within earshot of others.

4. If necessary, instruct the patient to change appropriately for the exam, removing clothing and objects (e.g., jewelry, dentures, and braided hair) that may cast artifacts within the area of interest (Figs. 6-8 and 6-9).

5. Speak in a well-modulated voice while providing a clear and succinct explanation of the procedure, and address any questions or concerns of the patient. Obtain a short pertinent patient history of why the examination has been requested. The radiographer should explain that a number of different positions may be needed to evaluate the area of interest and may require palpation of bony landmarks and instructions to turn into various positions.

6. Radiography of most structures usually requires a minimum of two projections, usually at right angles to each other. Side-to-side (i.e., left/right) relationships are demonstrated in the frontal projection (Fig. 6-10A), whereas anterior/posterior relationships are seen in the lateral projection (Fig. 6-10B). This is especially important in localizing foreign bodies and tumors and demonstrating fracture displacement or alignment.

7. It is customary and economical to use the smallest size image receptor that will include all the necessary information. Therefore, the smallest possible anatomic area (consistent with a diagnostic examination) will be irradiated to keep patient dose to a minimum. Use radiation protective shielding, as needed or when the examination allows.

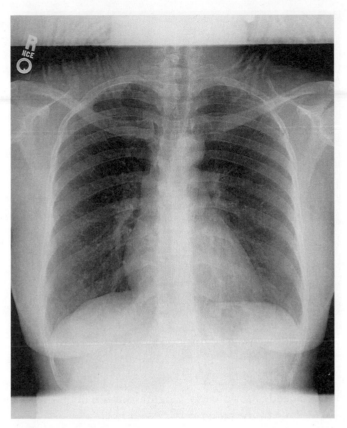

Figure 6-8. The posteroanterior projection of the chest is fairly well positioned and exposed, but observe the braids of hair that extend past the neck and superimpose on the pulmonary apices. Braided hair should be pinned up or otherwise removed from superimposition on thoracic structures. (Photo contributor: Stamford Hospital, Department of Radiology.)

8. In radiography of the long bones, every effort should be made to include both articulations associated with the injured bone, but it is essential to include at least the articulation nearest to the injury.

9. To ensure accurate diagnosis, supplemental images of any anatomic part may be required, for example, *oblique, axial, tangential, erect,* or *decubitus.* Exposure factors must be correctly adjusted for each change of position.

10. Each image must be accurately labeled with patient information such as name or identification number, institution name, date of examination, and side marker. Other information may be included according to institution policy.

IMMOBILIZATION AND RESPIRATION

Motion obliterates recorded detail; thus, it is essential that the radiographer be able to reduce patient motion as much as possible. There are two types of motion that can impact radiographic images: *involuntary* and *voluntary.* Although there are several methods that can be used to reduce motion unsharpness due to both voluntary motion and involuntary motion, good *patient communication* is paramount because it is required before any other method can be effective.

Skeletal Motion Terminology

The following terms are used to indicate anatomic *motion*:

- *Supination:* Turning of the body or arm so that the palm faces forward, with the thumb away from the midline of the body
- *Pronation:* Turning of the body or arm so that the palm faces backward, with the thumb toward the midline of the body
- *Abduction:* Movement of a part away from the body's MSP
- *Adduction:* Movement of a part toward the body's MSP
- *Flexion:* Bending motion of an articulation, decreasing the angle between associated bones
- *Extension:* Bending motion of an articulation, increasing the angle between associated bones
- *Eversion:* A turning outward or lateral motion of an articulation, sometimes with external tension or stress applied
- *Inversion:* A turning inward or medial motion of an articulation, sometimes with external tension or stress applied
- *Rotation:* Movement of a part about its central or long axis
- *Circumduction:* Movement of a limb that produces circular motion; circumscribes a small area at its proximal end and a wide area at the distal end

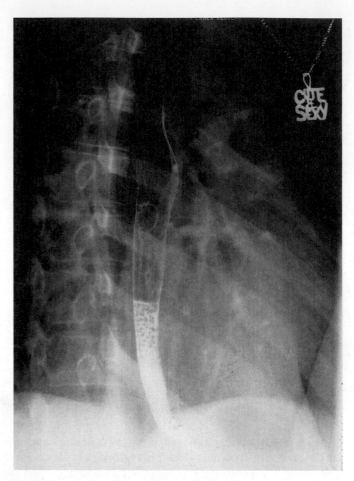

Figure 6-9. Left posterior oblique image of the esophagus with a jewelry artifact near the area of interest. The patient must remove clothing and other objects such as jewelry from the area to be examined before donning the dressing gown. (Photo contributor: Stamford Hospital, Department of Radiology.)

The single most important method to reduce *involuntary* motion is to use the *shortest possible exposure time*. Various types of *immobilization devices* can also be used to effectively reduce motion. Motion from muscular tremors as a result of anxiety or pain is involuntary and can be greatly minimized with good communication, a carefully placed positioning sponge or sandbag, and the use of the shortest exposure time possible.

Suspension of patient respiration for parts other than the extremities is an effective method of reducing *voluntary* motion; patient understanding and cooperation are required, thus making good *communication* the *most effective method of reducing voluntary motion*. The phase of respiration on which an exposure is made can be essential to the diagnostic quality of the radiographic image. Chest radiography, for example, normally requires that the exposure be made on inspiration (the second inspiration for better filling of the lungs). Most abdominal examinations are exposed on expiration. The phase of respiration on which the exposure is made can also make a significant difference in the required exposure (discussed in Part IV).

COMPREHENSION CHECK

Congratulations! You have completed your review of this chapter. If you are able to answer the following group of comprehensive questions, you can feel confident that you have mastered this section. You are then ready to go on to the "registry-type" questions that follow. For greatest success, do not go to the multiple-choice questions without first completing the following short-answer questions:

1. Discuss how knowledge of anatomy and pathologic conditions relates to positioning skills (p. 89).

2. Identify the sagittal and midsagittal, coronal and midcoronal, and transverse (horizontal) planes; describe their relationship with each other (p. 91).

3. Identify the four types of body habitus, and list physical characteristics of each (p. 91, pp. 93–95).

4. Name, identify, and describe the quadrants and nine regions of the abdomen (p. 94).

5. Identify surface anatomic localization points and their corresponding vertebrae (p. 95, 96).

6. Define and identify various skeletal movement terms (p. 97).

7. Discuss the importance of establishing an orderly sequence of preparation for performing radiologic examinations (p. 96, 97).

8. Explain the importance of obtaining two images at right angles to each other for most radiologic examinations (p. 96, 99).

9. Discuss the inclusion of articulations in radiography of the extremities (p. 97).

10. List the information that must be included on the radiographic image (p. 96, 97).

11. What is the most effective method of reducing *voluntary* and *involuntary* motions (p. 97, 98)?

12. Why/when might the radiographer be required to modify the routine projections (p. 100)?

CHAPTER REVIEW QUESTIONS

1. The plane that passes vertically through the body dividing it into anterior and posterior halves is termed the
   - (A) midsagittal plane
   - (B) midcoronal plane
   - (C) sagittal plane
   - (D) transverse plane

2. The position of the asthenic stomach, as compared with the position of the sthenic stomach, is more
   - (A) superior and lateral
   - (B) superior and medial
   - (C) inferior and lateral
   - (D) inferior and medial

3. What is the relationship between the midsagittal and midcoronal planes?
   - (A) Parallel
   - (B) Perpendicular
   - (C) 45°
   - (D) 70°

4. With the patient recumbent with feet positioned at a level lower than the head, the patient is said to be in the
   - (A) Trendelenburg position
   - (B) Fowler position
   - (C) decubitus position
   - (D) Sims position

5. Prior to x-ray examinations of the skull and cervical spine, the patient should remove
   1. dentures
   2. earrings
   3. necklaces
   - (A) 1 only
   - (B) 1 and 2 only
   - (C) 2 and 3 only
   - (D) 1, 2, and 3

6. Image identification markers should include
   1. patient's name and/or ID number
   2. date
   3. a right or left marker
   - (A) 1 only
   - (B) 1 and 2 only
   - (C) 1 and 3 only
   - (D) 1, 2, and 3

7. The radiographer should be able to
   1. take a short patient history prior to the examination
   2. modify routine protocol to obtain similar images of patients who are unable to move
   3. evaluate patient condition and needs
   - (A) 1 only
   - (B) 1 and 2 only
   - (C) 1 and 3 only
   - (D) 1, 2, and 3

8. The best way to control voluntary motion is
   - (A) immobilization
   - (B) careful explanation
   - (C) short exposure time
   - (D) physical restraint

9. Before bringing the patient into the radiographic room, the radiographer should
   1. be certain that the x-ray room is clean and orderly
   2. check that all necessary accessories are available in the room
   3. check that x-ray table is clean and pillowcases are fresh
   - (A) 1 only
   - (B) 1 and 2 only
   - (C) 2 and 3 only
   - (D) 1, 2, and 3

10. The lower portion of the costal margin is approximately at the same level as that of the
    - (A) midthorax
    - (B) umbilicus
    - (C) xiphoid tip
    - (D) third lumbar vertebra

Answers and Explanations

1. (B) The *midsagittal* (or median sagittal) plane (MSP) passes vertically through the midline of the body, dividing it into left and right halves. Any plane parallel to the MSP is termed a *sagittal* plane. *The midcoronal plane is perpendicular to the MSP* and divides the body into anterior and posterior halves. A *transverse* plane passes across the body, also perpendicular to a sagittal plane. These planes, especially the MSP, are very important reference points in radiographic positioning.

2. (D) The position, shape, and motility of various organs can differ greatly from one body habitus to another. The positions of the diaphragm, lungs, stomach, gallbladder, and large and small intestines vary greatly with body habitus. The individuals with small extreme habitus (*asthenic*) have structures *lower* and *more medial,* whereas these structures in individuals of the large extreme habitus (*hypersthenic*) are *high* and *lateral* (Figs. 6-4 and 6-5).

3. (B) The *midsagittal* plane passes vertically through the midline of the body, dividing it into left and right halves. Any plane parallel to the MSP is termed a *sagittal* plane. The *midcoronal* plane is *perpendicular* to the MSP and divides the body into anterior and posterior halves. The *transverse* plane passes across the body, also *perpendicular* to a sagittal plane. These planes, especially the MSP, are very important reference points in radiographic positioning.

4. (B) When the patient is in the recumbent position with his or her head *lower* than the feet, the patient is said to be in the *Trendelenburg* position. In the *Fowler* position, the patient's head is positioned *higher* than his or her feet. The *decubitus* position is used to describe the patient as in the recumbent position (prone, supine, or lateral), with the central ray directed horizontally. The *Sims* position is the left anterior oblique position assumed for enema tip insertion.

5. (D) The patient must remove any metallic objects that are within the area of interest. Dentures, earrings, necklaces, and braided hair can obscure bony details in the skull or cervical spine. The radiographer must be certain that the patient's belongings are cared for properly and returned following the examination (Figs. 6-8 and 6-9).

6. (D) Correct and complete patient information about every radiograph is of paramount importance. Each radiographic image must be accurately labeled with such patient information as *name* or *identification number, institution name, date of examination,* and *side marker.* Other information may be included according to institution policy.

7. (D) The acquisition of pertinent *clinical history* is one of the most valuable contributions to the diagnostic process. Because the diagnostic radiologist rarely has the opportunity to speak with the patient, this is a crucial responsibility of the radiographer. As the radiographer obtains a brief pertinent clinical history, the radiographer also *assesses the patient's condition* by observing and listening. To provide safe and effective care, the radiographer must be able to assess the severity of a traumatized patient's injury, his or her degree of motor control, the need for support equipment, or radiographic accessories. When caring for patients severely injured or too ill to move, the radiographer should be capable of modifying routine positions to obtain images with the required anatomic part/information.

8. (B) Motion obliterates recorded detail; it is therefore essential that the radiographer be able to reduce patient motion as much as possible. Even the slightest movement can cause severe degradation of the radiographic image. Suspension of patient respiration for parts other than the extremities is an effective method of reducing *voluntary* motion; patient understanding and cooperation are required, thus making good *communication* the most effective method of reducing *voluntary* motion. The single most important method to reduce *involuntary* motion is to use the *shortest possible exposure time.*

9. (D) A patient will naturally feel more comfortable and confident if brought into a clean, orderly x-ray room that has been prepared appropriately for the examination to be performed. A disorderly, untidy room and a disorganized radiographer would hardly inspire confidence; more likely, they will increase anxiety and apprehension.

10. (D) Surface landmarks, prominences, and depressions are useful to the radiographer in locating anatomic structures not visible externally. The *lower costal margin* is at about the same level as L3. The *umbilicus* is at the same approximate level as the L3–L4 interspace. The *xiphoid tip* is at about the same level as T10. The fourth lumbar vertebra is at the same approximate level as the *iliac crest.*

Anatomy, Positioning, and Pathology

OBJECTIVES

At the conclusion of this chapter, the student will be able to:

- Identify human anatomy as displayed on illustrations and x-ray images.
- Explain accurate positioning details for routine imaging of body parts/systems.
- Assess and critique x-ray images for positioning accuracy and quality.
- Discuss ways in which routine imaging can be modified for trauma, mobile imaging, pediatric, and other nonroutine circumstances.

THE SKELETAL SYSTEM

General radiography involves a great deal of bone imaging; therefore, radiographers are required to have a good knowledge of osteology and related pathology. *Osteology* is the study of bones; there are 206 bones in the human adult skeleton. The skeletal system serves several functions: Bones form the *supporting* framework of the body, as a *reservoir for minerals* such as calcium and phosphorus, storing them until the body requires them, and provides *protection* to the underlying critical and delicate structures.

Most bones have prominences (projections, processes, protuberances) and/or cavities (depressions) that have either *articular* or *attachment* functions. If their function is *articular*, they provide a surface for articulation, that is, joint formation. If their function is *nonarticular*, they serve as attachment for muscles, providing leverage for movement. There are many terms that describe the size, shape, location, or function of various processes and cavities.

- *Process:* a bony elevation; also called protuberance, prominence, or projection
- *Condyle:* a rounded process for attachment
- *Coracoid:* a beak-like process
- *Coronoid:* a crown-like process
- *Epicondyle:* smaller projection superior to a condyle
- *Facet:* small smooth process for articulation
- *Malleolus:* a club-shaped process
- *Spine or spinous process:* a sharp projection
- *Styloid:* a long pointed process
- *Trochanter:* a very large rounded process for attachment
- *Tubercle:* a small rounded process for attachment
- *Tuberosity:* a large rounded process for attachment

Bone tissue, or *osseous* (*os* = bone) tissue, is a specialized type of dense connective tissue. This tissue consists of bone cells (*osteocytes*) embedded in a nonliving matrix composed of calcium and collagen fibers. There are two types of osseous tissue: *cancellous* (spongy) and *compact* (hard, cortical) (Fig. 7-1A).

The structural unit of *compact* bone tissue is the haversian (osteon) system. One haversian system, or osteon, consists of a central haversian canal surrounded by concentric cylinders of osteocytes within the calcium matrix.

Cancellous, or spongy, bone tissue has a reticular or latticework-type structure. This network of lattice-like bone is called *trabeculae.* These trabeculae form little spaces/septa filled with red bone marrow.

The site of close approximation of two or more bones is an *articulation,* or *joint.* The study of bony articulations is termed *arthrology.* There are three classifications of bony articulations. *Synarthrotic* joints are *immovable;* because fibrous tissues connect the bony contiguous surfaces, they are also described as *fibrous* articulations. The sutures of the cranium are examples of synarthrotic joints. *Amphiarthrotic* joints, also described as *cartilaginous,* are *partially* movable. The intervertebral joints (between vertebral bodies) and the symphysis pubis are examples of amphiarthrotic joints. *Diarthrotic* joints, also described as *synovial,* are *freely movable.* The majority of human articulations are the diarthrotic/synovial type, and there are several *types* of diarthrotic articulations (their names describe their movements). The following table identifies types of diarthrotic joints, describes their movement(s), and gives examples of each:

Cavity: A Bony Depression

- *Antrum:* a nearly enclosed cavity
- *Groove:* a shallow, linear depression
- *Fissure:* a narrow slit
- *Foramen:* a hole in a bone
- *Fossa:* a furrow or shallow depression for articulation
- *Fovea:* a ditch or cup-like depression, usually for attachment
- *Meatus* or *canal:* a tube-like passageway
- *Sinus:* a nearly enclosed cavity
- *Sulcus:* a furrow

Functions of Skeletal System

- Support
- Reservoir for minerals
- Muscle attachment/movement
- Protection
- Hematopoiesis

Bone Tissue Types

- Cortical (hard, compact)
- Cancellous (spongy)

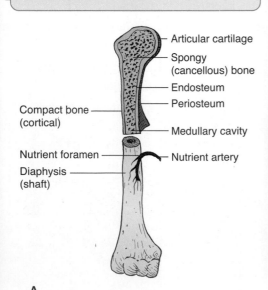

A

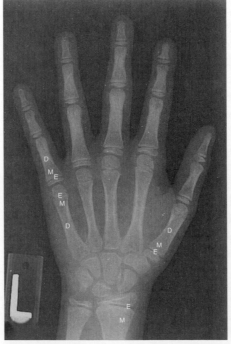

B

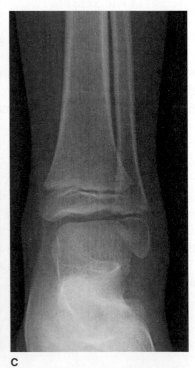

C

Figure 7-1. (A) Long bone anatomy. **(B)** Child's hand, with epiphyses (E), metaphyses (M), and diaphyses (D) indicated. **(C)** Child's ankle, demonstrating epiphyseal plates of distal tibia and fibula. (Photo contributor: Stamford Hospital, Department of Radiology.)

Joint Classifications

Joint Type	Range of Motion	Example(s)	
Gliding (plane)	Simplest motion, least movement; smooth/sliding motion	Intercarpal and intertarsal joints, acromioclavicular, and costovertebral joints	Plane joint (intercarpal) — Carpal bones
Pivot (trochoid)	Permits rotation around a single axis	Proximal radioulnar joint and atlantoaxial joint	Pivot joint (radioulnar) — Radius — Ulna
Hinge (ginglymus)	Permits flexion and extension	Elbow, interphalangeal joints, and ankle	Humerus — Hinge joint (humeroulnar) — Ulna
Ball-and-socket (spheroid)	Permits flexion, extension, adduction, abduction, rotation, and circumduction with more motion distally and less proximally	Shoulder and hip	Ball-and-socket joint (humeroscapular) — Head of humerus — Scapula
Condyloid (ellipsoid)	Permits flexion, extension, abduction, adduction, and circumduction (no axial)	Radiocarpal joint and metacarpophalangeal joints (2–5)	Condylar joint (metacarpophalangeal) — Metacarpal bone — Phalanx
Saddle (sellar)	Permits flexion, extension, abduction, adduction, and circumduction (no rotation)	First carpometacarpal joint (thumb)	Saddle joint (trapeziometacarpal) — Carpal bone — Metacarpal bone
Bicondylar (biaxial)	Principal motion in one direction; limited rotation motion	Temporomandibular joint (TMJ), knee	Bicondylar (biaxial) — Condyles

Articular Classifications

Category	Structure	Function
Synarthrotic	Fibrous	Immovable
Amphiarthrotic	Cartilaginous	Partially moveable
Diarthrotic	Synovial	Freely moveable

Arthritis is defined as inflammation of a joint; it is a common affliction involving damage to articular cartilage and is often accompanied by pain, swelling, stiffness, and/or deformity. The causes and variations of arthritis are numerous. The most common type of arthritis is *osteoarthritis,* or *degenerative arthritis.* The incidence of osteoarthritis increases with age but is not considered a normal part of aging.

The term *osteoporosis* describes a condition characterized by loss of bone mass, which predisposes bones to fracture. Throughout life, healthy bone undergoes cycles of growth and resorption—at appropriate times and in appropriate places, as the bones adapt themselves to muscular activity, growth, mechanical pressures, and so on. In osteoporosis, this remodeling fails to occur normally, and more bone is resorbed than is replaced; thus, the skeleton loses strength as a result of demineralization. Among the *risk factors* for osteoporosis are being female, postmenopausal, Caucasian, or Asian, and having a small skeletal frame; a family history of osteoporosis; and a sedentary lifestyle.

THE APPENDICULAR SKELETON

The *appendicular* skeleton (Fig. 7-2; shaded areas) consists of the *limbs* (appendages or extremities), arms, legs, and shoulder and pelvic girdles. Most of these bones contain locations for the *attachment* of muscles, thereby creating leverage for movement. Surfaces of adjacent bones connect to form bony articulations that promote movement.

Bones are classified as *long, short, flat,* and *irregular.* Many of the bones comprising the limbs are long bones. Long bones have a *shaft* (*diaphysis* or *body*) and *two extremities* (proximal and distal ends). The shaft (or *diaphysis*) (Fig. 7-1B) of long bones is the *primary ossification center* during bone development. It is composed of compact tissue and covered with a membrane called *periosteum.* The *epiphyses* of long bones are located at the extremities of the long bone and are the *secondary ossification centers* (Fig. 7-1B and C).

Within the shaft of a long bone is the *medullary cavity,* containing *bone marrow* and lined with a membrane called *endosteum.* In adults, yellow marrow occupies the shaft, and red marrow is found within the *proximal* and *distal* extremities of long bones. Bone marrow, particularly red, is important in the production of blood cells—a process called *hematopoiesis.*

The secondary ossification center, the epiphysis, is separated from the diaphysis in early life by a layer of cartilage known as the *epiphyseal plate.* As bone growth takes place, the epiphysis becomes part of the larger portion of bone. Once the epiphyseal plate disappears, a characteristic line remains and is thereafter recognizable as the *epiphyseal line.* The *metaphysis* is the wider portion of bone adjacent to the epiphyseal plate (Fig. 7-1B and C). The metaphysis includes the connecting cartilage that enables bony growth during childhood bone development; it disappears in adulthood. An *apophysis* is a normal outgrowth of a bone that eventually becomes a bony prominence for muscle/tendon attachment.

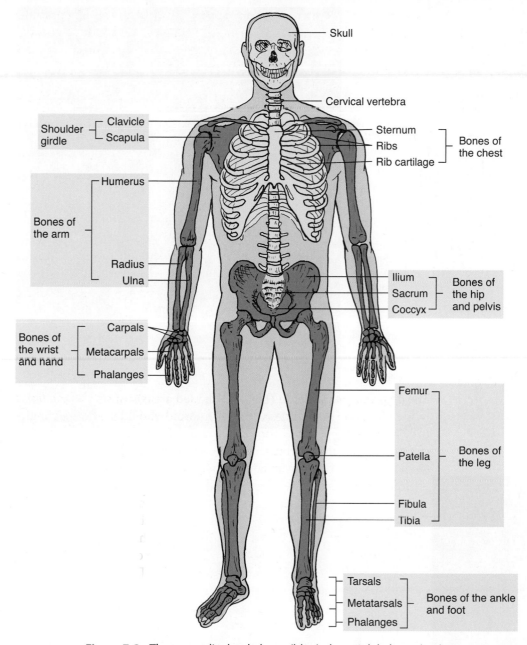

Figure 7-2. The *appendicular* skeleton (blue); the *axial* skeleton (tan).

The articular ends of bones are covered with *hyaline cartilage.* Hyaline cartilage is the most abundant type of cartilage. This tough, glossy material covers the articular surfaces of long bones and forms the anterior ends of the ribs (costal cartilage). It is also found in the bronchi, trachea, and larynx. The membranous covering of hyaline cartilage is *perichondrium.*

Upper Limb and Shoulder Girdle

Hand, Fingers, and Thumb. The hand (Fig. 7-3A and B) is composed of 5 *metacarpal* bones, corresponding to the palm of the hand, and 14 *phalanges,* the fingers. The second through fifth fingers have three

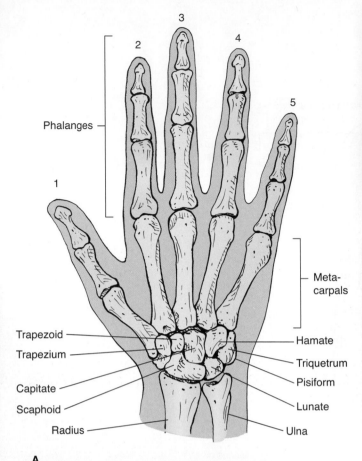

Phalanges

Trapezoid
Trapezium
Capitate
Scaphoid
Radius

Meta-
carpals

Hamate
Triquetrum
Pisiform
Lunate
Ulna

A

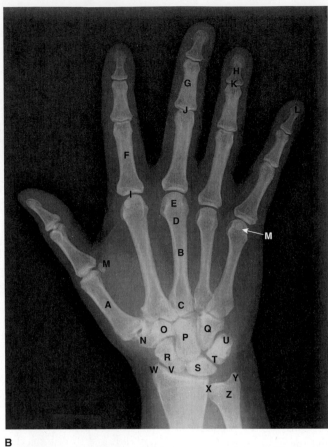

B

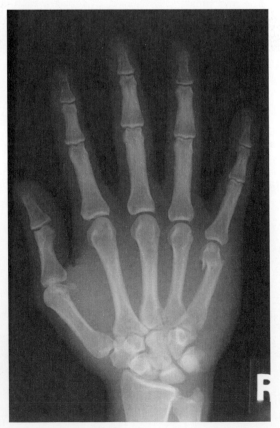

C

Figure 7-3. **(A)** Posterior aspect of the right hand and the wrist. **(B)** PA projection of the hand; note that an oblique projection of the first metacarpal and phalanges is obtained. A, metacarpal (shaft/body), first digit (thumb/pollex); B, third metacarpal (shaft/body); C, base of the third metacarpal; D, neck of the third metacarpal; E, head of the third metacarpal; F, proximal phalanx, second digit; G, middle phalanx, third digit; H, distal phalanx, fourth digit; I, second metacarpophalangeal joint; J, proximal interphalangeal joint, third digit; K, distal interphalangeal joint, fourth digit; L, ungual tuft, fifth digit; M, sesamoid bones; N, trapezium/greater multangular; O, trapezoid/lesser multangular; P, capitate/os magnum; Q, hamate/unciform; R, scaphoid; S, lunate/semilunar; T, triquetrum/triangular; U, pisiform; V, radiocarpal (wrist) joint; W, radial styloid process; X, distal radioulnar articulation; Y, ulnar styloid process; Z, head of ulna. **(C)** Boxer fracture (neck of the fifth metacarpal). (Boxer fracture image courtesy of David Sack, BS, RT(R), CRA, FAHRA.)

phalanges each (proximal, middle, and distal rows), and the first digit, or thumb (*pollex*), has two phalanges (proximal and distal). The rows of phalanges articulate with each other, forming proximal and distal *interphalangeal joints* (IPJs) (hinge/ginglymus joints), permitting flexion and extension motion.

The *bases* of the proximal row of phalanges articulate with the heads of the metacarpals to form the (condyloid/ellipsoid) *metacarpophalangeal* (MCPs) *joints,* which permit flexion and extension, abduction and adduction, and circumduction. The bases of the metacarpals articulate with each other and the distal row of carpals at the *carpometacarpal joints.* The first carpometacarpal joint (thumb) is a saddle/sellar joint, permitting flexion and extension, abduction and adduction, and circumduction.

Traumatic *fractures* of the hand and wrist are common. Fractures of the distal (ungual) phalangeal tufts usually occur from crushing injuries, such as being closed in car doors or struck with a hammer. Metacarpal and phalangeal fractures are common fractures and are often accompanied by dislocations of the MCP joint and IPJ. In fractures of the metacarpal shafts, the bony fragments are often displaced posteriorly and can be rotated as well.

A type of hand fracture occasionally seen is a *boxer's fracture*. A boxer's fracture involves the distal end (neck) of the fourth or fifth metacarpal and often includes posterior displacement/angulation of the fractured metacarpals' proximal structures (Fig. 7-3C). The fracture is termed "boxer" because it is usually caused by the blow of a clenched fist (as in boxing) against a hard, unyielding object such as a muscular/bony body part or a structure such as a wall.

Wrist. The wrist, as seen in the posteroanterior (PA) projection of the hand (Fig. 7-3A and B), is composed of eight carpal bones arranged in two rows (proximal and distal). The proximal row consists of, from lateral to medial, the *scaphoid,* the *lunate/semilunar,* the *triangular/triquetrum,* and the *pisiform.* The distal row, from lateral to medial, consists of the *trapezium/greater multangular,* the *trapezoid/lesser multangular,* the *capitate/os magnum* (the largest carpal), and the *hamate/unciform* (which has a hook-like process, the hamulus).

The joints of the wrist include the articulations between the carpals (*intercarpal joints*), which provide a gliding motion, and the *radiocarpal joint* (between the distal radius and the scaphoid), which provides flexion and extension, as well as abduction and adduction.

Most carpal fractures involve the scaphoid and often result from a fall onto an outstretched dorsiflexed hand. Symptoms include tenderness and swelling over the "anatomic snuff box." Special projections can be used to detect scaphoid hairline fractures (see Fig. 7-12B). The second most commonly fractured carpal is the triquetrum. Delayed union or nonunion of these fractures can be a result of damage to the nutrient artery during the initial trauma event. Unstable fractures, or cases of nonunion, may be treated with open reduction and internal fixation of the displaced/ununited fracture.

Carpal tunnel syndrome is a painful condition of the wrist. If the anteroposterior (AP) diameter of the tunnel is diminished, the

Carpal Bones

Proximal Row, Lateral to Medial
- Scaphoid
- Lunate/semilunar
- Triquetrum/triangular
- Pisiform

Distal Row, Lateral to Medial
- Trapezium/greater multangular
- Trapezoid/lesser multangular
- Capitate/os magnum
- Hamate/unciform

median nerve, which passes through the tunnel, is impinged upon, thus causing severe pain and disability in the affected hand and the wrist. Surgical decompression of the carpal tunnel can provide significant relief.

Forearm. The bones of the forearm, or antebrachium (Fig. 7-4), consist of the *radius* (laterally) and *ulna* (medially), which participate in the formation of the elbow joint proximally and the wrist distally.

The distal ulna presents a *head* and *styloid process* and articulates with the distal radius to form the *distal radioulnar joint.* The ulna is slender distally but enlarges proximally and becomes the larger of the two bones of the forearm. At its proximal end, the ulna presents the *olecranon process* (posteriorly) and the *coronoid process* (anteriorly) that are joined by a large articular cavity, the *semilunar,* or *trochlear, notch.* The coronoid process fits into the humeral *coronoid fossa* during flexion, and the olecranon process fits into the humeral *olecranon fossa* during extension. Just distal and lateral to the semilunar notch is the

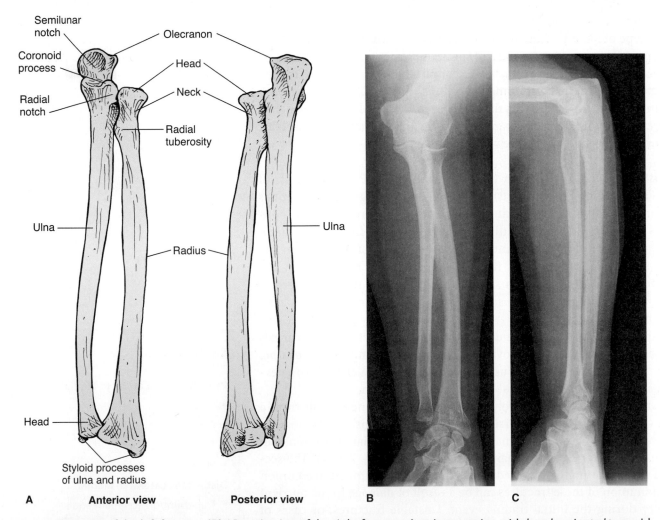

Figure 7-4. **(A)** Bones of the left forearm. **(B)** AP projection of the right forearm. Arm in extension with *hand supinated* to avoid overlap of the radius and ulna. **(C)** Lateral projection of the right forearm. Elbow flexed 90°, with the hand and wrist in lateral position; humeral epicondyles are superimposed (interepicondylar line ⊥). (Photo contributor: Conrad P. Ehrlich, MD.)

radial notch, which provides articulation for the radial head to form the *proximal radioulnar articulation.* Just as the ulna is the principal bone associated with the elbow joint, the radius is the principal bone associated with the wrist joint.

Distal radius fractures are one of the most common skeletal fractures, and the radius is the most commonly fractured bone of the arm. The distal radius presents a *styloid process* laterally; the *ulnar notch* is located medially, helping form the *distal radioulnar articulation.* The distal surface of the radius (carpal articular surface) is smooth for accommodating the scaphoid and lunate in the formation of the *radiocarpal joint.* The proximal radius has a cylindrical *head* with a medial surface that participates in the *proximal radioulnar joint;* its superior surface articulates with the capitulum of the humerus.

Fractures of the radial head and neck frequently result from a fall onto an outstretched hand with the elbow *partially flexed.* Severe fractures are often accompanied by posterior dislocation of the elbow joint.

Colles fractures (named after the Irish surgeon/anatomist who first described it: Abraham Colles) of the distal radius usually result from a fall onto an outstretched hand with the arm *extended.* Typically, the radius exhibits a transverse fracture with posterior displacement; this fracture is often accompanied by a fracture of the ulnar styloid process. Factors that increase the risk of Colles fractures include being aged 60 years or older, and having osteoporosis. Fractures of the ulnar styloid, when present, usually occur as a result of hyperabduction of the hand. Surgical repair of Colles fractures can involve either internal fixation via stainless steel/titanium metal pins, or with the use of plate and screws (Fig. 7-5).

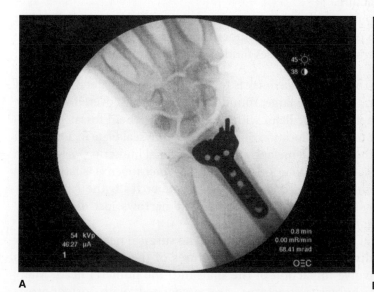
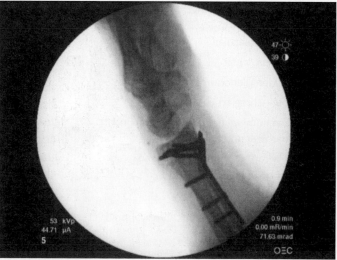

A   **B**

Figure 7-5. Colles fracture with plate and screw fixator in place. PA **(A)** and lateral **(B)**. Note scaphoid fracture also seen in panel A. (Photo contributor: Maryjane Hatch.)

Elbow. The distal *humerus* articulates with the radius and ulna to form the elbow joint (Fig. 7-6). The lateral aspect of the distal humerus presents a raised, smooth, rounded surface, the *capitulum,* which articulates with the superior surface of the *radial head.* The *trochlea* is on the medial aspect of the distal humerus and articulates with the semilunar notch of the ulna. Just proximal to the capitulum and trochlea are the *lateral* and *medial epicondyles;* the medial is more prominent and palpable. The *olecranon fossa* is found on the posterior distal humerus and functions to accommodate the olecranon process with the elbow in extension (Figs. 7-6 and 7-7).

Lateral epicondylitis (tennis elbow) is a painful condition caused by prolonged rotary motion of the forearm. *Dislocations* of the elbow can also occur from a fall onto an outstretched hand, sending the force to the elbow. If there is also a turning motion during a fall, the elbow can dislocate. One or both bones of the forearm can be involved; a posterior dislocation is the most common and is frequently accompanied by a radial head fracture. Rotation of the radial head can be palpated on the posterior lateral surface of the elbow, with the elbow in extension.

There are three important *fat pads* associated with the elbow. The anterior and posterior fat pads are located on the corresponding portions of the distal humerus, superimposed but separated by a membranous portion of the joint capsule. The anterior fat pad (composed of two small radial and coronoid fat pads) fills the shallow coronoid fossa and is readily visualized in the lateral projection of the normal elbow. The posterior fat pad fills the deeper olecranon fossa and is therefore *not* visualized in the normal lateral elbow projection. In the presence of injury and joint effusion, the anterior fat pad is displaced anteriorly and upward, whereas the posterior fat pad is displaced posteriorly. The classic "sail sign" or "spinnaker sail sign" (i.e., billowing sail) seen anteriorly in a lateral elbow radiograph often indicates a radial head or neck fracture.

The supinator fat pad/stripe is located at the proximal radius just anterior to the head, neck, and tuberosity. This fat pad can also become more apparent if injury causes fluid buildup to displace it.

Humerus. The *deltoid tuberosity* is found on the anterolateral surface of the humeral shaft. The large, round *humeral head* is covered with hyaline cartilage and articulates with the scapula's glenoid fossa. The *anatomic neck* marks the location of the fused epiphyseal plate in adults and separates the head and metaphysis. The proximal humerus presents two protuberances on its anterior surface: the *greater tubercle* is lateral, and the *lesser tubercle* is medial. Between the tubercles is the *bicipital,* or *intertubercular, groove.* The humeral shaft narrows just distal to the tubercles at the point of the *surgical neck.*

Humeral *fractures* most often affect the surgical neck region rather than the distal end of the bone. Fractures of the proximal humerus usually involve impaction of the shaft into the humeral head. Many traumatic humerus fractures are associated with osteoporosis or other pathologies. Fractures of the greater tubercle can result from a direct blow or as a consequence of forcible pull of the associated muscles.

Articulation Summary: Upper Limb and Shoulder Girdle

- Acromioclavicular
- Sternoclavicular
- Shoulder (glenohumeral)
- Elbow—three articulations:
  - b/w humeral trochlea and semilunar/trochlear notch
  - b/w capitulum and radial head
  - proximal radioulnar joint
- Distal radioulnar
- Radiocarpal (distal radius with scaphoid and lunate)
- Intercarpal
- Carpometacarpal
- Metacarpophalangeal
- Interphalangeal

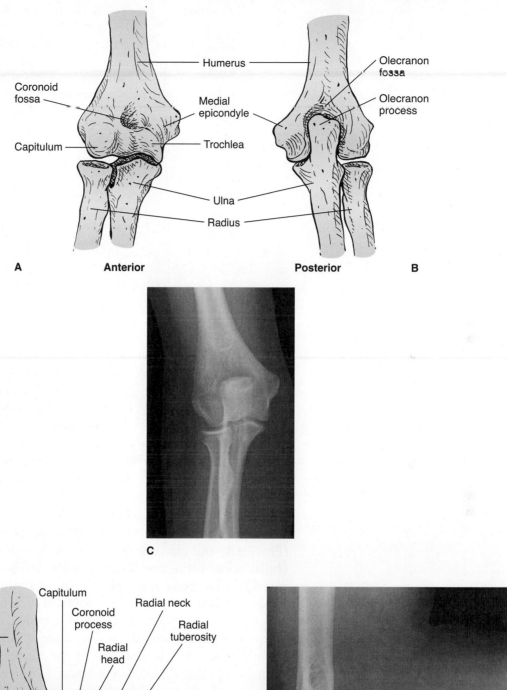

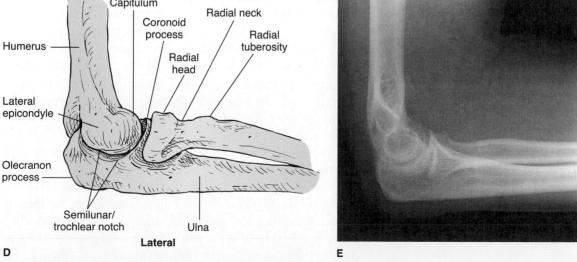

Figure 7-6. **(A)** Anterior and **(B)** posterior aspects of the bony articulation of the right elbow joint. **(C)** AP projection of the elbow. (Photo contributor: Conrad P. Ehrlich, MD.) **(D)** and **(E)**. Medial and lateral aspects of the bony articulation of the right elbow joint. (Photo contributor: Stamford Hospital, Department of Radiology.)

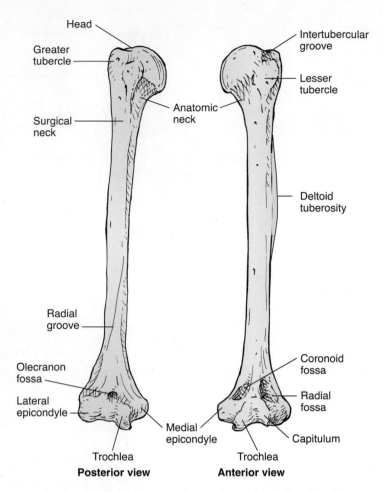

Figure 7-7. The humerus (posterior and anterior views).

Shoulder. The shoulder (pectoral) girdle consists of the scapulae (Fig. 7-8A) and clavicles (Fig. 7-9). Although the S-shaped *clavicle* (collar bone) is the first bone to ossify (5th week of gestation), it is usually the last bone to completely fuse at approximately 22–25 years of age and is one of the most commonly fractured bones in young people. Clavicular fractures are usually treated nonoperatively; good outcome is most often achieved by using a shoulder sling or figure-of-eight brace. The medial end of the clavicle articulates with the sternum to form the *sternoclavicular joint;* the clavicle articulates laterally with the scapula's acromion process, forming the *acromioclavicular joint.* Superior *dislocation* of the *acromioclavicular joint* is a common athletic injury.

The *scapula* is a flat bone, shaped like a triangle, with a *costal surface* that lies against the upper posterior rib cage. The scapula has a *superior* (or *medial*) *angle,* a *superior border,* a *medial* (or *vertebral*) *border,* a *lateral* (or *axillary*) *border,* and an *inferior angle,* or *apex.* Its superior border presents a *scapular notch,* and projecting anteriorly just medial to the humeral head is the palpable *coracoid process.* The *scapular spine* divides the posterior surface into a *supraspinatus fossa* and an *infraspinatus fossa;* the *acromion process* is the lateral extension of the scapular spine. The *glenoid fossa* is on the lateral aspect of the scapula and, with

Rotator Cuff Muscles

- Supraspinatus
- Infraspinatus
- Teres minor
- Deltoid
- Subscapularis

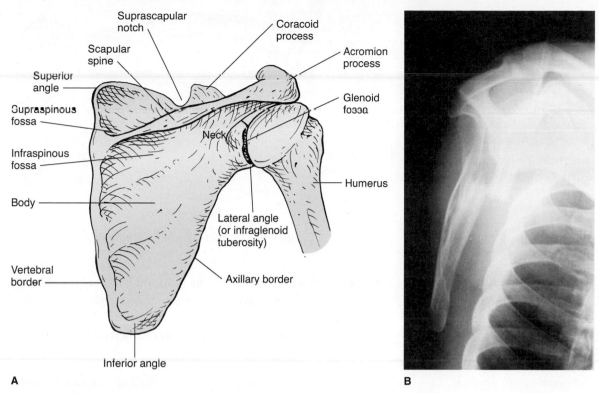

Figure 7-8. (A) Posterior aspect of the right scapula. **(B)** Scapular neck fracture, lateral projection. (Photo contributor: David Sack, BS, RT(R), CRA, FAHRA.)

its articulation with the humeral head, forms the (ball-and-socket) *shoulder joint.* The shoulder *labrum* is a ring of fibrocartilage that extends from the rim of the glenoid cavity, acting like a suction cup and deepening the joint "socket." Labral injuries of the shoulder often involve a tear, particularly SLAP tears (i.e., superior labrum anterior to posterior). SLAP tears can occur from a fall or blow to the shoulder, but most frequently occur as a result of throwing injuries, for example, in baseball pitchers.

Scapular fractures are uncommon because of the scapula being protected by the surrounding muscles. Of those fractures that do occur, two-thirds of them involve the scapular neck (Fig. 7-8B) and do not involve the articular surfaces. Most scapular fractures are a result of direct trauma to the shoulder region, very often as a result of motor vehicle accident (MVA). Scapular fractures can also be related to injuries to the clavicle, sternum, or ribs.

The *rotator cuff* is largely responsible for abduction and internal rotation movements and is composed of the supraspinatus, infraspinatus, teres minor, deltoid, and subscapularis muscles. *Rotator cuff injuries* are often a result of acute injury or chronic wear and tear. Injuries to the rotator cuff include tendonitis, impingement, and tears. Long-standing tendonitis can lead to calcification: *calcific tendonitis.*

The articular capsule of the shoulder is loose, not only permitting a great range of movement but also making it susceptible to *dislocation.* The majority of shoulder dislocations are anterior, almost always

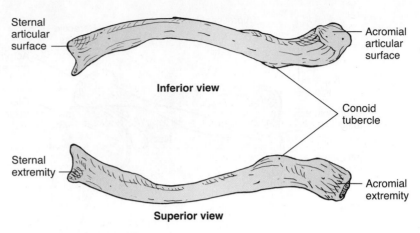

Figure 7-9. The right clavicle (inferior and superior views).

List of Abbreviations and Symbols Used in the Tables

AC	Acromioclavicular
∠	Angle
ASIS	Anterior superior iliac spine
AP	Anteroposterior
≈	Approximately (about)
b/w	Between
CMC	Carpometacarpal joint
CR	Central ray
°	Degrees
DIP	Distal interphalangeal joint
Dist	Distal
EAM	External auditory meatus
Fx	Fracture
>	Greater than
"	Inch(es)
IOML	Infraorbitomeatal line
IPJ	Interphalangeal joint
IPL	Interpupillary line
IR	Image receptor
Jt	Joint
kV	Kilovolt
Lat	Lateral
LAO	Left anterior oblique
LML	Lips-meatal line
LPO	Left posterior oblique
<	Less than
MCP	Metacarpophalangeal joint
MML	Mentomeatal line
MTP	Metatarsophalangeal joint
MSP	Midsagittal plane
m/w	Midway
OID	Object-to-image receptor distance
Obl	Oblique
OML	Orbitomeatal line
∥	Parallel to
⊥	Perpendicular to
PA	Posteroanterior
PIP	Proximal interphalangeal joint
Proj	Projection
Prox	Proximal
RAO	Right anterior oblique
RPO	Right posterior oblique
SID	Source-to-image receptor distance
w/	With
w/o	Without

associated with trauma. As the humeral head is forced anteriorly from the glenoid fossa, it is also often associated with injury to the joint capsule and detachment of the labrum from the glenoid fossa. Fracture of the humeral head, neck, or greater tuberosity can also occur with dislocations.

Positioning. Positioning of the upper limb and shoulder girdle requires a thorough knowledge of the anatomy concerned, as well as an awareness of possible pathologic conditions and their impact on *positioning limitations* and *technical factors*.

Radiopaque objects such as watches, bracelets, and rings should be removed whenever possible because they can obscure important anatomic information. The patient must be instructed regarding the importance of remaining still, and immobilization devices such as sandbags or sponges should be used as required. The shortest possible exposure time should be used, especially when involuntary motion can be a problem, as in patients with trauma, pediatric, or geriatric patients.

Most distal upper limb examinations are more comfortably and accurately positioned with the patient seated at the end of the x-ray table, with the forearm and elbow resting on the x-ray table. Imaging of the distal upper limb can be performed at the tabletop (i.e., without a Bucky grid); however, the proximal upper limb, including the humerus, shoulder, clavicle, and scapula usually require the use of a grid. *Suspended respiration* is suggested for radiography of the proximal portion of the upper limb and shoulder girdle. Patients must be adequately *shielded*.

The use of just a few important bony landmarks and their correct placement with respect to the image receptor (IR) are the basis for accurate positioning. Rotation of the arm and placement of the humeral epicondyles in correct relationship to the IR are the foundation of forearm, elbow, and shoulder positioning. Positioning of the wrist and hand uses the radial and ulnar styloid processes; bending maneuvers (i.e., radial and ulnar flexion); and MCP, DIP, and PIP joints.

Tables 7-1 through 7-11 provide a summary of routine and frequently performed special positions/projections of the upper limb and shoulder girdle.

TABLE 7-1. The Hand

Hand	Position of Part	Central Ray Directed	Structures Included/Best Seen
PA	· Hand pronated · Elbow flexed 90° · Fingers extended slightly apart	· ⊥ Third MCP	· PA carpals, metacarpals, phalanges, their articulations (Fig. 7-10A) · Obl proj of the thumb
This proj is often performed to include the wrist for *bone age* studies; 30″ SID is sometimes recommended, with the CR entering the head of the third metacarpal.			
PA obl proj	· Elbow flexed 90° · Hand and forearm 45° obl	· ⊥ Third MCP	· Obl proj of the carpals, metacarpals, phalanges, their articulations · Use of "finger sponge" places jts ‖ IR and opens jt spaces (Fig. 7-10B)
AP bilateral obl/ Norgaard method/ball-catcher's position	· Elbows extended · Hands and forearms supinated, 45° AP obl · 45° sponges placed under each hand for support · Thumbs abducted to prevent superimposition	· ⊥ Midpoint between both hands at the fifth MCP jts	· Both hands in 45° AP obl position · Used for evidence of rheumatoid arthritis
Lat (fan)/ lateromedial proj	· Elbow flexed 90° · Fingers extended and spread to create a "fan" position · Wrist lat, ulnar surface down	· ⊥ MCPs	· Superimposed carpals, metacarpals, and their articulations · Phalanges in true lat position, ‖ to the IR, free of superimposition
Lat *in extension*	· Elbow flexed 90° · Fingers extended · Wrist lat, ulnar surface down	· ⊥ MCPs	· Superimposed carpals, metacarpals, phalanges, their articulations · Decrease 10 kV for foreign body
Lat *in flexion*	· Elbow flexed 90° · Fingers slightly flexed and superimposed	· ⊥ MCPs	· Superimposed carpals, metacarpals, phalanges, their articulations · *Shows anterior/posterior fx displacement*

Lower Limb and Pelvis

Foot and Toes. The bones of the foot (Fig. 7-20) include the 7 *tarsal bones,* 5 *metatarsal bones,* and 14 *phalanges.* The *calcaneus* (os calcis), or heel bone, is the largest tarsal. It serves as an attachment for the Achilles tendon posteriorly, articulates anteriorly with the *cuboid bone,* presents three articular surfaces superiorly for its articulation with the *talus,* and has a prominent shelf on its anteromedial edge called the *sustentaculum tali.*

The inferior surface of the *talus* (*astragalus*) articulates with the superior calcaneus to form the three-faceted *subtalar* (*talocalcaneal*) *joint.* The talus also articulates anteriorly with the navicular bone. Articulating anteriorly with the navicular bone are the three *cuneiform bones:* medial/first, intermediate/second, and lateral/third. The navicular bone articulates laterally with the cuboid. The sinus tarsus (see Figs. 7-28 and 7-31) is part of the subtalar/talocalcaneal joint, separating its posterior portion from its anterior and middle portions, and is located on the lateral side of the foot. *Sinus tarsi syndrome* is a condition frequently associated with an inversion sprain of the ankle, with ligament injury resulting in subtalar joint instability. The sinus tarsus is usually well demonstrated in the medial oblique projection of the foot and sometimes seen in the lateral projection.

Tarsal Bones

- Calcaneus/os calcis
- Talus/astragalus
- Navicular
- Cuboid
- First/medial cuneiform
- Second/intermediate cuneiform
- Third/lateral cuneiform

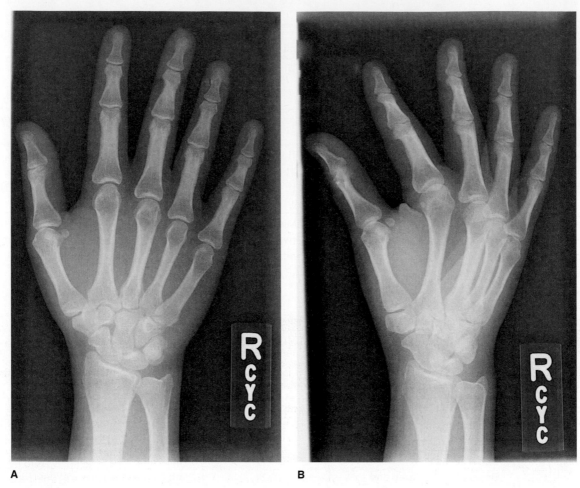

Figure 7-10. PA **(A)** and oblique **(B)** projections of the hand. (Photo contributor: Stamford Hospital, Department of Radiology.)

TABLE 7-2. The Thumb

Thumb	Position of Part	Central Ray Directed	Structures Included/Best Seen
AP	· Dorsal surface adjacent and ‖ IR	· ⊥ MCP	· AP proj of the first digit · *Three articulations should be seen:* CMC, MCP, and IPJ
PA	· Palmar surface ‖ IR · *OID is increased*	· ⊥ MCP	· PA proj of the first digit · *Three articulations should be seen:* CMC, MCP, and IPJ
The PA proj of the thumb can be used if the patient is unable to be positioned for the AP proj. It is important to note that due to increased OID, the PA proj results in a slight loss of detail.			
Lat	· Lat surface adjacent to the IR · Fingers elevated and resting on the sponge	· ⊥ MCP	· Lat proj of the first digit · *Three articulations should be seen:* CMC, MCP, and IPJ
PA obl, medial rotation	· Palmar surface adjacent and ‖ IR · Abduct thumb slightly to 45° obl position	· ⊥ MCP	· Obl proj of the first digit · *Three articulations should be seen:* CMC, MCP, and IPJ

TABLE 7-3. The Fingers

Fingers	Position of Part	Central Ray Directed	Structures Included/Best Seen
PA *Finger only*	· Hand pronated · Fingers extended · Elbow flexed 90°	· ⊥ PIP	· PA of the prox, middle, and dist phalanges of the affected finger
PA *Entire hand*	· Hand pronated · Fingers extended · Elbow flexed 90°	· ⊥ PIP	· PA of the prox, middle, and dist phalanges of the entire hand
Lat	· Elbow flexed 90° · Forearm lat · Finger(s) extended and ‖ IR	· ⊥ PIP	· Lat of the prox, middle, and dist phalanges · Second and third digits are done with the *radial side down* · Fourth and fifth digits are done with the *ulnar side down* · *Three articulations should be seen*: MCP, PIP, and DIP
PA obl Med or Lat rotation	· Elbow flexed 90° · Hand and forearm 45° obl	· ⊥ PIP	· Obl proj of the finger(s) · Use of "finger sponge" places jts ‖ IR and opens jt spaces (see Fig. 7-10B made w/o sponge)

TABLE 7-4. The Wrist

Wrist	Position of Part	Central Ray Directed	Structures Included/Best Seen
PA	· Hand pronated w/ MCPs slightly flexed · Elbow flexed 90°	· ⊥ Midcarpal region	· PA carpals, prox metacarpals, dist radius, and ulna (Fig. 7-11A) · *Flexion of MCPs reduces OID*
Lat	· Elbow flexed 90°, ulnar surface down · Radius and ulna superimposed	· ⊥ Midcarpal region	· Lat superimposed carpals, prox metacarpals · Superimposed dist radius and ulna (Fig. 7-11B)
PA obl, lat rotation	· Elbow flexed 90° · Wrist 45° obl to the IR, ulnar surface down	· ⊥ Midcarpal region	· Scaphoid and other *lat carpals* (trapezium and trapezoid) *and their interspaces* (Fig. 7-11C) · *Magnification* imaging can be useful to demonstrate scaphoid hairline fx (Fig. 7-12B)
PA obl, medial rotation	· Arm extended 45° to the IR · Ulnar surface down	· ⊥ Midcarpal region	· Pisiform, triquetrum, hamate · *Medial carpals and their interspaces*
PA proj, ulnar deviation	· Position as PA wrist · Evert hand (laterally) w/o moving the forearm	· ⊥ Scaphoid	· Scaphoid and other lat carpal interspaces · *Reduces foreshortening of scaphoid*
PA proj, radial deviation	· Position as PA wrist · Move elbow toward the body w/o moving the hand/wrist · Invert hand (medially) w/o moving the forearm	· ⊥ Midcarpal region	· Demonstrated *medial* carpal interspaces (Fig. 7-12)
Scaphoid/PA axial (*Stecher*)	· Forearm (a) pronated *or* (b) pronated and elevated 20°	· (a) 20° toward the elbow · (b) ⊥ Scaphoid	· Scaphoid w/o *foreshortening* and self-superimposition
Carpal canal/ tangential carpal canal (*Gaynor–Hart*)	· Hyperextend wrist w/ palm vertical	· 25°–30° into the long axis of the hand	· Carpal canal (*tunnel*) · Trapezium, scaphoid, capitate, triquetrum, and pisiform

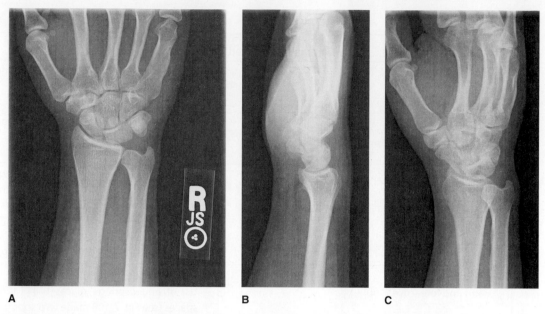

A   B   C

Figure 7-11. **(A)** PA projection of the wrist. Flexion of the metacarpophalangeal joints reduces OID. **(B)** Lateral projection of the wrist. **(C)** Semipronation oblique projection of the wrist. (Photo contributor: Conrad P. Ehrlich, MD.)

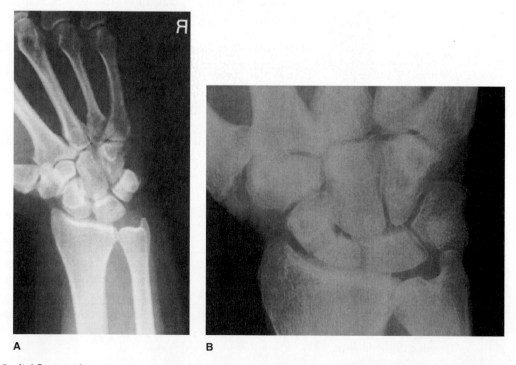

A   B

Figure 7-12. **(A)** Radial flexion/deviation maneuver of the left wrist. Radial flexion/deviation is used to better demonstrate the medial carpals (pisiform, triangular, hamate, and medial aspects of capitate and lunate). (Photo contributor: Stamford Hospital, Department of Radiology.) **(B)** Magnification image of the fractured carpal scaphoid. (Photo contributor: David Sack, BS, RT(R), CRA, FAHRA.)

TABLE 7-5. The Forearm

Forearm	Position of Part	Central Ray Directed	Structures Included/Best Seen
AP	· Forearm supinated and extended · Interepicondylar line ‖ IR · *Shoulder and elbow on the same plane*	· ⊥ Midforearm	· AP radius and ulna, including wrist and elbow jts (Fig. 7-13A) · *Forearm must be supinated* to avoid overlap of the radius and ulna
Lat	· Elbow flexed 90° · Epicondyles superimposed and interepicondylar line ⊥ the IR · Hand lat, *shoulder, and elbow on the same plane*	· ⊥ Midforearm	· Radius and ulna superimposed distally · Lat proj of the radius, ulna, elbow, wrist jts (Fig. 7-13B)

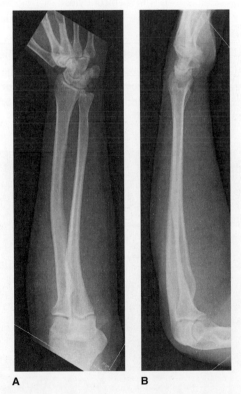

A   B

Figure 7-13. **(A)** AP projection of the forearm. The hand must be supinated to avoid overlap of the proximal radius and ulna. **(B)** Lateral projection of the forearm. Humerus should be on the same plane as the forearm to superimpose humeral epicondyles. (Photo contributor: Conrad P. Ehrlich, MD.)

TABLE 7-6. The Elbow

Elbow	Position of Part	Central Ray Directed	Structures Included/Best Seen
AP	· Forearm supinated and extended · Interepicondylar line ∥ IR	· ⊥ Elbow jt m/w b/w epicondyles	· AP elbow jt (Fig. 7-14A) · AP prox radius and ulna, dist humerus · Radial head and tuberosity partially superimposed on the ulna
Note: An elbow in AP partial flexion, unable to be extended, *requires two projs* to achieve an AP elbow: (1) *humerus* is placed ∥ the IR (with the elbow still in partial flexion) and the CR is ⊥ the elbow jt; (2) *forearm* is placed ∥ the IR (with the elbow still in partial flexion) and the CR is ⊥ the elbow jt. Thus, an AP of the dist humerus and prox forearm are obtained separately. A greater degree of elbow flexion can require a 5°–10° ∠ into the jt. (An AP with the CR directed ⊥ the flexed elbow demonstrates a "closed" jt space.)			
AP partial flexion	· Forearm supinated and extended ∥ IR with elbow partially flexed · Humerus supinated and extended ∥ IR with elbow partially flexed, place support under wrist and forearm	· ⊥ Elbow jt m/w b/w epicondyles	· Prox radius and ulna visualized on proj with forearm ∥ IR · Dist humerus visualized on proj with humerus ∥ IR · Distortion visible dependent on degree of flexion
Lat	· Elbow flexed 90° · Interepicondylar line ⊥ IR · Forearm and wrist lat	· Elbow jt at the epicondyles	· Lat elbow jt, prox radius, ulna, dist humerus · *Radial head partially superimposed on the ulna* · Olecranon process in profile (Fig. 7-14B)
AP obl, medial/internal rotation	· Arm extended, palm down · Interepicondylar line 45° to the IR	· ⊥ Elbow jt midway b/w epicondyles	· Obl elbow jt · *Coronoid process in profile* (Fig. 7-14C)
AP obl, lat/external rotation	· Forearm extended and rotated laterally · Radial surface down · Interepicondylar line 45° to the IR	· ⊥ Elbow jt midway b/w epicondyles	· Obl elbow jt · Radial head, neck, and tuberosity free from superimposition of the ulna
Trauma axial lats (*Coyle*)	· Elbow flexed 90°, hand pronated · Elbow flexed 80°, hand pronated	· To elbow, at 45° *toward* the shoulder · *From* shoulder *to* elbow, at 45°	· These replace lat and medial obl projs when the patient is unable to extend the arm · For radial head · For coronoid process

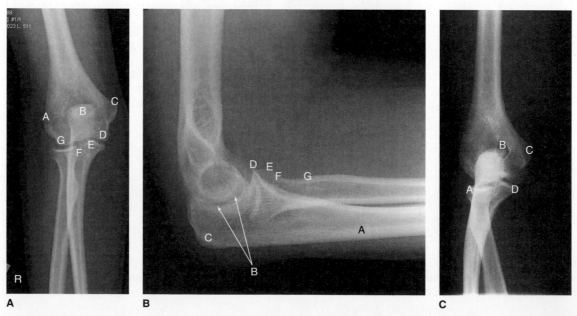

Figure 7-14. (A) AP projection of the elbow; radial head and tuberosity have correct partial superimposition on the ulna. A, lateral epicondyle; B, olecranon process; C, medial epicondyle; D, trochlea; E, coronoid process; F, proximal radioulnar articulation (or radial notch of the ulna); G, capitulum. (Photo contributor: Conrad P. Ehrlich, MD.) **(B)** Lateral projection elbow, elbow flexed 90°, and humeral epicondyles superimposed. A, shaft of ulna; B, semilunar/trochlear notch; C, olecranon process; D, coronoid process; E, radial head; F, radial neck; G, radial tuberosity. (Photo contributor: Stamford Hospital, Department of Radiology.) **(C)** Medial (internal) oblique view of the elbow; the coronoid process is seen free of superimposition. A, radial head; B, olecranon fossa; C, medial epicondyle; D, coronoid process. (Photo contributor: Stamford Hospital, Department of Radiology.)

TABLE 7-7. The Humerus

Humerus	Position of Part	Central Ray Directed	Structures Included/Best Seen
AP (external rotation)	· Arm extended and supinated; interepicondylar line ‖ IR	· ⊥ Midhumerus	· AP humerus, includes both jts · *Greater tubercle in profile*
Lat (internal rotation)	· Elbow flexed 90° · Interepicondylar line ⊥ IR	· ⊥ Midhumerus	· Lat humerus, includes both jts · *Lesser tubercle in profile*
Neutral	· Arm extended alongside at rest, hand facing thigh · Epicondyles approx. 45° to IR	· ⊥ Midhumerus	· Used for trauma when rotation not possible
Transthoracic lat	· Erect lat · Affected surgical neck centered to the IR · Unaffected arm over the head	· ⊥ Affected surgical neck	· Lat shoulder, prox humerus · Projected through the thorax

TABLE 7-8. The Shoulder

Shoulder	Position of Part	Central Ray Directed	Structures Included/Best Seen
AP neutral	· Arm extended · Interepicondylar line ≈45° IR	· ⊥ Shoulder jt; approx. ³/₄″ inferior and lat to coracoid process	· Used for trauma when rotation is contraindicated; includes both jts · Can demonstrate calcium deposits in soft-tissue structures
AP, internal and external rotation	· Arm extended and 1. supinated, w/ interepicondylar line ‖ IR 2. palm against thigh, interepicondylar line 45° to the IR 3. elbow slightly flexed, back of the hand against the thigh	· ⊥ Coracoid process	1. External rotation: true AP humerus, shows the greater tubercle in profile (Fig. 7-15A) 2. Neutral position: good for calcific deposits, trauma 3. Internal rotation: lat humerus, shows the lesser tubercle in profile
Note: In case of trauma, the humerus and shoulder must be examined in a neutral position to avoid unnecessary pain and additional injury.			
AP obl proj RPO or LPO Grashey method	· RPO or LPO (erect or recumbent) · MSP 35°–45° to the affected side · Scapula ‖ IR · Suspend respiration	· ⊥ 2″ medial and 2″ inferior to the superior and lat shoulder	· Glenohumeral jt and glenoid cavity (Fig. 7-15B)
Transthoracic lat	· Erect lat · Affected surgical neck centered to the IR · Unaffected arm over the head	· ⊥ Affected surgical neck	· Lat shoulder, prox humerus · Projected through the thorax
PA obl *scapular Y*	· RAO or LAO (erect or recumbent) · Affected shoulder centered to the IR · MCP 45°–60° to the IR (rotate to superimpose superior ∠ of scapula with AC jt)	· ⊥ Shoulder jt	· Glenohumeral jt · Especially for demonstration of dislocations (Fig. 7-16), fx prox humerus
Supraspinatus outlet *(Neer)*	· RAO or LAO (erect or recumbent) · Affected shoulder centered to the IR · MCP 45°–60° to the IR (rotate to superimpose superior ∠ of scapula with AC jt)	· 10°–15° caudal to superior margin of humeral head	· Prox humerus superimposed over body of scapula · Lat scapula · Open supraspinatus outlet
Inferosuperior axial (nontrauma) Lawrence method	· Supine w/ the shoulder elevated ≈2″ above the tabletop · Arm abducted 90°, in external rotation	· Horizontally to the axilla	· Lat of prox humerus, glenohumeral jt; coracoid process · Lesser tubercle in profile

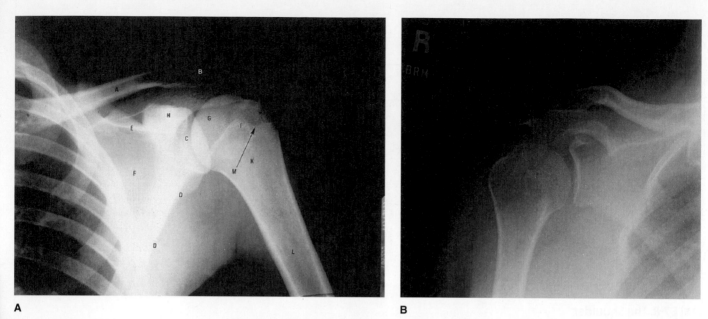

A   B

Figure 7-15. **(A)** Shoulder in external rotation places humerus in a true AP position and places the greater tubercle (J) in profile. A, shaft of clavicle; B, acromioclavicular joint; C, glenoid cavity; D, lateral/axillary border of scapula; E, scapular spine; F, body of scapula; G, head of humerus; H, coracoid process; I, lesser tubercle; J, greater tubercle; K, surgical neck of humerus; L, shaft of humerus; M, anatomic neck of humerus. (Photo contributor: Bob Wong, RT.) **(B)** Posterior oblique (Grashey method) for glenoid cavity. (Photo contributor: Stamford Hospital, Department of Radiology.)

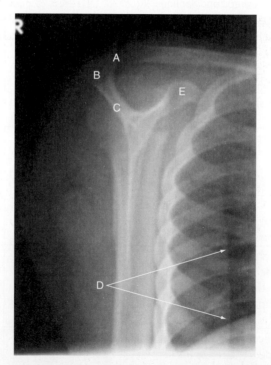

Figure 7-16. PA oblique projection; scapular Y view of the shoulder. Useful for the demonstration of dislocations. Humeral head displaced inferior to the coracoid process indicates *anterior dislocation,* whereas humeral head displaced inferior to the acromion process indicates *posterior dislocation.* A, acromioclavicular joint; B, acromion process; C, scapular spine; D, medial/vertebral border of scapula; E, coracoid process. (Photo contributor: Stamford Hospital, Department of Radiology.)

TABLE 7-9. The Clavicle

Clavicle	Position of Part	Central Ray Directed	Structures Included/Best Seen
PA or AP	· Recumbent or erect · Affected clavicle centered to the IR · Less OID in PA proj	· ⊥ Midshaft	· Entire length of the clavicle · Both articulations (Fig. 7-17A)
AP axial	· Recumbent or erect · Posterior shoulder against IR/Bucky/table · Affected clavicle centered to the IR	· To supraclavicular fossa 15°–30° cephalad	· AP axial proj of the clavicle · For fxs not seen in direct PA or AP (Fig. 7-17B)
PA axial	· Patient positioned erect with anterior thorax against IR/Bucky · Affected clavicle centered to the IR	· To supraclavicular fossa 15°–30° caudad	· PA axial proj of the clavicle · For fxs not seen in direct PA or AP (Fig. 7-17B) · *PA position is best for optimum detail (less OID)*

TABLE 7-10. The Acromioclavicular Joints

Acromioclavicular Joints	Position of Part	Central Ray Directed	Structures Included/Best Seen
AP Bilateral, with and w/o weights	· AP erect, MSP to mid-IR · Arms at sides (bilateral for comparison) · Two images in the same position: one w/o and one w/ *weights* · Images must be properly identified	· ⊥ Midline at the level of AC jts · 72″ SID recommended to improve detail and permit both joints to be included on one image	· AP proj of AC jt and soft tissues · Demonstrates *dislocation/separation* when performed in an erect position (see Fig. 7-18)

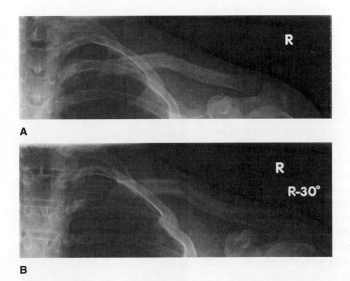

Figure 7-17. (A) AP projection of the fractured clavicle. **(B)** AP axial projection of the fractured clavicle, better illustrating extent of fracture. (Photo contributor: Conrad P. Ehrlich, MD.)

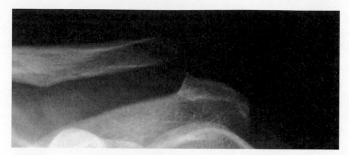

Figure 7-18. Acromioclavicular separation. The examination must be performed in the erect position (in the recumbent position, small separations may not be seen). (Reproduced with permission from Haig SV, Flores CR. *Orthopedic Emergencies: A Radiographic Atlas*. New York, NY: McGraw-Hill; 2005.)

TABLE 7-11. The Scapula

Scapula	Position of Part	Central Ray Directed	Structures Included/Best Seen
AP	· AP upright or recumbent · Scapula centered w/ arm abducted, elbow flexed	· ⊥ Midscapula, ≈2″ inferior to the coracoid process	· AP scapula with lat portion away from ribs · Exposure made during quiet breathing to blur lung markings (see Fig. 7-19A)
Lat proj erect RAO or LAO	· Erect PA 45°–60° w/ the affected anterior side *toward* the IR and · Arm across the chest for acromion and coracoid processes or · Palpate scapular borders and rotate the body to superimpose	· ⊥ Midvertebral border	· Lat scapula · Acromion and coracoid processes · Superimposed vertebral and axillary borders (Fig. 7-19B)
Lat proj recumbent RPO or LPO	· Recumbent obl · Affected posterior surface *away* from the IR · Palpate scapular borders and rotate till borders superimposed	· ⊥ Midaxillary border	· Lat scapula · Medial and lat borders superimposed · Humerus away from the scapula

Figure 7-19. (A) AP projection of the scapula. Note that arm abduction moves the scapula away from the rib cage, revealing a greater portion of the scapular body. A, acromion process; B, humeral head; C, glenoid fossa; D, scapular spine; E, clavicle (shaft); F, supraspinatus fossa; G, acromioclavicular articulation; H, scapular notch; I, coracoid process; J, inferior angle/apex of scapula; K, body/costal surface of scapula; L, axillary/lateral border scapula; M, superior border of scapula. (Photo contributor: Bob Wong, RT.) **(B)** Lateral projection of the scapula. It is taken with the arm elevated and the forearm resting on the head. It demonstrates the scapular body with the vertebral and axillary borders exactly superimposed. (Photo contributor: Stamford Hospital, Department of Radiology.)

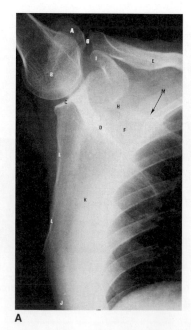

A

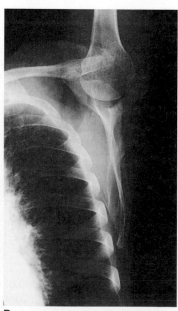

B

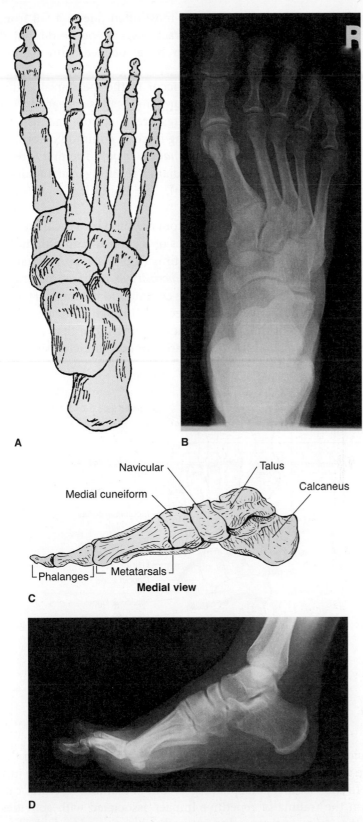

A

B

C   **Medial view**

Navicular   Talus

Medial cuneiform   Calcaneus

Phalanges   Metatarsals

D

Figure 7-20. **(A)** Bones of the foot (dorsal view). **(B)** Dorsoplantar projection of the foot. **(C)** Bones of the foot (medial view). **(D)** Mediolateral projection of the foot. (Photo contributor: Conrad P. Ehrlich, MD.)

Fractures of the calcaneus can occur, most often due to a fall from height directly onto the heel; these fractures can be comminuted and impacted. The calcaneus can also be associated with painful *spur* formation.

Stress (fatigue, march) fractures can occur in the metatarsal shafts; x-ray examination can "miss" these fractures until callus appears during bony repair process. Phalangeal fractures are common and usually occur as a result of a stubbing or crushing force. A common deformity of the first metatarsophalangeal joint is *hallux valgus*. The first (great) toe, called the *hallux*, slowly adducts (medially), resulting in an inflamed first metatarsophalangeal joint (*bunion*). The condition is relieved surgically.

The metatarsals and phalanges of the foot are similar to the metacarpals and phalanges of the hand. The bases of the fourth and fifth metatarsals articulate with the cuboid. The fifth (most lateral) metatarsal projects laterally and presents a large *tuberosity* at its base, making it susceptible to fracture. *Stress fractures* are common to the metatarsals.

The *hallux* has *two* phalanges; the second through fifth toes have *three* phalanges each. The phalanges of the toes are shorter than those of the fingers. The articulations of the foot are named/numbered similarly to those of the hand.

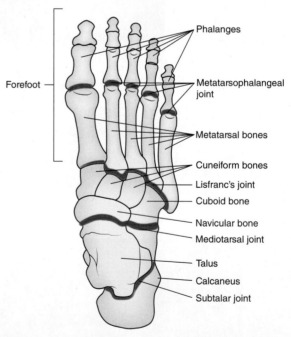

Articulations of the foot

Sesamoid bones are small, smooth bones formed in tendons. In the foot, there are two sesamoid bones located within the flexor tendon just proximal to the first metatarsophalangeal joint. Sesamoid fractures can occur from the trauma of repetitive impact associated with activities such as hiking and running, and sports such as tennis and basketball.

Ankle. The ankle joint (*mortise*) is formed by the articulation of the talus and distal portions of the tibia and fibula (see Fig. 7-32). The medial and lateral malleoli are the most frequently *fractured* components of the ankle joint; severe fractures can disrupt the integrity of the joint and lead to permanent instability and/or arthritis. Foot and/or ankle fractures can result from falls, twisting injuries, or direct impact.

Lower Leg. The *tibia* and *fibula* (Fig. 7-21) compose the bones of the lower leg. The tibia is larger and is situated medially. It articulates superiorly with the femur and inferiorly with the talus, forming a portion of the ankle joint. The tibia consists of a shaft/body and two expanded extremities. Its distal extremity has a prominence, the *medial malleolus,* which also participates in the formation of the ankle *mortise.* The fibular notch provides articulation for the fibula to form the *distal tibiofibular joint.*

The proximal end of the tibia presents a *medial* and a *lateral condyle,* on whose *superior* surfaces there are facets for articulation with the femur. The articular facets form a smooth surface called the *tibial plateau,* which provides attachment for the cartilaginous *menisci* of the knee joint. Between the two articular surfaces is a raised prominence, the *intercondylar eminence* (*tibial spine*).

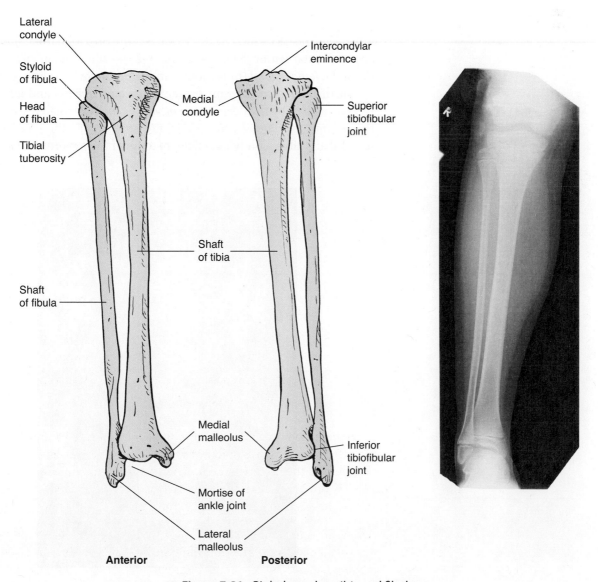

Figure 7-21. Right lower leg, tibia and fibula.

The proximal *anterior* surface of the tibia presents the *tibial tuberosity*, which provides attachment for the patellar ligament. *Osgood–Schlatter disease* is a chronic *epiphysitis* of the tibial tuberosity that occurs in some active young adults. Not really a disease, it is an overuse condition that results from repetitive impact trauma such as that occurs in jumping and kicking activities. Its symptoms include pain and tenderness at the tibial tuberosity and is manifested radiographically by bony separation at the epiphysis.

The fibula is the slender, lateral non–weight-bearing bone forming the lower leg; it also consists of a shaft/body and two expanded extremities. The bulbous *distal* end, known as the *lateral malleolus* (projects more distally than the medial), helps form the ankle joint and has a facet for articulation with the tibia (*distal tibiofibular joint*). The expanded *proximal* portion of the fibula is the *head*, which articulates with the lateral tibial condyle, forming the *proximal tibiofibular joint*. A *styloid* process extends *superiorly* from the head of the fibula. The *neck* is the constricted portion just distal to the fibular head. The fibula is most commonly fractured at the malleolus, just above the ankle joint.

Knee. The knee is formed by three bones—the proximal tibia, the patella, and the distal femur (Figs. 7-22 and 7-23)—which form *two articulations*, the *femorotibial* (hinge joint) and *femoropatellar* (gliding joint).

The distal posterior femur presents two large *medial* and *lateral condyles* separated by the deep *intercondylar fossa.* Two small prominences, the *medial* and *lateral epicondyles,* are superior to the condyles. The femoral and tibial condyles articulate to form the *femorotibial joint.*

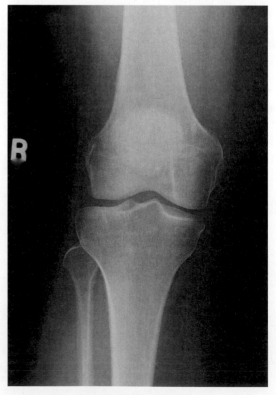

Figure 7-22. AP knee.

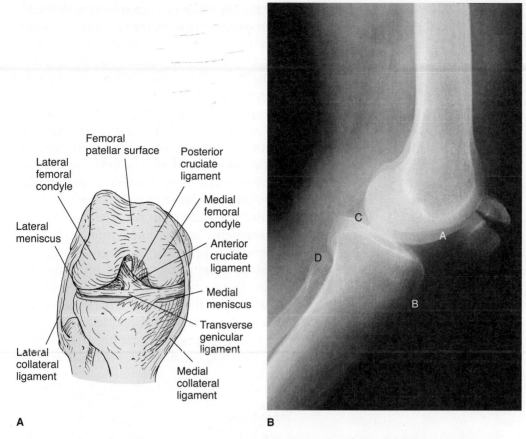

A   **B**

Figure 7-23. **(A)** Ligaments of the knee joint. **(B)** The knee should be flexed no more than 10° when transverse fracture of the patella is known or suspected; flexion can cause pain, fragment separation, and/or complication. The CR can be angled 5° cephalad to superimpose the magnified medial femoral condyle on the lateral condyle to permit better visualization of the joint space; angulation was not used in this projection, and the joint space is obscured by the magnified medial femoral condyle. A, medial femoral condyle; B, tibial tuberosity; C, tibial plateau; D, head of fibula. (Photo contributor: Stamford Hospital, Department of Radiology.)

The menisci are semilunar cartilages that lie medially and laterally between these articulating bones, and together with the *cruciate* and *collateral ligaments*, help form the *articular capsule* of the knee (Fig. 7-23A).

The *patella* is a triangular bone with its *base* superior and *apex* inferior. The *patella* is the largest *sesamoid* bone in the human body. It is attached to the tibial tuberosity by the patellar ligament and glides over the patellar surface of the distal femur (femoropatellar joint) during flexion and extension of the knee. Simple patellar fractures are usually *transverse* (Fig. 7-23B). Fractures of the patella can also be *stellate* or comminuted. Patellar fractures can require surgical internal fixation via figure-of-eight or tension band wiring; more complex fractures require partial patellectomy.

The congenital anomaly, *bipartite or multipartite patella*, can be misinterpreted as a fracture. Bipartite and multipartite patellae occur in a very small percentage of the population (about 1%) and are usually asymptomatic. Just opposite the *patellar surface*, on the posterior distal femur, is the smooth *popliteal surface*, which accommodates the popliteal artery.

Femur. The *femur* (Fig. 7-24) is the longest and strongest bone in the body. The femoral *shaft/body* is bowed slightly anteriorly. The proximal end of the femur consists of a *head,* which is received by the *acetabulum* of the pelvis. The femoral head has a small notch, the *fovea capitis femoris,* for ligament attachment. The ligament of the femoral head, or *ligamentum teres,* connects the fovea capitis femoris to the acetabulum. The *femoral neck,* which joins the head and shaft, angles upward approximately 120° and forward (in *anteversion*) approximately 15°. The *greater* (lateral) and *lesser* (medial) *trochanters* are large processes on the posterior proximal femur. The greater trochanter is a prominent positioning landmark that lies in the same transverse plane as the pubic symphysis and coccyx. The (posterior) *intertrochanteric crest* runs obliquely between the trochanters; the (anterior) *intertrochanteric line* runs anteriorly parallel to the crest. The femoral shaft presents a long narrow ridge posteriorly called the *linea aspera.*

Its distal anterior portion presents the *patellar surface*—a triangular depression over which the patella glides during flexion and extension motions.

The distal posterior surface presents the *popliteal surface*—a depression that houses the popliteal artery. The medial and lateral femoral condyles are very prominent posterior structures and between them is the deep intercondylar fossa. The medial and lateral femoral epicondyles are just above the condyles.

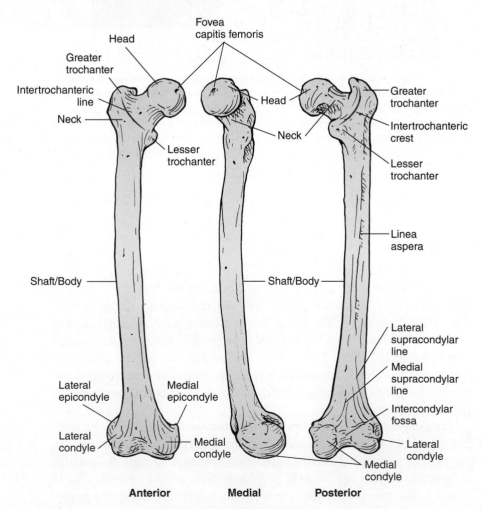

Figure 7-24. The right femur.

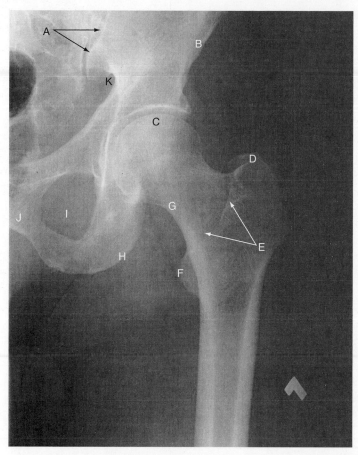

Figure 7-25. AP projection of the left hip. Leg is internally rotated, placing femoral neck parallel to the IR. A, SI joint; B, anterior inferior iliac spine; C, femoral head; D, greater trochanter; E, intertrochanteric crest; F, lesser trochanter; G, femoral neck; H, ischial tuberosity; I, obturator foramen; J, pubis; K, greater sciatic notch. (Photo contributor: Stamford Hospital, Department of Radiology.)

The articulation of the femoral head with the pelvic acetabulum forms the *hip joint*. The femoral neck (Figs. 7-24 and 7-25) is the most commonly *fractured* portion of the femur. In young people, hip fractures are most often a result of high-impact and/or high-velocity trauma. In the elderly, they are most often the result of a fall.

Fractures of the femoral shaft are usually the result of a direct blow; fracture *displacement* is dependent on muscular pull and traumatic impact. Dislocations of the hip joint are fairly uncommon because of the very strong pelvic and hip musculature. Disturbance of the fovea capitis femoris or disruption of the nutrient arteries supplying the femoral neck can result in *avascular necrosis* of the femoral head.

Pelvis. *Pelvis*, the Latin word for "basin," was originally named for its shape. The pelvic girdle consists of two *innominate* (hip or *coxal*) bones, one on each side of the sacrum. Each innominate bone consists of three fused bones: the *ilium*, *ischium*, and *pubis* (Fig. 7-26).

Parts of these three bones contribute to the formation of the *acetabulum* (Latin word for "little vinegar cup")—the socket articulation for the femoral head. The *labrum* is a ring of fibrocartilage along the outer rim of the acetabulum that acts like a suction cup, deepening the acetabulum and increasing contact between the articular surfaces of the

Hip Fracture Classifications

- Subcapital: common, inferior to femoral head
- Transcervical: across the femoral neck
- Basicervical: at the base of the femoral neck
- Intertrochanteric: common, between the trochanters

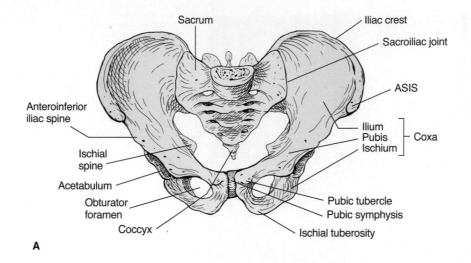

A

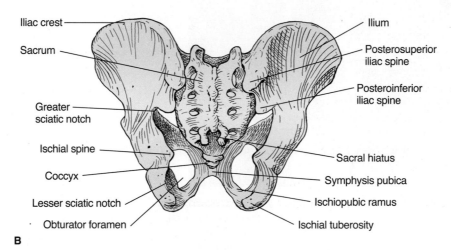

B

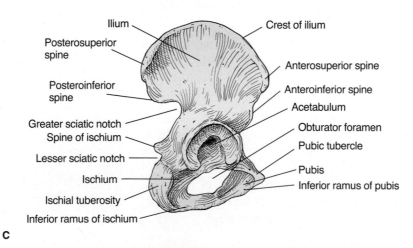

C

Figure 7-26. **(A)** The pelvis (anterior view). **(B)** The pelvic girdle (posterior view). **(C)** The right hip bone (lateral view) showing the acetabulum. (*Continued*)

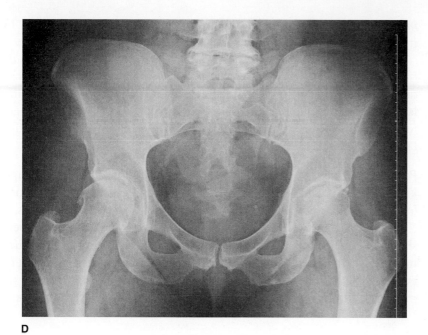

D

Figure 7-26. (*Continued*) **(D)** AP projection of the pelvis. The femoral necks are seen in their entirety: Internal rotation of the feet/legs places them parallel to the IR. Note fractures of the pubic and ischial rami on the left. (Photo contributor: Stamford Hospital, Department of Radiology.)

acetabulum and the femoral head. Any tear or other injury to the labrum causes hip or groin pain, stiffness, clicking, or "catching" sensation. Labral injuries can be degenerative or traumatic.

The *ilia* are the large, superior bones whose medial auricular surfaces form the sacroiliac (*SI*) *joints* bilaterally. The broad, flat portion of each ilium is the *ala*, or wing; the upper part of the ala forms a ridge of bone called the *iliac crest*, which terminates in *anterior* and *posterior iliac spines*. The *arcuate line* of the ilium is a smooth, rounded border on the internal surface of the ilium. It is immediately inferior to the *iliac fossa*.

The *ischium* forms the posteroinferior portion of the pelvis. The posterior part of the ischium forms the major portion of the *greater* and *lesser sciatic notches* separated by the *ischial spine*. The most inferior portion is the *ischial tuberosity*—a large, rough prominence that provides attachment for posterior thigh muscles. The inferior *ramus* of the ischium extends medially from the tuberosities to unite with the inferior ramus of the pubis.

The *pubic* bones form the anterior portion of the pelvis. Their bodies unite to form the *pubic symphysis;* just lateral to each superior margin of the symphysis are the prominent *pubic tubercles*. The superior pubic *ramus* fuses with the ilium and the inferior pubic *ramus* with the ischium to form the large *obturator foramen*. The *pectineal line* of the pubis is a ridge on the superior rami of the pubic bones. In combination with the *arcuate line*, it comprises the *iliopectineal line*.

The superior circumference of the *lesser pelvis* forms the *brim* of the pelvis, or the *pelvic inlet*. The *edge* of the inlet is known as the *pelvic brim*. The terms are often used interchangeably.

Most pelvic fractures are result of trauma (MVA, falls, sports injuries) and carry a significant risk of serious pelvic bleeding. Pelvic fractures can cause disturbance of the urinary bladder or urethra; an

Normal Male/Android Pelvis

- Narrower, more vertical
- Deeper from anterior to posterior
- Pubic angle 50°–60° (less than 90°)
- Pelvic inlet narrower and heart-shaped/round

Normal Female/Gynecoid Pelvis

- Wider, more angled toward horizontal
- Shallower from anterior to posterior
- Pubic angle 80°–85° (approximately 90°)
- Pelvic inlet larger and rounder

intravenous urogram or abdominopelvic computed tomography (CT) may be required to diagnose any urinary leakage.

The normal *female* (*gynecoid*) *pelvis* differs from the normal *male* (*android*) *pelvis* in that it is shallower and its bones are generally more delicate. In females, the pelvic outlet is wider and more circular; the ischial tuberosities and acetabula are further apart, and the angle formed by the pubic arch is also greater. All these bony characteristics facilitate the birth process (Fig. 7-27).

Positioning. Positioning of the lower limb and pelvis requires a thorough knowledge of the skeletal anatomy and an awareness of possible pathologic conditions and their impact on positioning and technical factors.

Clothing having radiopaque objects such as buttons, snaps, or zippers should be removed if possible. Bulky or bunched clothing can produce undesirable radiographic artifacts and should therefore be removed whenever possible and replaced with a hospital dressing gown. Elastic waist garments can contribute to nonuniform density on abdominal radiographs.

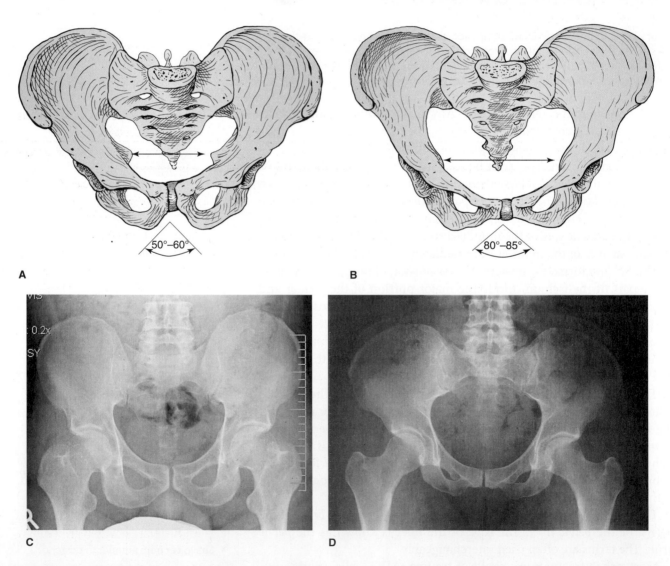

Figure 7-27. Architectural differences in the **(A)** male and **(B)** female pelves. **(C)** AP projection of the male pelvis. **(D)** AP projection of the female pelvis. Femoral necks are parallel to the IR and greater trochanters are seen in profile. (Photo contributor: Stamford Hospital, Department of Radiology.)

The patient must be instructed about the importance of remaining still, and immobilization devices such as radioparent (transparent to x-rays) sponges and sandbags should be used as required. The shortest possible exposure time should be used, especially when involuntary motion is a potential problem.

Many distal lower limb examinations can be performed at the table-top (i.e., non-Bucky); the knee frequently requires a grid, and femur, hip, and pelvis almost always do. *Suspended respiration* is suggested for radiography of the proximal portion of the lower limb and the pelvis. Patients must always be appropriately *shielded*.

Some of the lower leg projections can be performed in either AP or PA position, depending on the condition and comfort of the patient. Lateral projections can be easily obtained by using a horizontal (cross-table lateral) beam when limb or patient movement is contraindicated.

Tables 7-12 through 7-22 provide a summary of routine and frequently performed special positions/projections of the lower limb and the pelvis.

TABLE 7-12. The Foot

Foot	Position of Part	Central Ray Directed	Structures Included/Best Seen
AP or AP axial dorsoplantar	· Knee flexed ≈45° · Plantar surface on the IR	· ⊥ or 10° toward the heel to the base of the third metatarsal	· Frontal proj of tarsals (except calcaneus and part of the talus) · Frontal proj of metatarsals, phalanges and their articulations
AP axial weight-bearing	· Patient erect · Full weight evenly distributed on feet · Plantar surface on the IR	· 15° toward the heel to the base of the third metatarsal	· Frontal proj of tarsals (except calcaneus and part of the talus) · Frontal proj of metatarsals, phalanges and their articulations · Demonstration of longitudinal arches
AP obl medial rotation	· Start as dorsoplantar · Rotate medially 30°–40°Plantar surface and IR are 30°–40°	· ⊥ Base of the third metatarsal	· Most tarsals and metatarsals (except the most medial), their articulations · Sinus tarsi, tuberosity of fifth metatarsal (see Fig. 7-28)
AP obl lat rotation	· Start as dorsoplantar · Rotate laterally 30° · Plantar surface and IR are 30°	· ⊥ Base of the third metatarsal	· First and second metatarsals and interspaces · First and second cuneiforms and interspaces · Navicular well visualized
Lat (*mediolateral or lateromedial*)	· Recumbent lat · Patella ⊥ tabletop · Foot slightly dorsiflexed · Plantar surface ⊥ IR · The lat proj is more *accurately* obtained in the *lateromedial* (rather than mediolateral) position	· ⊥ Metatarsal bases	· Lat foot, ankle jt, dist tibia and fibula · Superimposed tarsals, tibia, and fibula (see Fig. 7-29)
Lat weight-bearing	· Weight-bearing lat · Patella ⊥ IR · Plantar surface ⊥ IR	· ⊥ Metatarsal bases	· Lat foot, ankle jt, dist tibia and fibula · Superimposed tarsals, tibia, and fibula (see Fig. 7-29) · Demonstrates the status of the plantar arches

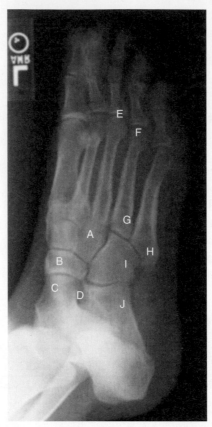

Figure 7-28. Medial oblique view of the left foot, demonstrating articulations of the cuboid with the calcaneus, fourth and fifth metatarsals, and lateral cuneiform. The talonavicular articulation and sinus tarsi are also demonstrated. A, lateral/third cuneiform; B, navicular bone; C, talus/astragalus; D, sinus tarsi; E, third metatarsophalangeal joint; F, head of the fourth metatarsal; G, base of the fourth metatarsal; H, base/tuberosity of the fourth metatarsal; I, cuboid; J, calcaneus/os calcis. (Photo contributor: Stamford Hospital, Department of Radiology.)

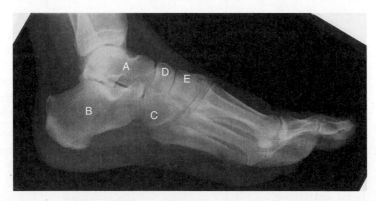

Figure 7-29. Lateral projection of the foot, demonstrating superimposed tarsals, metatarsals, and phalanges; a little more of the distal tibia and fibula should be visualized. A, talus/astragalus; B, calcaneus/os calcis; C, cuboid; D, navicular bone; E, medial/first cuneiform. (Photo contributor: Stamford Hospital, Department of Radiology.)

TABLE 7-13. The Toes

Toes	Position of Part	Central Ray Directed	Structures Included/Best Seen
AP or AP axial (dorsoplantar)	· Knee flexed ≈45° · Plantar surface on the IR	· ⊥ or 10° toward the heel, to second MTP	· Phalanges, their articulations, dist metatarsals in frontal proj
AP, entire forefoot (dorsoplantar)	· Knee flexed ≈45° · Plantar surface on the IR	· ⊥ or 10°–15° toward the heel, centered to the third MTP jt	· Phalanges, their articulations, dist metatarsals in frontal proj of entire forefoot
AP obl, medial rotation	· Start as dorsoplantar · Rotate medially 30°–45°	· ⊥ Third MTP	· Obl proj of phalanges, their articulations, dist metatarsals
Lat	· Turn to the side that brings affected toe(s) closest to the IR · Unaffected toes may be taped back	· ⊥ Prox IPJ	· Lat proj of toe(s) and associated articulations
Sesamoids (*tangential*)	· Prone, *foot* dorsiflexed 15°–20° · Toes dorsiflexed 15°–20°, resting on IR	· ⊥ or ≈10° caudad to the IR to first MTP	· Sesamoids in profile, free of superimposition

TABLE 7-14. The Calcaneus

Calcaneus (Os Calcis)	Position of Part	Central Ray Directed	Structures Included/Best Seen
Plantodorsal, axial	· Seated on table with the leg extended · Plantar surface ⊥ tabletop · Immobilize w/ strip of tape/gauze held by the patient	· 40° *cephalad* to the base of the third metatarsal	· Axial proj of calcaneus · Includes the trochlear process, sustentaculum tali, talocalcaneal jt (see Fig. 7-30)
Dorsoplantar, axial	· Prone, plantar surface ⊥ tabletop · IR placed against the plantar surface	· 40° *caudally* to the level of base of second metatarsal	· Axial proj of calcaneus · Includes the trochlear process, sustentaculum tali, talocalcaneal jt
Lat	· Recumbent on the affected side · Patella ⊥ tabletop · Foot and ankle lat	· ⊥ Midcalcaneus	· Lat calcaneus, talus, navicular, ankle jt, and sinus tarsi (see Fig. 7-31)

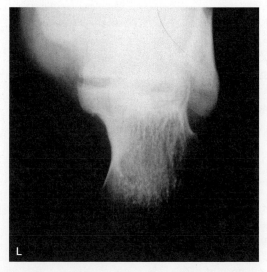

Figure 7-30. Plantodorsal projection of calcaneus; sustentaculum tali, trochlear process, and calcaneal tuberosity are well visualized. (Photo contributor: Stamford Hospital, Department of Radiology.)

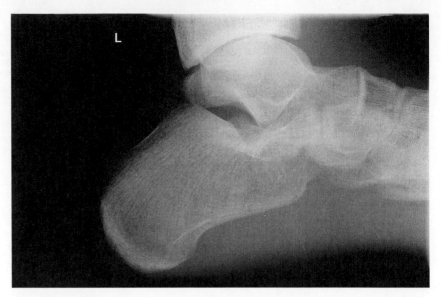

Figure 7-31. Lateral calcaneus; sinus tarsi are well visualized. (Photo contributor: Stamford Hospital, Department of Radiology.)

Long Bone Measurement. Accurate measurement of long bones, usually the lower limbs, is occasionally required to evaluate abnormal growth patterns in children or lower back disorders in adults (see Table 7-20). Gait abnormalities are frequently associated with leg length inequality and can lead to degenerative arthritis of the lumbar spine and/or the lower limb.

Arthrography. *Arthrography* is a contrast examination performed to evaluate soft-tissue joint structures such as articular cartilages, menisci, ligaments, and bursae. It can be performed by using conventional or digital fluoroscopic imaging, or more commonly, with magnetic resonance imaging (MRI) or CT.

TABLE 7-15. The Ankle

Ankle	Position of Part	Central Ray Directed	Structures Included/Best Seen
AP	· Leg extended AP · Plantar surface ⊥ IR	· ⊥ Midway b/w malleoli through tibiotalar jt	· AP ankle jt, dist tibia/fibula, talus (see Fig. 7-32A)
AP obl Mortise jt Medial rotation	· Leg extended AP · Rotated 15°–20° medially · Intermalleolar plane ‖⊥to IR	· ⊥ Midway b/w malleoli, ⊥ intermalleolar plane	· AP ankle mortise · Talotibial, talofibular jts well seen · All three aspects of the mortise jt seen in profile (see Fig. 7-32B)
AP obl, medial rotation	· Leg extended AP · Rotated 45° medially	· ⊥ Midway b/w malleoli, ⊥ to IR	· Dist tibiofibular jt, minimal to no overlap · Lat malleolus free of superimposition · Lat aspect of talus with minimal superimposition
Lat (*mediolateral or lateromedial*)	· Recumbent on the affected side · Patella ⊥ tabletop · Foot dorsiflexed (≈90°) · The lat proj is more *accurately* obtained in the *lateromedial* (rather than mediolateral) position	· ⊥ Ankle jt	· Lat dist tibia/fibula, ankle jt · Lat talus, calcaneus, navicular

TABLE 7-15. The Ankle—Cont'd

Ankle	Position of Part	Central Ray Directed	Structures Included/Best Seen
AP stress projs, inversion and eversion	· Leg extended, ankle true AP · Foot dorsiflexed · Plantar surface ⊥ · one exposure w/ jt in stressed inversion · one exposure w/ jt in stressed eversion	· ⊥ Midway b/w malleoli	· AP ankle jt in inversion and eversion · Evaluates jt separation, ligament tear
AP weight-bearing	· Patient erect in AP position against upright Bucky or IR · Full weight distributed on both feet · Feet placed facing straight ahead and ‖	· ⊥ Midway b/w malleoli through tibiotalar jt	· Weight-bearing AP ankle jt, dist tibia/fibula, talus
Lat weight-bearing	· Patient erect in lat position against upright Bucky or IR · Legs separated, affected ankle placed closest to the Bucky or IR in mediolateral position · Unaffected side placed posterior and out of the field of view	· ⊥ Ankle jt	· Weight-bearing lat dist tibia/fibula, ankle jt · Weight-bearing lat talus, calcaneus, navicular

Note: If someone (e.g., the MD) must hold the ankle in position for the stress views, appropriate radiation precautions are provided.

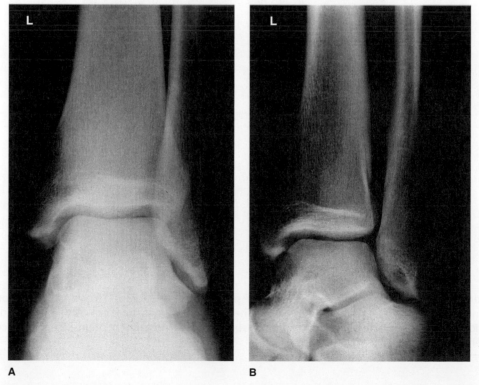

A   B

Figure 7-32. (A) AP projection of the ankle joint. (Photo contributor: Stamford Hospital, Department of Radiology.) **(B)** The 15°–20° medial oblique projection of the ankle is used to demonstrate the ankle mortise. An oblique projection of the distal tibia/fibula, proximal talus, and their articular surfaces is also demonstrated. (Photo contributor: Stamford Hospital, Department of Radiology.)

TABLE 7-16. The Lower Leg (Tibia/Fibula)

Lower Leg (*Tibia/Fibula*)	Position of Part	Central Ray Directed	Structures Included/Best Seen
AP	· Leg extended AP · No pelvic rotation · Foot dorsiflexed	· ⊥ Midshaft tibia	· AP lower leg · Both jts included (Fig. 7-33A)
Lat	· Recumbent on the affected side · Patella ⊥ tabletop · Ankle and foot lat	· ⊥ Midshaft	· Lat tibia/fibula · Both jts included (Fig. 7-33B)
AP obl (*medial and lat rotation*)	· Leg extended w/ foot dorsiflexed · Leg rotated 45° medially or laterally	· ⊥ Midshaft tibia	· Medial rotation shows prox and dist tibiofibular articulations

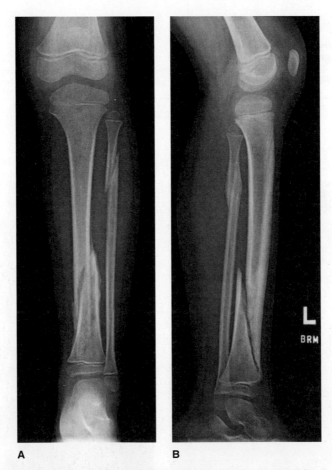

A   **B**

Figure 7-33. Fractures and their degree of displacement. **(A)** AP projection of the tibia and fibula. **(B)** Lateral projection of the tibia and fibula. Both joints should be included whenever possible. These images demonstrate how AP/PA projections demonstrate medial/lateral relationships and how lateral projections demonstrate anterior/posterior relationships. (Photo contributor: Stamford Hospital, Department of Radiology.)

TABLE 7-17. Knee

Knee	Position of Part	Central Ray Directed	Structures Included/Best Seen

AP	· Leg extended AP
	· No pelvic rotation
	· Leg may be rotated 3°–5° internally
		· To ½" below patellar apex (knee jt)
		· Direction of the CR depends on distance b/w the ASIS and the tabletop:
		  · up to 19 cm (thin pelvis) 3°–5° caudad
		  · 19–24 cm 0° CR
		  · >24 cm (thick pelvis) 3°–5° cephalad
			· AP knee jt, dist femur, and prox tibia/fibula
			· Patella seen through the femur

Lat	· Recumbent on the affected side · Patella ⊥ tabletop · Knee flexed 20°–30°	· 5° cephalad to knee jt	· Lat proj of the knee and femoropatellar jts · Superimposed femoral condyles · *Knee should not be flexed >10° with known or suspected patellar fx (see Fig. 7-23B)*
AP *weight-bearing* *(bilateral)*	· AP erect against upright Bucky · Weight evenly shared on legs	· ⊥ CR midway b/w knees at the level of patellar apices	· AP weight-bearing knee jts · Particularly useful for evaluation of *arthritic conditions* (see Fig. 7-40C)
AP obl proj, medial rotation	· Patient supine with long axis of knee centered to IR · Knee rotated internally 45°	· ⊥ IR · Directed ½" dist to patellar apex	· Dist femur, prox tibia/fibula · Lat femoral and tibial condyles, and fibular head free of superimposition · Prox tibiofibular jt well demonstrated · Patella superimposed over medial femoral condyle
AP obl proj, lat rotation	· Patient supine with long axis of knee centered to IR · Knee rotated externally 45°	· ⊥ IR · Directed ½" dist to patellar apex	· Dist femur, prox tibia/fibula · Medial femoral and tibial condyles in profile · Patella superimposed over lat femoral condyle
PA axial Intercondylar fossa (*Camp–Coventry*)	· PA recumbent · Knee flexed, so tibia forms 40° w/ the tabletop · Foot resting on the support	· CR 40° caudad (⊥ long axis of tibia) to the knee jt	· *PA axial* (superoinferior) proj · Shows intercondylar fossa, tibial plateau, and eminences · "Tunnel view" (see Fig. 7-34A and B)
AP axial Intercondylar fossa (*Bècleré*)	· AP w/ knee flexed ≈20°–30° · Resting on supported IR	· CR cephalad (⊥ long axis of tibia) to the knee jt	· *AP axial* (inferosuperior) proj · Shows intercondylar fossa, tibial plateau, and eminences; "tunnel view"
PA axial Intercondylar fossa (*Holmblad*)	· Patient kneeling on IR/tabletop · Knee flexed 60°–70°, body supported on unaffected knee	· CR ⊥ IR and tibia · CR directed to midpopliteal crease	· *PA axial* (superoinferior) proj · Shows intercondylar fossa, tibial plateau, and eminences

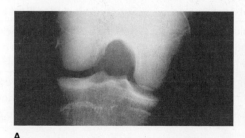
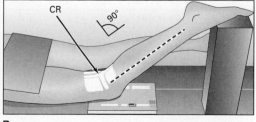

A   B

Figure 7-34. (A) Intercondylar fossa, using the Camp–Coventry method. The tibial plateau and eminences are well visualized. (Photo contributor: Stamford Hospital, Department of Radiology.) **(B)** Patient and CR positioning for the Camp–Coventry method.

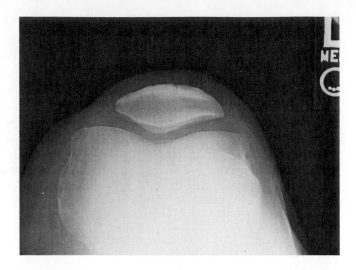

Figure 7-35. Tangential "sunrise" (Settegast) projection of the patella. The femoropatellar joint is well demonstrated. (Photo contributor: Stamford Hospital, Department of Radiology.)

TABLE 7-18. Patella

Patella	Position of Part	Central Ray Directed	Structures Included/Best Seen
PA patella	· Prone position · **Leg rotated ≈5°–10° laterally to place patella || tabletop**	· ⊥ **Patella (enters the popliteal region)**	· PA patella, including the knee jt · **Better detail than the AP position (less OID)**
Lat patella	· Recumbent on the affected side · Patella ⊥ tabletop · Knee flexed 20°–30°	· ⊥ Patella	· Lat proj of femoropatellar jt · Superimposed femoral condyles · *Knee should not be flexed >10° with known or suspected patellar fx (see Fig. 7-23B)*
Tangential (*Settegast*)	· Prone (or seated) on the x-ray table · Knee flexed at least 90°	· CR directed to midfemoropatellar jt ; 15°–20° ∠ may be required	· *Tangential* proj of the patella, femoropatellar articulation · Useful for demonstrating *vertical* fx · *Must not be attempted* in known or suspected transverse fx of the patella
Tangential (*Merchant*)	· Supine (or seated) on the x-ray table · Knee flexed ≈45° · IR ~12″ dist to the knees	· Directed 30° caudal midway between patellae · 6″ SID to reduce magnification	· *Tangential* proj of the patellae (Fig. 7-35) and intercondylar sulci · Open patellofemoral articulations—demonstrates *vertical* fx · *Must not be attempted* in known or suspected transverse patellar fx

Note: It has been suggested that the *Settegast method* be modified to *lesser degrees of flexion,* in order that the patella not be pulled into the femoropatellar groove.

TABLE 7-19. The Femur

Femur	Position of Part	Central Ray Directed	Structures Included/Best Seen
AP	· Supine, affected femur centered to IR · Leg internally rotated 15°	· ⊥ Midfemoral shaft (to include hip and possibly knee jt)	· AP proj of the femur, including hip jt · Leg rotation *overcomes anteversion* of the femoral neck and places neck || IR
Lat (*mediolateral*)	· Recumbent lat w/ the affected leg centered to the IR · Patella ⊥ tabletop	· ⊥ Midshaft	· Lat proj of the femur, from knee jt up · May be performed w/ horizontal *beam if suspected fx or pathologic disease*

Note: If an orthopedic appliance is present, the x-ray image should include the entire appliance and the articulation closest to it.

TABLE 7-20. Long Bone Measurement

Long Bone Measurement	Position of Part	Central Ray Directed	Structures Included/Best Seen
AP (leg)/long bone measurement	· Supine · Leg extended and centered to the IR · Metal ruler taped alongside · One exposure each at hip, knee, and ankle jts (on one IR)	· ⊥ Hip, knee, ankle jts	· Tightly collimated AP proj of hip, knee, and ankle jts · With (metallic) ruler alongside

Note: For bilateral examination, the ruler is placed b/w legs; there must be no rotation, and if one knee is somewhat flexed, the other must be identically flexed for the exposure.

Note: Starting in 2021, the National Council on Radiation Protection and Measurements (NCRP) advises against the use of gonadal shielding during pelvic and abdominal examinations. Reasons for the discontinuation of gonadal shielding during these examinations include the overall reduction in exposure factors used to acquire general x-ray examinations, unnecessary repeats due to improper shield placement, and the tendency for automatic exposure control (AEC) to administer more radiation than necessary when lead shields are in the collimated field.

The physician or patient may request the use of protective shielding. Any protective shields must be carefully placed; superimposition on diagnostically important anatomic structures can cause retakes and exposure to unnecessary radiation. In addition, if gonadal shields are used during pelvic and abdominal examinations, it is crucial that the radiographer manually selects their technique factors; AEC will attempt to penetrate the lead shield if it is within the collimated field, causing overexposure. By practicing manual technique selection, over-irradiation will be avoided.

TABLE 7-21. Pelvis

Pelvis	Position of Part	Central Ray Directed	Structures Included/Best Seen
AP pelvis	· Supine, MSP ⊥ tabletop · No pelvic rotation · Legs rotated internally 15°	· ⊥ Midline at a point midway b/w the ASIS and pubic symphysis; top of IR ≈1″–2″ above the iliac crest	· AP proj of the pelvis and upper femora · Femoral necks, greater trochanters free of superimposition (Fig. 7-36)
AP pelvis, bilateral frog leg (nontrauma, modified Cleaves)	· Supine · Knee(s) and hip(s) acutely flexed · Thigh(s) abducted 40°	· *Unilateral:* ⊥ femoral neck of the affected side centered to IR · *Bilateral:* 3″ below the ASIS	· Hip structures and prox third of the femur · Greater trochanter should be seen superimposed on the femoral neck (see Fig. 7-37)
Note: Starting in 2021, the National Council on Radiation Protection and Measurements (NCRP) advises against the use of gonadal shielding during pelvic and abdominal examinations. Reasons for the discontinuation of gonadal shielding during these examinations include the overall reduction in exposure factors used to acquire general x-ray examinations, unnecessary repeats due to improper shield placement, and the tendency for automatic exposure control (AEC) to administer more radiation than necessary when lead shields are in the collimated field.			
AP pelvis, axial anterior pelvic bones (outlet/inlet)	· Supine · No pelvic rotation	· Outlet: CR to pubic symphysis/greater trochanter at 20°–35° cephalad (males), 30°–45° cephalad (females) · Intlet: CR 40° caudad, entering m/w between ASISs	· Outlet: shows ischial body and ramus, pubic superior and inferior rami · Inlet: shows entire (upper) pelvic inlet
AP obl ilium	· Supine · Sagittal plane passing through hip jt of affected side centered to IR · Obl to 40° toward the affected side	· ⊥ CR enters the sagittal plane 2″ medial to ASIS at level m/w b/w crest and greater trochanter	· AP obl proj of ilium and sciatic notches · Part obliquity opens the ilium by placing it ‖ to the IR

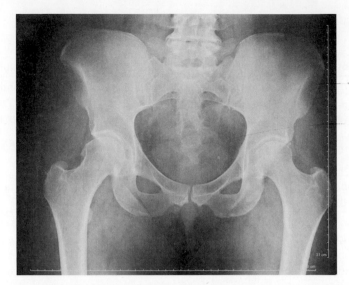

Figure 7-36. AP projection of the pelvis. The femoral necks are seen in their entirety: Internal rotation of the feet/legs places them parallel to the IR. Note fractures of the pubic and ischial rami on the left. (Photo contributor: Stamford Hospital, Department of Radiology.)

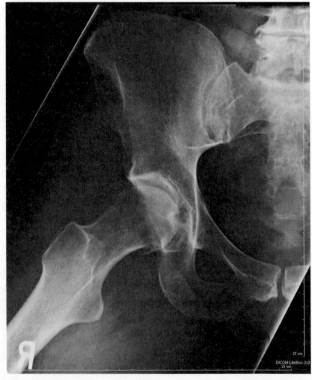

Figure 7-37. AP oblique (modified Cleaves) view of the hip. The femoral neck and the greater and lesser trochanters are well defined; the lesser trochanter is seen medially.

TABLE 7-22. Hip

Hip	Position of Part	Central Ray Directed	Structures Included/Best Seen
AP	· Supine, sagittal plane 2″ medial to ASIS centered to IR · No pelvic rotation · Leg rotated 15° internally	· Sagittal plane 2″ medial to the ASIS at the level of greater trochanter	· AP hip jt, femoral neck and prox femur · A portion of the pelvic bones is included · *The greater trochanter should be seen in profile*
Note: Another method of hip localization is to bisect the ASIS and pubic symphysis: This is the peak of the femoral head. A point ≈2.5″ dist and ⊥ to the midpoint of the femoral neck (see Fig. 7-25).			
Note: Leg inversion must never be forced and is contraindicated in cases of known or suspected fx or destructive disease.			
AP hip, frog leg (nontrauma, modified Cleaves)	· Supine, ASIS of the affected side centered to the IR · Knee and hip acutely flexed · Thigh(s) abducted 40°	· ⊥ to the femoral head	· AP obl proj of the hip jt · Lesser trochanter should be seen on the medial aspect of the femur (see Fig. 7-37)
Axiolateral inferosuperior/ cross-table lat hip (*horizontal beam lat; Danelius–Miller*)	· Supine, unaffected leg elevated · Leg rotated internally 15° (*see note below*) · Grid/IR placed against affected thigh, ‖ femoral neck	· ⊥ Femoral neck and IR	· Lat proj of the prox femur and its articulation with the acetabulum · The lesser trochanter will be prominently seen on the posterior aspect of the femur
Note: Leg inversion must never be forced and is *contraindicated* in cases of known or suspected fx or destructive disease.			
Modified axiolateral (*Clements– Nakayama*)	· Supine, legs extended · Affected side to the *edge* of the table (Bucky side) · Cassette placed on the extended Bucky tray and tilted back ≈15°–20°, CR ⊥	· CR angled 15°–20° posteriorly, entering prox medial thigh, ⊥ midfemoral neck	· Lat obl of prox femur, hip jt
Posterior obl pelvis, acetabulum (*Judet*)	· Semisupine recumbent · 45° posterior obl	· If affected side *down,* CR ⊥ pubic symphysis · If affected side *up,* CR ⊥ 2″ dist to the (upside) ASIS	· *Downside* shows the anterior rim of the acetabulum · *Upside* shows the posterior rim of the acetabulum

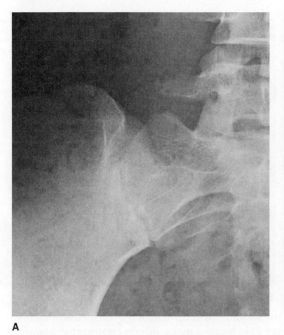
A

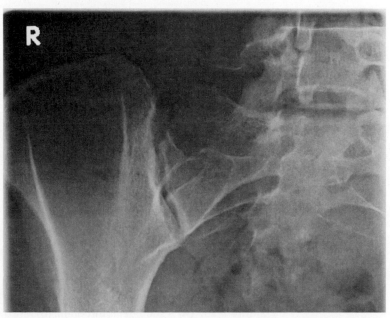
B

Figure 7-38. **(A)** AP right SI joint with perpendicular CR. **(B)** LPO right SI joint with perpendicular CR; 25° obliquity opens SI joint nicely. (Photo contributor: Conrad P. Ehrlich, MD.)

The conventional x-ray examination is most often performed as *double* contrast, with a *positive contrast agent* (water-soluble iodinated) coating the structures and a *negative* contrast agent (air) filling the joint cavity. Fluoroscopic images are obtained during the examination while applying various *stress maneuvers.* Overhead radiographs could be requested as supplemental images.

In MRI or CT arthrography, contrast media is first introduced into the joint space under fluoroscopy. The MRI contrast medium is typically gadolinium, whereas the CT contrast medium is generally a water-soluble iodinated medium. Joint manipulation can be performed and fluoroscopic images obtained before the patient is escorted to the MRI or CT department for further imaging.

The knee is the most common joint to be examined in this way, although the hip, wrist, shoulder (Fig. 7-39A), and TMJ can also be evaluated with contrast arthrography.

Terminology and Pathology. Some of the radiologically significant skeletal disorders or conditions of the upper and lower limbs with which the student radiographer should be familiar are listed as follows:

• Acromegaly
• Battered child syndrome
• Bone metastases
• Bursitis
• Carpal tunnel syndrome
• Epicondylitis
• Fracture (see Figs. 7-17, 7-23, 7-33, and 7-42)
• Gout
• Osgood–Schlatter disease
• Osteoarthritis (Fig. 7-40B)
• Osteochondroma
• Osteomalacia
• Osteomyelitis
• Osteoporosis
• Paget disease (Fig. 7-40A)
• Rickets
• Slipped femoral capital epiphysis
• Subluxation
• Talipes
• Tendonitis

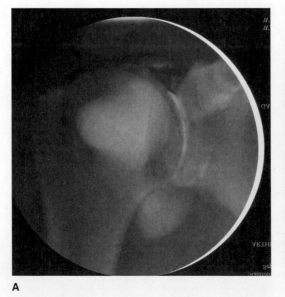

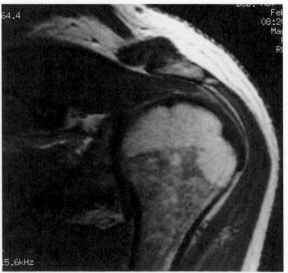

A   B

Figure 7-39. (A) A shoulder arthrogram. **(B)** MRI of the shoulder is accomplished noninvasively and provides visualization of structures having subtle differences in tissue density. (Photo contributor: Stamford Hospital, Department of Radiology.)

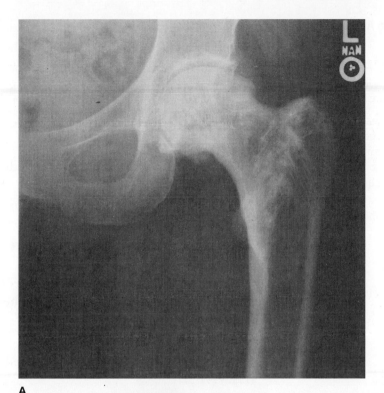

A

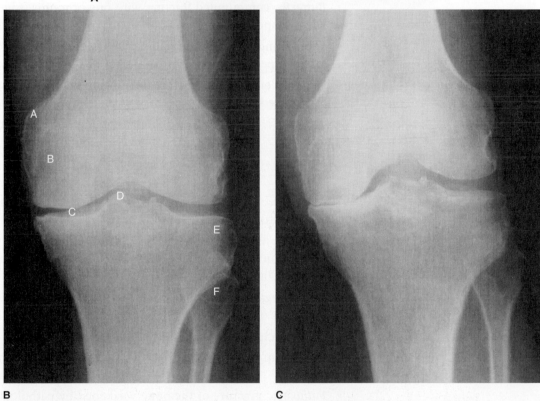

B   C

Figure 7-40. **(A)** AP projection of the hip and proximal femur demonstrates Paget disease. Early lytic changes are seen throughout the bone; observe the beginning of typical "cotton wool" appearance in the region of the head and trochanters. The hip is well positioned, the femoral neck is parallel to the IR (not foreshortened), and the greater trochanter is seen in profile. (Photo contributor: Stamford Hospital, Department of Radiology.) **(B)** AP knee joint, recumbent. **(C)** The same knee joint taken weight-bearing. Note demonstration of significant joint narrowing. A, medial femoral epicondyle; B, medial femoral condyle; C, tibial plateau; D, medial intercondylar tubercle/tibial intercondylar eminence; E, lateral tibial condyle; F, head of fibula. (Reproduced with permission from Miller TT, Schweitzer ME. *Diagnostic Musculoskeletal Imaging.* New York, NY: McGraw-Hill; 2005.)

Some Conditions Requiring Adjustment in Exposure

Decrease in Exposure Factors	Increase in Exposure Factors
Arthritis	Acromegaly
Ewing sarcoma	Chronic gout
Osteomalacia	Multiple myeloma
Osteoporosis	Osteochondroma
Rickets	Osteopetrosis
Thalassemia	Paget disease (osteitis deformans)

Types of Fractures (Fig. 7-41)

- *Simple:* an undisplaced fracture (Fig. 7-41A)
- *Displaced:* fractured ends of the bone are out of alignment (Fig. 7-41B)
- *Compound:* fractured end of the bone has penetrated skin (open fracture)
- *Incomplete:* fracture does not traverse the entire bone; little or no displacement
- *Greenstick:* break of cortex only on one side of bone; found in infants and children (Fig. 7-41D)
- *Torus/buckle* (Fig. 7-42): greenstick fracture with one cortex buckled/compacted and the other intact
- *Stress/fatigue:* response to repeated strong, powerful force (e.g., jogging, marching)
- *Avulsion:* small bony fragment pulled from bony prominence as a result of forceful pull of the attached ligament or tendon (chip fracture)
- *Hairline:* faint undisplaced fracture
- *Comminuted:* one fracture composed of several fragments (Fig. 7-41C)
- *Butterfly:* comminuted fracture with one or more wedge or butterfly wing–shaped pieces
- *Spiral:* long fracture encircling a shaft; result of torsion (twisting force); especially lower leg (distal tibia and proximal fibula)
- *Oblique:* longitudinal fracture forming an angle (~45°) with the long axis of the shaft
- *Transverse:* fracture occurring at right angles to the long axis of the bone
- *Boxer:* fracture of the neck of the fourth or fifth metacarpal (Fig. 7-3C)
- *Monteggia:* fracture of the proximal third of the ulnar shaft with anterior dislocation of the radial head
- *Colles:* transverse fracture of distal third of the radius with posterior angulation and associated avulsion fracture of the ulnar styloid process (Fig. 7-4B)
- *Trimalleolar:* fracture of the lateral malleolus, fracture of the medial malleolus on medial and posterior surfaces
- *Jones:* fracture of the base of the fifth metatarsal
- *Pott:* fracture of the distal tibia and fibula with dislocation of the ankle joint
- *Pathologic:* fracture of the bone weakened by pathologic condition, for example, metastatic bone disease

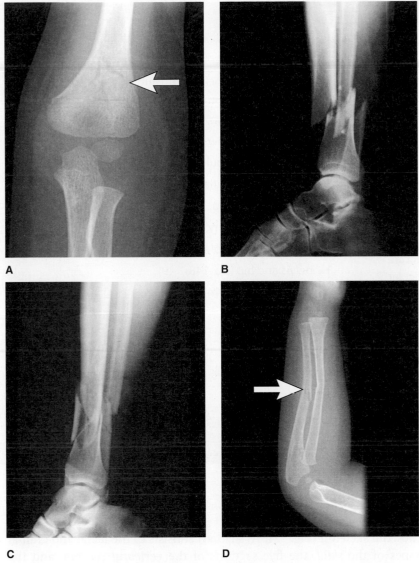

A

B

C

D

Figure 7-41. **(A)** Nondisplaced fracture, **(B)** displaced fracture, **(C)** comminuted fracture, and **(D)** greenstick fracture. (From Saladin K. Anatomy & Physiology: The Unity of Form and Function. 9th ed. New York, NY: McGraw-Hill Education; 2014.)

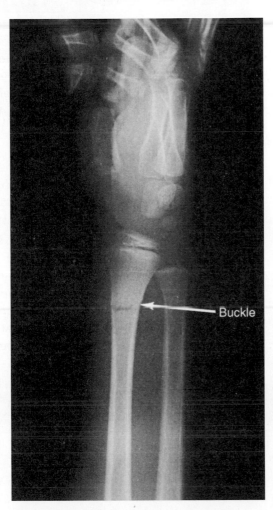

Buckle

Figure 7-42. Torus/buckle-type greenstick fracture. (Reproduced with permission from Simon RS, Koenigsknecht SJ. *Emergency Orthopedics: The Extremities*. 3rd ed. East Norwalk, CT: Appleton & Lange; 1995.)

Congratulations! You have completed a large portion of this chapter. If you are able to answer the following group of very comprehensive questions, you should feel confident that you have really mastered this section. You can refer back to the indicated pages to check your answers and/or review the subject matter.

1. Identify the bony structures composing the appendicular skeleton; be prepared to discuss and answer questions relevant to anatomy and pathology of the appendicular skeleton, bone structure and development, characteristics, and articular classifications.

2. Describe the (a) method of positioning, (b) direction and point of entry of the CR, (c) principal structures visualized, and (d) pertinent traumatic or pathologic conditions and any technical adjustments they may necessitate relative to the appendicular skeleton, including routine and special views of the

   A. hand and wrist (pp. 120–122)
   B. forearm and elbow (pp. 123–124)
   C. humerus and shoulder (p. 125–126)
   D. clavicle and scapula (pp. 127–128)
   E. foot and ankle (pp. 139–143)
   F. lower leg, knee, and patella (pp. 144–146)
   G. femur and long bone measurement (pp. 146–147)
   H. pelvis and hip (pp. 148–149)
   I. arthrography (p. 142, 150)

Neural/Vertebral Arch

Composed of
- Two pedicles
- Two laminae

Encloses
- Vertebral foramen

Supports Seven Processes
- Two superior articular processes
- Two inferior articular processes
- Two transverse processes
- One spinous process

THE AXIAL SKELETON

The axial skeleton (Fig. 7-43A; shaded) consists of the facial and cranial bones of the *skull*, the five sections of the *vertebral column*, and the sternum and ribs of the *thorax*.

Vertebral Column

The vertebral column (Fig. 7-43B) is composed of 33 bones divided into 7 cervical, 12 thoracic, 5 lumbar, 5 (fused) sacral, and 4 (fused) coccygeal regions, with each region having its own characteristic shape. The vertebral bodies gradually increase in size through the lumbar region. The vertebrae are joined by ligaments and cartilage; the first 24 are separate and movable, whereas the last 9 are fixed. *Intervertebral disks* between the vertebral bodies form *amphiarthrotic* joints.

The cervical and lumbar regions form *lordotic* (convex anteriorly) curves; the thoracic and sacral regions form *kyphotic* (convex posteriorly) curves (Fig. 7-43B; lateral). An exaggerated thoracic curve is called *kyphosis* (hunchback); an exaggerated lumbar curve is called *lordosis* (sway-back). Lateral curvature of the vertebral column is called *scoliosis*.

Approximately 1 in 20 children has some degree of deformity of his or her vertebral column. Scoliosis is most often idiopathic (i.e., has no known cause), but a familial tendency is often noted. Scoliosis has female predominance and is not associated with any symptoms of back pain or fatigue. Scoliosis surveys are performed for a number of

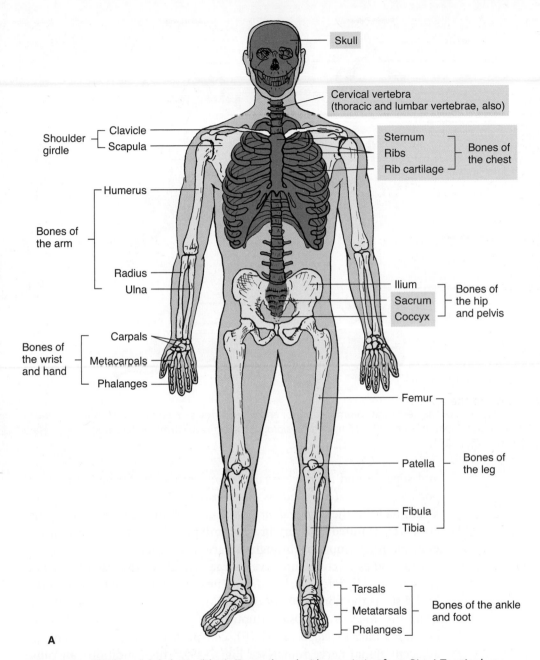

Skull

Cervical vertebra
(thoracic and lumbar vertebrae, also)

Shoulder
girdle
— Clavicle
— Scapula

Sternum
Ribs
Rib cartilage
— Bones of
the chest

Humerus

Bones of
the arm

Radius
Ulna

Ilium
Sacrum
Coccyx
— Bones of
the hip
and pelvis

Bones of
the wrist
and hand
Carpals
Metacarpals
Phalanges

Femur

Patella
— Bones of
the leg

Fibula
Tibia

Tarsals

Metatarsals
— Bones of the ankle
and foot

Phalanges

A

Figure 7-43. **(A)** The axial skeleton (blue). (Reproduced with permission from *Rice J. Terminology With Human Anatomy*. 3rd ed. East Norwalk: Appleton & Lange/McGraw Hill LLC; 1995.) (*continued*)

reasons. They help determine degree of severity and skeletal maturity, too much or progression, and ensure adequacy of treatment.

The typical vertebra has a *body* and a *neural/vertebral arch* surrounding the *vertebral foramen*. The neural arch is composed of two *pedicles*, two laminae that support four articular processes, two transverse processes, and one spinous process. The pedicles are short, thick processes extending back from the posterior aspect of the vertebral body, each one sustaining a *lamina*. The laminae extend posteriorly to the midline and join to form the *spinous process* (lack of union, or malunion, results in *spina bifida*). Each pedicle has notches superiorly and inferiorly (*superior* and *inferior vertebral notches*) that—with adjacent vertebrae—form the *intervertebral foramina*, through which the spinal nerves pass. The neural arch also has lateral *transverse processes* for muscle attachment

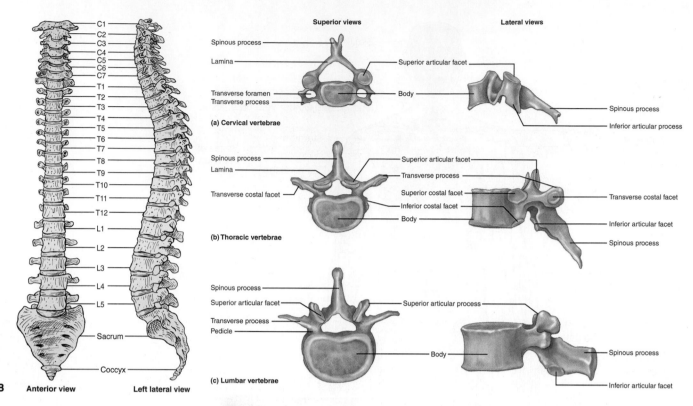

Figure 7-43. (*Continued*) **(B)** AP and lateral views of the vertebral column; superior and lateral views of a typical vertebra from each vertebral section. (Reproduced with permission from Saladin K. *Anatomy and Physiology: The Unity of Form and Function.* 7th ed. New York: McGraw-Hill Education; 2015, Figure 8.25, p. 251.)

Articulation Summary: *Vertebral*

- Occipitoatlantal
- Atlantoaxial
- Costovertebral
- Costotransverse
- Lumbosacral
- Sacroiliac
- Sacrococcygeal
- Intervertebral
- Zygapophyseal/interarticular

and *superior* and *inferior articular processes* for the formation of *zygapophyseal joints* (classified as *diarthrotic*). The consecutive vertebral foramina form the *vertebral, or spinal,* canal—through which the spinal cord is transmitted. The vertebral column permits flexion, extension, lateral, and rotary motions through its various articulations.

The bodies of consecutive vertebrae articulate with each other and are separated by *intervertebral disks.* The outer portion of the intervertebral disks is the fibrous *annulus fibrosus,* which encloses a central portion, the *nucleus pulposus.* Rupture of the intervertebral disk, or *herniated nucleus pulposus* (HNP), can push into the spinal canal or adjacent spinal nerve roots (see Fig. 7-49). This condition can cause back pain and even loss of neurologic function in the areas where the affected spinal nerves are distributed.

Cervical Spine. There are seven cervical vertebrae (Fig. 7-44). The *atlas* (C1) is a ring-shaped bone having no body and no spinous process; it is composed of an *anterior arch and a posterior arch,* two *lateral masses,* and two *transverse processes.*

The anterior arch has a *tubercle* at its midpoint and has a *facet* on its posterior surface for articulation with the anterior portion of the odontoid process/dens. The posterior arch has a tubercle as well. The lateral masses have *superior articular processes* that articulate with the skull at the *atlanto-occipital joint,* where flexion and extension occur. Its lateral masses articulate inferiorly with the *axis* (C2).

The axis (C2) has a superior projection, the *dens,* or *odontoid process.* The axis articulates superiorly with the atlas at the *atlantoaxial joint,* a

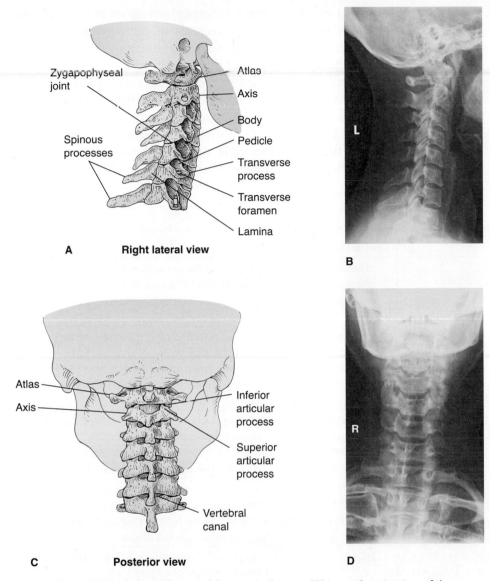

Figure 7-44. (A) Right lateral view of the cervical spine. **(B)** Lateral projection of the cervical spine. (Photo contributor: Conrad P. Ehrlich, MD.) **(C)** Posterior view of the cervical spine. **(D)** AP projection of the cervical spine. (Photo contributor: Conrad P. Ehrlich, MD.)

pivot joint where rotation of the head takes place, and inferiorly with C3 at the zygapophyseal articulation. The dens has a *facet* on its anterior surface for articulation with the posterior aspect of the anterior arch of C1. The spinous process of C2 is particularly large and strong.

The typical cervical vertebra is small and has a *transverse foramen* in each transverse process for passage of the vertebral artery and vein. The cervical laminae are thin and narrow; they meet at midline to form a short spinous process. Cervical spinous processes are almost horizontal and usually *bifid*. The spinous process of C7 (*vertebra prominens*) is not bifid, is larger and more horizontal, and is a useful positioning landmark.

Fractures and/or dislocations of the cervical spine are usually owing to acute *hyperflexion* or *hyperextension* as a result of indirect trauma. *Whiplash* injury is caused by a sudden, forced movement in one direction and then the opposite direction (as in rear-end automobile impacts). Whiplash symptoms frequently include neck pain and stiffness, headache, and pain and numbness of the upper limbs. Whiplash is often evidenced radiographically by straightening or reversal of the normal lordotic curve. Lateral projections of the cervical spine are sometimes performed to evaluate whiplash injury by demonstrating the degree of anterior and posterior motions.

Osteoarthritis is characterized in the cervical and lumbar spine by chronic, progressive degeneration of cartilage and *hypertrophy* of bone along the articular margins, characterized radiographically by narrowed joint spaces, and *osteophytes*. Osteoarthritis is often observable in the articulations of the fingers, toes, hips, and knees as well.

Table 7-23 provides a summary of positions/projections of the cervical spine.

TABLE 7-23. Cervical Spine

Cervical Spine	Position of Part	Central Ray Directed	Structures Included/Best Seen
AP axial	· Supine or erect · MSP ⊥ IR · Adjust flexion so the mastoid tip and occlusal plane are aligned	· 15°–20° cephalad to thyroid cartilage	· AP of *lower five* cervical vertebrae and intervertebral disk spaces
AP open mouth/ *atlas and axis*	· Supine or erect · MSP ⊥ IR · Mouth open, adjust flexion, so the mastoid tips and upper occlusal plane are aligned ⊥ IR (‖ CR)	· ⊥ Center of the opened mouth	· AP proj of C1 and C2 (Fig. 7-45A) and their articulations · *Too much flexion* superimposes teeth on odontoid · *Too much extension* superimposes base of the skull on odontoid
AP dens (*Fuchs*)	· Supine · MSP ⊥ IR · MML ⊥ to IR (as close as possible), angles of mandible equidistant to IR	· Angled as needed to bring ‖ to MML · Centered to IR	· AP proj of dens, C1, and C2 (Fig. 7-45A) and their articulations · *Must not be attempted if upper cervical fx or degenerative disease is suspected*
Note: If the upper portion of the odontoid process is not seen, PA (Judd) proj may be attempted *if upper cervical fx or degenerative disease is not suspected.* The PA is similar to a Waters position. The odontoid is seen projected within the foramen magnum. *Because extension of the neck is required, this position must not be attempted if upper cervical fx or degenerative disease is suspected.*			
Lat	· Erect w/ L side adjacent to IR · Chin slightly elevated, shoulders depressed · MSP ‖ IR · Centered at the level of C4; just dist to mastoid tip	· ⊥ C4	· Lat proj all seven vertebrae (Fig. 7-45B) · Shows intervertebral jt spaces, zygapophyseal jts, spinous processes, bodies · Owing to unavoidable OID, a 72″ SID should be used
Lat flexion and extension	· Erect w/ L side adjacent to IR · MSP ‖ IR · Flexion: depress chin as much as possible · Extension: elevate chin as much as possible	· ⊥ C4	· Lat proj in flexion and/or extension (Fig 7-46) · Shows intervertebral jt spaces, zygapophyseal jts, spinous processes, bodies · Owing to unavoidable OID, a 72″ SID should be used · *Often used in cases of whiplash injury*
Cross-table (horizontal beam) lat	· Supine w/ L side adjacent to IR · Do not manipulate head or neck · Do not remove cervical collar If present · MSP ‖ IR, as close as possible w/o manipulation · Must be performed as the first radiograph for patients with *trauma* or suspected *subluxation*	· ⊥ C4 · ⊥ IR	· Lat proj all seven vertebrae (Fig. 7-45B) · Shows intervertebral jt spaces, zygapophyseal jts, spinous processes, bodies · Owing to unavoidable OID, a 72″ SID should be used if possible

TABLE 7-23. Cervical Spine—Cont'd

Cervical Spine	Position of Part	Central Ray Directed	Structures Included/Best Seen
PA axial obls (*LAO and RAO*)	· PA erect, MSP 45° to IR · Centered to C4 (upper margin of the thyroid cartilage) · Chin slightly raised	· 15°–20° caudad to the center of the IR	· Obl cervical · Best view of intervertebral foramina *closest* to the IR
AP axial obls (*LPO and RPO*)	· AP erect, MSP 45° to IR · Centered to C4 (upper margin of the thyroid cartilage) · Chin slightly raised	· 15°–20° cephalad to the center of the IR/C4	· Obl cervical · Best view of intervertebral foramina *farthest* from the IR
Note: Axial obl cervical spine proj may be performed in the *recumbent position* on patients whose trauma prohibits movement.			
Lat cervicothoracic/ *swimmer's*	· Erect or recumbent lat · *Midaxillary line* centered to the IR, MSP ∥ IR · Arm adjacent to the IR over the head · Depress opposite shoulder farthest from the IR	· ⊥ T2	· Lat proj of the lower cervical and upper thoracic vertebrae · Particularly useful for individuals with broad shoulders

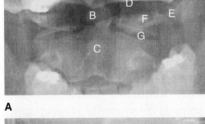
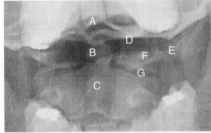
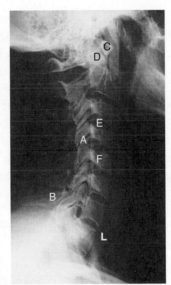
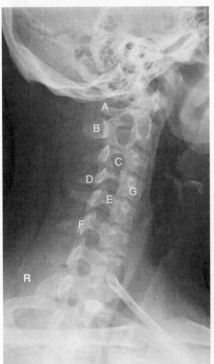

Figure 7-45. (A) Open-mouth projection of C1–C2. Locate and identify the bony structures shown particularly well in this projection. A, occlusal plane/maxillary incisors; B, odontoid process/dens; C, body, C2/axis; D, base of skull; E, transverse process, C1; F, body, C1; G, atlantoaxial articulation. **(B)** Lateral projection of the cervical spine. A, zygapophyseal articulation; B, spinous process C7/vertebra prominens; C, tubercle of anterior arch, C1; D, odontoid process/dens; E, intervertebral joint/disk space; F, vertebral body, C5. **(C)** An RPO cervical spine. Locate and identify the bony structures shown particularly well in each projection. A, posterior arch, C1; B, spinous process, C2; C, intervertebral foramen, C3; D, spinous process, C4; E, pedicle, C5; F, transverse process, C4; G, body, C4. (Photo contributor: Conrad P. Ehrlich, MD.)

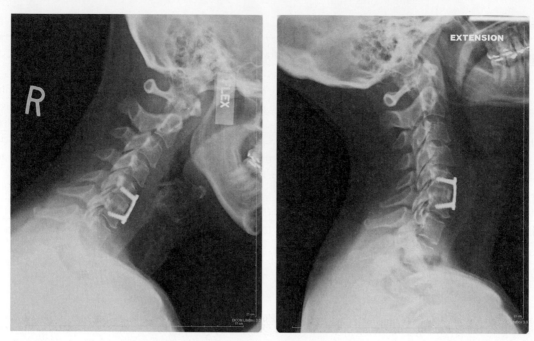

Figure 7-46. Lateral projections of the cervical spine in flexion and extension—used to demonstrate degree of anterior and posterior motion. (Photo contributor: Conrad P. Ehrlich, MD.)

Thoracic Spine. There are 12 thoracic vertebrae, which are larger in size than cervical vertebrae and which increase in size as they progress inferiorly toward the lumbar region. Thoracic spinous processes are fairly long and sharply angled caudally (T8 usually has the longest vertical spinous process). The bodies and transverse processes have *articular facets* for the *diarthrotic* rib articulations (Fig. 7-47).

A common metabolic bone disorder frequently noted in radiographic examinations of the thoracic spine is osteoporosis. *Osteoporosis* is characterized by bone demineralization and can result in compression fractures of the vertebrae. The condition is most common in sedentary and postmenopausal women.

Table 7-24 provides a summary of positions/projections of the thoracic spine.

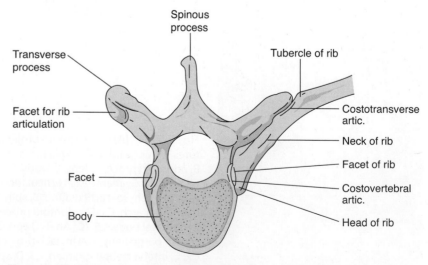

Figure 7-47. Thoracic vertebra and its articulation with the rib (superior view).

TABLE 7-24. The Thoracic Spine

Thoracic Spine	Position of Part	Central Ray Directed	Structures Included/Best Seen
AP	· Supine, MSP ⊥ tabletop/IR · Top of IR 1″ above shoulders	· ⊥ T7	· AP proj of the thoracic vertebrae and intervertebral spaces · It is helpful to use the anode heel effect and/or compensating filtration to provide more uniform density (see Fig. 7-48A)
Note: To demonstrate *zygapophyseal jts, 70° obl images* are obtained.			
Lat, breathing	· L lat recumbent · Midaxillary line centered to the table · Arms ⊥ long axis of the body · Top of IR 1″ above shoulders · Utilize orthostatic breathing technique to blur ribs and lung markings; use 2–3 s exposure	· 5°–15° cephalad (⊥ long axis of the spine)	· Lat proj of thoracic vertebrae · Especially bodies, intervertebral spaces and foramina (see Fig. 7-48B)
Lat, expiration	· L lat recumbent · Midaxillary line centered to the table · Arms ⊥ long axis of the body · Top of IR 1″ above shoulders · Take exposure on suspended full inspiration for uniform density of vertebrae above diaphragm	· 5°–15° cephalad (⊥ long axis of the spine)	· Lat proj of thoracic vertebrae · Especially bodies, intervertebral spaces and foramina (see Fig. 7-48B)

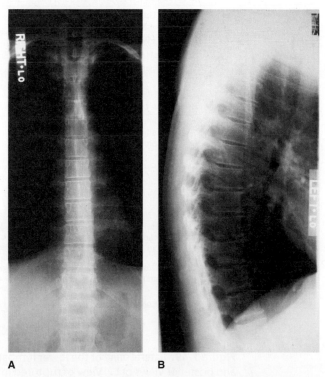

A   B

Figure 7-48. **(A)** AP projection of the thoracic spine. Note density difference between upper and lower spine; this can be improved by using the anode heel effect to advantage (placing cathode over lower spine). **(B)** Lateral projection of thoracic spine. "Breathing technique" has helped blur pulmonary vascular markings and provided good visualization of nearly all the thoracic vertebrae. (Photo contributor: Stamford Hospital, Department of Radiology.)

Lumbar Spine. The five lumbar vertebrae are the largest of the vertebral column and increase in size toward the sacral region. The spinous processes are short and horizontal and serve as an attachment for strong muscles (Fig. 7-49). The causes of lumbar pain are numerous, including trauma, fracture, spasm of the paralumbar muscles, herniated intervertebral disk, and osteoarthritis.

Some of the disorders that can be detected radiographically include *osteoarthritis, spondylolysis, spondylolisthesis,* and *ankylosing spondylitis.* Myelography and especially MRI are used to evaluate *herniated intervertebral disks.*

Transitional vertebrae occur at the junction between spinal sections. The lumbar and sacral areas of the vertebral column are the sections most commonly associated with transitional vertebrae. *Lumbarization* is the assimilation of S1 into what appears to be L6.

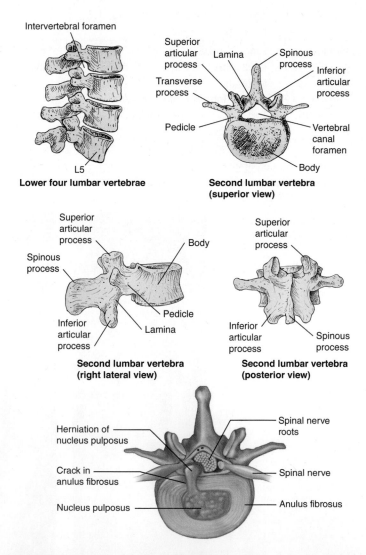

Figure 7-49. Lateral view of the lower lumbar vertebrae. Superior, right lateral, and posterior views of L2. View of ruptured intervertebral disk, or *HNP,* can push into the spinal canal or adjacent spinal nerve roots. HNP can cause back pain and loss of neurologic function. (Lowermost figure: Reproduced with permission from Saladin K. *Anatomy and Physiology: The Unity of Form and Function.* 7th ed. New York : McGraw-Hill Education; 2015.)

Sacralization, more common than lumbarization, is the assimilation of L5 to the sacrum.

Table 7-25 provides a summary of positions/projections of the lumbar spine.

Sacrum. There are five fused sacral vertebrae (Fig. 7-53A); the fused *transverse processes* form the *alae.* The anterior and posterior *sacral foramina* transmit spinal nerves. The *sacrum* articulates superiorly with the fifth lumbar vertebra, forming the L5–S1 articulation, and inferiorly with the *coccyx* to form the *sacrococcygeal joint.*

Tables 7-26 through 7-28 provide a summary of positions/projections of the sacrum, SI joints, coccyx, and scoliosis series.

TABLE 7-25. The Lumbar Spine

Lumbar Spine	Position of Part	Central Ray Directed	Structures Included/Best Seen
AP (or PA)	· Supine, MSP ⊥ tabletop · Knees flexed, feet flat on the table	· ⊥ L3	· AP proj of lumbar vertebrae L1–L4 · Intervertebral spaces, transverse processes · *Flexion of the knees reduces lumbar curve and OID (see Fig. 7-50)*
Note: The *AP proj* of the lumbar spine is most comfortable for very thin patients and those with low back pain. The *PA proj* has the advantages of delivering lower gonadal dose and of placing the intervertebral jts more closely ‖ with the divergent x-ray beam.			
AP axial L5–S1	· Supine, MSP ⊥ tabletop · Legs extended	· To MSP at 30°–35° cephalad to MSP, ≈1½″ above the pubic symphysis	· AP of lumbosacral articulation not seen on AP lumbar
AP obl proj (*RPO and LPO*)	· AP recumbent · Obl 45° w/ the spine centered to the IR	· ⊥ L3	· Obl proj of lumbar vertebrae (see Fig. 7-51) · Especially for zygapophyseal articulations (L1–L4) of the side *adjacent* to the IR
PA obl proj (*RAO and LAO*)	· PA recumbent · Obl 45° w/ the spine centered to the IR	· ⊥ L3	· Obl proj of lumbar vertebrae (see Fig. 7-51) · Especially for zygapophyseal articulations (L1–L4) of the side *farthest* from the IR
Note: This proj demonstrates the characteristic "Scotty dog" (see Fig. 7-51).			
Note: L5–S1 zygapophyseal articulations shown in 35° obl.			
Lat	· L lat recumbent · Midcoronal line centered to the IR	· 5°–8° caudad to L3	· Lat proj · Especially for vertebral bodies, interspaces, intervertebral foramina, spinous processes · *If MSP adjusted ‖ tabletop, CR is vertical (Fig. 7-52A)*
Note: Lat lumbar spine in flexion and extension and/or AP with R and L bending are often used to demonstrate the presence or absence of motion in area(s) of spinal fusion.			
Lat (L5–S1)	· L lat recumbent · Center MCP to the IR · Adjust MSP ‖ tabletop	· CR ⊥ IR 1½″ inferior to the crest and 2″ posterior to the ASIS	· Lat proj L5–S1 · *If MSP not adjusted ‖ tabletop, CR is ∠5°–8° caudad (Fig. 7-52B)*
AP right and left bending	· Erect or recumbent · MSP ⊥ IR · Bottom edge of IR 1″–2″ below iliac crest · Patient bent laterally as far as possible	· CR ⊥ IR · CR centered to IR	· Demonstrates thoracic and lumbar vertebrae in lat bending positions · 1″–2″ of iliac crests

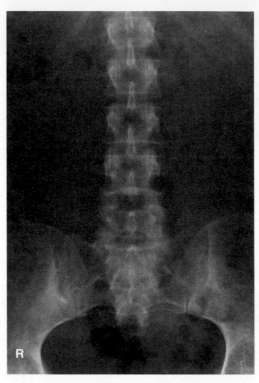

Figure 7-50. AP projection of the lumbar spine. Flexion of the knees reduces the lumbar curve and OID and relieves strain on lower back muscles; patients are most comfortable with sponge or pillow support placed under knees. (Photo contributor: Stamford Hospital, Department of Radiology.)

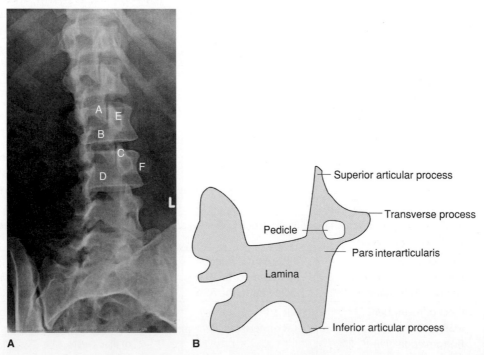

A   **B**

Figure 7-51. Oblique lumbar spine **(A)**, illustrating the lumbar zygapophyseal joints. Anatomy corresponds to "Scotty dog" seen in **(B)**. Structures seen in panel A are as follows: Scotty's "ear" (C) corresponds to the *superior articular process,* its "nose" to the *transverse process* (F), its "eye" is the *pedicle* (E), its "neck" the *pars interarticularis* (B), its "body" is the *lamina* (D), and its "front leg" is the *inferior articular process* (A). (Photo contributor: Stamford Hospital, Department of Radiology.)

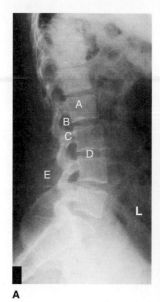

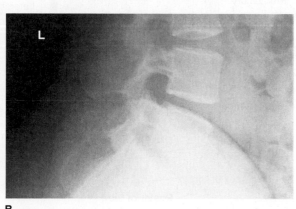

Figure 7-52. (A) Lateral projection of the lumbar spine. If MSP is adjusted parallel to tabletop, CR angulation is unnecessary. A, body, L2; B, intervertebral foramen; C, pedicle; D, intervertebral disk space; E, spinous process, L4. **(B)** Lateral projection L5–S1. (Photo contributor: Stamford Hospital, Department of Radiology.)

TABLE 7-26. The Sacrum and Coccyx

Sacrum and Coccyx	Position of Part	Central Ray Directed	Structures Included/Best Seen
AP axial sacrum	· AP supine · MSP ⊥ tabletop	· 15° cephalad to the midline to point 2″ superior to the pubic symphysis	· AP proj of the sacrum · CR ‖ the sacral curve providing less distorted visualization (see Fig. 7-53B)
AP axial coccyx	· AP supine · MSP ⊥ tabletop	· 10 caudad to the midline to point 2″ above the pubic symphysis	· AP proj of the coccyx · CR ‖ the coccygeal curve providing less distorted visualization (see Fig. 7-53C)
Lat sacrum or coccyx, separate	· L lat recumbent · Knees flexed for support	· Sacrum: ⊥ a point 3″–4″ posterior to the ASIS · Coccyx: ⊥ a point 3″–4″ posterior and 2″ dist to the ASIS	· Sacrum: Lat proj of the sacrum · Coccyx: Lat proj of coccyx and its articulation with the sacrum
Lat sacrum and coccyx, combined	· L lat recumbent · Knees flexed for support	· ⊥ a point 3″–4″ posterior to the upper ASIS, centered to the IR	· Lat proj of the sacrum and coccyx in their entirety

TABLE 7-27. The Sacroiliac Joints

Sacroiliac Jts	Position of Part	Central Ray Directed	Structures Included/Best Seen
AP axial	· Supine, MSP centered	· 30°–35° cephalad, to the midline ~2″ below the level of ASIS	· Sacrum, SI jts, and L5–S1 articulation
AP obl proj *(LPO and RPO)*	· Supine · Obliqued 25°–30° *affected side up* · Sagittal plane passing 1″ medial to the ASIS centered to the IR	· ⊥ a point 1″ medial to ASIS	· SI jt of the elevated side · Opposite obl is similarly obtained; SI jt is placed ⊥ IR (see Fig. 7-38A and B)
PA obl proj *(LAO and RAO)*	· Prone · Obliqued 25°–30° *affected side down* · Sagittal plane passing 1⊥ medial to the ASIS centered to the IR	· ⊥ a point 1″ medial to the ASIS	· SI jt of the "down" side · Opposite obl is similarly obtained; SI jt is placed ⊥ IR—35° cephalad

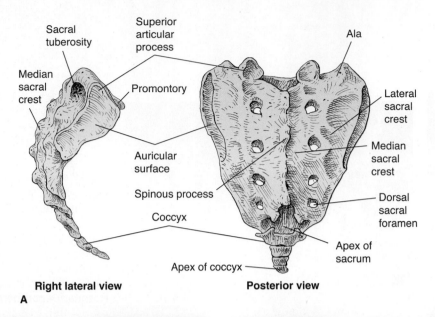

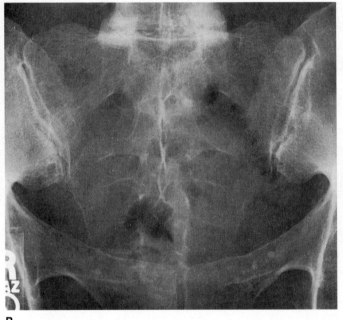

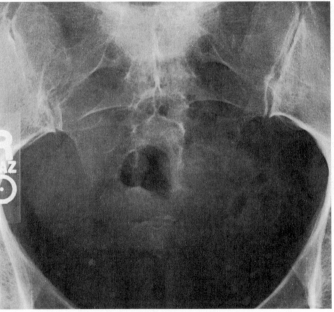

Figure 7-53. (A) Sacrum and coccyx. **(B)** AP projection of the sacrum. Cephalad angulation "opens" the sacral foramina. **(C)** AP projection of the coccyx. Caudal angulation "opens" the coccygeal curve. (Photo contributor: Stamford Hospital, Department of Radiology.)

Coccyx (See Table 7-26). There are four or five fused coccygeal vertebrae (see Fig. 7-53A). Fracture of the coccyx usually results from a fall onto it, landing in a seated position. Fracture displacement is fairly common and occasionally requires removal of the fractured fragment to relieve the painful symptoms.

Scoliosis Series. See Table 7-28 for positioning for a scoliosis series.

Thorax

Sternum and Sternoclavicular Joints (See Tables 7-29 and 7-30). The bones of the *thorax* (sternum, ribs, and thoracic vertebrae; Fig. 7-56) function to protect the heart, lungs, and major blood vessels. Minor trauma to

Articulation Summary: *Thorax*

- Sternoclavicular
- Sternochondral
- Costochondral
- Costovertebral
- Costotransverse

TABLE 7-28. Scoliosis Series

Scoliosis Series	Position of Part	Central Ray Directed	Structures Included/Best Seen

PA bending	· 14" × 17" or 14" × 36" IR
	· Vertebrae to include 1" of the iliac crest/L5–S1
	· Four exposures made:
	  · PA recumbent
	  · PA erect
	  · PA bending L
	  · PA bending R
		· ⊥ center of IR	· Radiation dose is reduced when gonadal, breast, and thyroid shields are used and when examination is performed PA rather than AP (Fig. 7-54)

PA or AP (Ferguson method)	· 14" × 17" or 14" × 36" IR · Vertebrae to include 1"–2" of the iliac crest/L5–S1 · Patient in AP or PA position against Bucky or IR	· ⊥ center of the IR	· Clear visualization of thoracic and lumbar vertebrae In AP or PA · Protective shielding is recommended
Lat	· 14" × 17" or 14" × 36" IR · Vertebrae to include 1"–2" of the iliac crest/L5–S1 · Patient in left lat position	· ⊥ center of the IR	· Clear visualization of thoracic and lumbar vertebrae in lat position · Protective shielding utilize is recommended

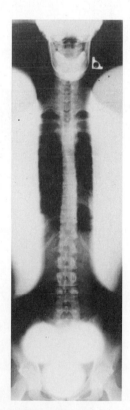

Figure 7-54. AP scoliosis series with protective shielding in place. (Photo contributor: Nuclear Associates.)

TABLE 7-29. The Sternum

Sternum	Position of Part	Central Ray Directed	Structures Included/Best Seen
PA Obl proj (RAO position)	· 15°–20° RAO position · Greater obliquity for thin patients · Sternum centered to the midline of the table/grid	· ⊥ Midsternum	· Sternum visualized in RAO position · Projects sternum into heart shadow for *uniform exposure*
Note: A long exposure can be used during quiet breathing to blur pulmonary vascular markings, or exposure can be made on expiration (Fig. 7-55).			
Lat	· Erect L lat · Shoulders rolled back · MSP vertical · IR top 1.5″ above the manubrial notch	· ⊥ Midsternum	· Lat proj of the sternum free of superimposition of ribs · Exposure made on deep inspiration to move the sternum away from ribs

TABLE 7-30. The Sternoclavicular Joints

Sternoclavicular Joints	Position of Part	Central Ray Directed	Structures Included/Best Seen
PA	· Prone, MSP centered to the IR · IR centered at T3 (suprasternal notch)	· ⊥ T3	· Bilateral PA proj of sternoclavicular jts visualized through superimposed vertebrae and ribs
PA Obl proj (*LAO and RAO positions*)	· Prone, MSP centered to the IR · Rotate ≈15° *affected side down*	· ⊥ Affected jt	· Obl proj of the sternoclavicular jt *closest to the IR* · Similar results obtained w/ ⊥ MSP and CR ∠15° toward midline from the affected side

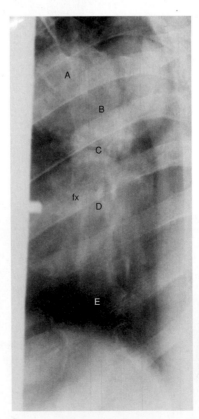
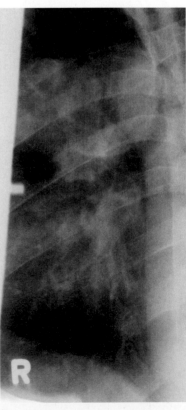

Figure 7-55. (A) RAO sternum. A, medial extremity of clavicle; B, manubrium; C, sternal angle; D, body/gladiolus; E, xyphoid process; fracture (fx) site of the displaced fracture. "Breathing technique" helps blur superimposed structures and permits improved visualization of the bony sternum. **(B)** RAO of the same sternum, exposed on suspended respiration. (Photo contributor: David Sack, BS, RT(R), CRA, FAHRA.)

A   B

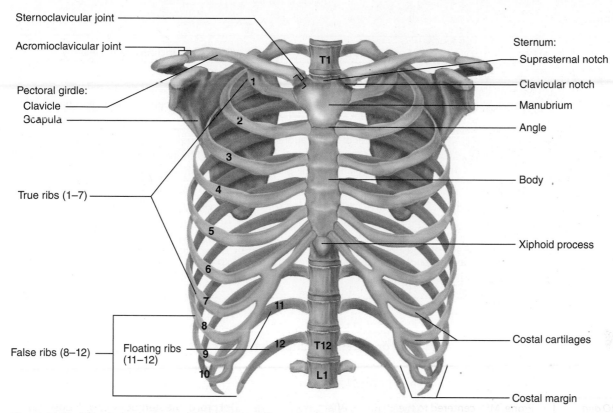

Figure 7-56. The thoracic cage and pectoral girdle, anterior aspect. (Reproduced with permission from Saladin K. *Anatomy and Physiology: The Unity of Form and Function*. 7th ed. New York : McGraw-Hill Education; 2015.)

the thorax can result in uncomplicated lacerations, contusions, or simple rib fracture. However, more significant trauma, such as those often associated with MVAs, can have more serious consequences as a result of numerous rib fractures causing injury to the mediastinum, pleural cavity, and/or heart and great blood vessels. The *sternum* forms the anterior central portion of the thorax and is composed of three major divisions: the *manubrium, body,* and *xiphoid process.* The articulation between the manubrium and the body is the *sternal angle* (angle of Louis), which coincides with the location of the second rib. Sternal fractures are uncommon; when they do occur, fracture displacement is rare but the possibility of traumatic injury to the heart must still be considered.

Ribs (See Table 7-31). The *rib cage* (see Fig. 7-56) consists of 12 pairs of ribs. Ribs 1–7 articulate with thoracic vertebrae and the sternum and are called *vertebrosternal* or "true" ribs. The first pair of ribs lies under the clavicles and is not palpable; the remaining 11 pairs of ribs are usually palpable. Ribs 8–10 articulate with thoracic vertebrae and the superjacent costal cartilage to form the *anterior costal margin* and are called *vertebrochondral* or *false ribs.* The last two pairs of false ribs articulate only with thoracic vertebrae and are called *floating ribs.* The lower edge of the rib cage forms the *inferior costal margin.* The spaces between the ribs are called *intercostal spaces* and are occupied by two sets of intercostal muscles.

Rib fractures are a common injury in thoracic trauma owing to their relative thinness and exposed position. Their fracture may be

Radiographically Significant Skeletal Disorders and Conditions of the Axial Skeleton

Achondroplasia

Ankylosing spondylitis

Cervical rib

Degenerative disk disease

Flail chest

Herniated disk

Hydrocephalus

Kyphosis

Lordosis

Osteophyte

Osteoporosis

Pectus excavatum

Scoliosis

Spina bifida

Spondylolisthesis

Spondylolysis

Transitional vertebra

Whiplash

TABLE 7-31. The Ribs

Ribs	Position of Part	Central Ray Directed	Structures Included/Best Seen
AP or PA, above and below diaphragm	· Recumbent or erect AP or PA · MSP ⊥ midline of the table · Top of IR 1″ above the shoulder	· ⊥ Center of the IR, about the level of T7	· AP or PA proj · Upper posterior ribs best delineated · Do PA for better detail of anterior ribs
PA obl projs (*LAO, RAO*)	· Prone or erect PA · Rotate 45°, *unaffected side down*	· ⊥ Center of the IR, about the level of T7 (at T10–T12 for below-diaphragm ribs)	· Obl shows *axillary* portions of ribs · RAO shows left ribs · LAO shows right ribs
AP obl projection (*LPO, RPO position*)	· Supine or erect AP · Rotate to 45° affected side toward the IR	· ⊥ Center of the IR, about the level of T7 (at T10–T12 for below-diaphragm ribs)	· LPO shows *left* posterior ribs and their axillary portions · RPO shows *right* posterior ribs and their axillary portions

Note: Above-diaphragm ribs are exposed on deep *inspiration* or during quiet breathing (long exposure). *Below-diaphragm* ribs are best demonstrated when exposed on *complete expiration.*

complicated by *pneumothorax, hemothorax,* liver laceration (right lower ribs), or spleen laceration (left lower ribs).

Head and Neck

Skull. The *skull* has two major parts: the *cranium,* which is composed of 8 bones and houses the brain, and the 14 irregularly shaped *facial bones* (Figs. 7-57 and 7-58). The eight cranial bones are the paired *parietal* and *temporal* bones and the unpaired *frontal, occipital, ethmoid,* and *sphenoid* bones. The 14 facial bones include the paired *nasal, lacrimal, palatine, inferior nasal conchae, maxillae,* and *zygomatic* bones and the unpaired *vomer* and *mandible.*

The average-shaped skull is termed *mesocephalic* (petrous pyramids and midsagittal plane [MSP] form an angle of ≈47°), the broad skull is termed *brachycephalic* (petrous pyramids and MSP form an angle of ≈54°), and the elongated skull is termed *dolichocephalic* (petrous pyramids and MSP form an angle of ≈40°). These deviations are readily observable in axial CT scan and magnetic resonance images. The inner and outer compact tables of the skull are separated by cancellous tissue called *diploë.* The internal table has a number of branching *meningeal grooves* and larger *sulci* that house blood vessels.

The bones of the skull are separated by immovable (*synarthrotic*) joints called *sutures.* The major sutures of the cranium are the *sagittal,* which separates the parietal bones; the *coronal,* which separates the frontal and parietal bones; the *lambdoidal,* which separates the parietal and occipital bones; and the *squamosal,* which separates the temporal and parietal bones (see Figs. 7-57 and 7-58). The articular surfaces of these bones have serrated edges with small projecting bones called *wormian* bones that fit together to form the articular sutures.

The sagittal and coronal sutures meet at the *bregma,* which corresponds to the fetal anterior fontanel. The sagittal and lambdoidal sutures meet posteriorly at the *lambda,* which corresponds to the fetal posterior fontanel. The parietal, frontal, and sphenoid bones meet at the *pterion* (see Fig. 7-57), the location of the anterolateral fontanel. The highest point of the skull is called the *vertex.*

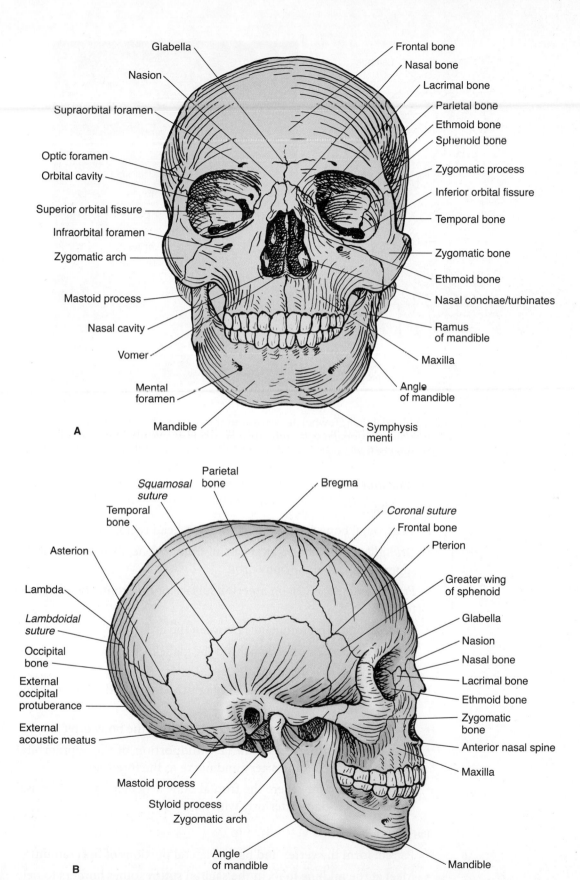

Figure 7-57. **(A)** Anterior view of the skull, labeled. **(B)** Lateral view of the skull, labeled.

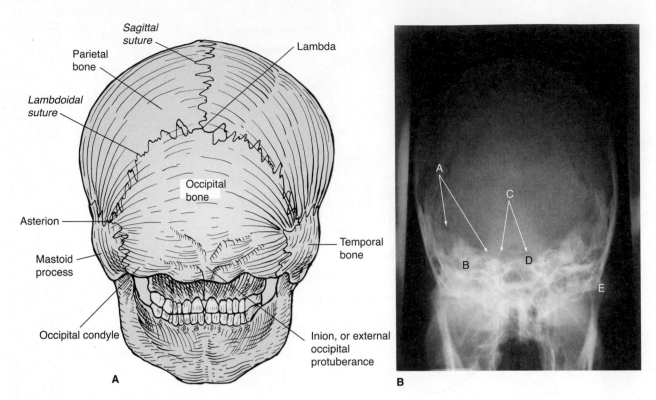

Figure 7-58. (A) Posterior view of the skull, labeled. **(B)** AP axial skull (Towne) demonstrates the occipital bone. A, petrous ridge; B, petrous portion of the temporal bone; C, foramen magnum; D, dorsum sella and posterior clinoid processes; E, mandibular condyle. (Photo contributor: Stamford Hospital, Department of Radiology.)

Cranial Bones (8)

Frontal (1)

Parietal (2)

Temporal (2)

Occipital (1)

Ethmoid (1)

Sphenoid (1)

Cranial Bones

Frontal Bone

- The frontal bone corresponds to the forehead region (Fig. 7-57).
- *Orbital plates* (2): horizontal part of frontal bone; forms much of the superior aspect of the bony orbit
- *Frontal eminences* (2): on anterior surface of the frontal bone, lateral to MSP
- *Glabella:* smooth prominence between the eyebrows
- *Frontal sinuses* (2): directly behind the glabella, between the tables of the skull
- *Superciliary arches/ridges* (2): ridge of the bone under the eyebrow region
- *Supraorbital margins* (2): upper border/rim of the bony orbit
- *Supraorbital notches/foramina* (2): midportion of the supraorbital margin; passage for the artery and nerve to the forehead
- *Frontonasal suture:* where the frontal bone articulates with the nasal bones (corresponds exteriorly with *nasion*)

Parietal Bones

- Paired; form the vertex and part of lateral portions of the cranium
- Meet at the midline to form the sagittal suture; other borders to help form coronal, squamosal, and lambdoidal sutures (Fig. 7-58)
- *Parietal eminences:* rounded prominence on the lateral surface of each parietal bone

Ethmoid Bone

- Located between the orbits; helps form parts of the nasal and orbital walls (see Figs. 7-57 and 7-59)
- *Cribriform plate:* porous, passage for olfactory nerves; horizontal portion between orbital plates of the frontal bone
- *Crista galli:* extends superiorly from the midportion of the cribriform plate
- *Perpendicular plate:* extends downward from crista galli to form the major portion of the nasal septum
- *Superior and middle nasal turbinates/conchae:* cartilaginous; within nasal cavity, attached to the perpendicular plate
- *Ethmoidal labyrinths/lateral masses:* help form the medial wall of the orbit; ethmoidal sinuses within

Sphenoid Bone

- Wedge- or bat-shaped bone located between the frontal and occipital bones (Figs. 7-59–7-61)
- Anchor for eight cranial bones
- Forms small part of the lateral cranial wall and part of the skull base
- Consists of body, two lesser wings, two greater wings, two pterygoid plates/processes, and hamuli

---

Types of Fractures

Linear fracture

A skull fx, straight and sharply defined

Depressed fracture

A comminuted skull fx, with one or more portions pushed inward

Hangman fracture

Fx of C2 with anterior subluxation of C2 on C3; result of forceful hyperextension

Compression fracture

Especially of spongy (cancellous) bone; diminished thickness or width as a result of compression-type force (e.g., vertebral body)

Blowout fracture

Fx of the orbital floor as a result of a direct blow

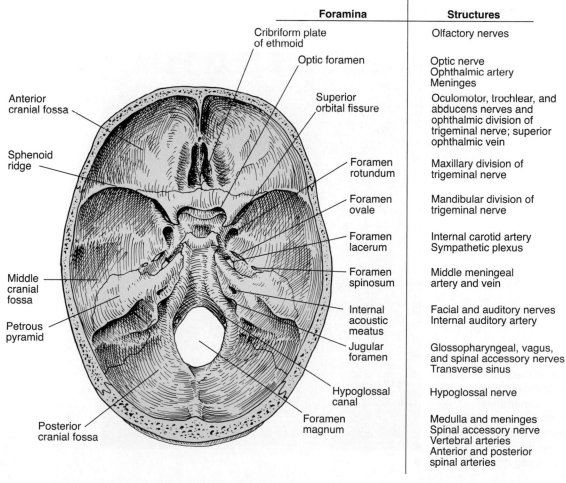

Foramina	Structures
Cribriform plate of ethmoid	Olfactory nerves
Optic foramen	Optic nerve Ophthalmic artery Meninges
Superior orbital fissure	Oculomotor, trochlear, and abducens nerves and ophthalmic division of trigeminal nerve; superior ophthalmic vein
Foramen rotundum	Maxillary division of trigeminal nerve
Foramen ovale	Mandibular division of trigeminal nerve
Foramen lacerum	Internal carotid artery Sympathetic plexus
Foramen spinosum	Middle meningeal artery and vein
Internal acoustic meatus	Facial and auditory nerves Internal auditory artery
Jugular foramen	Glossopharyngeal, vagus, and spinal accessory nerves Transverse sinus
Hypoglossal canal	Hypoglossal nerve
Foramen magnum	Medulla and meninges Spinal accessory nerve Vertebral arteries Anterior and posterior spinal arteries

Labels on figure: Anterior cranial fossa, Sphenoid ridge, Middle cranial fossa, Petrous pyramid, Posterior cranial fossa

Figure 7-59. Base of the skull showing the fossae and principal foramina (superior view).

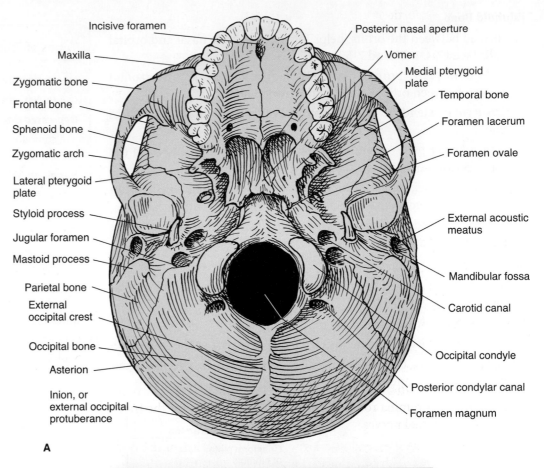

Incisive foramen

Maxilla

Zygomatic bone

Frontal bone

Sphenoid bone

Zygomatic arch

Lateral pterygoid plate

Styloid process

Jugular foramen

Mastoid process

Parietal bone

External occipital crest

Occipital bone

Asterion

Inion, or external occipital protuberance

Posterior nasal aperture

Vomer

Medial pterygoid plate

Temporal bone

Foramen lacerum

Foramen ovale

External acoustic meatus

Mandibular fossa

Carotid canal

Occipital condyle

Posterior condylar canal

Foramen magnum

A

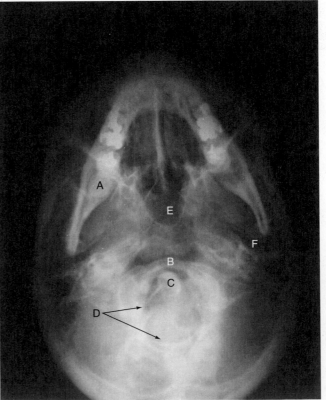

Figure 7-60. (A) Basal view of the skull (external aspect, inferior view). **(B)** SMV skull demonstrates the base of the skull. A, mandible; B, anterior arch, C1; C, odontoid process/dens; D, foramen magnum; E, sphenoid sinuses; F, auditory canal. (Photo contributor: Stamford Hospital, Department of Radiology.)

B

- *Body:* central portion; midline of the skull base; anterior part joins the ethmoid bone; contains the two sphenoid sinuses

- *Lesser (minor) wings:* anterior portion, articulate with orbital plates; contain optic canals for the passage of optic nerves and ophthalmic arteries

- *Anterior clinoid processes:* formed by the medial aspect of lesser wings

- *Tuberculum sellae:* ridge of the bone between anterior clinoid processes; anterior boundary of sella turcica

- *Optic (chiasmic) groove:* horizontal depression crossing the body of bone in front of sella turcica, where optic nerves cross

- *Optic foramen and canal:* passage for the optic nerve and ophthalmic artery at the orbit's apex

- *Sella turcica:* deep depression in the sphenoid bone; houses the pituitary gland

- *Dorsum sellae:* posterior boundary/wall of sella turcica

- *Posterior clinoid processes:* extend laterally from dorsum sellae

- *Clivus:* basilar portion; slopes down and posteriorly from dorsum sellae; articulates with basilar portion of the occipital bone

- *Superior orbital fissures:* large spaces between the greater and lesser wings; for passage of four cranial nerves

- *Greater (major) wings:* larger, posterior portion of the sphenoid bone; contains the foramina rotundum, ovale, and spinosum for the transmission of cranial nerves

- *Pterygoid processes:* extend inferiorly from the junction of the body with great wing; each has a medial and lateral *plate* that articulates with the posterior part of adjacent maxillae

- *Inferior orbital fissures:* large openings, lie between the greater wings and the maxilla

Occipital Bone

- Forms part of the posterior wall and the inferior part of the cranium (see Figs. 7-58A and B and 7-59)

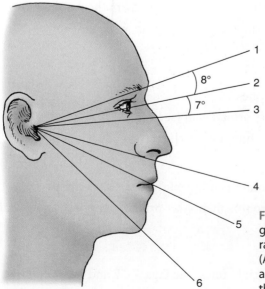

Figure 7-61. Four fundamental baselines used in skull radiography: 1, the glabellomeatal (GML); 2, the orbitomeatal (OML) (also known as canthomeatal or radiographic baseline); 3, the infraorbitomeatal (IOML); 4, the acanthiomeatal (AML); 5, the lips-meatal line (LML); and 6, the mentomeatal line (MML). There is approximately a 7° difference between the OML and the IOML and an 8° between the OML and the GML.

Facial Bones (14)

Nasal (2)

Lacrimal (smallest) (2)

Palatine (2)

Inferior nasal conchae (2)

Zygomatic/malar (2)

Maxillae (2)

Vomer (1)

Mandible (largest; only movable) (1)

- Upper portion of each side articulates with parietal bones to form the lambdoidal suture
- *Basilar portion:* articulates anteriorly with basilar portion (clivus) of the sphenoid bone
- *Lateral portions* (2): bilateral to foramen magnum; occipital condyles, hypoglossal canals, and jugular foramina located here
- *Foramen magnum:* large opening; transmits inferior portion of the brain (medulla oblongata), which is continuous with the spinal cord
- *Squamosal portion:* posterior, superior portion; presents the external occipital protuberance (inion, occiput)

Temporal Bones

- Irregularly shaped bones forming lateral aspects of the cranium
- Located between greater wings of the sphenoid bone and the occipital bone (see Figs. 7-57 and 7-60A and B)
- Dense, *petrous portions* form ridges and contain the organs of hearing
- Contain internal auditory meati and carotid canals
- *Zygomatic processes:* extend from flat, squamous portion; articulate with zygomatic (facial) bones
- *Mandibular fossae:* articulate with mandibular condyles to form TMJs
- *Temporal styloid processes:* sharp, slender processes extending anteriorly and inferiorly to mastoid processes
- *External auditory meatus (EAM):* external openings of the ear canal
- *Mastoid processes:* inferior to EAM; contain numerous air cells; communicate with the tympanic cavity (middle ear) at mastoid antrum

Facial Bones

Nasal Bones

- Small, rectangular (see Fig. 7-57)
- Form bridge of the nose
- Movable part of the nose is composed of cartilage
- Articulate with each other at the midline to form the nasal suture
- Frontonasal suture: formed by articulation with the frontal bone; corresponds to nasion externally

Lacrimal Bones

- Smallest of the facial bones
- Form part of the medial orbital wall (see Fig. 7-57)
- Lacrimal groove: accommodates lacrimal (tear) duct

Zygomatic (Malar) Bones

- Inferior and lateral to outer canthus of the eye; cheek bones
- Have four processes: frontosphenoidal, orbital, temporal, and maxillary (see Fig. 7-57)

Maxillae

- Second largest of the facial bones (see Figs. 7-57 and 7-60)
- Articulate with each other to form most of the upper jaw (hard palate)

- *Palatine processes:* plates of the bone that articulate at the midline to form two-thirds of the hard palate
- Form most of the roof of mouth (hard palate) and the floor of nasal cavity
- Contain the maxillary sinuses (maxillary antra; antra of Highmore) just superior to bicuspid teeth; the thin floor of the maxillary sinus is formed by the alveolar process
- *Alveolar ridge/process:* contains sockets for teeth; spongy ridge of bone
- *Anterior nasal spine:* corresponds to *acanthion* externally
- *Infraorbital foramen:* located below the orbit, lateral to the nasal cavity

Palatine Bones

- Small bones; form posterior one-third of the hard palate (see Fig. 7-60)
- L-shaped; have vertical and horizontal processes
- *Horizontal parts:* articulate with palatine processes of maxillae to complete the hard palate
- *Vertical parts:* project superiorly from the horizontal part to articulate with the sphenoid bones

Inferior Conchae (Nasal Turbinates)

- Completely osseous (see Fig. 7-57)
- Placed inferiorly on each lateral wall of the nasal cavity

Vomer

- Inferior to the perpendicular plate of the ethmoid bone
- Forms posterior bony septum (Fig. 7-57A)
- *Choanae:* posterior opening into nasopharynx; separated by the posterior portion of vomer

Mandible

- U-shaped bone; largest facial bone (Fig. 7-57)
- Only movable facial bone
- *Mandibular symphysis:* where two halves fuse after birth
- *Mental tubercles:* prominences at the inferolateral margin of symphysis
- *Mental protuberance:* protuberance at the lower portion of symphysis
- *Alveolar process/ridge:* spongy ridge of the bone with sockets for teeth
- *Body:* horizontal position
- *Ramus:* posterior vertical portion
- *Angle:* junction of the vertical and horizontal parts; corresponds to external landmark: *gonion*
- *TMJ:* articulation of the head of condyle with mandibular fossa of the temporal bone; only movable articulation in the skull
- *Coronoid process:* extends anterior and superior from the ramus and has no articulation; serves as muscle attachment

- *Mandibular notch:* deep notch between the condyloid and coronoid processes
- *Mental foramen:* small opening on the outer surface of the body, approximately below the second premolar; passage for the mandibular nerve
- *Mandibular foramen:* opening on the inner side of ramus for the mandibular nerve

Tables 7-32 through 7-38 provide a summary of positions/projections of the cranium and all facial bones.

TABLE 7-32. The Cranium

Cranium	Position of Part	Central Ray Directed	Structures Included/Best Seen
PA	· Prone, MSP ⊥ midtable · OML ⊥ IR (see Fig. 7-62)	· ⊥ Nasion	· PA proj of the skull · Petrous pyramids should fill the orbits · Demonstrates frontal bone, lat cranial walls, frontal sinuses, crista galli (see Fig. 7-62)

Note: General survey cranium can be obtained with CR ∠15° caudad to the nasion (ridges fill lower one-third orbits). *Similar projs* of the same structures may be obtained AP with OML vertical if the CR is directed in the opposite direction. Anterior structures will be somewhat *magnified* and *eye/lens dose will be greater.*

PA axial *(Caldwell)*	· PA, MSP centered to the IR · OML ⊥ IR · IR centered to the nasion	· 15° caudad to the nasion	· PA axial of the cranium · Petrous portions in the lower third of orbits · Frontal and ethmoid sinuses seen (see Fig. 7-70) · 20°–25° ∠ projects petrous pyramids just below orbital margin; will better demonstrate superior orbital fissures
AP axial *(Towne)*	· Supine, MSP ⊥ midtable · OML vertical, ⊥IR · Top of IR 1.5″ below the vertex	· 30° caudad to a point ≈2.5″ above the glabella (or 37° to IOML)	· AP axial of the skull · Especially for the *occipital bone* · Symmetrical proj of petrous pyramids · Projects dorsum sella and posterior clinoid processes w/ in the foramen magnum (Fig. 7-63A)

Notes:
· Excessive tube ∠ or neck flexion will project posterior arch of C1 into the foramen magnum.
· Similar results can be obtained in the PA position (*PA axial; Haas* method) with the CR ∠25° cephalad to the OML; the CR enters 1½″ below the inion and exits 1½″ above the nasion; it is particularly useful for hypersthenic or kyphotic patients, although some magnification of the occipital bone must be expected.
· An AP axial of the *zygomatic arches* can be obtained by directing the CR to the glabella and decreasing the technical factors.

Lat	· Skull MSP ‖ IR · Interpupillary line vertical · IOML ⊥ front edge of the IR	· ⊥ a point 2″ superior to EAM	· Lat proj of the skull · Demonstrates superimposed cranial and facial structures · Anterior and posterior clinoid processes should be superimposed · Supraorbital margins and greater wings of the sphenoid should be superimposed (see Fig. 7-63B)
Submentovertical (SMV) proj	· Supine or seated AP · Neck hyperextended to place IOML ‖ IR · CR and MSP ⊥ IR	· ⊥ IOML and IR, enters MSP m/w b/w mandibular angles at the level of sella turcica (¾″ ant. to EAM)	· Full basal proj of the skull, useful for many foramina (spinosum, ovale, carotid canals · Sphenoid and maxillary sinuses seen · Dens seen through the foramen magnum · Symmetrical proj of petrous pyramids w/ mandibular condyles projected anterior to petrosae · Mandibular symphysis superimposed on the frontal bone (see Figs. 7-60B and 7-64)

TABLE 7-32. The Cranium—Cont'd

Cranium	Position of Part	Central Ray Directed	Structures Included/Best Seen
Note: A decrease of 10 kV will demonstrate a bilateral axial proj of the zygomatic arches (see Figs. 7-64B and 7-65).			
Trauma AP	· Supine, MSP ⊥ midtable · OML ⊥ IR	· ⊥ Nasion	· AP proj of skull · Petrous pyramids should fill the orbits
Trauma AP axial (reverse Caldwell)	· AP, MSP centered to the IR · OML ⊥ grid/IR · IR centered to the nasion	· 15° cephalad to the nasion	· AP axial of the cranium · Petrous portions in the lower third of orbits · Facial structures somewhat magnified
Trauma AP axial (Towne)	· Supine, MSP ⊥ midtable · IOML vertical, ⊥ IR · Top of IR 1.5″ below the vertex	· 37° caudad to a point ≈1.5″ above the glabella	· AP axial of the skull · Especially for the *occipital bone* · Symmetrical proj of petrous pyramids · Projects dorsum sella and posterior clinoid processes w/ in the foramen magnum
Lat *(trauma)*	· Supine, dorsal decubitus · Head supported on the sponge · Grid IR vertical and adjacent to the side of interest · MSP ⊥ CR and ‖ IR · Interpupillary line ⊥ IR	· ⊥ IR, 2″ superior to EAM	· Lat proj of the skull in the dorsal decubitus position · Can demonstrate sphenoid sinus effusion as the only sign of basal skull fx

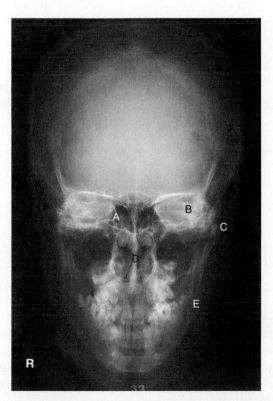

Figure 7-62. PA skull radiograph; the correct amount of flexion places the petrous pyramids within the orbits. A, ethmoid sinuses; B, petrous portion of temporal bone; C, mastoid air cells/process; D, vomer; E, mandibular angle. (Photo contributor: Stamford Hospital, Department of Radiology.)

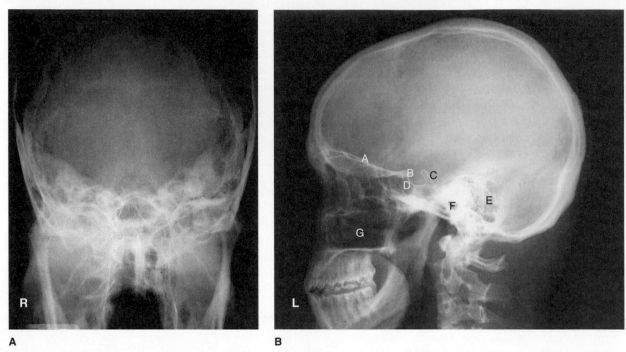

Figure 7-63. **(A)** AP axial (Towne method) projection of the skull; demonstrates the dorsum sella and posterior clinoid processes within the foramen magnum; useful for demonstration of the occipital bone. **(B)** Lateral projection of the skull. A, supraorbital margins; B, anterior clinoid processes; C, dorsum sella; D, sphenoid sinus; E, mastoid air cells; F, external auditory meatus; G, maxillary sinus. (Photo contributor: Stamford Hospital, Department of Radiology.)

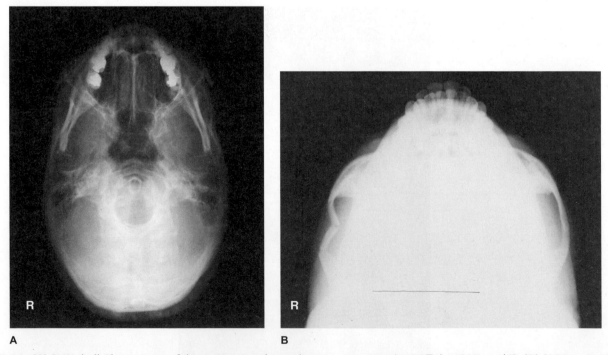

Figure 7-64. **(A)** SMV skull. The success of this projection depends on positioning the CR ⊥ the IOML and IR. **(B)** SMV projection of the skull, collimated and exposure factors adjusted to demonstrate zygomatic arches. Note fracture of the right zygomatic arch. (Photo contributor: Stamford Hospital, Department of Radiology.)

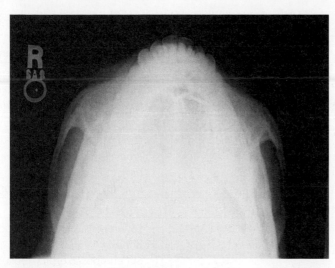

Figure 7-65. SMV projection of bilateral zygomatic arches. (Photo contributor: Stamford Hospital, Department of Radiology.)

Orbits. The orbital cavities are formed by seven bones (frontal, sphenoid, ethmoid, maxilla, palatine, zygoma/malar, and lacrimal). The orbital walls are fragile, and the orbital floor is subject to traumatic *blowout* fractures—the second most common facial fracture (nasal fracture is number one). Orbital fractures can be accompanied by injury to adjacent structures—bone, muscle, other soft tissue. Leakage of air from the adjacent maxillary sinuses can cause orbital edema. Orbital floor fractures can be demonstrated by using the *parietoacanthial* (*Waters*) projection; CT is often indicated for further evaluation (see Table 7-33).

Paranasal Sinuses. There are four paired *paranasal sinuses: frontal, ethmoidal, maxillary,* and *sphenoidal* (Fig. 7-69); they vary greatly in size and shape. The left and right frontal sinuses are usually asymmetrical. They are located behind the glabella and superciliary arches of the frontal bone. The frontal sinuses are not present in young children and reach their adult size in the 15th or 16th year. The ethmoidal sinuses are composed of 6–18 thin-walled air cells that occupy the bony labyrinth of the ethmoid bone. The ethmoidal sinuses of children are very small and do

TABLE 7-33. The Orbits

Orbits	Position of Part	Central Ray Directed	Structures Included/Best Seen
Parietoacanthial proj (*modified Waters*)	· MSP PA w/ MSP ⊥, head resting on extended chin · OML is 55° to the IR	· ⊥ IR, through mid-orbits	· Entire orbits · Petrous pyramids Projected below orbits · *Used for foreign body location*
Note: X-ray beam may be collimated to the orbital region, with the CR passing through MSP, and exiting midorbits.			
PA axial	· PA, skull MSP centered to the IR · OML ⊥ IR · IR centered ¾″ dist to nasion	· 30° caudad to ¾″ dist the nasion	· PA axial of orbits, nasal septum, maxillae, and zygomas · Petrous pyramids are seen just *below* the *orbits* · *Used for foreign body location*

TABLE 7-34. The Facial Bones

Facial Bones	Position of Part	Central Ray Directed	Structures Included/Best Seen
Parietoacanthial *(Waters)*	· PA, MSP ⊥ centered to IR · Chin extended, OML is 37° to the IR · MML is ⊥ plane of IR	· ⊥ Parietal region, exiting at the acanthion	· Axial proj of facial bones, especially orbits, zygomas, and maxillae · Best single proj for *facial bones*
Modified parietoacanthial *(modified Waters)*	· PA w/ MSP ⊥ and centered to the IR · Chin extended so OML is 55° to the IR	· ⊥ Parietal region, exiting at the acanthion	· Orbital floors ⊥ ⊥ IR · *Produces less distortion of the orbital rims* · *Used to demonstrate blowout fx*
Note: Patient should be upright to demonstrate air/fluid levels.			
Lat	· Skull MSP ∥ table/IR · Interpupillary line ⊥ · IOML ⊥ front edge of the IR	· ⊥ Zygoma, m/w b/w EAM and outer canthus	· Lat proj of superimposed facial bones · Superimposed orbital roofs, sella turcica, mandible
PA axial *(Caldwell)*	· PA, MSP centered to the IR · OML ⊥ IR · IR centered to the nasion	· 15° caudad to the nasion	· PA axial of facial bones · Petrous portions in lower the third of orbits
AP axial *trauma* *(reverse Waters)*	· Supine, MSP ⊥ midtable	· CR cephalad, ∥ MML and entering the acanthion	· Axial, but *magnified*, proj of facial bones
Lat *trauma*	· Supine, dorsal decubitus · Use "cross-table," horizontal beam	· CR enters 2″ superior to EAM; IR placed adjacent to lat aspect of the patient skull	· Lat proj of facial bones in the dorsal decubitus position · Can demonstrate sphenoid sinus effusion as the only sign of basal skull fx

TABLE 7-35. The Nasal Bones

Nasal Bones	Position of Part	Central Ray Directed	Structures Included/Best Seen
Lat, R and L	· MSP of skull ∥ table · Interpupillary line ⊥ · IOML ∥ transverse axis of the IR	· ⊥ a point ½″ dist to the nasion; include nasofrontal suture through the anterior nasal spine of the maxilla	· Lat proj of superimposed nasal bones · Their associated soft tissue (see Fig. 7-66)
PA Axial (Caldwell)	· MSP ⊥ IR · Tuck chin to bring OML ⊥ IR	· 15° caudad to exit at nasion	· PA axial of facial bones, nasal septum, and anterior nasal spine · Petrous portions in lower the third of orbits
Parietoacanthial *(Waters)*	· PA, MSP ⊥ centered to IR · Chin extended, so OML is 37° to the IR	· ⊥ Parietal region, exiting at the acanthion	· Axial proj of facial bones, especially orbits, zygomas, and maxillae · Best single proj for *facial bones*

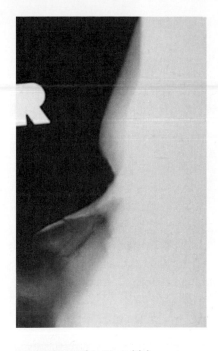

Figure 7-66. Lateral nasal bones demonstrating fracture. (Photo contributor: Stamford Hospital, Department of Radiology.)

TABLE 7-36. The Mandible

Mandible	Position of Part	Central Ray Directed	Structures Included/Best Seen
PA	· PA, MSP of skull ⊥ · Head resting on nose and chin · IR centered to level of lips	· ⊥ Lips	· PA proj of mandible, especially body (Fig. 7-67A)
PA axial	· PA, MSP of skull ⊥ · Head resting on forehead and nose · IR centered to the acanthion	· 20°–25° cephalad to the acanthion	· PA axial mandible, especially for rami and condyles
Axiolateral obl	· MSP of skull ∥ · IR centered to mandible · For ramus: true lat position · For body: head rotated 30° toward IR · For symphysis: head rotated 45° toward IR	· 25° cephalad, through ROI	· Axiolateral of mandible portions · Rotate MSP 15° forward to better demonstrate the body (see Fig. 7-67B)
AP axial *(Towne)*	· Supine, MSP of skull ⊥ IR · OML ⊥ IR	· CR enters 1″ superior to glabella at 30° caudad (or 37° to the IOML)	· AP axial of mandibular rami, especially for mandibular condyles
Submentovertical proj (SMV)	· Supine or seated AP · Neck hyperextended to place IOML ∥ IR · CR and MSP ⊥ IR	· ⊥ IOML and IR, enters MSP at level of sella	· Full basal proj of the skull · Symmetrical proj of petrous pyramids w/ mandibular condyles projected anterior to petrosae and symphysis superimposed on the frontal bone (see Fig. 7-64) · Also useful for the odontoid process through the foramen magnum
Parietoacanthial/PA (modified Waters)	· PA w/ MSP ⊥ and centered to the IR · Chin extended, so the OML is ≈55° to the IR	· ⊥ Parietal region, exiting at the acanthion	· Axial proj of facial bones, especially orbits, zygomas, maxillae, and mandible

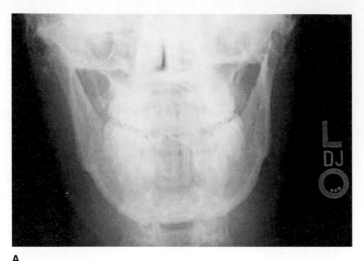
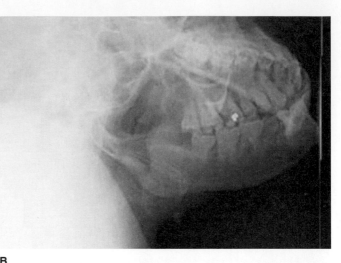

A **B**

Figure 7-67. (A) PA mandible. **(B)** Axiolateral mandible, projects the body and ramus for visualization. (Photo contributor: Stamford Hospital, Department of Radiology.)

TABLE 7-37. The Temporomandibular Joint (TMJ)

TMJ	Position of Part	Central Ray Directed	Structures Included/Best Seen
AP axial (modified *Towne*)	· AP, MSP ⊥ mid-IR · OML ⊥ IR	· 35° caudad, enters ≈3″ above the nasion	· AP axial proj of condyloid processes and their articulations · *Unless contraindicated,* another exposure is made with the *mouth open* (Fig. 7-68)
Axiolateral (modified *Schüller*)	· Skull MSP ‖ IR · IPL ⊥ TP · Center point ½″ anterior to EAM to IR	· 25° caudad, exiting the lowermost TMJ · CR enters about ½″ anterior and 2″ superior to upper EAM	· Axiolateral TMJ of side down · *Unless contraindicated, a second exposure is made with the mouth open*
Axiolateral obl (*Schüller*)	· skull in true lat position, with point ½″ anterior to EAM centered to IR · Rotate MSP down 15° *toward* the IR · adjust IPL ⊥то IR	· 15° caudad, enters 1½″ superior to the uppermost EAM, exiting the lowermost TMJ	· Axiolateral TMJ of side down · *Unless contraindicated, a second exposure is made with the mouth open*

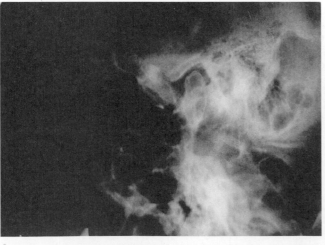
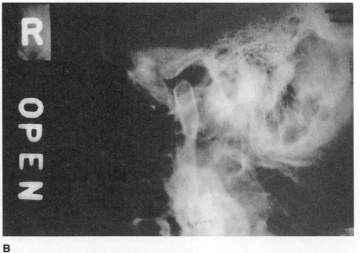

A **B**

Figure 7-68. (A) Radiograph demonstrates the oblique lateral projection of the TMJ in the closed-mouth position. **(B)** The open-mouth position. (Photo contributor: Stamford Hospital, Department of Radiology.)

TABLE 7-38. The Paranasal Sinuses

Paranasal Sinuses	Position of Part	Central Ray Directed	Structures Included/Best Seen
PA axial (Caldwell), horizontal beam	· Erect or seated PA · Skull MSP ⊥ and centered to the IR · Tilt grid to 15° ∠ · or · Elevate chin to place OML 15° w/ horizontal · MSP and OML ⊥ to the IR	· ⊥ Nasion	· PA axial of frontal and anterior ethmoid sinuses · Petrous pyramids are seen in the lower one-third of the orbits (see Fig. 7-70)
Parietoacanthial (Waters)	· Erect or seated PA · Skull MSP ⊥ and centered to the IR · Head resting on chin and OML 37° to the IR (MML is approx. ⊥) · Centered to the acanthion	· ⊥ Enters the parietal region and exits the acanthion	· Parietoacanthial proj of maxillary sinuses · Projected above petrous pyramids (see Fig. 7-71)

Note: Insufficient neck extension results in petrosae superimposed on the floor of maxillary sinus; distorted proj of the frontal and ethmoid sinuses.

A modification of the parietoacanthial proj made with the *mouth open* will demonstrate the *sphenoid sinuses* through the open mouth.

Lat	· Erect or seated · Skull MSP ∥ IR; IOML ⊥ to front edge of IR · Interpupillary line ⊥ IP · Center ½″–1″ posterior to the outer canthus	· ⊥ Mid-IR, enters ½″–1″ posterior to the outer canthus	· Lat proj of all paranasal sinuses (see Fig. 7-72)
Submentovertical (full basal, SMV)	· Erect or seated AP · Neck hyperextended to place IOML ∥ IR · CR ⊥ IR	· ⊥ IOML and IR, enters MSP at the level of sella turcica	· Basal proj of the sphenoid and ethmoid sinuses · Mandibular symphysis should be superimposed on the frontal bone (see Fig. 7-73)

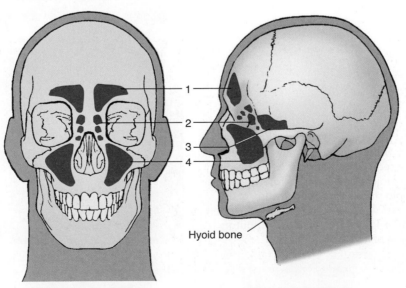

Anterior view of skull   **Lateral view of skull**

Hyoid bone

Figure 7-69. The paranasal sinuses, AP and lateral views. 1, Frontal sinuses; 2, ethmoid sinuses; 3, sphenoid sinuses; and 4, maxillary sinuses.

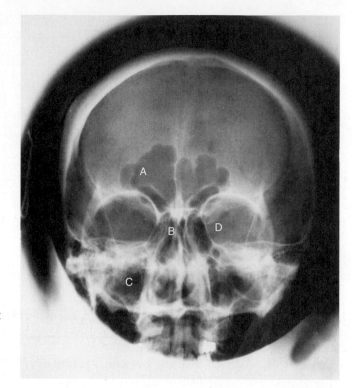

Figure 7-70. PA axial projection (Caldwell position) of the frontal and anterior ethmoid sinuses. The caudal angulation is somewhat excessive because the petrous pyramids are seen at the lowermost portion of the orbits. Correct angulation places the petrous pyramids in the lower one-third of the orbits. A, frontal sinuses; B, ethmoid air cells/sinuses; C, maxillary sinus; D, superior orbital fissure. (Photo contributor: Stamford Hospital, Department of Radiology.)

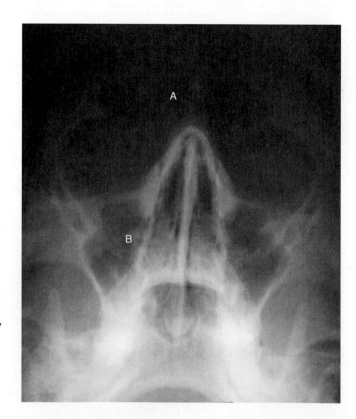

Figure 7-71. Parietoacanthial projection (Waters method). The sinuses are centered to the IR. The chin is adequately extended, and the petrous pyramids are seen below the floor of the maxillary sinuses. The parietoacanthial projection provides a foreshortened view of the frontal and ethmoid sinuses. In a modification of this projection, the sphenoid sinuses would be seen through the open mouth. A, frontal sinuses; B, maxillary sinus. (Photo contributor: Stamford Hospital, Department of Radiology.)

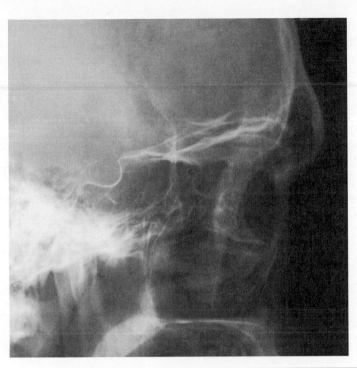

Figure 7-72. Lateral projection of the paranasal sinuses. All paranasal sinuses are demonstrated on the lateral projection. (Photo contributor: Stamford Hospital, Department of Radiology.)

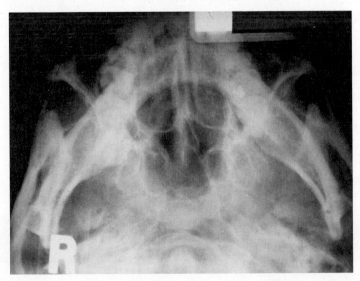

Figure 7-73. SMV projection of paranasal sinuses. Sphenoid and posterior ethmoid are demonstrated.

not fully develop until after the 14th year. The maxillary sinuses (maxillary antra/antra of Highmore) are the largest of the paranasal sinuses and are located in the body of the maxillae. The *maxillary* antra are particularly prone to infection and collections of stagnant mucus. The maxillary antra reach their adult size around the 12th year. The sphenoidal sinuses are located in the body of the sphenoid bone and are usually asymmetrical. They generally reach adult size by the 14th year.

Radiography of the paranasal sinuses must be performed in the erect position so that any *fluid levels* may be demonstrated and to distinguish between fluid and other pathology such as *polyps*.

To demonstrate air/fluid levels, *the CR must always be directed parallel to the floor,* even if the patient is not in a completely erect position (just as in chest radiography). If the CR is angled to parallel the plane of the body, any fluid levels will be distorted or actually obliterated (see Table 7-38).

COMPREHENSION CHECK

Congratulations! You have completed a large portion of this chapter. If you are able to answer the following group of very comprehensive questions, you should feel confident that you have really mastered this section. You can refer back to the indicated pages to check your answers and/or review the subject matter.

1. Identify the bony structures comprising the axial skeleton; be prepared to discuss and answer questions relevant to anatomy and pathology of the axial skeleton, bone structure and development, characteristics, and articulations.

2. Describe the (a) method of positioning, (b) direction and point of entry of the CR, (c) principal structures visualized, and (d) pertinent traumatic and pathologic conditions and any technical adjustments they may necessitate relative to the axial skeleton, including routine and special views of the following:

A. cervical spine (pp. 158–160)

B. thoracic spine (p. 161)

C. lumbar spine (pp. 162–165)

D. sacrum, coccyx (pp. 165–166)

E. scoliosis series (p. 167)

F. sternum, SC joints and ribs (p. 168)

G. ribs (p. 170)

H. orbits and facial bones (p. 181, 182)

I. nasal bones (p. 182)

J. mandible and TMJs (p. 183, 184)

K. paranasal sinuses (pp. 185–187)

BODY SYSTEMS

Respiratory System

Introduction. The respiratory system includes the nose, pharynx (throat), larynx (voice box), trachea (windpipe), bronchi, and lungs. The nose, pharynx, and larynx make up the *upper respiratory system* (Figs. 7-74 and 7-75), whereas the trachea, bronchi, and lungs make up the *lower respiratory system*. The functions of the respiratory system include supplying oxygen to the blood and relieving the body of carbon dioxide (Fig. 7-76). Pulmonary function depends on the processes of *ventilation* and *alveolar gas exchange*.

The external openings of the *nose* are the nostrils, or *nares;* its internal/posterior openings are the *choanae* or *internal nares*. The external visible portion of the nose consists of hyaline cartilage, muscle, and skin—whereas its inner surface is lined with mucous membrane and receives olfactory nerve endings for the sense of smell. The internal nose structures function to warm, moisten, and filter incoming air and to detect smell.

The *pharynx* is divided into three portions: the *nasopharynx*, the *oropharynx*, and the *laryngopharynx*. The pharynx is just posterior to the oral cavity; it begins at the choanae and terminates at the level of the cricoid cartilage. The pharynx functions as part of the digestive system, as well as the respiratory system, because it serves as passageway for both food and air. As part of the digestive system, the pharynx aids in *deglutition* (swallowing); it also houses the pharyngeal *tonsils*, which have immunologic functions.

The auditory tubes open into the nasopharynx; the oropharynx and the laryngopharynx are the pharyngeal portions common to both the respiratory and digestive systems; the laryngopharynx opens into the larynx anteriorly and the esophagus posteriorly.

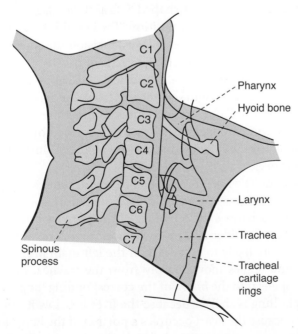

Figure 7-74. Anatomy of the neck, especially structures demonstrated in the soft-tissue study.

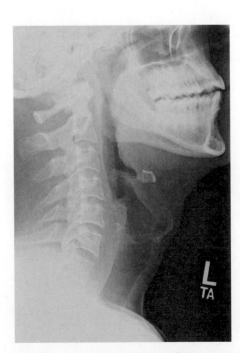

Figure 7-75. Lateral projection, soft-tissue neck study (see Table 7-39).

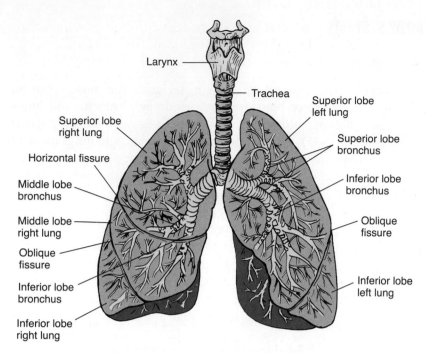

Figure 7-76. Trachea and bronchi (anterior view).

The *larynx* lies in the anterior neck at about the level of C4–C6; it connects the laryngopharynx and the trachea. The laryngeal walls are composed of nine cartilages. Three of the cartilages are *single/unpaired;* they are the *thyroid* cartilage, the *epiglottis,* and the *cricoid* cartilage. Three of the cartilages are *paired:* the *arytenoid,* the *cuneiform,* and the *corniculate* cartilages. The paired cartilages are principally concerned with speech.

The thyroid cartilage, also called the laryngeal prominence or Adam's apple, is the most superior cartilage and forms the anterior laryngeal wall. The epiglottis is a leaf-shaped (elastic) cartilage that covers the glottis (vocal folds) during deglutition. The cricoid (hyaline) cartilage is the most inferior of the nine cartilages; incision for emergency tracheotomy is made just below the cricoid cartilage.

The *trachea* (windpipe) is a cylindrical cartilaginous tube, approximately 4½ inches in length, extending from the larynx (~C6) to the primary bronchi (~T5). Its ciliated mucosa functions to protect against mucus, dust, and pathogens. The trachea is formed by *16–20 C-shaped* cartilaginous (hyaline) rings that can be palpated through the skin of the anterior neck.

At about the level of T5, the trachea divides into the right and left *mainstems,* or primary, *bronchi;* at the bifurcation is a ridge called the *carina,* which separates the openings of the primary bronchi. The right main bronchus is wider and more vertical; therefore, aspirated foreign bodies are more likely to enter it than the left main bronchus, which is narrower and angles more sharply from the trachea. Each mainstem bronchus opens into the *hilum* of the corresponding lung.

The right lung is shorter because the liver is below it; the left lung is narrower because the heart occupies a portion of the lung's left side. The lungs have a somewhat conical shape; their narrow upper portion is called the *apex,* and their wide *base* is defined by the *diaphragmatic*

Divisions of Pharynx

- Nasopharynx
- Oropharynx
- Laryngopharynx

Laryngeal Cartilages (Nine)

Three single/unpaired:
- Thyroid
- Epiglottis
- Cricoid

Three paired:
- Arytenoid
- Cuneiform
- Corniculate

surface. Structures such as the mainstem bronchi and pulmonary artery and veins enter and leave the lungs at the *hilum.* The *right lung* has *three lobes:* The upper and middle lobes are separated by the *horizontal fissure,* and the middle and lower lobes are separated by the *oblique fissure.* The *left lung* has *two lobes:* The upper and lower lobes are separated by the *oblique fissure* (Fig. 7-76).

The lungs are enclosed in a serous membrane, the *parietal pleura.* The *visceral pleura* lines the inner thoracic wall and covers the superior surface of the diaphragm; the potential space between the two layers of the pleura is the *pleural cavity.*

Pneumothorax is the presence of air in the pleural cavity. A large pneumothorax is usually accompanied by a partial or complete collapse of the lung (atelectasis). Radiographic indications of atelectasis include *elevation of the hemidiaphragm of the affected side* and an *increase in tissue* density of the collapsed lung. *Thoracentesis* is the procedure required to remove significant amounts of air, blood, or other fluids in the pleural cavity.

One of the most diagnostically useful and frequently performed radiographic examinations is the chest x-ray. During the course of their illness and recovery, patients often need successive chest examinations to monitor their progress, and reproduction of quality images is an important part of quality control. Accurate positioning and selection of technical factors are critical to the diagnostic value of the radiographic images (Fig. 7-77A). *Even slight rotation or leaning can cause significant distortion of the size and shape of the heart.* Consistent and accurate positioning is essential to radiographic quality.

The radiographer must take careful note of each patient's apparel, body type, and clinical information. Important considerations include removal of any radiopaque clothing and accessories, placing the IR

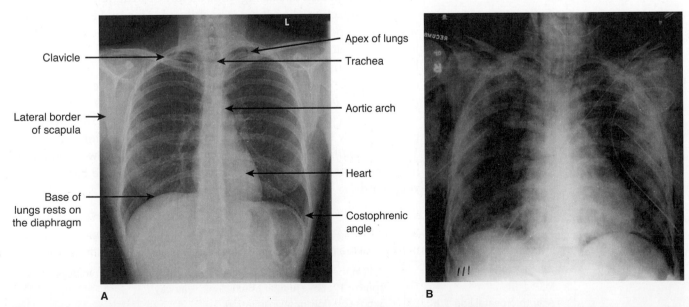

A   B

Figure 7-77. **(A)** Normal PA chest image. Accurate positioning and selection of technical factors are critical to the diagnostic value of the radiographic image. (From Peart O. *Lange Radiographic Positioning Flashcards.* New York, NY: McGraw-Hill Education; 2014.) **(B)** Mobile AP chest radiograph. Observe an endotracheal tube and ECG leads, one chest tube on the right and two on the left. The patient has extensive soft-tissue emphysema. Radiographers must exercise particular care when working around various patient tubes. (From the American College of Radiology (ACR) Learning File. Photo contributor: ACR.)

transversely for broad-chested individuals (to include the *costophrenic angles*—blunting of the costophrenic angles is often a result of pleural effusion), instructing female patients with large breasts to move them up and laterally for the PA projection, exposing on the second inspiration for hypersthenic individuals, and adjusting exposure factors for various pathologic conditions. Appropriate radiation protection measures must always be provided.

Mobile chest radiography often brings the radiographer into contact with seriously ill patients. The radiographer must be very cautious when positioning these patients, for there are often numerous tubes (e.g., chest tubes, endotracheal tubes, electrocardiographic [ECG] leads, Swan–Ganz lines, urinary catheters) associated with maintaining the patient's airway or reinflating a collapsed lung, removing fluid or air from the pleural cavity, administering medications, measuring central venous pressure, or measuring urine output (Fig. 7-77B). The variety of wires and/or tubes can interfere with visualization of anatomic structures needed for optimum diagnostic value. Whenever possible, and with appropriate knowledge and caution, it is helpful to have these moved away from areas of interest.

Tables 7-40 and 7-41 provide a summary of routine projections and frequently performed special projections of the respiratory structures.

Soft-Tissue Neck. The *upper airway* (see Fig. 7-74 and Table 7-39) can be examined in the *AP* and *lateral* positions. These projections are used to demonstrate hypertrophy of the pharyngeal tonsils or adenoids. It is desired to see the nasopharynx *filled with air* to provide adequate contrast; therefore, the exposure must be made on *slow nasal inspiration*.

Airway. AP and lateral projections of the airway and larynx are occasionally required to rule out *foreign body, polyps, tumors,* or any other condition suspected of causing some airway obstruction.

In AP projection, the patient is positioned as for an AP cervical spine, with the CR perpendicular to the *laryngeal prominence*. In lateral projection, the patient is positioned as for a lateral cervical spine and centered to the coronal plane passing through the trachea (anterior to the cervical spine) at the level of the laryngeal prominence. *Exposures are made on slow inspiration* to visualize air-filled structures.

Depending on the structure(s) of interest being examined, these positions may be used with barium and/or during performance of the *Valsalva/modified Valsalva maneuver*. Phonation of vowel sounds can help demonstrate more superior structures such as the larynx and/or vocal cords.

TABLE 7-39. The Upper Airway/Soft-Tissue Neck

Upper Airway	Position of Part	Central Ray Directed	Structures Included/Best Seen
AP upper airway	· AP supine or erect · MSP ⊥ IR · Acanthiomeatal line ⊥ IR	· ⊥ IR at the level of T1–T2, i.e., approx. 1″ above jugular notch · Expose on slow nasal inspiration	· Air-filled nasopharynx/upper airway
Lat upper airway	· Lat, preferably erect · MSP ∥ IR	· ⊥ IR at the level of C6–C7; expose on slow nasal inspiration	· Air-filled nasopharynx/upper airway (Fig. 7-75)

TABLE 7-40. The Chest: PA and Lateral

Chest	Position of Part	Central Ray Directed	Structures Included/Best Seen
PA	· Erect PA, MSP exactly ⊥ IR · Shoulders depressed and rolled forward · Top of the IR 1.5″–2″ above shoulders	· ⊥ T7	· PA proj of thoracic viscera and skeletal anatomy · *Inspiration* demonstrates air-filled trachea and lungs, 10 posterior ribs · *Expiration* shows pulmonary vascular markings · *Inspiration and expiration* are done for pneumothorax, foreign body, diaphragm excursion, and atelectasis (Fig. 7-78A)

Notes:
· Chest radiography is performed in the *erect* position whenever possible to demonstrate air/fluid levels.
· AP proj maybe used, especially for mobile studies, but PA offers best cardiac detail.
· The MSP must be exactly vertical; any *rotation can cause significant distortion* and misrepresentation of the visceral structures (see Fig. 7-79A).
· Rotation is detected on the PA image by asymmetrical distance between the sternal ends of the clavicles and the center of the adjacent thoracic vertebral body.
· Shoulders are rolled forward to remove the scapulae from superimposition on the lung fields.
· Superiorly, the pulmonary apices must be seen; inferiorly, the costophrenic angles must be seen in their entirety.
· *Inspiration* must be adequate to demonstrate 10 posterior above-diaphragm ribs.
· A 72″ SID is recommended to decrease magnification of the heart.
· *Obl projs* of the chest are occasionally performed as supplemental views. The LAO and RAO positions are performed with the MSP at 45° to the IR.

Chest	Position of Part	Central Ray Directed	Structures Included/Best Seen
AP supine	· AP supine, MSP exactly ⊥ IR · If possible, raise head of bed/stretcher to place patient in semierect position · Shoulders relaxed and rolled forward · Top of the IR 1.5″–2″ above shoulders	· Angled caudad to bring CR ⊥ long axis of thorax at level of T7	· AP proj of thoracic viscera and skeletal anatomy · *Inspiration* demonstrates air-filled trachea and lungs, 10 posterior ribs · *Expiration* shows pulmonary vascular markings · *Inspiration and expiration* are done for pneumothorax, foreign body, diaphragm excursion, and atelectasis
Lat	· Erect L lat, MSP ∥ IR · Arms over the head · Top of IR 1.5″–2″ above shoulders	· ⊥ IR, enters at the level of midthorax/T7	· Lat proj of the chest particularly useful for the heart, aorta, L lung and its fissures, and other left-sided structures/pathology; L lat usually done to place the heart closer to the IR (Fig. 7-78B)

Notes:
· MSP must be *exactly vertical;* any lat leaning can cause significant distortion and misrepresentation of the visceral structures.
· *Rotation* is detected on the lat radiograph by superimposition of ribs on sternum or vertebrae.
· Pulmonary apices and angles must be visualized (see Fig. 7-79B).

Terminology and Pathology. The following is a list of radiographically significant conditions and devices with which the student radiographer should be familiar:

- Asthma
- Atelectasis
- Bronchiectasis
- Bronchitis
- Central venous pressure line
- Chest tube (Fig. 7-77)
- Chronic obstructive pulmonary disease
- Cystic fibrosis
- Dextrocardia (Fig. 7-80)
- Emphysema (Figs. 7-77 and 7-81)
- Empyema

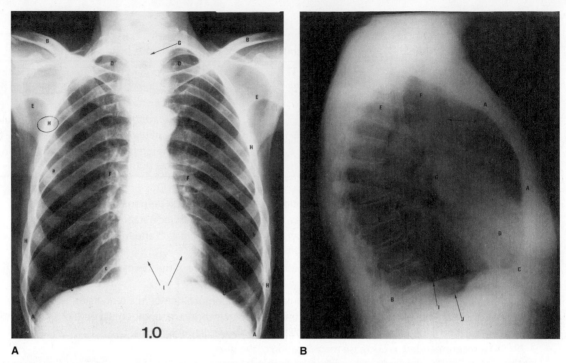

A   B

Figure 7-78. (A) PA projection of the chest. Identify the lettered structures. A, costophrenic angle; B, clavicle; C, diaphragmatic domes; D, pulmonary apices; E, scapula; F, rib—eighth posterior; G, air-filled trachea; H, fourth rib—axillary portion; I, heart; a, sixth rib; b, axillary portion—eighth rib; c, vertebral/floating rib. **(B)** Lateral projection of the chest. A, sternum; B, intervertebral foramen; C, apex of heart; D, heart; E, thoracic vertebra; F, pulmonary apices; G, hilar region; H, air-filled trachea; I and J, L and R hemidiaphragms. (Photo contributor: Bob Wong, RT.)

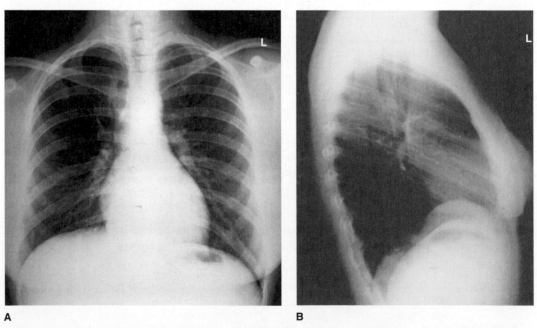

A   B

Figure 7-79. (A) PA projection of the chest of a normal, healthy adult *demonstrating the importance of positioning accuracy*. Slight rotation has made the manubrium visible at the site of the right sternoclavicular joint, *providing a density very similar to that created by a paraspinous or mediastinal mass*. **(B)** Lateral projection of the same chest and without rotation. The sternum is seen free of superimposed ribs; the thoracic and lumbar vertebral spinous processes are seen. (From the ACR Learning File. Photo contributor: ACR.)

TABLE 7-41. The Chest: Axial and Decubitus

Chest	Position of Part	Central Ray Directed	Structures Included/Best Seen
AP lordotic/axial (lordotic)	· Erect AP · MSP ⊥, standing about 12″ away from IR and leaning back 15°–20° against it · Top of IR about 3″ above shoulders	· ⊥ Point about 3″–4″ below jugular notch	· AP axial (lordotic) proj of entire pulmonary apices projected below clavicles · With individuals unable to lean backward, the CR can be directed 15°–20° cephalad
Lat decubitus (R or L)	· Recumbent lat on the affected or unaffected side as indicated by history · Anterior or posterior surface adjacent to the IR · MSP ⊥ mid-IR w/ top of IR 1.5″ above shoulders	· ⊥ Mid-IR; enters about 3″ below jugular notch	· Frontal (AP or PA) proj of the chest · Useful for demonstration of air or fluid levels

Note: If free air is suspected, it is best demonstrated with affected side up; if fluid is suspected, it is best demonstrated with affected side down.

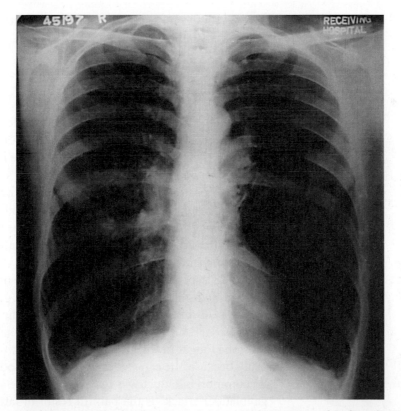

Figure 7-80. PA chest radiograph demonstrating the characteristic irreversible trapping of air found in emphysema, which gradually increases and overexpands the lungs, thus producing the *characteristic flattening of the diaphragm* and *widening of the intercostal spaces.* The increased air content of the lungs requires a compensating decrease in technical factors.

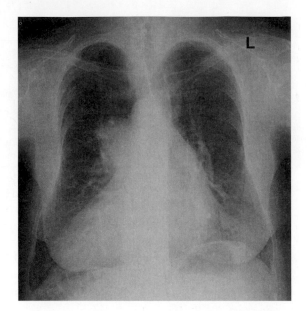

Figure 7-81. PA chest radiograph demonstrating dextrocardia. Dextrocardia is often associated with other heart defects.

- Endotracheal tube (see Fig. 7-77)
- Hemothorax
- Hickman catheter
- Pneumoconiosis
- Pneumonia pneumothorax
- Swan–Ganz catheter
- Thoracentesis
- Tuberculosis

Biliary System

Introduction. The biliary tree consists of the left and right hepatic ducts, common hepatic duct, cystic duct, common bile duct, and gallbladder (GB) (Fig. 7-82). The hepatic ducts leave the liver and join to form the *common hepatic duct.* The short *cystic duct* continues to the GB. The common hepatic and cystic ducts unite to form the long *common bile duct,* which joints with the pancreatic duct to form the short *hepatopancreatic ampulla (of Vater).* The ampulla opens into the descending duodenum through the *duodenal papilla* that is surrounded by the *hepatopancreatic sphincter (of Oddi).*

The *GB* is located in a shallow fossa on the inferior surface of the liver between its right and quadrate lobes. Small gallstones are able to pass from the GB through the cystic duct; those that are too large irritate the GB mucosa, resulting in *cholecystitis. Gallstones* can also lodge in ducts. If a stone lodges in the cystic duct, cholecystitis without *jaundice* is the result, because bile can still drain into the duodenum. A stone lodged in the common bile duct will result in jaundice as well as cholecystitis. A "gallbladder attack" is the painful result of fatty chyme stimulating the release of *cholecystokinin,* which elevates pressure within the stone-laden GB.

The GB of the average-build patient is located between the 10th and 12th ribs on the right, midway between the vertebral column and lateral border of the body. In *hypersthenic* individuals, it is usually found approximately 2 inches higher and more lateral, whereas in *asthenic* individuals, it is usually 2 inches lower and more midline. In the *erect* position, the GB of an asthenic patient can be as low as the iliac fossa.

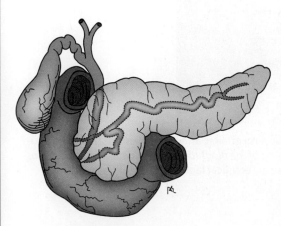

Figure 7-82. Illustration of main hepatic and biliary ducts, GB, and pancreas within the duodenal loop.

TABLE 7-42. Surgical and ERCP Imaging

Surgical Cholangiography	Position of Part	Central Ray Directed	Structures Included/Best Seen
AP	· Supine	· ⏐ Center of the IR	· AP of the biliary tree and gallbladder area
			· To evaluate the hepatopancreatic ampulla and biliary tree for calculi or other pathology (following injection of contrast into the common bile duct) (Fig. 7-84C)

Note: Can be performed RPO with L side elevated 15°–20° and R upper quadrant centered to the IR.

ERCP	Position of Part	Central Ray Directed	Structures Included/Best Seen
AP LPO	· Recumbent · Part LPO	· ⊥ Biliary tree/common bile duct	· Fluoroscopy and spot images to evaluate the biliary tree · Contrast media injected through hepatopancreatic ampulla of Vater · Rotation of part/equipment required to visualize the entire biliary tree

Radiographic examinations of the biliary system (Table 7-42) no longer include *oral cholecystography*; however, *operative cholangiography*, *T-tube cholangiography*, and *endoscopic retrograde cholangiopancreatography* (*ERCP*) are often performed. Each of these examinations requires the use of a contrast agent. ERCPs and operative cholangiographies are often performed in conjunction with sonographic imaging (Fig. 7-83).

Operative cholangiography is used to examine the bile ducts and frequently follows a *cholecystectomy*. An iodinated contrast agent is introduced into the common bile duct to evaluate biliary and hepatopancreatic ampulla patency. Any calculi can be detected and removed before completion of surgery.

Occasionally, a T-shaped tube is left in the common bile duct for postsurgical drainage. T-tube cholangiography is performed by

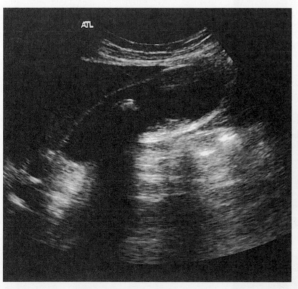

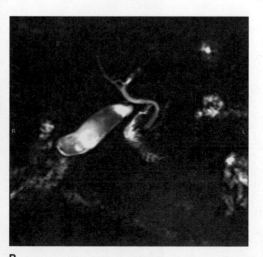

A   B

Figure 7-83. **(A)** A sonogram of the GB demonstrating the presence of gallstones. (Photo contributor: Stamford Hospital, Department of Radiology.) **(B)** Magnetic resonance image (coronal T2) of biliary system. (Photo contributor: Conrad P. Ehrlich, MD.)

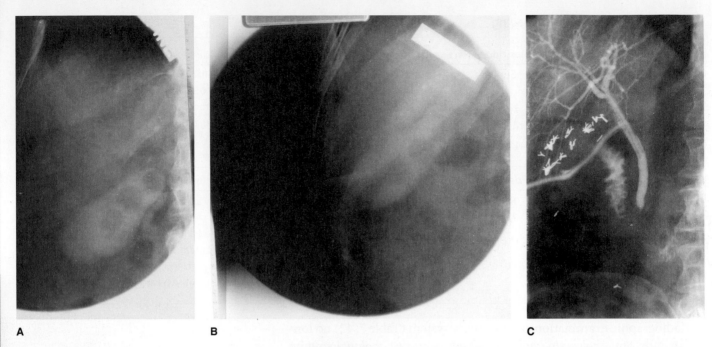

A   B   C

Figure 7-84. **(A)** PA projection of GB (with gallstones). **(B)** LAO of the same GB. Oblique position moves the GB away from vertebrae. **(C)** T-tube cholangiogram. (Photo contributor: Stamford Hospital, Department of Radiology.)

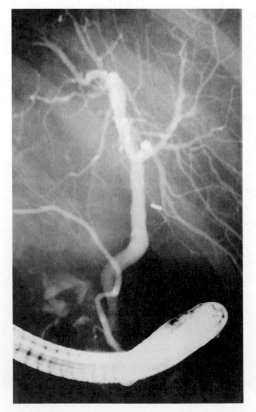

Figure 7-85. Fluoroscopic image of normal ERCP. The pancreatic and common bile ducts are clearly delineated. (Photo contributor: Stamford Hospital, Department of Radiology.)

injecting a contrast agent through the tube to detect any remaining calculi and evaluate the biliary tree patency.

ERCP is a specialized procedure used to evaluate suspected biliary and/or pancreatic conditions. An *endoscope* is passed through the mouth, esophagus, and stomach and into the descending duodenum to the orifice of the hepatopancreatic ampulla. Following *canalization* of the hepatopancreatic ampulla, fluoroscopic images are obtained in the AP and/or LPO positions. Contrast material is injected into the common bile duct for evaluation of the biliary system. Table 7-42 addresses surgical imaging and ERCP. The imaging procedure should immediately follow the injection because under normal conditions, contrast will empty from the biliary ducts in approximately 5 min (Fig. 7-85).

Terminology and Pathology. The following is a list of radiographically significant conditions with which the student radiographer should be familiar:

- Cholecystitis
- Hepatitis
- Cholelithiasis
- Jaundice
- Cirrhosis
- Pancreatitis

Digestive System

Introduction. The major portion of the gastrointestinal (GI) tract lies within the abdominopelvic cavity. Its principal functions are the chemical breakdown and absorption of nutrients. The digestive system (Fig. 7-86A and B) consists of the *GI tract* and *accessory organs*. The *GI tract,* or *alimentary canal,* is a continuous tube of varying dimensions consisting of the esophagus, stomach, and small and large intestines. The teeth, tongue, salivary glands, liver, GB, and pancreas are *accessory organs* that aid in the mechanical and chemical breakdown of food.

The lobulated salivary glands encircle the entrance to the oropharynx. The largest of the salivary glands is the *parotid* gland, which is located just anterior to the ear, above the mandibular angle, and is emptied by the Stenson duct. The *submandibular* glands are located near the inner surface of the mandibular body and empty their digestive juices into the mouth via the Wharton duct. The *sublingual* gland is located in the floor of the mouth and opens into the mouth by way of multiple ducts of Rivinus—the largest of these is the Bartholin duct.

Salivary glands can be investigated radiographically (termed *sialography*) via injection of (water-soluble iodinated) contrast material for demonstration of glandular disorders such as tumors, calculi, or fistula formation following trauma to the area. Sialography involves cannulation of the ostium of the parotid duct (Stenson) or the submandibular duct (Wharton). Figure 7-87 illustrates submandibular sialography.

The *esophagus* functions to propel a food bolus toward the stomach through *peristaltic* motion. Stroke, multiple sclerosis, dementia, and esophageal cancer are some of the conditions that can cause swallowing dysfunction or difficulty in swallowing (dysphagia). A swallowing/deglutition study (Table 7-43) can be performed to demonstrate and/or evaluate the swallowing mechanism. The *cardiac sphincter* is located at the distal end of the esophagus. "Heartburn" is an inflammation of the esophageal *mucosa* as a result of gastric *reflux* of acidic material into the

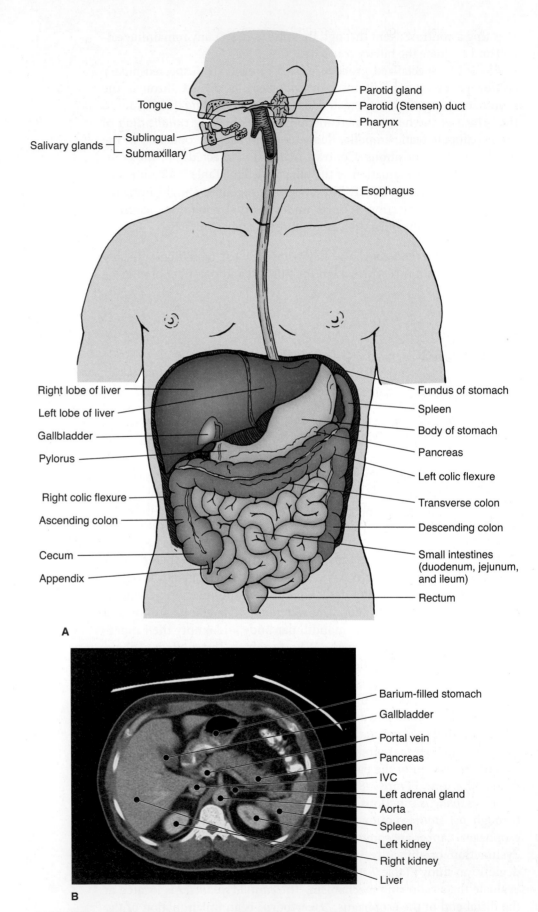

Figure 7-86. (A) The digestive system. **(B)** Axial CT scan of the abdomen demonstrating many digestive and circulatory structures.

TABLE 7-43. Swallowing/Deglutition Dysfunction Study

Swallowing	Position of Part	Central Ray	Structures Included/Best Seen
AP	· Erect, upper esophagus centered to the IR	· ⊥ IR	· AP proj used to check for symmetry
Lat	· Erect, upper esophagus centered to the IR	· ⊥ IR	· Fluoroscopic images to demonstrate deglutition mechanism in cases of dysphagia, aspiration, globus sensation · Lat is the single best proj

esophagus. *Esophageal varices* are dilated, *tortuous* veins directly beneath the esophageal mucosa. A *hiatal hernia* is a herniation of the stomach through the esophageal hiatus of the diaphragm, producing a sac-like dilatation above the diaphragm (Fig. 7-88A and B). The presence of reflux, varices, or herniation can be detected radiographically with the use of barium sulfate.

From the lower esophagus through the anal canal, the GI tract has the same four tissue layers. The innermost lining layer is the *mucosa;* mucous membranes line cavities that directly open to the exterior. This mucous membrane is composed of a layer of epithelium, whose cells are shed and are replaced every 5–7 days. The two other layers of the mucosa are the lamina propria and a thin muscular layer. They assist in immunity and in forming gastric folds (rugae), respectively.

The *submucosa* is highly vascular (blood and lymphatic vessels), contains a broad complex of neurons, and can also include glands and lymphatic tissue.

The *muscular* layer of structures through the esophagus consists of skeletal muscle, which permits the voluntary muscular actions of chewing and swallowing. Skeletal muscle is also found at the anal sphincter, permitting defecation. The remainder of the GI tract muscular layer is smooth/involuntary muscle that functions to mix and propel digestive secretions and food content.

The *serosa*/serous membrane is the outermost layer of the GI tract. Serous membranes line body cavities and cover organs that do not directly open to the exterior. Serous membranes produce a lubricating serous fluid that allows organs to glide over one another without friction. The serous membrane of the thoracic cavity is the double-walled pleura; the serous membrane of the abdominal cavity is the double-walled *peritoneum.*

Salivary Glands and Their Ducts

- Parotid: Stenson duct
- Submandibular: Wharton duct
- Sublingual: Bartholin duct

GI Tract Tissue Layers

Inner to outer:
- Mucosa
- Submucosa
- Muscular
- Serosa

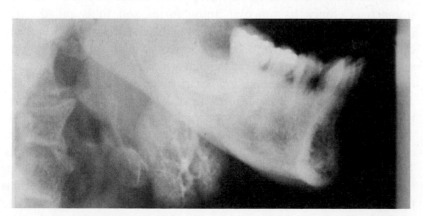

Figure 7-87. Submandibular sialogram. (Photo contributor: Stamford Hospital, Department of Radiology.)

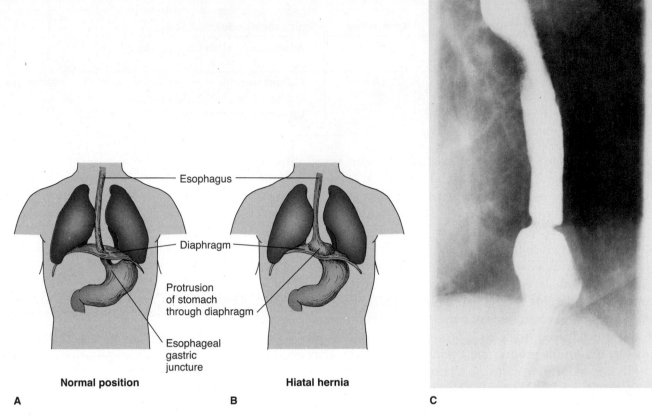

Figure 7-88. **(A)** Normal position of the stomach. **(B)** Note protrusion of the stomach through esophageal hiatus (hiatal hernia). **(C)** Esophagram demonstrating hiatal hernia (with Schatzki ring). (Photo contributor: Stamford Hospital, Department of Radiology.)

Five Major Peritoneal Folds

- *Greater omentum:* an apron of fat over transverse colon and small bowel
- *Lesser omentum:* suspends stomach and duodenum from liver; contains some biliary vessels
- *Mesentery:* binds jejunum and ileum to posterior abdominal wall; fan-shaped
- *Mesocolon:* binds transverse and sigmoid colon to posterior abdominal wall

Stomach

- Fundus
- Body
- Pylorus

The peritoneum has an outer parietal layer that lines the abdominal cavity. Its inner visceral layer is reflected over and between the abdominal organs, forming large folds between the viscera; these folds attach the organs both to the abdominal cavity and to each other. These folds also house nerves, as well as blood and lymphatic vessels. There are five major peritoneal folds: the greater omentum, the lesser omentum, the mesentery, the falciform ligament, and the mesocolon.

The *stomach* is the dilated, sac-like portion of the GI tract. When the stomach is empty, its mucosal lining forms soft folds called *rugae* (Fig. 7-89A). *Gastritis* is an inflammation of the gastric mucosa that can be caused either by excessive secretion of acids or by ingestion of irritants such as aspirin or corticosteroids. Exteriorly, it presents a *greater curvature* on its lateral surface and a *lesser curvature* on its medial surface. The proximal opening of the stomach, at the *gastroesophageal junction*, is the *cardiac sphincter*; the *pyloric sphincter* is located at its distal end. The portion of the stomach around the distal esophagus is called the *cardia*; the portion superior to the esophageal juncture is the *fundus*. The sharp angle between the esophagus and the fundus is the *cardiac notch*. The major portion of the stomach is the *body*; the distal portion is the *pylorus*. The *incisura angularis* is located on the lesser curvature and marks the beginning of the pylorus. The distal portion of the pylorus is marked by the *pyloric sphincter*.

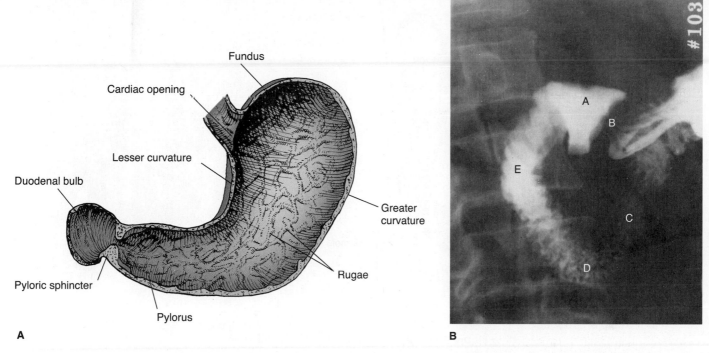

Figure 7-89. (A) Stomach (internal aspect). **(B)** Barium-filled duodenal loop; duodenal bulb and descending, transverse, and ascending duodenum are well demonstrated. A, duodenal bulb; B, pyloric valve; C, ascending duodenum; D, transverse duodenum; E, descending duodenum. (Photo contributor: Stamford Hospital, Department of Radiology.)

The *small intestine* is composed of the duodenum, jejunum, and ileum. The *duodenum* is the shortest portion. It begins just beyond the pyloric sphincter and is divided into four portions: the duodenal cap or bulb, descending duodenum, transverse duodenum, and ascending duodenum. These portions form a C-shaped loop (*duodenal loop*) that is occupied by the head of the pancreas (Fig. 7-89B). The descending portion receives the hepatopancreatic ampulla and the duodenal papilla (see the "Biliary System" section). The ascending portion terminates at the duodenojejunal flexure (angle of Treitz). Although the position of the short (9 inches) duodenum is fixed, the *jejunum* (9 feet) and the *ileum* (13 feet) are very mobile. Twisting of the small intestine is called *volvulus* and can cause compression of blood vessels, leading to loss of blood supply, *ischemia*, and *infarct* of the affected area. The small intestine terminates at the *ileocecal valve*. The lengths of intestine usually quoted are those present at autopsy and can be up to 50% longer than the actual size because of loss of muscle tone following death.

The approximately 5-foot long *large intestine (colon)* (Fig. 7-90A) functions in the formation, transport, and evacuation of feces. The colon begins at the terminus of the small intestine; its first portion is the dilated, sac-like *cecum*, located inferior to the ileocecal valve (Fig. 7-90A and B). Projecting posteromedially from the cecum is the short (~3.5 inches) *vermiform appendix*. Its lumen is particularly narrow in adolescents and young adults and may become occluded by a fecalith and result in inflammation (appendicitis).

The *ascending colon* is continuous with the cecum and is located along the right side of the abdominal cavity. It bends medially and anteriorly in the right hypochondrium, forming the *right colic (hepatic) flexure*. The colon traverses the abdomen as the *transverse colon* and bends

Small Intestine

- Duodenum: ~10 inches (9–12 inches at autopsy)
- Jejunum: ~3–6 feet (up to 9 feet at autopsy)
- Ileum: ~6–12 feet (up to 13 feet at autopsy)

Large Intestine (~5 feet)

- Cecum
- Ascending colon
- Transverse colon
- Descending colon
- Sigmoid colon
- Rectum

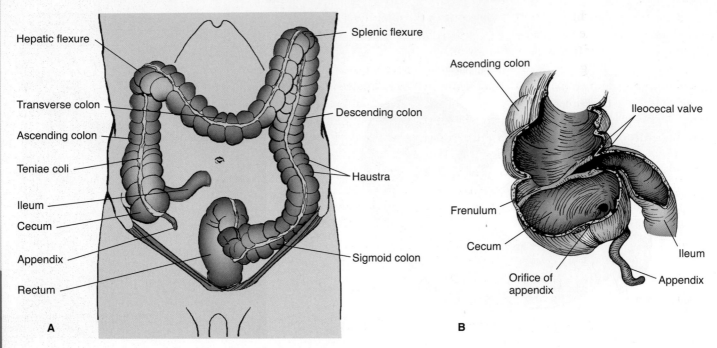

Figure 7-90. **(A)** The colon. **(B)** The ileocecal valve.

posteriorly and inferiorly in the left hypochondrium, forming the *left colic (splenic) flexure.* The *descending colon* continues down the left side of the abdominal cavity and, at about the level of the pelvic brim, the colon moves medially to form the S-shaped *sigmoid colon.* The *rectum* is that part of the large intestine, approximately 5 inches in length, between the sigmoid and the anal canal.

Diverticula are small saccular protrusions of the intestinal mucosa through the intestinal wall. They are most commonly associated with the sigmoid colon and can become occluded by fecaliths and subsequently inflamed (diverticulitis). If an inflamed diverticulum perforates, it can result in severe bleeding and peritonitis.

Patient Preparation. Preliminary patient preparation is generally required of patients undergoing radiographic examinations of various portions of the digestive system. The upper GI tract (stomach and small intestine) must be empty and the lower tract (large intestine) must be cleansed of any gas and fecal material. Patients should be questioned about their preparation and have a preliminary "scout" image taken to check abdominal contents and for any radiopaque (e.g., gallstones, residual barium) material.

Radiography of the digestive system often requires the use of artificial contrast media (barium sulfate suspension or water-soluble iodine) coupled with air to make up for the lack of subject contrast. *Double-contrast studies* of the stomach and large intestine are frequently conducted. Barium sulfate functions to coat the organ with radiopaque material, whereas air inflates the structure. This permits visualization of the shape of the structure as well as *visualization of pathology within its lumen.* Thus, conditions such as *polyps* can be seen projecting within the air-filled lumen. A barium-filled *lumen* would make visualization of anything but the organ shape virtually impossible.

The speed with which barium sulfate passes through the alimentary canal depends on the patient habitus (hypersthenic usually fastest) and the concentration of the barium suspension.

When performing examinations on patients suspected or known to have stomach or intestinal perforation, *water-soluble* iodinated contrast media should be used instead of barium sulfate. Water-soluble contrast media are excreted more rapidly than barium sulfate preparations, and if leaked through a perforation into the peritoneal cavity, will simply be absorbed and excreted by the kidneys.

These studies are far from pleasant for patients, and the radiographer should make every effort to fully explain the procedure while endeavoring to expedite the examination and make the patient as comfortable as possible.

Currently, with the increased use of digital fluoroscopy, fewer "overhead" radiographs are obtained. Tables 7-44 through 7-47 provide a summary of the most frequently performed positions/projections of the upper and lower GI tracts.

Abdomen. Abdominal pain is a common problem and is among the most routine symptoms presented in an emergency department. The term "acute abdomen" refers to the rapid onset of severe symptoms and can be an indication of life-threatening intra-abdominal pathology. Causes of abdominal pain include appendicitis, intestinal obstruction, paralytic ileus, diverticulitis, peptic ulcer disease, gastroenteritis, pelvic inflammatory disease, and so on. Radiologic investigation is often indicated.

A *three-way abdomen* study (AP recumbent, AP erect, and L lateral decubitus) may be requested or an *acute abdomen survey* (AP

TABLE 7-44. The Abdomen

Abdomen	Position of Part	Central Ray Directed	Structures Included/Best Seen
AP supine	· Supine · MSP centered to the IR · IR centered to the iliac crest (see Fig. 7-91)	· ⊥ Midline at the level of crest	· AP proj often used as "scout" image preliminary to contrast studies · Shows size and shape of the kidneys, liver, and spleen, psoas muscles, as well as any calcifications or masses
PA erect/ upright	· PA erect (or AP) · MSP centered to the IR · IR centered ≈2″ above the iliac crest	· ⊥ Mid-IR	· PA erect proj used to demonstrate air/fluid levels; both hemidiaphragms should be included (see Fig. 7-92A and B)
Lat decubitus	· Patient lat recumbent (AP or PA) MSP ⊥ and centered to the upright IR, cassette centered ≈2″ above the iliac crest	· Horizontal and ⊥ mid-IR	· Usually, *left* lat decubitus of abdomen to demonstrate air/fluid levels in patients unable to assume the erect position; both hemidiaphragms should be included
Dorsal decubitus	· Patient supine with right or left side against IR · Patient's arms above head and out of field of view · Center IR ≈2″ above iliac crest	· Horizontal and ⊥ mid-IR	· Lat view of the abdomen · Diaphragm and as much of the lower abdomen demonstrated as possible · Air/fluid levels in bowel loops present

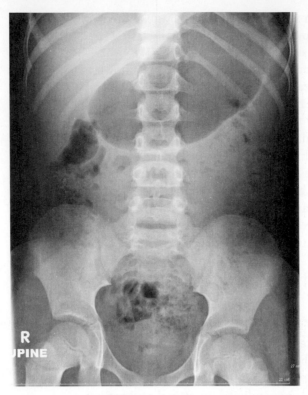

Figure 7-91. AP projection of the abdomen. (Photo contributor: Conrad P. Ehrlich, MD.)

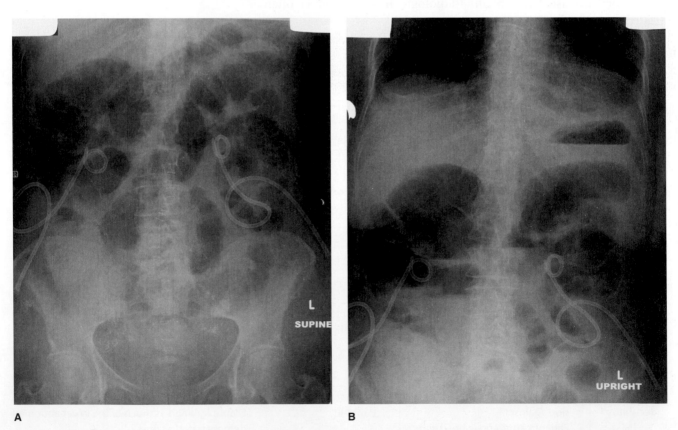

A **B**

Figure 7-92. Abdominal pain is among the most common symptoms presented in an emergency department. *Acute abdomen* involves rapid onset of severe symptoms and can be an indication of life-threatening intra-abdominal pathology. An *acute abdomen survey,* AP recumbent **(A)**, AP erect **(B)** or L lateral decubitus, and erect PA chest are often used to evaluate possible obstruction or free air/fluid under the diaphragm/within the abdomen. Note the air levels seen in the upright abdomen **(B)** above.

TABLE 7-45. The Esophagus

Esophagus	Position of Part	Central Ray Directed	Structures Included/Best Seen
AP (or PA)	· Supine, MSP centered and ⊥ table · IR top 1″–2″ above shoulders · Barium swallowed during (<0.1 s) exposure	· ⊥ Mid-IR, ≈T6–T7, approx. 3″ below jugular notch	· Barium-filled esophagus in AP (or PA) proj
RAO or LAO	· Prone obl, 35°–40° · RAO or LAO, IR top 1″–2″ above shoulders · Barium swallowed during exposure	· ⊥ Mid-IR, ≈T6–T7	· RAO: barium-filled esophagus in RAO proj demonstrated b/w the vertebrae and heart · LAO: barium-filled esophagus in LAO proj demonstrated b/w lungs and T spine · RAO is the best single proj of barium-filled esophagus (see Fig. 7-94)
Left lat	· Recumbent lat, MCP centered to the IR · Top of the IR just above shoulders · Barium swallowed during exposure	· ⊥ Mid-IR	· Barium-filled esophagus in lat proj · *May be taken in right lat position if necessitated by patient condition*

Notes:
· Esophagus for the demonstration of *varices* best demonstrated in the *recumbent* position, table slightly Trendelenburg, and/or performance of the Valsalva maneuver.
· Exposure times of 0.1 s or less should be used to avoid motion.
· Respiration normally stops during and shortly after the act of swallowing, so patients need not be instructed to stop breathing.

recumbent, AP erect or L lateral decubitus, and erect PA chest) to evaluate possible obstruction (Fig. 7-93) or free air and fluid within the abdomen/under the diaphragm (see Table 7-40 and Fig. 7-92A and B). Patients with these conditions usually experience severe pain and nausea. The radiographer must be caring, skilled, and efficient.

Esophagus. The *esophagus* (Table 7-45) functions to propel a food bolus toward the stomach through peristaltic motion. The cardiac sphincter, also known as the lower esophageal sphincter, is located at the distal end of the esophagus. "Heartburn" is an inflammation of the esophageal mucosa as a result of *reflux* of acidic gastric material into the esophagus. Esophageal *varices* are dilated, tortuous veins lying directly beneath the esophageal mucosa. A *hiatal hernia* is herniation of a portion of the stomach through the diaphragm's esophageal hiatus, producing a dilatation above the diaphragm (Fig. 7-88A and B). The presence of reflux, varices, or herniation can be detected radiographically with the use of barium sulfate (Fig. 7-94).

Stomach and Small Intestine. Radiologic examination of the stomach and/or the small bowel generally begins with fluoroscopic examination. The fluoroscopist observes the swallowing mechanism, mucosal lining (rugae) of the stomach, and the filling and emptying mechanisms of the stomach and proximal small bowel while the patient is turned and rotated in various positions to visualize all aspects of the stomach and any abnormalities, such as hiatal hernia (see Fig. 7-88C). Double-contrast examinations of the upper GI system (Fig. 7-95) are performed frequently. Occasionally, glucagon or another similar drug will be given to the patient (IV or IM) prior to the examination to relax the GI tract

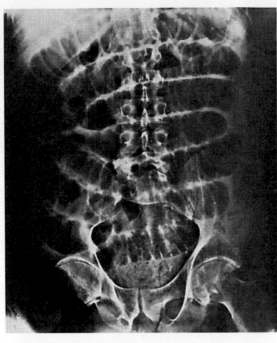

Figure 7-93. Small bowel obstruction indicated by the dilated bowel loops having a ladder-like pattern. The patient is recumbent; therefore, air/fluid levels are not demonstrated. (Reproduced with permission from Doherty GM, ed. *Current Surgical Diagnosis & Treatment*. 12th ed. New York, NY: McGraw-Hill; 2006:666.)

and permit more complete filling. The fluoroscopist will obtain the necessary images, and the radiographer may take supplemental "overhead" projections. *Small bowel series* examinations require that successive images of the abdomen be obtained at specified intervals; an additional fluoroscopic image is obtained when barium reaches the *ileocecal valve*.

Contrast material (usually water soluble) may occasionally be instilled through a GI tube for visualization of the GI tract. GI tubes can be used therapeutically to siphon gas and fluid from the GI tract or diagnostically, by using contrast agent, to locate the site of obstruction or pathology (see Table 7-46).

Barium sulfate is *contraindicated* if a *perforation* is suspected somewhere along the course of the GI tract (e.g., a perforated diverticulum or gastric ulcer); a water-soluble (absorbable) iodinated contrast medium is generally used instead. *Enteroclysis* is a procedure in which the contrast medium is administered through a patient's nasogastric tube for the purpose of locating and studying any site of obstruction.

Large Intestine. The lower GI tract is most often examined by *retrograde* filling with barium sulfate and, frequently, air. The fluoroscopist observes filling of the large bowel in various positions and obtains images as indicated. Much of the barium is then drained from the intestine, and air is introduced. The objective is to coat the bowel with barium and then distend its lumen with air. The double-contrast method is ideal for demonstration of intraluminal lesions such as polyps.

The success of the barium enema (BE) examination depends on several factors, but without proper patient preparation, a diagnostic examination is often impossible. *Poor preparation resulting in retained fecal material in the colon can mimic or conceal pathologic conditions.*

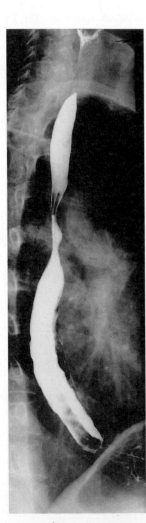

Figure 7-94. RAO of a barium-filled esophagus. The esophagus has three normal constrictions at the levels of the cricoid cartilage, the left bronchus, and the esophageal hiatus of the diaphragm. (Photo contributor: Stamford Hospital, Department of Radiology.)

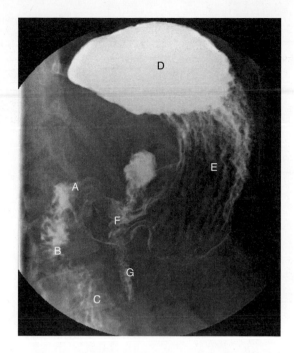

Figure 7-95. LPO of the stomach. In this position, air replaces the barium that drains from the duodenal bulb and pylorus, thus providing double-contrast visualization of these structures. A, duodenal bulb; B, descending duodenum; C, transverse duodenum; D, fundus; E, body/gastric mucosa; F, pylorus; G, ascending duodenum. (Photo contributor: Stamford Hospital, Department of Radiology.)

TABLE 7-46. The Stomach and Small Bowel

Stomach	Position of Part	Central Ray Directed	Structures Included/Best Seen
AP or PA	· Supine or prone, MSP centered to IR, at level of L2	· ⊥ Mid-IR (at the level of L2)	· AP or PA proj of transversely spread stomach · Demonstrates contours, greater and lesser curvatures (Fig. 7-97)
Note: Hypersthenic patients frequently have high, transverse stomachs with indistinguishable curvatures. The adult hypersthenic stomach can be "opened" and its *contours* made readily visible by angling the CR 35°–45° cephalad. The top edge of a lengthwise 14" × 17" IR is placed level with the patient's chin and the CR directed to mid-IR.			
LPO	· Supine, obliqued ≈40° to left · Centered midway b/w vertebrae and L abdominal wall at the level of L1	· ⊥ Mid-IR (at the level of L1)	· Barium-filled fundus · Good position for *double-contrast* study of the body, pylorus, and duodenal bulb (see Fig. 7-95)
Note: As the fundus is the most *posterior* portion of stomach, it readily fills w/ barium in AP position and moves more superiorly.			
Right lat	· Recumbent lat · Center m/w b/w MCP and anterior abdominal wall to the IR at the level of L2	· ⊥ Mid-IR (at the level of L2)	· Lat stomach and prox small bowel · Demonstrates anterior and posterior aspects of the stomach, retrogastric space, pyloric canal, and duodenal loop (see Fig. 7-96)
Note: This proj provides the best visualization of the pyloric canal and duodenal bulb in the hypersthenic patient.			
RAO	· Recumbent PA obliqued 40°–70° · Centered m/w b/w vertebrae and lat abdominal wall at the level of L2	· ⊥ Mid-IR (at the level of L2)	· Right PA obl proj of the stomach, barium-filled pyloric canal and duodenal loop · Demonstrates stomach's emptying mechanism, because *peristaltic activity is greatest in this position*
Small bowel AP/PA	· Prone, MSP centered to the IR · IR centered to the level of L2	· ⊥ Mid-IR	· AP or PA proj of the dist esophagus area, stomach, and prox small bowel · Can demonstrate hiatal hernia w/ patient in the Trendelenburg position

Continued

TABLE 7-46. The Stomach and Small Bowel—Cont'd

Stomach	Position of Part	Central Ray Directed	Structures Included/Best Seen
Scout image can be taken in AP position is patient cannot tolerate PA position.			
PA (follow through)	· Prone, MSP centered to the IR · 15–30 min intervals: IR centered 2" above Iliac crest · Hourly intervals: IR centered to iliac crest	· ⊥ Mid-IR	· 15–30 min: PA proj of entire stomach and small bowel · Hourly: PA proj of entire small bowel · Prone position aids with compression of abdomen and separation of bowel loops
Ileocecal spots	· Supine or prone; department preference · Performed under fluoroscopy or general x-ray · Radiolucent paddles are often used to separate bowel loops and target ileocecal valve	· ⊥ Mid-IR	· Barium-filled ileocecal valve free of superimposition · Most often taken 2–3 h after barium is ingested

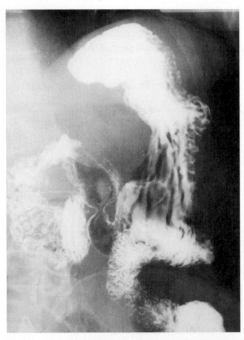

Figure 7-96. Lateral projection demonstrates the anterior and posterior stomach surfaces and the retrogastric space. (Photo contributor: Stamford Hospital, Department of Radiology.)

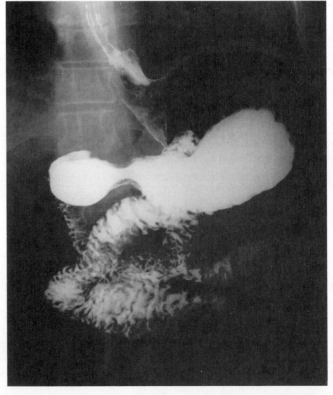

Figure 7-97. PA projection of the stomach. Note barium in the body and pylorus. (Photo contributor: Stamford Hospital, Department of Radiology.)

TABLE 7-47. The Large Intestine

Contrast Enema	Position of Part	Central Ray Directed	Structures Included/Best Seen
AP	· Supine, MSP centered to the IR at the level of the iliac crest	· ⊥ Mid-IR	· AP proj of the entire contrast-filled large intestine

Notes: The large intestine of hypersthenic patients is high and around the periphery of the abdomen; hence, they may require that the AP and PA be done on two 14″ × 17″ IRs placed crosswise in the Bucky tray. In contrast, the colon of the asthenic patient is low, redundant, and more midline.

PA	· Prone, MSP centered to the IR at the level of the iliac	· ⊥ Mid-IR	· PA proj of the entire contrast-filled large intestine · AP or PA erect may be used to demonstrate double-contrast *flexures*
AP axial obl (sigmoid)	· Supine, MSP centered to the IR · 30°–40° LPO rotation	· 30°–40° cephalad to midline at the level of ASIS	· AP obl axial proj of *sigmoid colon* · Angulation opens the length of the S-shaped colon (see Fig. 7-98)

Note: PA axial may be performed to show similar structures; CR is directed 35°–40° caudad.

RAO and LAO	· PA, obl ≈35°–40°, centered to the midline · RAO: IR centered to the level of the iliac crest, 1″ left from MSP · LAO: IR centered 1″–2″ above the iliac crest, 1″ right from MSP	· ⊥ Mid-IR	· RAO: Right PA obl proj of the colon; demonstrates *ascending colon and hepatic flexure* (see Fig. 7-99) · LAO: left PA obl proj of the colon; demonstrates *descending colon and splenic flexure* · LPO and RPO
LPO and RPO	· AP, obl ≈35°–40°, centered to the midline · LPO: IR centered to the level of the iliac crest, 1″ right from MSP · RPO: IR centered 2–3 inches above the iliac crest, 1″ left from MSP	· ⊥ Mid-IR	· RPO: Right PA obl proj of the colon; demonstrates splenic flexure, open descending colon · LPO: left AP obl proj of the colon; demonstrates hepatic flexure, open ascending and rectosigmoid colon
Left lat rectum	· Lat recumbent, MCP centered to the IR · IR centered at the level of ASIS	· ⊥ Mid-IR	· L lat proj · Especially for the *rectum* and the *rectosigmoid* area · This proj may also be performed cross-table
Lat decubitus (R and L)	· Lat recumbent (AP or PA) · MSP ⊥ and centered to the upright IR · At the level of the iliac crest	· Horizontal and ⊥ mid-IR	· Air rises to provide double-contrast delineation of lat walls of the colon · Both decubitus are routinely performed (see Fig. 7-100)
PA or AP postevacuation	· Supine or prone · MSP ⊥ and centered to the IR · At the level of the iliac crest	· ⊥ Mid-IR	· Entire large intestine visualized; residual contrast medium present · Demonstrates large bowel mucosa

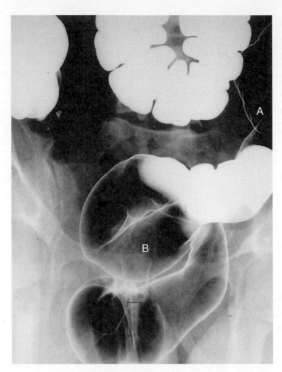

Figure 7-98. Double-contrast PA axial projection of the rectum and sigmoid. The caudal tube angulation serves to "open" the redundant S-shaped sigmoid colon. Similar results may be obtained in the AP position with a cephalad tube angle. A, descending colon; B, sigmoid colon. (Photo contributor: Stamford Hospital, Department of Radiology.)

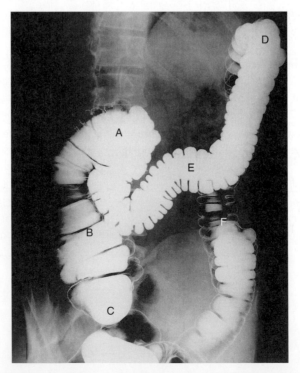

Figure 7-99. RAO of the barium- and air-filled large bowel. Note that the hepatic flexure is "opened" for better visualization. An LPO would provide similar results. The opposite oblique images (LAO, RPO) are used to demonstrate the splenic flexure and descending colon. A, right colic/hepatic flexure; B, ascending colon; C, cecum; D, left colic/splenic flexure; E, transverse colon; F, descending colon. (Photo contributor: Stamford Hospital, Department of Radiology.)

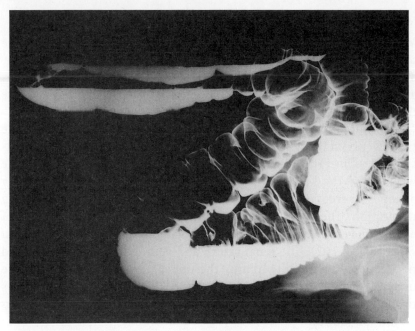

Figure 7-100. Right lateral decubitus view of the air- and barium-filled colon. The heavier barium sulfate moves toward the dependent side, whereas air rises to fill the remainder of the barium-coated lumen. Thus, the *right lateral decubitus demonstrates double-contrast visualization of the "left-sided walls" of the ascending and descending colons* (i.e., lateral side of the descending colon and medial side of the ascending colon). (Photo contributor: Stamford Hospital, Department of Radiology.)

The BE is most easily tolerated and retained by the patient if it is cool or actually cold (≈40°F–45°F). There is probably no radiographic examination that causes more embarrassment and anxiety than the BE and air-contrast procedure. The radiographer must be sensitive to the concerns and needs of the patient both by providing a complete explanation of the procedure and by ensuring the patient's modesty as much as possible.

Table 7-47 summarizes frequently performed BE projections taken following the fluoroscopic procedure.

Terminology and Pathology. The following is a list of radiographically significant abdominal and digestive conditions and devices with which the student radiographer should be familiar:

- Achalasia
- Appendicitis
- Ascites
- Colostomy
- Crohn disease
- Diverticulitis
- Diverticulosis
- Dysphagia
- Enteritis
- Esophageal reflux
- Esophageal varices
- Gastroenteritis
- Hiatal hernia (see Fig. 7-88)
- Ileostomy
- Intussusception
- Irritable bowel syndrome
- Peptic ulcer
- Peritonitis
- Polyp
- Pyloric stenosis
- Ulcerative colitis
- Volvulus

Urinary System

Introduction. Two of the functions of the urinary system (Fig. 7-101) are to *remove wastes from the blood* and *eliminate them in the form of urine.* The tiny units within the renal substance that perform these functions are called *nephrons.* The major components of the urinary system are the *kidneys, ureters,* and *bladder.*

The paired *kidneys* are *retroperitoneal* and embedded in adipose tissue between the vertebral levels of T12 and L3. Because of the position of the liver, the right kidney is usually 1–2 inches lower than the left kidney. The kidneys move inferiorly 1–3 inches when the body assumes an erect position; they move inferiorly and superiorly during respiration. The slit-like opening on the medial concave surface of each kidney is the *hilum,* which opens into a space called the *renal sinus* (Fig. 7-102). The renal artery and vein, lymphatic vessels, and nerves pass through the hilum. The upper, expanded portion of the ureter is called the *renal pelvis,* or *infundibulum,* and also passes through the hilum; it is continuous with the major and minor *calyces* within the kidney.

Within each kidney, the renal *parenchyma* is divided into two parts: the outer *cortex* and the inner *medulla.* The cortex is compact and has a grainy appearance as a result of the many *glomeruli* within its tissues. The medulla contains 10–14 *renal pyramids* with a characteristic striated appearance that is owing to the *collecting tubules* within (see Fig. 7-102).

The proximal portion of each *ureter* is at the renal pelvis. As the ureter passes inferiorly, three normal constrictions can be observed: at the ureteropelvic junction, at the pelvic brim, and at the ureterovesicular junction. The ureters lie in a plane anterior to the kidneys; ureteral filling with contrast media is best achieved by using the prone position. Urine is carried through the ureters by peristaltic activity. If a ureter is obstructed by a kidney stone, *hydronephrosis* occurs. The ureters enter the *urinary bladder* posteroinferiorly (Fig. 7-103). The base of the bladder rests on the pelvic floor. The triangular-shaped area formed by the *ureteral* and *urethral orifices* is called the *trigone.* Micturition is the

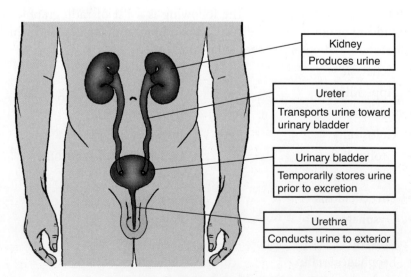

Figure 7-101. Components of the urinary system.

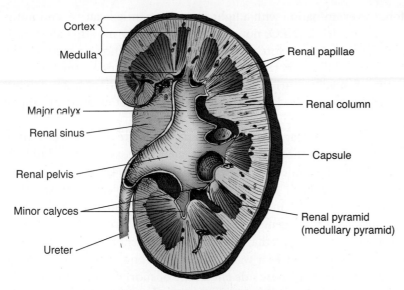

Figure 7-102. Section through the left renal pelvis.

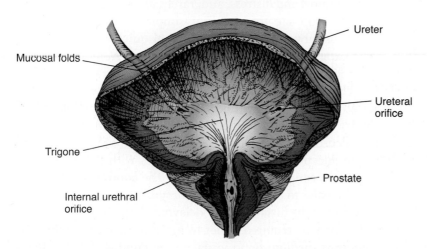

Figure 7-103. Bladder trigone (anterior portion of the bladder removed).

process of emptying the urinary bladder of its contents through the *urethra*. The male urethra is approximately 7–8 inches long and is divided into prostatic, membranous, and penile portions. The female urethra is approximately 1.5 inches in length.

A common complication of regional enteritis or diverticular disease is the formation of a *fistula* between the urinary bladder and the small or large intestine. Fistulous tracts may often be evaluated radiographically with contrast media.

Routine radiographic procedures of the urinary system are generally performed via the IV route. When performed in the retrograde manner, *cystoscopy* is required.

Although the numbers of urinary system x-ray examinations have been steadily decreasing, and are infrequently performed in many institutions now, a review of these examinations is as follows.

Patient Preparation and Procedure. Investigation of the urinary tract requires patient preparation sufficient to rid the intestinal tract of gas and fecal material. Typical preparation usually begins the evening

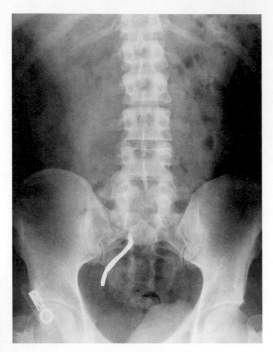

Figure 7-104. A preliminary or "scout" image of the abdomen is taken before the start of an intravenous urogram. The radiograph is checked for residual barium from previous contrast studies, patient preparation (including barium from previous studies; note residual barium in the patient's appendix), location of kidneys, technical factors, and any calcifications. (Photo contributor: Stamford Hospital, Department of Radiology.)

before the examination with a light dinner, a gentle laxative, and nothing to eat or drink (NPO; non per os [nothing by mouth]) after midnight. Immediately before beginning the intravenous urogram, the patient must be instructed to empty his or her bladder; this prevents dilution of opacified urine in the bladder. If the patient has a urinary catheter, it is generally clamped just before the injection and unclamped before the postvoid image. The intravenous urogram is preceded by a preliminary scout image of the abdomen to evaluate patient preparation and reveal any calcifications (renal or gallstones), position of kidneys, and accuracy of technical factor selection (Fig. 7-104).

Because the urinary structures have so little subject contrast, artificial contrast material must be used for better visualization of these structures. Contrast agents used for urographic procedures can have unpleasant and (rarely) lethal side effects. Intravenous injection of contrast frequently produces a warm, flushed feeling, a bitter or metallic taste, or mild nausea. These side effects are of short duration and usually pass as quickly as they come. More serious side effects include *urticaria*, respiratory discomfort and distress, and, rarely, *anaphylaxis*. An *antihistamine* is the appropriate treatment of simple side effects, but the radiographer must always be prepared to deal quickly and efficiently with patients experiencing more serious reactions. *Nonionic* contrast agents are far less likely to produce side effects. Contrast agents and their side effects are more thoroughly discussed in Chapter 5.

The selected contrast agent is injected intravenously, and successive radiographs are obtained at specified intervals. A time interval marker must be included on each image to indicate the elapsed postinjection time. Injection and postinjection protocol varies with the institution, radiologist, patient condition, and diagnosis. The contrast may be rapidly injected in a *bolus* to obtain a 30-s *nephrogram*.

Compression over the distal ureters (delaying contrast or urine travel to the bladder) may be required either to more completely fill the kidneys with contrast medium or to visualize the contrast-filled kidneys for a longer period of time (Fig. 7-105). Maximum concentration of the contrast material usually occurs at 15–20 min after injection but varies with the degree of patient hydration.

Radiographs collimated to the kidneys (11 × 14–inch crosswise) may be required at 1, 3, and 5 min to evaluate a diagnosis of renal hypertension. Both oblique images may be required to evaluate a suspected tumor or lesion. AP and oblique kidney, ureter, and bladder (KUB) images are usually required at 10–15 min after injection. A prone KUB image is frequently requested at 20 min. Because the ureters lie in a plane anterior to the kidneys, *ureteral filling* with contrast media is best achieved by using the PA projection (Fig. 7-106).

Types of Examinations. Routine IV procedures are most correctly called *intravenous urography* (*IVU*), or *excretory urography,* although they are still commonly called intravenous *pyelography* (IVP) (*pyel* refers only to renal *pelvis*). Intravenous procedures demonstrate *function* of the urinary system, hence the term *excretory* urography. Retrograde studies demonstrate only the *structure* of the part and are generally conducted to evaluate the lower urinary tract (lower ureters, bladder, and urethra).

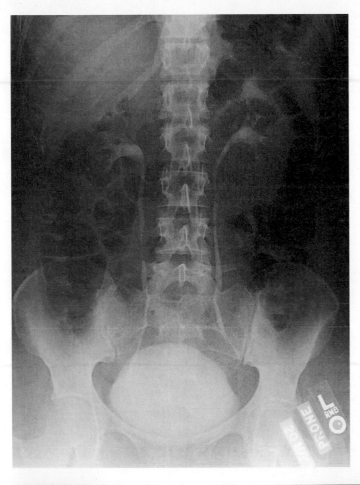

Figure 7-105. PA projection of IVU demonstrating contrast-filled ureters. Because the ureters lie in a plane that is anterior to that of the kidneys, they are best demonstrated as contrast-filled structures in the *PA position*. The contrast material, which is heavier than urine, gravitates to fill the anterior ureters. (Photo contributor: Stamford Hospital, Department of Radiology.)

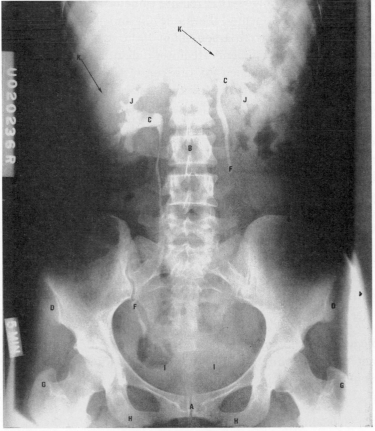

Figure 7-106. This KUB image is a 5-min intravenous urogram. Good collimation is evident and the kidneys, ureters, and bladder are included in their entirety. A, pubic symphysis; B, body, L3; C, renal pelvis; D, ASIS; E, iliac crest; F, ureter; G, greater trochanter; H, ischium; I, bladder; J, renal collecting system/calyces; K, renal cortex. (Photo contributor: Bob Wong, RT.)

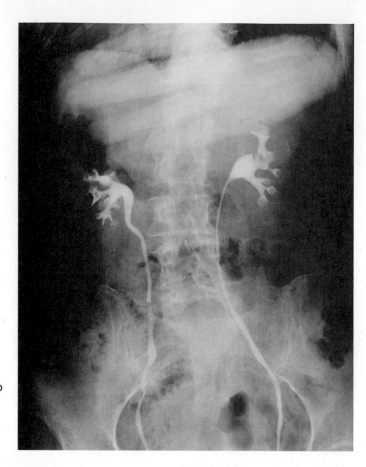

Figure 7-107. When positioning the abdomen, it is important to position the patient's hands at his or her side or resting high on the chest. Note the position of the patient's right hand in this retrograde urogram. (From the ACR Learning File. Photo contributor: ACR.)

Retrograde urograms (Fig. 7-107) require catheterization of the ureter(s). Radiographs that include the kidney(s) and ureter(s) in their entirety are obtained after retrograde filling of the structures. A cystogram or (voiding) *cystourethrogram* requires only urethral catheterization. Radiographs are obtained of the contrast-filled bladder and frequently of the contrast-filled urethra during voiding. *Cystoscopy* is required for the location and catheterization of the vesicoureteral orifices.

Excretory urography and retrograde urography involve accurate positioning of the abdomen to include the kidneys, ureters, and bladder. If these structures cannot fit on a single image, a second radiograph is generally taken for the bladder. Tables 7-48 through 7-51 provide a review of abdomen/KUB and bladder positioning for IVU.

The PA projection will best demonstrate *contrast-filled ureters* (see Fig. 7-107).

The 30° oblique KUB projection places the kidney of the *up* side *parallel* to the IR and the ureter of the side *down* parallel to the IR. Figure 7-109 is an RPO projection that places the left kidney and the right ureter parallel to the IR.

Terminology and Pathology. The following is a list of radiographically significant urinary conditions and devices with which the student radiographer should be familiar:

- Cystitis
- Double-collecting system
- Double ureter
- Fistula

TABLE 7-48. Intravenous Urography

Intravenous Urography	Position of Part	Central Ray Directed	Structures Included/Best Seen
AP, scout, and series	· Supine · MSP centered to IR · IR positioned to include kidneys in their entirety *and* symphysis pubis	· ⊥ Midline at the level of the crest	· Entire urinary system including symphysis pubis visualized · Demonstration of kidneys marked by presence of upper renal shadows · Potential for separate view of the bladder for hypersthenic patients
RPO and LPO	· Supine, rotated 30° to right or left side · IR centered to vertebral column	· ⊥ Midline at the level of the crest	· Demonstrates upside kidney and downside ureter
Postvoid	· Erect AP or prone · MSP centered to IR · IR positioned to include symphysis pubis	· ⊥ Midline at the level of the crest · Centering lower may be necessary to include bladder, depending on habitus	· Entire urinary system including symphysis pubis visualized, residual contrast medium seen

TABLE 7-49. Retrograde Urography

Retrograde Urography	Position of Part	Central Ray Directed	Structures Included/Best Seen
AP scout	· Supine · MSP centered to IR · IR positioned to include kidneys in their entirety · Patient's knees will be flexed over stirrups for contrast administration; this will help reduce lumbar curvature	· ⊥ Midline at the level of the crest	· Kidneys visualized with presence of unilateral or bilateral ureter catheterization · Demonstration of kidneys marked by presence of upper renal shadows
AP pyelogram	· Supine · MSP centered to IR · IR positioned to include kidneys and ureters in their entirety · Patient's knees will be flexed over stirrups for contrast administration; this will help reduce lumbar curvature	· ⊥ Midline at the level of the crest · Exposure taken on full expiration	· Complete filling of renal pelves, calyces, and ureters with contrast · Demonstration of kidneys marked by presence of upper renal shadows
The radiologist may require a 10°–15° Trendelenburg table position to prevent contrast from flowing into the ureters.			
AP ureterogram	· Supine · MSP centered to IR · IR positioned to include kidneys and ureters in their entirety · Patient's knees will be flexed over stirrups for contrast administration; this will help reduce lumbar curvature	· ⊥ Midline at the level of the crest · Exposure taken on full expiration	· Complete filling of renal pelves and ureters with contrast · Demonstration of kidneys marked by presence of upper renal shadows
The radiologist may require the foot of the table to be lowered 35°–40° to demonstrate ureter tortuosity and kidney mobility.			

TABLE 7-50. Cystourethrography

Cystourethrography	Position of Part	Central Ray Directed	Structures Included/Best Seen
AP voiding cystourethrogram female	· Supine or erect, MSP ⊥ and centered to the IR · IR centered to the pubic symphysis	· ⊥ Midline at the level of the pubic symphysis	· AP proj of the bladder and prox urethra · A 5° ∠ caudad can be used for the female to place bladder neck and urethra below the pubis
RPO voiding cystourethrogram male	· Supine or erect AP · 30° rotation RPO · Legs slightly separated	· ⊥ Midline at the level of the symphysis pubis	· Contrast-filled urethra projected over right thigh (Fig 7-108)

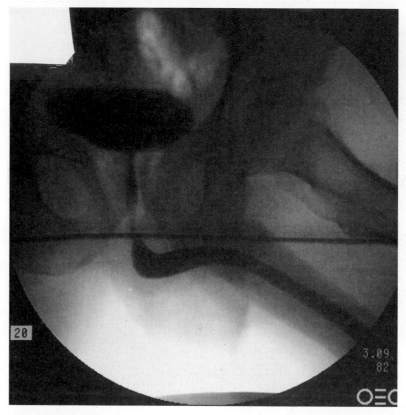

Figure 7-108. Voiding cystourethrogram. (Photo contributor: Stamford Hospital, Department of Radiology.)

- Foley catheter
- Horseshoe kidney
- Hydronephrosis
- Hydroureter
- Incontinence
- Nephroptosis
- Nephrostomy tube
- Pelvic kidney
- Polycystic kidney
- Prostatic hypertrophy

- Pyelonephritis
- Renal calculi
- Renal hypotension
- Staghorn calculus (see Fig. 7-110)
- Supernumerary kidney
- Uremia
- Ureteral stent
- Ureterocele
- Vesicoureteral reflux

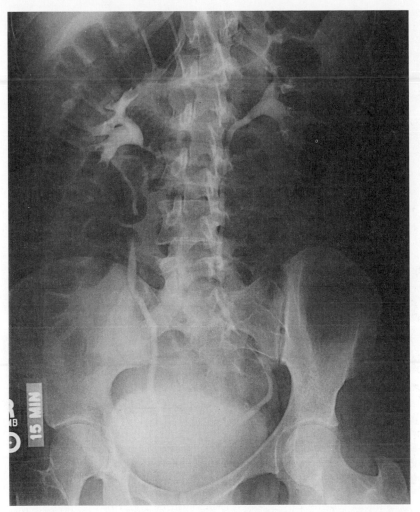

Figure 7-109. A 15-min RPO during IVU, demonstrating the left kidney and right ureter parallel to the IR. The 30° oblique KUB projection places the *kidney* of the *up* side *parallel* to the IR, and the *ureter* of the side *down* parallel to the IR. (Photo contributor: Stamford Hospital, Department of Radiology.)

Female Reproductive System

Introduction. The female reproductive system consists of the ovaries, oviducts, and uterus. The broad, suspensory, round, and ovarian ligaments are all associated with support of the reproductive organs.

The *ovaries* are the female gonads that function to release ova (female reproductive cells) during ovulation and produce various female hormones, including estrogen and progesterone. The *oviducts,* or Fallopian tubes, are 3–5 inches long, arise from the uterine cornua (angles), and extend laterally to arch over each ovary. The oviduct lateral extremities are broader than their medial ends and are bordered by motile *fimbriae* (see Figs. 7-111 and 7-112). The fimbriae sweep over the ovary and function to collect the liberated ovum. *Fertilization* of the ovum usually occurs in the outer portion of the oviducts. Ova are propelled through the oviduct by peristaltic motion. *Salpingitis* is possibly the most common cause of female sterility; if fertilization does occur, the zygote is unable to traverse the oviduct owing to its scarred or narrowed condition. Occasionally, a fertilized ovum will become implanted in the oviduct, a condition known as ectopic, or tubal, pregnancy. This condition

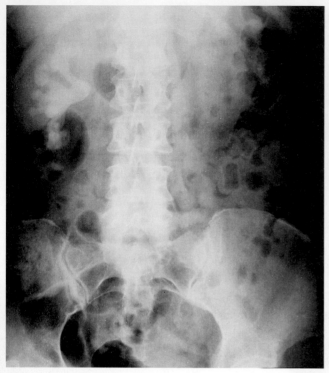
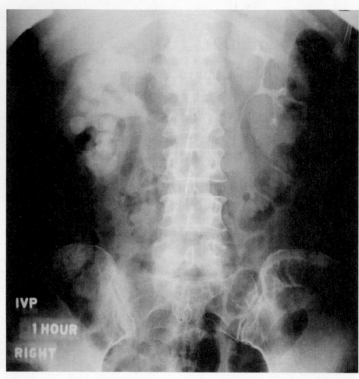

A   **B**

Figure 7-110. Although radiograph **(A)** may appear to be part of an intravenous urogram, no contrast agent is associated with the opaque right kidney; the opaque area is a result of the formation of a *staghorn calculus*. Radiograph **(B)** is a 1-h intravenous urogram demonstrating both collecting systems. Staghorn calculi are usually associated with chronic infection and alkaline urine. They may be associated with a single calyx or an entire renal pelvis and may be unilateral or bilateral. Whenever possible, staghorn (named for their shape, resembling a stag's antlers) calculi are removed because they can cause partial obstruction of the calyces and/or ureteropelvic junction. (From the ACR Learning File. Photo contributor: ACR.)

is a gynecologic emergency because, if left untreated, the patient can die from internal hemorrhage.

The most superior, arched, portion of the *uterus* is the fundus. The angle on each side is the cornu and marks the point of entry of the oviducts. The *body* is the large central region, and the narrow inferior portion is the *cervix*.

Hysterosalpingogram. The most commonly performed radiologic examination of the reproductive system is hysterosalpingography, which is used for evaluation of the uterus, oviducts, and ovaries of the female reproductive system. The procedure serves to delineate the position, size, and shape of the structures and demonstrates pathology such as *polyps, tumors,* and *fistulas.* However, it is most often used to demonstrate *patency* of the oviducts in cases of *infertility* and is sometimes therapeutic in terms of opening a blocked oviduct.

TABLE 7-51. Hysterosalpingogram

HSG	Position of Part	Central Ray Directed	Structures Included/Best Seen
AP	· Supine, MSP centered to the IR · A point 2″ above the pubic symphysis centered to the IR	· ⊥ Mid-IR	· AP proj of the uterus and oviducts · 30° obl images may be obtained as required (see Fig. 7-112A and B)

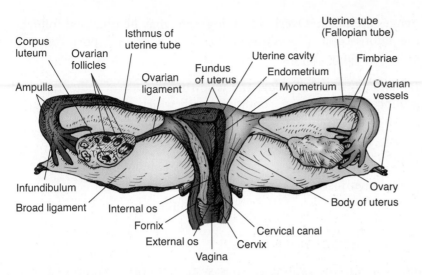

Figure 7-111. Uterus, uterine tubes (oviducts), and ovaries.

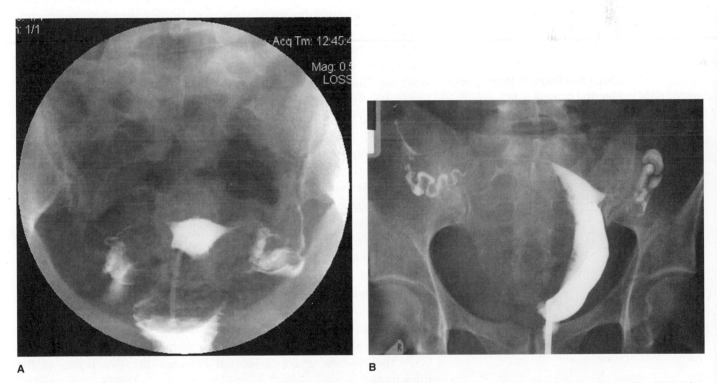

A

B

Figure 7-112. (A) AP projection of hysterosalpingogram study. Contrast-filled uterus and oviducts are shown, with spillage into the pelvic cavity. (Photo contributor: Stamford Hospital, Department of Radiology.) **(B)** Large mass distorting the uterus.

Hysterosalpingograms should be *scheduled* approximately 10 days after the start of menstruation. This is the time just *before* ovulation, when there should be little chance of irradiating a newly fertilized ovum.

After the cervical canal is cannulated, an iodinated contrast agent is injected via the cannula into the uterine cavity. If the oviducts are patent, contrast will flow through them and into the peritoneal cavity. Fluoroscopy is performed during injection and spot

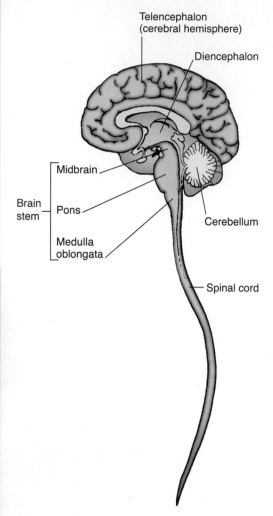

Figure 7-113. The CNS: brain and spinal cord.

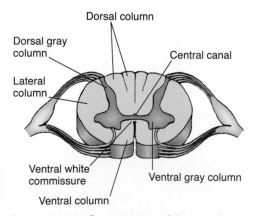

Figure 7-114. Cross-section of the spinal cord.

images are taken. Overhead radiographs may be obtained following the fluoroscopic procedure. Table 7-51 addresses positioning for hysterosalpingography.

Terminology and Pathology. The following is a list of radiographically significant reproductive conditions with which the student radiographer should be familiar:

- Bicornuate uterus
- Ectopic pregnancy
- Endometriosis
- Infertility
- Leiomyoma
- Pelvic inflammatory disease
- Placenta previa
- Salpingitis

Central Nervous System

Introduction. The central nervous system (CNS) is composed of the *brain* and the *spinal cord* (Fig. 7-113), enclosed within the bony skull and vertebral column, respectively. The brain consists of the cerebrum (largest part), *cerebellum, pons varolii,* and *medulla oblongata.* The *gray matter* of the brain consists of neuron cell bodies; the *white matter* consists of tracts (pathways) of axons. In transverse section, the spinal cord is seen to have an H-shaped configuration of gray matter internally, surrounded by white matter (Fig. 7-114). The brain and the spinal cord work together in the perception of sensory stimuli, in integration and correlation of stimuli with memory, and in neural actions resulting in coordinated motor responses to stimuli.

The CNS is enclosed within three tissue membranes, the *meninges.* The *pia mater* is the innermost vascular membrane, which is closely attached to the brain and the spinal cord. The *arachnoid mater* is a thin layer outside the pia mater and attached to it by web-like fibers. The *subarachnoid space* is between the pia and arachnoid mater and is filled with cerebrospinal fluid (CSF). The brain and the spinal cord float in CSF, which acts as a shock absorber.

Cerebral artery hemorrhage will leak blood into the CSF. *Lumbar puncture* is performed (between L3 and L4 or L4 and L5) to remove small quantities of CSF for testing and to introduce contrast medium during myelography. The *dura mater* is a double-layered fibrous membrane outside the arachnoid mater. The *subdural space* is located between the arachnoid and dura mater; it does not contain CSF. The *epidural space* is located between the two layers of the dura mater.

The cylindrical spinal cord is a continuation of the medulla oblongata, extending through the foramen magnum and the spinal canal to its termination at the *conus medullaris* (about the level of L1). The lumbar and sacral nerves have long roots that extend from the spinal cord as the *cauda equina* (horse's tail).

Procedures. Routine radiographic examination of the bony components of the CNS includes studies of the skull and the vertebral column. CT and MRI have replaced many plain radiographic procedures in the diagnosis and management of traumatic injuries and pathologic processes of the brain and the spinal cord.

Myelogram. Nevertheless, *myelography* remains a valuable diagnostic tool to demonstrate the site and extent of *spinal cord tumors* and *herniated intervertebral disks*. The intervertebral disk can rupture as a result of trauma or degeneration. The *nucleus pulposus* protrudes posteriorly through a tear in the *annulus fibrosus* and impinges on nerve roots (Fig. 7-115). More than 90% of disk ruptures occur at the L4–L5 and L5–S1 interspaces. Narrowing of the affected disk space may often be detected radiographically, and the defects caused by the rupture can generally be demonstrated through myelography, CT, or MRI.

Water-soluble nonionic iodinated contrast agents are the most widely used contrast media for myelography. Advantages of water-soluble contrast agents (over non–water-soluble) include better visualization of the nerve roots (see Fig. 7-116) and absorption properties that allow the contrast agents to be left in the subarachnoid space after the examination (because these are easily absorbed by the body). However, the use of water-soluble contrast agents for myelography does require that radiographs be obtained accurately and without delay because these are absorbed fairly quickly.

Foot and shoulder supports must be securely attached to the x-ray table. The patient should receive a complete explanation of the examination and must be instructed about the importance of keeping his or her chin extended when the table is lowered into the Trendelenburg position.

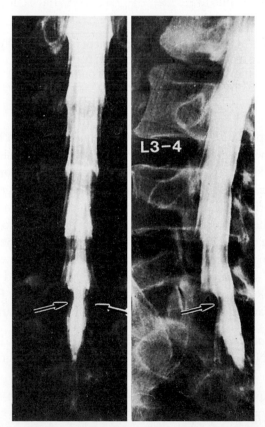

Figure 7-115. Myelograms demonstrating herniated L4–L5 disk. (Reproduced with permission from deGroot J. *Correlative Neuroanatomy*. 21st ed. East Norwalk, CT: Appleton & Lange; 1991.)

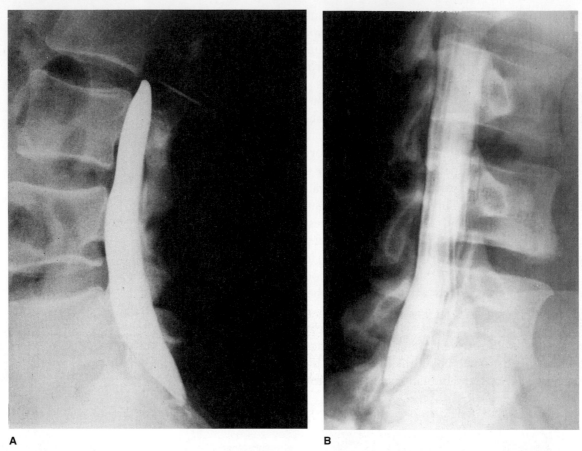

A   **B**

Figure 7-116. (A) Oil-base contrast myelography. (Photo contributor: Stamford Hospital, Department of Radiology.) **(B)** Water-soluble contrast myelography; observe improved visualization of nerve roots seen at the level of each pedicle as linear radiolucencies within the small inferolateral extensions of the contrast agent. (From the ACR Learning File. Photo contributor: ACR.)

A lumbar puncture is performed (usually at the fourth intervertebral space with the patient in the prone or flexed lateral position), a small quantity of CSF is removed from the subarachnoid space and sent to the laboratory for testing, and an equal amount of contrast agent is injected intrathecally (i.e., into the subarachnoid space of the spinal canal). The position of the contrast column will change according to gravitational forces, and its movement is observed fluoroscopically as the x-ray table is angled to varying degrees of the Trendelenburg and Fowler positions. Fluoroscopic spot images are taken as needed, followed by overhead radiographs. Routine protocol generally includes an AP or PA view and a horizontal beam (cross-table) lateral view of the vertebral area examined.

Terminology and Pathology. The following is a list of radiographically significant CNS conditions with which the student radiographer should be familiar:

- Degenerative disk disease
- Herniated nucleus pulposus
- Hydrocephalus
- Meningioma
- Parkinson disease
- Meningitis
- Meningomyelocele
- Spondylosis

Circulatory System

Introduction. The circulatory system consists of the *heart* and vessels (arteries, capillaries, veins) that distribute blood throughout the body (see Fig. 7-117). The heart is the muscular pump, and the *arteries* carry oxygenated blood throughout the body. The *capillaries* are responsible

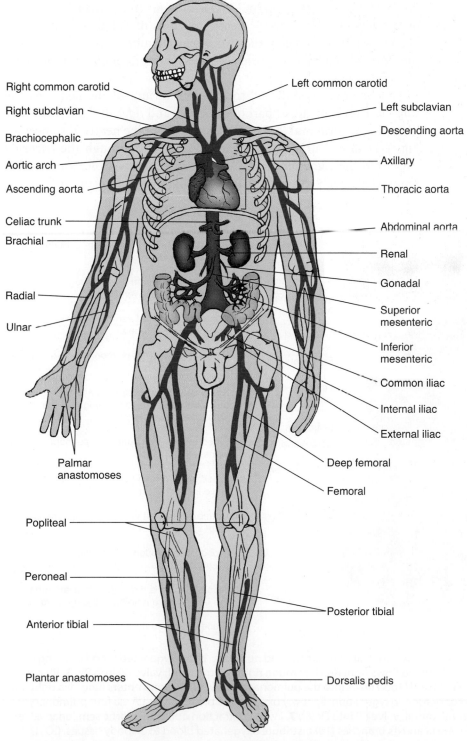

Figure 7-117. The major arteries of the cardiovascular system.

for diffusion of gases and exchange of nutrients and wastes. The *veins* collect deoxygenated blood and return it to the heart and lungs.

Contraction of the heart muscle as it pumps blood is called *systole*; relaxation is called *diastole*; these values are measured with a *sphygmomanometer*. Accompanying the contraction and expansion of the heart is contraction and expansion of arterial walls, called *pulse*.

The heart wall is made up of the external *epicardium*, the middle *myocardium*, and the internal *endocardium*. The *pericardium* is the fibroserous sac enclosing the heart and roots of the great vessels. The heart has four chambers. The two upper chambers are the *atria*, and the two lower chambers are the *ventricles*. The apex of the heart is the tip of the left ventricle.

Venous blood is returned to the right atrium of the heart via the *superior* (from the upper part of the body) and *inferior* (from the lower body) *venae cavae* and the *coronary sinus* (from the heart substance; see Fig. 7-118). On atrial systole, the blood passes through the *tricuspid valve* into the right ventricle. During ventricular systole, the blood is pumped through the *pulmonary semilunar valve* into the *pulmonary*

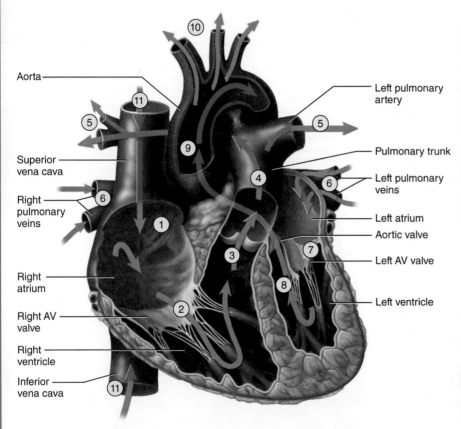

1. Blood enters right atrium from superior and inferior venae cavae.

2. Blood in right atrium flows through right AV valve into right ventricle.

3. Contraction of right ventricle forces pulmonary valve open.

4. Blood flows through pulmonary valve into pulmonary trunk.

5. Blood is distributed by right and left pulmonary arteries to the lungs, where it unloads CO_2 and loads O_2.

6. Blood returns from lungs via pulmonary veins to left atrium.

7. Blood in left atrium flows through left AV valve into left ventricle.

8. Contraction of left ventricle (simultaneous with step 3) forces aortic valve open.

9. Blood flows through aortic valve into ascending aorta.

10. Blood in aorta is distributed to every organ in the body, where it unloads O_2 and loads CO_2.

11. Blood returns to right atrium via venae cavae.

Figure 7-118. Cardiopulmonary circulation. Blood flow is indicated by arrows and numbers: **1,** deoxygenated blood entering RA (1) from superior and inferior venae cavae (11); **2,** blood flows from RA (1) through right AV (tricuspid) valve (2) into RV; **3,** RV contraction opens the pulmonary semilunar valve (3) and blood flows into the pulmonary artery (4); **4,** blood enters lungs via right and left pulmonary arteries (5), releases CO_2, and undergoes oxygenation; **5,** newly oxygenated blood enters LA via four pulmonary veins (6); **6,** blood flows from LA through left AV (mitral) valve (7) into LV (8); **7,** LV (8) contraction opens the aortic semilunar valve and blood flows into the ascending aorta (9). Aorta and its branches (10) distribute oxygenated blood to all body tissues. CO_2 is collected by the venous system, and deoxygenated blood is returned via the superior and inferior venae cavae (11) to the RA. (Reproduced with permission from Saladin K. *Anatomy and Physiology: The Unity of Form and Function.* 7th ed. New York : McGraw-Hill Education; 2015.)

artery (the only artery to carry deoxygenated blood) to the lungs for oxygenation.

Blood is returned via the *pulmonary veins* (the only veins to carry oxygenated blood) to the left atrium. During atrial systole, blood passes through the *mitral (bicuspid) valve* into the left ventricle. During ventricular systole, the oxygenated blood is pumped through the *aortic semilunar valve* into the aorta. When blood pressure is reported, as, for example, "130 over 85," the top number (130) represents the systolic pressure and the lower number (85) represents the diastolic pressure.

The *aorta* is the trunk artery of the body; it is divided into the ascending aorta, aortic arch (see Fig. 7-119), descending thoracic aorta, and abdominal aorta. Many arteries arise from the aorta to supply destinations throughout the body. The *superior* and *inferior venae cavae* and the *coronary sinus* are the major veins, collecting venous blood from the upper and lower body areas and heart substance, respectively. The formation of sclerotic plaques (as in *atherosclerosis*) and other conditions that impair the flow of blood can lead to *ischemia* and tissue *infarction*. Atherosclerosis of the coronary arteries can cause *angina pectoris* and *myocardial infarction*.

The *four divisions* of the aorta and *their major branches* are as follows:

Ascending Aorta

* Left and right coronary arteries

> **Pulmonary Circulation**
> * Unoxygenated blood from the right side of the heart is directed to the lungs for oxygenation and then to the left side of the heart
>
> **Systemic Circulation**
> * Oxygenated blood from the left side of the heart is pumped to the body tissues and then back to the right side of the heart

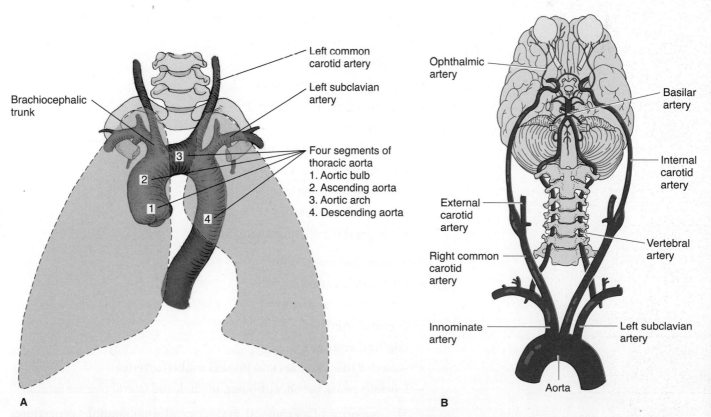

A   **B**

Figure 7-119. **(A)** Thoracic aorta illustrating major branches of the aortic arch. **(B)** Blood supply to the brain. (Reproduced with permission from Doherty GM, ed. *Current Surgical Diagnosis & Treatment*. 12th ed. New York : McGraw-Hill; 2006.)

Aortic Arch (Fig. 7-119A and B)

- Brachiocephalic (innominate) artery
- Right common carotid artery
- Right subclavian artery
- Left common carotid artery
- Left subclavian artery

Blood Supply to the Brain

- Internal carotid arteries (Fig. 7-119A and B)
  - Branch from common carotid arteries
  - Supply anterior brain
- Vertebral arteries
  - Branch from subclavian arteries
  - Supply posterior brain

Thoracic Aorta

- Intercostal arteries
- Superior phrenic arteries
- Bronchial arteries
- Esophageal arteries

Abdominal Aorta

- Inferior phrenic arteries
- Celiac (axis) artery/trunk gives rise to:
  - Common hepatic artery
  - Left gastric artery
  - Splenic artery
- Superior mesenteric artery
- Suprarenal arteries
- Renal arteries
- Gonadal arteries (testicular or ovarian)
- Inferior mesenteric artery
- Common iliac arteries give rise to:
  - Internal iliac arteries
  - External iliac (hypogastric) arteries

Arteries of the Lower Limb

- Internal iliac arteries
- External iliac arteries
- Femoral arteries
- Popliteal arteries
- Anterior tibial arteries and posterior tibial arteries
- Dorsalis pedis, peroneal/fibular, medial, and lateral plantar arteries

The majority of peripheral and visceral angiographic procedures are performed in a specially equipped angiographic suite by cardiovascular–interventional technologists (Figs. 7-120 and 7-121). Many cardiovascular suites nowadays use digital subtraction angiography (DSA). *Subtraction* is a technique that removes unnecessary structures such as bone from superimposition on contrast-filled blood vessels. DSA is subtraction achieved by means of a computer, which can also permit manipulation of contrast and other image characteristics by the technologist. The student radiographer, although not

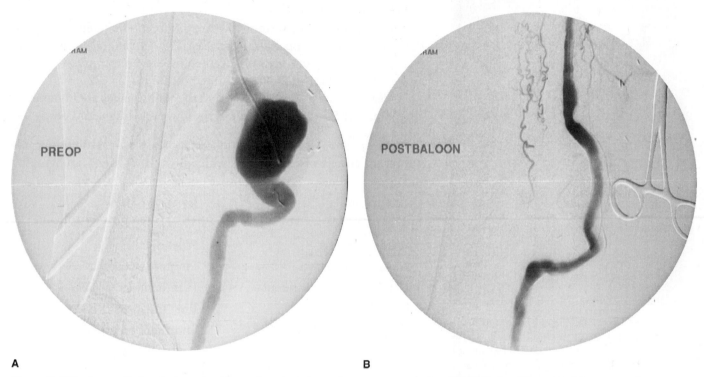

Figure 7-120. Lower limb arteriogram subtraction demonstrating *aneurysm, before* **(A)** and *after* **(B)** repair. (Photo contributor: Stamford Hospital, Department of Radiology.)

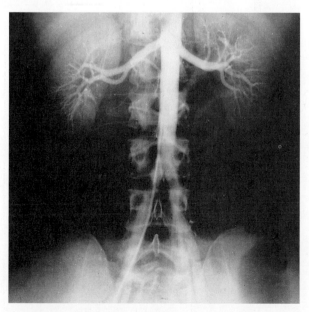

Figure 7-121. The renal arteriogram is one of many types of procedures performed by specially trained teams of health care professionals. (From the ACR Learning File. Photo contributor: ACR.)

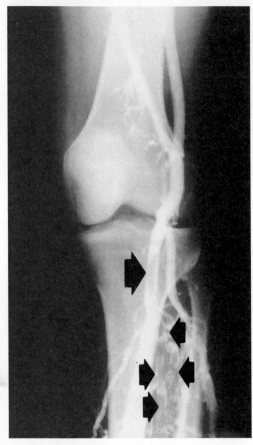

Figure 7-122. AP projection of a lower limb venography demonstrating multiple intraluminal filling defects. (Reproduced with permission from Way LW, ed. *Current Surgical Diagnosis & Treatment.* 10th ed. East Norwalk, CT: Appleton & Lange; 1994.)

performing most of these examinations, should be familiar with the names of the most common procedures and the conditions and disorders for which they are performed.

Venography. The one vascular procedure that might still be performed in general radiography is the lower limb *venography* (Fig. 7-122). This examination is generally performed to confirm a suspected deep vein thrombosis in an effort to avoid the complications of pulmonary embolism.

The patient should be examined on a radiographic table that can be tilted to a semierect position of at least 45°. Tourniquets are used to force contrast medium into the deep veins. Sterile technique must be rigorously maintained. An injection of 50–100 mL at 1–2 mL/s is usually given through a superficial vein in the foot. Images are obtained at approximately 5- to 10-s intervals of the lower leg, thigh, and pelvis.

Terminology and Pathology. The following is a list of radiographically significant circulatory conditions with which the student radiographer should be familiar:

- Aneurysm
- Angina pectoris
- Atherosclerosis
- Atrial septal defect
- Cerebrovascular accident (CVA)
- Coarctation of aorta
- Congestive heart failure
- Coronary artery disease
- Hypertension
- Myocardial infarction
- Phlebitis
- Pulmonary edema
- Pulmonary embolism
- Rheumatic heart disease
- Thrombophlebitis
- Ventricular septal defect

COMPREHENSION CHECK

Congratulations! You have completed the last section of this chapter. If you are able to answer the following group of very comprehensive questions, you should feel confident that you have really mastered this section. You can refer back to the indicated pages to check your answers and/or review the subject matter.

1. Identify the principal structures comprising the respiratory system and discuss their function(s) (p. 189).

2. Describe the (a) method of positioning, (b) direction and point of entry of the CR, (c) principal structures visualized, and (d) pertinent traumatic and pathologic conditions and any technical adjustments that may be required relative to the routine and special views of the chest (PA, lateral, oblique, lordotic, decubitus) and airway (pp. 193–195).

3. Identify the principal structures comprising the biliary system and discuss their function(s) (p. 196).

4. Describe the (a) method of positioning, (b) direction and point of entry of the CR, (c) principal structures visualized, and (d) pertinent traumatic and pathologic conditions and any technical adjustments that may be required relative to the routine and special views of the biliary system, including (p. 197, 198)

   A. surgical cholangiography

   B. ERCP

5. Identify the principal structures comprising the digestive system and discuss their function(s) (pp. 199–205).

6. Describe the (a) method of positioning, (b) direction and point of entry of the CR, (c) principal structures visualized, and (d) pertinent traumatic and pathologic conditions and any technical adjustments that may be required relative to the routine and special views of the digestive system, including

   A. swallowing dysfunction/deglutition study (p. 199)

   B. abdomen (p. 205)

   C. esophagus (p. 207)

   D. stomach and small intestine (p. 209, 210)

   E. large intestine (p. 211)

7. Identify the principal structures comprising the urinary system and discuss their function(s) (p. 214, 215).

8. Describe the (a) method of positioning, (b) direction and point of entry of the CR, (c) principal structures visualized, and (d) pertinent traumatic and pathologic conditions and any technical adjustments that may be required relative to the routine and special views of the urinary system, including

   A. KUB (p. 205)

   B. IVU (p. 219)

   C. retrograde examinations (p. 219)

   D. bladder (p. 220)

9. Identify the principal structures comprising the female reproductive system and discuss their function(s) (p. 221, 222).

10. Describe the (a) method of positioning, (b) direction and point of entry of the CR, (c) principal structures visualized, and (d) pertinent traumatic and pathologic conditions and any technical adjustments that may be required in *hysterosalpingography* (p. 223).

11. Identify the principal structures comprising the CNS and discuss their function(s) (p. 224, 225).

12. Describe the (a) indications for (b) principal structures visualized, and (c) pertinent traumatic and pathologic conditions and any technical adjustments that may be required in myelography (p. 225, 226).

13. Identify the principal structures comprising the circulatory system and discuss their function(s) (pp. 227–230).

14. List the kinds of specialized examinations that might be performed to demonstrate various traumatic and pathologic conditions of the circulatory system (p. 231, 232).

CHAPTER REVIEW QUESTIONS

Congratulations! You have completed this chapter. You may go on to the "registry-type" multiple-choice questions that follow. For greatest success, be sure to also complete the short-answer questions given at the end of each section of this chapter.

Questions 1–10 refer to the "Appendicular Skeleton" section.

1. In the AP projection of the knee, the
    1. patella is visualized through the femur
    2. CR is directed ½ inch distal to the patellar base
    3. CR is directed 3°–5° cephalad when the distance between the tabletop and the ASIS is 17 cm
    (A) 1 only
    (B) 1 and 2 only
    (C) 2 and 3 only
    (D) 1, 2, and 3

2. A Colles fracture usually involves the following:
    1. transverse fracture of the proximal radius
    2. posterior and outward displacement of the hand
    3. chip fracture of the ulnar styloid process
    (A) 1 only
    (B) 1 and 2 only
    (C) 2 and 3 only
    (D) 1, 2, and 3

3. Which of the following projections require(s) that the humeral epicondyles be superimposed?
    1. Lateral thumb
    2. Lateral wrist
    3. Lateral humerus
    (A) 1 only
    (B) 1 and 2 only
    (C) 2 and 3 only
    (D) 1, 2, and 3

4. In the 15°–20° mortise oblique position of the ankle, the
    1. talofibular joint is visualized
    2. talotibial joint is visualized
    3. plantar surface should be vertical
    (A) 1 only
    (B) 1 and 3 only
    (C) 2 and 3 only
    (D) 1, 2, and 3

5. The following projection(s) should not be performed until a transverse fracture of the patella has been ruled out:
    1. AP knee
    2. flexed lateral knee
    3. axial/tangential patella
    (A) 1 only
    (B) 1 and 2 only
    (C) 2 and 3 only
    (D) 1, 2, and 3

6. Which of the following best demonstrates the cuboid, sinus tarsi, and tuberosity of the fifth metatarsal?
    (A) Lateral foot
    (B) Lateral oblique foot
    (C) Medial oblique foot
    (D) Weight-bearing foot

7. The left SI joint is placed perpendicular to the IR when the patient is placed in a
    (A) left lateral position
    (B) 25°–30° RAO position
    (C) 25°–30° RPO position
    (D) 30°–40° RPO position

8. The proximal tibiofibular articulation is best demonstrated in which of the following positions?
    (A) Medial oblique
    (B) Lateral oblique
    (C) AP
    (D) Lateral

9. An axial projection of the clavicle is often helpful in demonstrating a fracture not visualized using a perpendicular central ray. When examining the clavicle in the AP axial projection, how should the central ray be directed?

   (A) Cephalad

   (B) Caudad

   (C) Medially

   (D) Laterally

10. The scapular Y projection of the shoulder demonstrates

    1. a lateral projection of the shoulder

    2. anterior or posterior dislocation

    3. an oblique projection of the shoulder

    (A) 1 only

    (B) 1 and 2 only

    (C) 2 and 3 only

    (D) 1, 2, and 3

Questions 11–20 refer to the "Axial Skeleton" section.

11. In the AP axial projection (Towne method) of the skull, with the central ray directed 30° caudad to the OML and passing midway between the external auditory meati, which of the following is best demonstrated?

    (A) Facial bones

    (B) Frontal bone

    (C) Occipital bone

    (D) Basal foramina

12. Which of the following is a functional study used to demonstrate the degree of AP motion present in the cervical spine?

    (A) Open-mouth projection

    (B) Moving mandible AP

    (C) Flexion and extension laterals

    (D) Right and left bending

13. The AP projection of the coccyx requires that the central ray be directed

    1. 15° cephalad

    2. 2 inches above the pubic symphysis

    3. midline at the level of the lesser trochanter

    (A) 1 only

    (B) 2 only

    (C) 1 and 2 only

    (D) 1 and 3 only

14. Which of the following is (are) demonstrated in the lateral projection of the thoracic spine?

    1. Intervertebral joints

    2. Zygapophyseal joints

    3. Intervertebral foramina

    (A) 1 only

    (B) 2 only

    (C) 1 and 2 only

    (D) 1 and 3 only

15. The thoracic vertebrae are unique in that they participate in the following articulations:

    1. costovertebral

    2. costotransverse

    3. costochondral

    (A) 1 only

    (B) 1 and 2 only

    (C) 2 and 3 only

    (D) 1, 2, and 3

16. To demonstrate undistorted air/fluid levels, the CR must always be directed

    (A) parallel with the long axis of the body/part

    (B) parallel with the floor

    (C) perpendicular to the long axis of the body/part

    (D) perpendicular to the floor

17. All of the following statements regarding the PA projection of the skull, with central ray perpendicular to the IR, are true, *except*

    (A) OML is perpendicular to the IR

    (B) petrous pyramids fill the orbits

    (C) MSP is parallel to the IR

    (D) central ray exits at the nasion

18. Which of the paranasal sinuses is composed of many thin-walled air cells?

    (A) Frontal

    (B) Sphenoid

    (C) Ethmoid

    (D) Maxillary

19. The intervertebral joints of the thoracic spine are demonstrated with the

    (A) midcoronal plane 45° to the IR

    (B) MSP 45° to the IR

    (C) midcoronal plane 70° to the IR

    (D) MSP parallel to the IR

20. Which of the following structures is subject to blowout fracture?

    (A) Ethmoid sinuses

    (B) Zygomatic arch

    (C) Mandibular condyle

    (D) Orbital floor

Questions 21–60 refer to the "Body Systems" section.

21. Aspirated foreign bodies in older children and adults are most likely to lodge in the

    (A) right main bronchus

    (B) left main bronchus

    (C) esophagus

    (D) proximal stomach

22. Which of the following is (are) important when positioning the patient for a PA projection of the chest?

    1. The patient should be examined in the erect position

    2. Clavicles should be brought above the apices

    3. Scapulae should be brought lateral to the lung fields

    (A) 1 only

    (B) 1 and 2 only

    (C) 1 and 3 only

    (D) 1, 2, and 3

23. Chest radiography should be performed by using 72-inch SID whenever possible to

    1. visualize vascular markings

    2. obtain better lung detail

    3. maximize magnification of the heart

    (A) 1 only

    (B) 1 and 2 only

    (C) 2 and 3 only

    (D) 1, 2, and 3

24. Blunting of the costophrenic angles seen on a PA projection of the chest can be an indication of

    (A) pleural effusion

    (B) ascites

    (C) bronchitis

    (D) emphysema

25. Which of the following conditions is characterized by "flattening" of the diaphragm?

    (A) Emphysema

    (B) Empyema

    (C) Atelectasis

    (D) Pneumonia

26. Inspiration and expiration projections of the chest may be performed to demonstrate

    1. pneumothorax

    2. presence of a foreign body

    3. bronchitis

    (A) 1 only

    (B) 1 and 2 only

    (C) 1 and 3 only

    (D) 1, 2, and 3

27. Which of the following criteria are used to evaluate a good PA projection of the chest?

    1. Ten posterior ribs should be visualized

    2. Sternoclavicular joints should be symmetrical

    3. Scapulae should be outside the lung fields

    (A) 1 and 2 only

    (B) 1 and 3 only

    (C) 2 and 3 only

    (D) 1, 2, and 3

28. All of the following statements regarding respiratory structures are true, *except*

    (A) the right lung has three lobes

    (B) the uppermost portion of a lung is its apex

    (C) the lobes of the left lung are separated by the horizontal fissure

    (D) the trachea bifurcates into mainstem bronchi

29. To demonstrate the pulmonary apices below the level of the clavicles in the AP position, the CR should be directed

    (A) perpendicular

    (B) 15°–20° caudad

    (C) 15°–20° cephalad

    (D) 40° cephalad

30. Radiographic indications of atelectasis include

    1. decreased radiographic density/increased brightness of the affected side

    2. elevation of the hemidiaphragm of the affected side

    3. flattening of the hemidiaphragm of the affected side

    (A) 1 only

    (B) 3 only

    (C) 1 and 2 only

    (D) 1 and 3 only

31. During IVU, the prone position is generally recommended to demonstrate

    1. filling of obstructed ureters

    2. the renal pelvis

    3. the superior calyces

    (A) 1 only

    (B) 1 and 2 only

    (C) 1 and 3 only

    (D) 1, 2, and 3

32. The contraction and expansion of arterial walls in accordance with forceful contraction and relaxation of the heart is called

    (A) hypertension

    (B) elasticity

    (C) pulse

    (D) pressure

33. Which of the following projections of the abdomen could be used to demonstrate air or fluid levels when the erect position cannot be obtained?

    1. AP Trendelenburg

    2. Dorsal decubitus

    3. Lateral decubitus

    (A) 1 only

    (B) 1 and 2 only

    (C) 2 and 3 only

    (D) 1, 2, and 3

34. Which of the following best describes the relationship between the esophagus and the trachea?

    (A) Esophagus is posterior to the trachea

    (B) Trachea is posterior to the esophagus

    (C) Esophagus is lateral to the trachea

    (D) Trachea is lateral to the esophagus

35. To demonstrate esophageal varices, the patient must be examined in the

    (A) recumbent position

    (B) erect position

    (C) anatomic position

    (D) Fowler position

36. The usual preparation for an upper GI series includes

    (A) clear fluids 8 h prior to examination

    (B) NPO after midnight

    (C) enemas until clear before examination

    (D) light breakfast at the day of examination

37. Which of the following positions would best demonstrate a double-contrast visualization of the left and right colic flexures?

    (A) Left lateral decubitus

    (B) AP recumbent

    (C) Right lateral decubitus

    (D) AP erect

38. In which of the following positions are a barium-filled pyloric canal and duodenal bulb best demonstrated during a GI series?

    (A) RAO

    (B) Left lateral

    (C) Recumbent PA

    (D) Recumbent AP

39. What position is frequently used to project the GB away from the vertebrae in the asthenic patient?

    (A) RAO

    (B) LAO

    (C) Left lateral decubitus

    (D) PA erect

40. Which of the following barium/air-filled anatomic structures is best demonstrated in the RAO position?

    (A) Splenic flexure

    (B) Hepatic flexure

    (C) Sigmoid colon

    (D) Ileocecal valve

41. In what order should the following studies be conducted?

    1. Barium enema

    2. Intravenous urogram

    3. Upper GI

    (A) 3, 1, 2

    (B) 1, 3, 2

    (C) 2, 1, 3

    (D) 2, 3, 1

42. All of the following statements regarding the urinary system are true, *except*

    (A) the left kidney is usually higher than the right

    (B) the kidneys move inferiorly in the erect position

    (C) the upper, expanded part of the ureter is the hilum

    (D) vessels, nerves, and lymphatics pass through the renal hilum

43. Which of the following examinations require(s) restriction of the patient's diet?

    1. GI series

    2. Abdominal survey

    3. Urogram

    (A) 1 only

    (B) 1 and 2 only

    (C) 1 and 3 only

    (D) 1, 2, and 3

44. During a GI examination, the AP recumbent projection of a stomach of average size and shape will usually demonstrate

    1. barium-filled fundus

    2. double-contrast visualization of distal stomach portions

    3. barium-filled duodenum and pylorus

    (A) 1 only

    (B) 1 and 2 only

    (C) 1 and 3 only

    (D) 1, 2, and 3

45. Which of the following examinations require(s) catheterization of the ureters?

    1. Retrograde urogram

    2. Cystogram

    3. Voiding cystogram

    (A) 1 only

    (B) 1 and 2 only

    (C) 2 and 3 only

    (D) 1, 2, and 3

46. Some common mild side effects of intravenous administration of water-soluble iodinated contrast agents include

    1. flushed feeling

    2. bitter taste

    3. urticaria

    (A) 1 only

    (B) 1 and 2 only

    (C) 1 and 3 only

    (D) 1, 2, and 3

47. Hysterosalpingograms may be performed for the following reason(s):

    1. demonstration of fistulous tracts

    2. investigation of infertility

    3. demonstration of tubal patency

    (A) 1 only

    (B) 1 and 2 only

    (C) 1 and 3 only

    (D) 1, 2, and 3

48. A postvoid image of the urinary bladder is usually requested at the completion of an intravenous urogram and may be helpful in demonstrating
    1. residual urine
    2. prostate enlargement
    3. ureteral tortuosity
    (A) 1 only
    (B) 1 and 2 only
    (C) 1 and 3 only
    (D) 1, 2, and 3

49. During routine IVU, the oblique position demonstrates the
    (A) kidney of the side up parallel to the IR
    (B) kidney of the side up perpendicular to the IR
    (C) urinary bladder parallel to the IR
    (D) urinary bladder perpendicular to the IR

50. To better demonstrate contrast-filled distal ureters during IVU, it is helpful to
    1. use a 15° AP Trendelenburg position
    2. apply compression to the proximal ureters
    3. apply compression to the distal ureters
    (A) 1 only
    (B) 2 only
    (C) 1 and 2 only
    (D) 1 and 3 only

51. The space located between the arachnoid and dura mater is the
    (A) subarachnoid space
    (B) subdural space
    (C) epidural space
    (D) epiarachnoid space

52. During a GI examination, the lateral recumbent projection of a stomach of average shape will demonstrate
    1. anterior and posterior aspects of the stomach
    2. medial and lateral aspects of the stomach
    3. double-contrast body and antral portions
    (A) 1 only
    (B) 1 and 2 only
    (C) 2 and 3 only
    (D) 1, 2, and 3

53. The method by which contrast-filled vascular images are removed from superimposition upon bone is called
    (A) positive masking
    (B) reversal
    (C) subtraction
    (D) registration

54. Indicate the correct sequence of oxygenated blood as it returns from the lungs to the heart.
    (A) Pulmonary veins, left atrium, left ventricle, aortic valve
    (B) Pulmonary artery, left atrium, left ventricle, aortic valve
    (C) Pulmonary veins, right atrium, right ventricle, pulmonary semilunar valve
    (D) Pulmonary artery, right atrium, right ventricle, pulmonary semilunar valve

55. In myelography, the contrast medium is generally injected into the
    (A) cisterna magna
    (B) individual intervertebral disks
    (C) subarachnoid space between the first and second lumbar vertebrae
    (D) subarachnoid space between the third and fourth lumbar vertebrae

56. The upper chambers of the heart are the
    (A) ventricles
    (B) atria
    (C) pericardia
    (D) myocardia

57. Myelography is a diagnostic examination used to demonstrate
    1. posterior protrusion of the herniated intervertebral disk
    2. anterior protrusion of the herniated intervertebral disk
    3. internal disk lesions
    (A) 1 only
    (B) 2 only
    (C) 1 and 2 only
    (D) 1 and 3 only

58. The four major arteries supplying the brain include the
    1. brachiocephalic artery
    2. common carotid arteries
    3. vertebral arteries
    (A) 1 and 2 only
    (B) 1 and 3 only
    (C) 2 and 3 only
    (D) 1, 2, and 3

59. Venous, or deoxygenated, blood is returned to the heart via the
    1. inferior vena cava
    2. superior vena cava
    3. coronary sinus
    (A) 1 only
    (B) 2 only
    (C) 1 and 2 only
    (D) 1, 2, and 3

60. The apex of the heart is formed by the
    (A) left atrium
    (B) right atrium
    (C) left ventricle
    (D) right ventricle

Answers and Explanations

1. (A) The AP projection of the knee requires the knee to be extended. There should be no pelvic rotation, although the leg may be rotated 3°–5° internally. The central ray is directed to ½ inch below patellar apex (location of the knee joint). The direction of the CR depends on the distance between the ASIS and the tabletop; that is, up to 19 cm (thin pelvis) angle 3°–5° caudad; 19–24 cm is 0° (perpendicular) CR; greater than 24 cm (thick pelvis) 3°–5° cephalad. This demonstrates an AP projection of the knee joint, distal femur, and proximal tibia/fibula. The patella is seen through the femur. The femoral condyles are superimposed in the lateral projection of the knee.

2. (C) A Colles fracture is often caused by a fall onto an outstretched hand in order to "brake" the fall. As a result, the wrist suffers an impacted transverse fracture of the distal inch of the radius, with displacement of the hand posteriorly (i.e., backward, ~30°) and outward, causing the characteristic "dinner fork" deformity seen on x-ray examination. This injury is usually accompanied by a chip fracture of the ulnar styloid process.

3. (C) For the lateral projections of the hand, wrist, forearm, and elbow, the elbow must be flexed 90° to superimpose the distal radius and ulna and humeral epicondyles. Although a lateral humerus projection can be performed with the elbow flexed, if flexion is not possible, the elbow may remain in the AP position and a transthoracic lateral projection of the upper one-half to two-thirds of the humerus may be obtained. Because a coronal plane passing through the epicondyles (interepicondylar line) is perpendicular to the IR in this position, the epicondyles will be superimposed. To obtain a lateral projection of the thumb (first digit), the patient's wrist must be somewhat internally rotated. Remember that an oblique projection of the thumb is obtained in a PA projection of the hand.

4. (D) The medial oblique projection (15°–20° mortise view) of the ankle is valuable because it demonstrates the tibiofibular joint as well as the talotibial joint, thereby visualizing all the major articulating surfaces of the ankle joint. To demonstrate maximum joint volume, it is recommended that the plantar surface be vertical.

5. (C) If a transverse fracture of the patella is present and the knee is *flexed,* there is a danger of *separation* of the fractured segments. Because both a lateral knee and an axial patella require knee flexion, they should be avoided until a transverse fracture is ruled out. When present, a transverse fracture may be seen through the femur on the AP projection. The axial (sunrise) projection of the patella is generally used for demonstrating *vertical* patellar fractures.

6. (C) To demonstrate many of the tarsals and intertarsal spaces, including the cuboid, third (lateral) cuneiform, sinus tarsi, and tuberosity of the fifth metatarsal, a *medial oblique* projection is required (plantar surface and IR form a 30° angle). The *lateral* oblique projection of the foot demonstrates the navicular bone and first (medial) and second (intermediate) cuneiforms. Weight-bearing lateral feet are used to demonstrate the longitudinal arches.

7. (C) SI joints lie obliquely in the pelvis and open anteriorly at an angle of 25°–30° to the MSP. A 25°–30° oblique position places the joints perpendicular to the IR. The left SI joint is demonstrated in the RPO and LAO positions, with little difference in magnification.

8. (A) With the femoral condyles of the affected side rotated *medially/internally* to form a 45° angle with the IR, the *proximal* tibiofibular articulation is placed parallel with the IR and the fibula is free of superimposition with the tibia. The lateral oblique projection completely superimposes the tibia and the fibula. The AP and lateral projections superimpose enough of the tibia and the fibula so that the tibiofibular articulation is "closed."

9. (A) With the patient positioned for an AP axial projection, the central ray is directed cephalad. The reverse is true when examining the clavicle in the prone position. This serves to project the pulmonary apices away from the clavicle. Patients having clavicular pain are more comfortably examined by using the PA erect or AP recumbent projection/position.

10. (C) The scapular Y projection requires that the coronal plane be approximately 60° to the IR, thus resulting in an oblique projection of the shoulder. The vertebral and axillary borders of the scapula are superimposed on the humeral shaft, and the resulting relationship between the glenoid fossa and the humeral head will demonstrate anterior or posterior dislocation. Lateral or medial dislocation is evaluated on the AP projection.

11. (C) The AP axial projection is obtained by angling the central ray 30° caudad to the OML (see Fig. 7-63A). This projects the anterior structures (frontal and facial bones) downward, thus permitting visualization of the *occipital bone* without superimposition (Towne method). The dorsum sella and posterior clinoid processes of the sphenoid bone should be visualized within the foramen magnum. The *frontal bone* is best shown in the PA projection with a perpendicular central ray. The parietoacanthial projection is the single best position for *facial bones. Basal foramina* are well demonstrated in the submentovertical (SMV) projection.

12. (C) The degree of anterior to posterior motion is occasionally diminished with a "whiplash"-type injury. Anterior (forward, flexion) and posterior (backward, extension) motion is evaluated in the lateral position, with the patient assuming flexion and extension positions as much as possible. Left and right bending images of the vertebral column are frequently obtained to evaluate scoliosis.

13. (B) The AP projection of the *coccyx* requires that the CR be directed 10° caudally and centered to a point 2 inches above the pubic symphysis. The AP projection of the *sacrum* requires a 15° cephalad angle of the CR, centered to a point midway between the pubic symphysis and the ASIS.

14. (D) Intervertebral joints are well visualized in the *lateral* projection of all the vertebral groups. Thoracic and lumbar intervertebral foramina are well demonstrated in the *lateral* projection. Thoracic and lumbar *zygapophyseal joints* are demonstrated in an *oblique* position—thoracic requires a 70° oblique projection and lumbar requires a 45° oblique projection.

15. (B) There are 12 thoracic vertebrae, which are larger in size than cervical vertebrae and which increase in size as they progress inferiorly toward the lumbar region. Thoracic spinous processes are fairly long and are sharply angled caudally. The bodies and transverse processes have *articular facets* for the *diarthrotic* rib articulations (see Fig. 7-48). These structures form the *costovertebral* (head of the rib with the body of vertebra) and *costotransverse* (tubercle of the rib with the transverse process of vertebra) articulations. The *costochondral* articulation describes where the anterior end of the rib articulates with its costal cartilage.

16. (B) Radiography of the paranasal sinuses, and other structures such as the chest, must be performed in the erect position so that any *air/fluid levels* may be demonstrated. In the paranasal sinuses, the erect position helps distinguish between fluid and other pathology such as *polyps.*

To demonstrate air/fluid levels, *the CR must always be directed parallel to the floor,* even if the patient is not completely in an erect position (just as in chest radiography). If the CR is angled to parallel the plane of the body, any fluid levels will be distorted or indeed obliterated.

17. (C) In the exact PA projection of the skull, the CR is perpendicular and exits the nasion. The petrous pyramids should *fill* the orbits. If the CR is angled caudally, the petrous pyramids are projected lower in the orbits; at approximately 25°–30° caudal angle, they are projected *below* the orbits. In the PA projection, the OML must be perpendicular to the IR, or the petrous pyramids will not fill the orbits. The MSP must be perpendicular to the IR, or the skull will be rotated and anatomic details will lose L–R symmetry. The MSP is parallel to the IR in the lateral projection of the skull.

18. (C) There are four paired paranasal sinuses: *frontal, ethmoidal, maxillary,* and *sphenoidal* (see Fig. 7-69). They vary greatly in their size and shape. The left and right *frontal* sinuses are usually asymmetrical. They are located behind the glabella and superciliary arches of the frontal bone. The *frontal* sinuses are not present in young children and generally reach their adult size in the 15th or 16th year. The *ethmoid* sinuses are composed of 6–18 *thin-walled air cells* that occupy the bony labyrinth of the ethmoid bone. The ethmoidal sinuses of children are very small and do not fully develop until after the 14th year. The *maxillary* sinuses (maxillary antra/antra of Highmore) are the largest of the paranasal sinuses and are located in the body of the maxillae. The maxillary antra are particularly prone to infection and collections of stagnant mucus. The maxillary antra reach their adult size around the 12th year. The *sphenoid* sinuses are located in the body of the sphenoid bone and are usually asymmetrical. They generally reach adult size by the 14th year.

19. (D) Intervertebral *joints* are well visualized in the *lateral* projection of all the vertebral groups. Thoracic and lumbar intervertebral *foramina* are well demonstrated in the *lateral* projection. Thoracic and lumbar *zygapophyseal joints* are demonstrated in an *oblique* position—thoracic requires a 70° oblique projection and lumbar requires a 45° oblique projection. Cervical articular facets (forming zygapophyseal joints) are 90° to the MSP and are therefore well demonstrated in the lateral projection. The cervical intervertebral foramina lie 45° to the MSP (and 15°–20° to a transverse plane) and are therefore demonstrated in the oblique position.

20. (D) The orbital cavities are formed by seven bones (frontal, sphenoid, ethmoid, maxilla, palatine, zygoma/malar, and lacrimal). The orbital walls are fragile, and the orbital floor is subject to traumatic *blowout* fractures—the second most common facial fracture (nasal fractures being number one). Orbital fractures can be accompanied by injury to adjacent structures—bone, muscle, and other soft tissues. Leakage of air from the adjacent maxillary sinuses can cause orbital edema. *Orbital floor* fractures can be demonstrated by using the *parietoacanthial* (*Waters*) projection; CT is often indicated for further evaluation.

21. (A) Because the right main bronchus is wider and more vertical, aspirated foreign bodies are more likely to enter it than to the left main bronchus, which is narrower and angles more sharply from the trachea. An aspirated foreign body does not enter the esophagus and/or stomach because they are digestive, not respiratory, structures.

22. (C) The chest should be examined in the erect position whenever possible to demonstrate any air or fluid levels. The shoulders should be relaxed and depressed to move the clavicles *below* the lung apices. The shoulders should be rolled forward to move the *scapulae* out of the lung fields.

23. (B) Chest radiographs are obtained in the erect position at 72-inch SID whenever possible. The long SID is easily achieved with a minimum patient exposure owing to the low density of the tissue being examined (ribs and lungs). The longer SID *minimizes* magnification of the heart and provides better visualization of pulmonary vascular markings.

24. (A) Fluid in the thoracic cavity between the visceral and parietal pleurae is called *pleural effusion*. In the erect position, fluid gravitates to the lowest point, settling in and "blunting" the costophrenic angles. *Ascites* is an accumulation of serous fluid in the peritoneal cavity. *Bronchitis* is an inflammation of the bronchial tubes. Pulmonary *emphysema* is a chronic pulmonary disease characterized by an increase beyond the normal in the size of air spaces distal to the terminal bronchiole and with destructive changes in the walls of the bronchioles.

25. (A) *Emphysema* is characterized by irreversible trapping of air, which gradually increases and overexpands the lungs, thus producing the characteristic *flattening of the diaphragm* and *widening of the intercostal spaces* (see Fig. 7-81). The increased air content of the lungs requires a compensating *decrease in technical factors*. *Empyema* describes pus in the pleural cavity as a result of an infec-

tion of the lungs. *Atelectasis* is a collapsed or airless lung. *Pneumonia* is an inflammation of the lung; there are more than 50 causes of pneumonia.

26. (B) Phase of respiration is exceedingly important in thoracic radiography; lung expansion and the position of the diaphragm strongly influence the appearance of the finished radiograph. Inspiration and expiration radiographs of the chest are taken to demonstrate air in the pleural cavity (pneumothorax), to demonstrate degree of diaphragm excursion, or to detect the presence of a foreign body. The expiration image will require a somewhat greater exposure (equivalent of 6–8 kV or more) to compensate for the diminished quantity of air in the lungs.

27. (D) To evaluate sufficient inspiration and lung expansion, 10 posterior ribs should be visualized. Sternoclavicular joints should be symmetrical; any loss of symmetry indicates rotation. Accurate positioning and selection of technical factors are critical to the diagnostic value of the radiographic images. Even slight rotation or leaning can cause significant distortion of the heart size and shape. To visualize maximum lung area, the shoulders are rolled forward to remove the scapulae from the lung fields.

28. (C) The trachea (windpipe) bifurcates into left and right mainstem bronchi, each entering its respective lung hilum. The left bronchus divides into two parts, one for each lobe of the left lung; the right bronchus divides into three parts, one for each lobe of the right lung. The lungs have a somewhat conical shape; their narrow upper portion is called the *apex,* and their wide lower portion is the *base.* Structures such as the mainstem bronchi and pulmonary artery and veins enter and leave the lungs at the *hilum.* The *right* lung has *three* lobes: The upper and middle lobes are separated by the horizontal fissure, and the middle and lower lobes are separated by the oblique fissure. The *left lung* has *two lobes:* The upper and lower lobes are separated by the *oblique fissure* (see Fig. 7-76).

29. (C) When the shoulders are relaxed, the clavicles are usually carried below the pulmonary apices. To examine the portions of lungs lying behind the clavicles, the CR is directed 15°–20° cephalad to project the *clavicles above the apices* when the patient is examined in the AP position.

30. (C) Pneumothorax is the presence of air in the pleural cavity. A large pneumothorax is usually accompanied by a partial or complete *atelectasis* (collapse of the lung).

Radiographic indications of atelectasis include an increase in *tissue* density of the collapsed lung (therefore, *decreased image density/increased brightness*) and elevation of the hemidiaphragm of the *affected* side. The procedure required to remove significant amounts of air, blood, or other fluids in the pleural cavity is thoracentesis.

31. (B) The kidneys lie obliquely in the posterior portion of the trunk, with their superior portions angled posteriorly and their inferior portions and ureters angled anteriorly. Therefore, to facilitate filling of the most anteriorly placed structures, the patient is examined in the prone position. Opacified urine then flows to the most dependent part of the kidney and ureter—the ureteropelvic region, inferior calyces, and ureters.

32. (C) As the heart contracts and relaxes while functioning to pump blood from the heart, those arteries that are large and those in closest proximity to the heart will feel the effect of the heart's forceful contractions in their walls. The arterial walls pulsate in unison with the heart's contractions. This movement may be detected with the fingers in various parts of the body and is called the *pulse*.

33. (C) Air or fluid levels will be clearly demonstrated only if the central ray is directed parallel to them. Therefore, to demonstrate air or fluid levels, erect or decubitus positions should be used. A "three-way abdomen" study is often conducted to evaluate possible obstruction or free air or fluid within the abdomen and usually consists of AP recumbent, AP erect, and left lateral decubitus projections of the abdomen.

34. (A) The trachea (windpipe) is a tube-like passageway for air that is supported by C-shaped cartilaginous rings. The trachea is part of the respiratory system and is continuous with the mainstem bronchi. The esophagus, part of the alimentary canal, is a hollow tube-like structure connecting the mouth and the stomach and lies posterior to the trachea. If one inadvertently aspirates food or drink into the trachea, choking occurs.

35. (A) Esophageal varices are tortuous dilatations of the esophageal veins. They are much less pronounced in the erect position and must always be examined with the patient in a recumbent position. The recumbent position affords more complete filling of the veins, as blood flows against gravity.

36. (B) The upper GI tract must be empty for best x-ray evaluation. Any food or liquid mixed with the barium sulfate suspension can simulate pathology. Preparation therefore is to withhold food and fluids for 8–9 h before the examination, typically after midnight, as fasting examinations are usually performed first thing in the morning.

37. (D) To demonstrate structures via double-contrast technique, the barium must be moved away from the area and replaced with air. The *AP erect position* will accomplish that for both the colic flexures. The erect position allows barium to move downward, whereas air rises to fill the flexures. The decubitus positions are useful to demonstrate the lateral and medial walls of the ascending and descending colon.

38. (A) The RAO position affords a good view of the pyloric canal and the duodenal bulb. It is also a good position for the barium-filled esophagus, projecting it between the vertebrae and the heart. The left lateral projection of the stomach demonstrates the left retrogastric space; the recumbent PA position is used as a general survey of the gastric surfaces, and the recumbent AP position with a slight left oblique affords a double-contrast study of the pylorus and the duodenum.

39. (B) There are four types of body habitus. Listed from largest to smallest, they are hypersthenic, sthenic, hyposthenic, and asthenic. The position, shape, and motility of various organs can differ greatly from one body type to another. The typical asthenic GB is situated low and medial, often very close to the midline. To move the GB away from the midline, the LAO position is used. The GB of hypersthenic individuals occupies a high lateral and transverse position.

40. (B) In the prone oblique positions (RAO/LAO), the flexure disclosed is the one closer to the IR. Therefore, the RAO position will open up the hepatic flexure. The AP oblique positions (RPO/LPO) demonstrate the side away from the IR.

41. (C) When scheduling patient examinations, it is important to avoid the possibility of residual contrast medium covering areas of interest on later examinations. The intravenous urogram should be scheduled first because the contrast medium used is excreted rapidly. The BE should be scheduled next. The GI series is scheduled last. Any barium remaining from the previous BE should not be enough to interfere with the stomach or duodenum, although a preliminary scout image should be taken in each case.

42. (C) The major components of the urinary system are the *kidneys, ureters,* and *bladder.* The tiny functional units within the renal substance are *nephrons.*

The kidneys are retroperitoneal structures held in position by adipose tissue. They are located between the vertebral levels of T12 and L3. The right kidney is usually 1–2 inches lower than the left because of the presence of the liver on the right. The kidneys move inferiorly 1–3 inches when the body assumes an erect position; they move inferiorly and superiorly during respiration. The slit-like opening on the medial concave surface of each kidney is the *hilum*, which opens into a space called the renal sinus (see Fig. 7-102). The renal artery and vein, lymphatic vessels, and nerves pass through the hilum. The upper, expanded portion of the ureter is called the *renal pelvis*, or *infundibulum*, and also passes through the hilum; it is continuous with the major and minor *calyces* within the kidney.

43. (C) A patient having a GI series is required to be NPO (nothing by mouth) for at least 8 h prior to the examination; food or drink in the stomach can simulate disease. A patient scheduled for a urogram must have the preceding meal withheld to avoid the possibility of aspirating vomitus in case of allergic reaction. An abdominal survey does not require the use of contrast medium, and no patient preparation is required.

44. (B) With the body in the AP recumbent position, barium flows easily into the fundus of the stomach, displacing it somewhat superiorly. The fundus, then, is filled with barium, whereas the air that had been in the fundus is displaced into the gastric body, pylorus, and duodenum, illustrating them in double-contrast fashion. Air-contrast delineation of these structures allows us to see through the stomach to retrogastric areas and structures. Barium-filled duodenum and pylorus are best demonstrated in the RAO position.

45. (A) Retrograde urograms require catheterization of the urethra and/or the ureter(s). Radiographs that include the kidney(s) and ureter(s) in their entirety are obtained after retrograde filling of the structures. A cystogram or (voiding) cystourethrogram requires only *urethral* catheterization. Radiographs of the contrast-filled bladder and frequently of the contrast-filled urethra during voiding are obtained. Cystoscopy is required for location and catheterization of the vesicoureteral orifices.

46. (B) Because the urinary structures have so little subject contrast, artificial contrast material must be used for better visualization of these structures. Contrast agents used for urographic procedures can have unpleasant, and (rarely) even lethal, side effects. Intravenous injection of contrast frequently produces a warm, flushed feeling, a bitter or metallic taste, or mild nausea. These side effects are of short duration and usually pass as quickly as they come. More serious side effects include urticaria, respiratory discomfort/distress, and, rarely, anaphylaxis. An antihistamine is the appropriate treatment of simple side effects, but the radiographer must always be prepared to deal quickly and efficiently with patients experiencing more serious reactions. Nonionic contrast agents are far less likely to produce side effects.

47. (D) The most commonly performed radiologic examination of the reproductive system is hysterosalpingography, which is used for evaluation of the uterus, oviducts, and ovaries of the female reproductive system. The procedure serves to delineate the position, size, and shape of the structures and demonstrate pathology such as polyps, tumors, and fistulas. However, it is most often used to demonstrate *patency* of the oviducts in cases of *infertility* and is sometimes therapeutic in terms of opening a blocked oviduct.

48. (B) An AP postvoid bladder image is usually required to detect any *residual urine* in the evaluation of *tumor masses* or *enlarged prostate glands*. An erect image is occasionally requested to demonstrate renal mobility and ureteral tortuosity.

49. (A) During IVU, both oblique positions are generally obtained. The 30° oblique KUB (kidney, ureters, bladder) projection places the kidney of the side *away* from the x-ray table *parallel* to the IR. The kidney closer to the x-ray table is placed perpendicular to the IR. The oblique positions provide an oblique projection of the urinary bladder.

50. (A) A 15°–20° AP Trendelenburg position during IVU is often helpful in demonstrating filling of the distal ureters and the area of the vesicoureteral orifices. In this position, the contrast-filled urinary bladder moves superiorly, encouraging filling of the distal ureters and superior bladder, and provides better delineation of these areas. The central ray should be directed perpendicular to the IR. Compression of the *distal* ureters is used to prolong filling of the renal pelvis and calyces. Compression of the *proximal* ureters is not advocated.

51. (B) The CNS is enclosed within three tissue membranes, the *meninges*. The pia mater is the innermost vascular membrane, which is closely attached to the brain and the spinal cord. The arachnoid mater is a thin layer outside the pia mater and attached to it by web-like fibers. The *subarachnoid space* is between the pia and arachnoid mater and is filled with CSF. The brain and spinal cord float in CSF, which acts as a shock absorber. The dura mater is a double-layered fibrous membrane outside the arachnoid mater. The *subdural space* is located between the arachnoid and dura mater; it does not contain CSF. The *epidural space* is located between the two layers of the dura mater.

52. (A) *Anterior and posterior aspects* of the stomach are visualized in the *lateral* position; medial and lateral aspects of the stomach are visualized in the AP projection. With the body in the AP recumbent position, *barium* flows easily into the *fundus* of the stomach, displacing the stomach somewhat superiorly. The fundus, then, is filled with barium, whereas *air* is displaced into the *gastric body, pylorus,* and *duodenum*, demonstrating them as double contrast. Air-contrast delineation of these structures allows us to see through the stomach up to the retrogastric areas and structures.

53. (C) Superimposition of bony details frequently makes angiographic demonstration of blood vessels less than optimal. The method used to remove these superimposed bony details is called *subtraction. Digital* subtraction can accomplish this through the use of a computer, but *photographic* subtraction may also be performed by using images from an angiographic series. *Registration* is the process of matching one series image exactly over another. A reversal image, or positive mask, is a reverse of the black and white radiographic tones.

54. (A) Deoxygenated blood is returned by way of the inferior and superior venae cavae to the right side of the heart. The blood is emptied into the right atrium, passes through the tricuspid valve, and enters the right ventricle. It is forced through the pulmonary semilunar valve into the pulmonary artery (by contraction of the right ventricle) and passes to the lungs for reoxygenation. From the lungs, it is collected by the *pulmonary* veins, which carry the oxygenated blood to the left atrium, where it travels through the mitral valve into the *left ventricle*. On contraction of the left ventricle, blood passes through the *aortic valve* into the aorta and to all parts of the body.

55. (D) Generally, contrast medium is injected into the subarachnoid space between the third and fourth lumbar vertebrae. Because the spinal cord ends at the level of the first or second lumbar vertebra, this is considered to be a relatively safe injection site. The cisterna magna can be used, but the risk of contrast entering and causing side effects increases.

56. (B) The heart wall is made up of the external epicardium, the middle myocardium, and the internal endocardium. The pericardium is the fibroserous sac enclosing the heart and roots of the great vessels. The heart has four chambers. The two *upper* chambers are the *atria,* and the two *lower* chambers are the *ventricles.* The apex of the heart is the tip of the left ventricle.

57. (A) An intervertebral disk can rupture as a result of trauma or degeneration. The nucleus pulposus protrudes *posteriorly* through a tear in the annulus fibrosus and impinges on nerve roots and can be demonstrated by placing positive or negative contrast media into the subarachnoid space. Internal disk lesions can be demonstrated only by injecting contrast into the individual disks. (This procedure is termed *diskography.*) Anterior protrusion of a herniated intervertebral disk does not impinge on the spinal cord and is not demonstrated in myelography.

58. (C) Major branches of the common carotid arteries (internal carotids) function to supply the anterior brain, whereas the posterior brain is supplied by the vertebral arteries (branches of the subclavian arteries). The brachiocephalic (innominate) artery is unpaired and is one of three branches of the aortic arch, from which the right common carotid artery is derived. The left common carotid artery comes directly off the aortic arch.

59. (D) Venous blood is returned to the right atrium of the heart via the *superior* (from upper body) and *inferior* (from lower body) *venae cavae* and the *coronary sinus* (from the heart substance; see Fig. 7-118). On atrial systole, the blood passes through the tricuspid valve into the right ventricle. During ventricular systole, the blood is pumped through the pulmonary semilunar valve into the pulmonary artery and then to the lungs for oxygenation. Blood is returned via the pulmonary veins to the left atrium. During atrial systole, blood passes through the mitral (bicuspid) valve into the left ventricle. During ventricular systole, the oxygenated blood is pumped through the aortic semilunar valve into the aorta.

60. (C) The heart wall is made up of the external epicardium, the middle myocardium, and the internal endocardium. The pericardium is the fibroserous sac enclosing the heart and roots of the great vessels. The heart has four chambers. The two upper chambers are the atria, and the two lower chambers are the ventricles. The *apex* of the heart is the tip of the left ventricle.

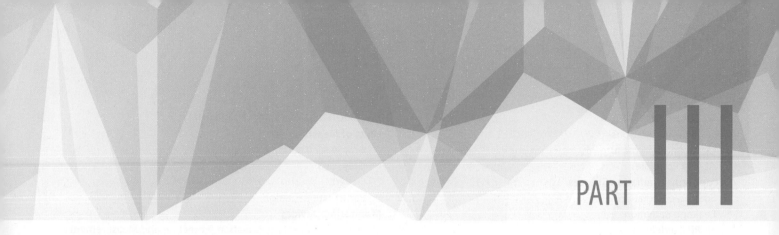

PART III

Safety

CHAPTER 8
Radiation Physics and Radiobiology

Ionizing Effects of X-Radiation
    Electromagnetic Radiation
    Production of X-rays at the Tungsten Target
    Interactions Between X-ray Photons and Matter
Dose–Response Relationships
    Dose–Response Curves
    Linear: Threshold and Nonthreshold
    Nonlinear: Threshold and Nonthreshold
    Late Effects
    Types of Risk
Biologic Effects of Ionizing Radiation
    Law of Bergonié and Tribondeau
    Radiation Weighting and Tissue Weighting Factors
    Linear Energy Transfer and Relative Biologic Effectiveness Versus
    Biologic Damage
    Molecular Effects of Ionizing Radiation
    Cellular and Relative Tissue Radiosensitivity
Genetic Effects
    Pregnancy
    Females
    Males
    Children
    Genetically Significant Dose
Somatic Effects
    Carcinogenesis
    Cataractogenesis
    Life-Span Shortening
    Reproductive Risks

    Embryologic/Fetal Effects
    Skin Effects
    Blood Cell Effects

CHAPTER 9
Patient Protection

Beam Restriction
    Purpose
    Types
    Light-Localization Apparatus
    Accuracy
Technical Factors
    Milliampere Seconds and Kilovoltage
    Generator Type
Filtration
    Inherent Filtration
    Added Filtration
    NCRP Guidelines
Shielding
    Rationale for Use
    Types and Placement of Shields
    Patient Position
Reducing Patient Exposure
    Patient Communication
    Positioning of Patient
    Automatic Exposure Control
Image Receptors
Grids and Air-Gap Technique
Fluoroscopy
NCRP Recommendations for Patient Protection

CHAPTER 10
Personnel Protection
General Considerations
Occupational Exposure
ALARA Principle
Occupational Radiation Sources
Scattered Radiation
Leakage Radiation
NCRP Guidelines
Fundamental Methods of Protection
Cardinal Rules
Inverse Square Law
Primary and Secondary Barriers
NCRP Guidelines
Protective Apparel and Its Care
Protective Accessories
Special Considerations
Pregnancy
Mobile Units
Fluoroscopic Units and Procedures

CHAPTER 11
Radiation Exposure and Monitoring
Units of Measurement
Gray in Air (Gy_a)
Gray (Gy_t)
Sievert
Particulate Radiation
Monitoring Devices
National Council on Radiation Protection and Measurements
(NCRP) Guidelines for Use
Optically Stimulated Luminescent Dosimeter
Film Badge Dosimeter
Thermoluminescent Dosimeter
Pocket Dosimeter
Direct Ion Storage Dosimeter
Evaluation and Maintenance of Records
NCRP Recommendations

Radiation Physics and Radiobiology

OBJECTIVES

At the conclusion of this chapter, the student will be able to:

- Define terminology related to the electromagnetic spectrum.
- Discuss human exposure to types of background radiation.
- Describe the two processes of x-ray production.
- Describe the two major interactions between x-ray photons and tissue in diagnostic x-ray.
- Distinguish between deterministic and probabilistic effects.
- Identify dose–response curves and discuss the application(s) of each.
- Identify the characteristics of cells/tissues that determine radiosensitivity.
- Describe the types of molecular effects of ionizing radiation.
- List examples of somatic versus genetic effects.

IONIZING EFFECTS OF X-RADIATION

Electromagnetic Radiation

A review of electromagnetic radiation and energy is essential to the study of x-rays and other forms of ionizing radiation. *Electromagnetic radiation* can be described as wave-like fluctuations of electric and magnetic fields. There are several kinds of electromagnetic radiation. Figure 8-1 illustrates that visible light, microwaves, and radio waves, as well as x-rays and gamma rays, are all part of the *electromagnetic spectrum.* All electromagnetic radiations have the same *velocity,* that is, 3×10^8 m/s (186,000 miles/s); however, they differ significantly in *wavelength* and *frequency.*

Wavelength refers to the distance between two consecutive wave crests (Fig. 8-2). *Frequency* refers to the number of cycles per second (cycles/s). Wavelength is measured in meters, whereas the unit of measurement for frequency is the hertz (Hz).

Frequency and wavelength are closely associated with the relative *energy* of electromagnetic radiations. More energetic radiations have shorter wavelength and higher frequency. The relationship among frequency, wavelength, and energy is graphically illustrated in Figure 8-1.

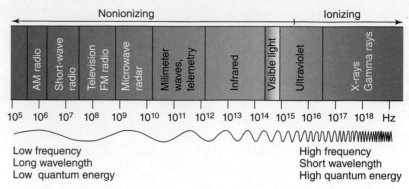

Figure 8-1. The electromagnetic spectrum. Frequency and photon energy are *directly* related; frequency and photon energy are *inversely* related to wavelength.

Some radiations are energetic enough to rearrange atoms in the materials through which they pass, and they can therefore be hazardous to living tissue. These radiations are called *ionizing radiations* because they have the energetic potential to break apart electrically neutral atoms, resulting in the production of negative and/or positive *ions*. X-ray photons, having the *dual nature* of both particles and electromagnetic waves, are highly energetic ionizing radiation. Diagnostic x-rays are extremely short, between 10^{-8} and 10^{-12} m in wavelength. The unit formerly used for such small dimensions was angstrom (Å); 1 Å = 10^{-10} m.

Humans have always been exposed to ionizing radiation. Some ionizing radiations (e.g., those emitted by uranium) occur naturally in the earth's crust and in its atmosphere (from the sun and cosmic reactions in space). These radiations are present in the structures in which we live and the food we consume; radioactive gas is present in the air that we breathe, and there are traces of radioactive materials in our bodies. These radiations are called external and internal sources of *natural background* (environmental) *radiation*. The levels of natural background radiation can vary greatly from one geographic location to

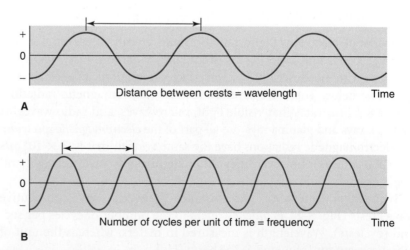

Figure 8-2. Wavelength (A) versus frequency (B). *Wavelength* is described as the distance between successive crests. The shorter the wavelength, the more are crests or cycles per unit of time (e.g., per second). Therefore, the shorter the wavelength, the greater is the *frequency* (number of cycles per second). Wavelength and frequency are *inversely* related.

another. Our largest sources of natural background radiation exposure are radon and thoron gases.

In addition to natural background radiation, we are also exposed to sources of radiation created by humans. *Artificial* or *man-made* radiation contributes to the dose received by the US population. According to the Biologic Effects of Ionizing Radiation (BEIR) VII report, medical and dental x-rays and nuclear medicine studies account for approximately 79% of the man-made radiation exposure in the United States. In addition, NCRP Report No. 160 states that medical radiation exposure now contributes to approximately 50% of the public's exposure to ionizing radiation (Fig. 8-3). Nuclear Regulatory Commission (NRC) regulations and radiation exposure limits are published in Title 10 of the Code of Federal Regulations (CFR), Part 20.

Substances in *consumer products* such as tobacco, the domestic water supply, building materials, commercial air travel, and, to a lesser extent, smoke detectors, televisions, and computer screens account for 2% of the man-made radiation exposure. Occupational exposures, fallout, and the nuclear fuel cycle comprise less than 1% of the man-made component.

X-ray *photons* are man-made infinitesimal bundles of energy that deposit some of their energy into matter as they travel through it. This deposition of energy and subsequent *ionization* has the potential to cause chemical and biologic damage. Although humans are exposed to ionizing radiation from both natural and man-made sources, very high doses of *man-made* ionizing radiation can cause tissue damage that can manifest within *days* after the exposure. Late effects such as cancer, which can occur after more ordinary doses, may take many *years* to develop.

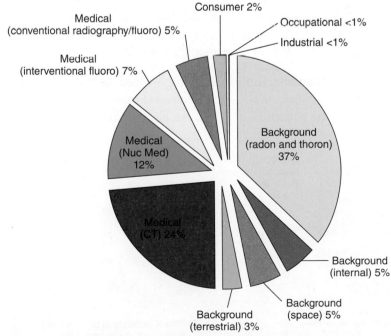

Figure 8-3. The population's exposure to natural background and medical sources of ionizing radiation. As a result of the rapid growth in use of medical radiation, public exposure to medical radiation has increased from 31% to 50% of their total exposure to ionizing radiation. Natural background radiations (the earth, the sun, building materials) comprise the other 50% of our exposure. Nuc Med, nuclear medicine.

Natural Background Radiation

37%: Radon and thoron gases

5%: Space radiation

5%: Internal sources

3%: Terrestrial sources

Medical Radiation

24%: Computed tomography

12%: Nuclear medicine

7%: Interventional fluoroscopy

5%: Conventional radiography and fluoroscopy

Other Radiation Sources

2%: Consumer sources

<1%: Industrial sources

<1%: Occupational sources

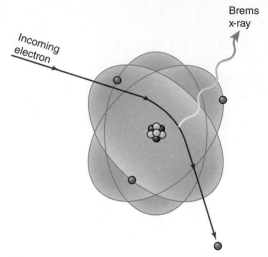

Figure 8-4. Production of bremsstrahlung (brems) radiation. A high-speed electron is deflected from its path and the loss of kinetic energy is emitted in the form of an x-ray photon.

The process of ionization in living material necessarily changes atoms/molecules at least briefly and, consequently, can damage cells. If cell damage does occur and is not effectively repaired, the cell may not (1) survive, (2) reproduce, or (3) perform its normal function. Alternatively, it can result in a working but *modified* cell. Once modified, *somatic* cells can become cancerous, whereas *germ* cells can lead to inherited/genetic diseases.

Production of X-rays at the Tungsten Target

The production of diagnostic x-rays occurs when high-speed *electrons* are suddenly decelerated by the tungsten target. The *source* of electrons is the heated cathode filament; the electrons are driven across to the anode's focal spot when thousands of volts (kilovolts) are applied. When the high-speed electrons are suddenly stopped at the focal spot, they interact with tungsten atoms and their kinetic energy is converted to heat and x-ray photon energy. X-ray production occurs through two mechanisms: *bremsstrahlung radiation* and *characteristic radiation*.

Bremsstrahlung (Brems) or "Braking" Radiation. A high-speed electron is accelerated toward a tungsten atom within the anode focal track. The negative electron is attracted by the positive nucleus of the tungsten atom and, as a result, pulled off course and redirected toward the nucleus. The electron's deflection from its original course caused by the "braking" (slowing down) results in a loss of energy. *This energy loss is given up in the form of an x-ray photon: bremsstrahlung (brems or braking) radiation* (Fig. 8-4). The electron might not give up all of its kinetic energy in one such interaction; it might go on to have several more interactions with tungsten atoms deeper in the target, each time giving up an x-ray photon having less and less energy. This is one reason the x-ray beam is heterogeneous (polyenergetic), that is, has a spectrum of energies. *Brems radiation comprises 70%–90% of the primary x-ray beam.*

Characteristic Radiation. In this case, a high-speed electron encounters a tungsten atom and ejects a K-shell electron (Fig. 8-5A), thereby leaving a vacancy in the K shell (Fig. 8-5B). An electron from a higher energy

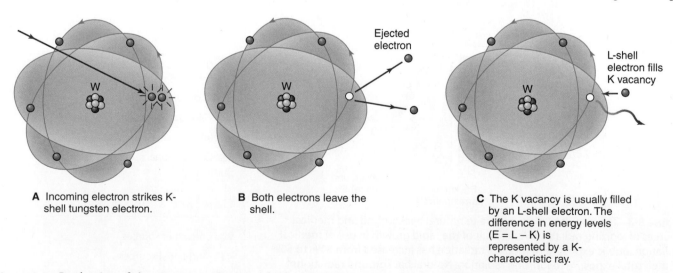

A Incoming electron strikes K-shell tungsten electron.

B Both electrons leave the shell.

C The K vacancy is usually filled by an L-shell electron. The difference in energy levels (E = L − K) is represented by a K-characteristic ray.

Figure 8-5. Production of characteristic radiation. A high-speed electron **(A)** ejects a tungsten K-shell electron, leaving a K-shell vacancy **(B)**. An electron from the L shell fills the vacancy and emits a K-characteristic ray **(C)**.

level shell (e.g., the L shell) fills the vacancy. In doing so, because of the difference in energy level between the K and L shells, a K-*characteristic x-ray photon* is emitted (Fig. 8-5C). The *energy of the characteristic ray* is equal to the difference in binding energy between the K and L shells. K-characteristic x-rays from a tungsten target x-ray tube have 69 keV energy. Characteristic radiation comprises the minor portion of the x-ray beam (10%–30%).

Interactions Between X-ray Photons and Matter

The gradual decrease in exposure rate as ionizing radiation passes through tissues is called *attenuation*. Attenuation is principally attributable to the two major types of interactions that occur between x-ray photons and tissue in the diagnostic x-ray range of energies: photoelectric effect and Compton scatter.

Photoelectric Effect. In *photoelectric effect,* a relatively *low*-energy (low-kV) x-ray photon interacts with tissue and expends *all* of its energy (true/total absorption) to eject an *inner shell* electron. This leaves an inner shell orbital vacancy. An electron from the shell above drops down to fill the vacancy and, in doing so, gives up energy in the form of a *characteristic ray* (Fig. 8-6).

The photoelectric effect is more likely to occur in absorbers having *high atomic number* (e.g., bone, positive contrast media) and with *low-energy photons*. The photoelectric effect contributes significantly to patient dose, as all the x-ray photon energy is absorbed by the tissue (and, therefore, contributes to the production of short-scale contrast). Its probability is Z^3/E^3 in the diagnostic energy range.

Compton Scatter. In *Compton scatter,* a fairly *high*-energy (high-kV) x-ray photon interacts with tissue atoms, giving up *some* of its energy to eject an *outer shell* electron (Fig. 8-7). The ejected electron is called a *recoil electron.* The scattered x-ray photon is deflected with somewhat

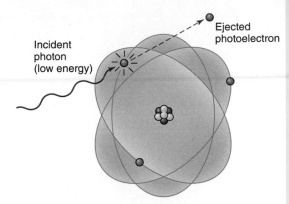

Figure 8-6. In photoelectric effect, the incoming (low-energy) photon releases *all* of its energy as it ejects an inner shell electron from the orbit.

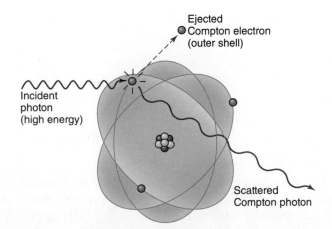

Figure 8-7. In Compton scatter, the incoming (high-energy) photon uses *part* of its energy to eject an outer shell electron; in doing so, the photon changes direction (scatters) but retains much of its original energy.

reduced energy (modified scatter). However, it retains much of its original energy and exits the body as an energetic scattered photon.

Because the scattered photon exits the body, it does not pose a radiation hazard to the patient. It can, however, contribute to scattered radiation *image fog* and pose a *radiation hazard to personnel* (as in fluoroscopic procedures).

Summary

- All of the radiations of the electromagnetic spectrum travel at the same velocity, 3×10^8 m/s, but differ in wavelength and frequency.

- Wavelength is the distance between two consecutive wave crests. The number of cycles and crests per second is frequency; its unit of measurement is hertz.

- Wavelength and frequency are inversely related.

- Speed of light = frequency × wavelength ($c = f\lambda$).

- The public's exposure to ionizing radiation is owing to two types of background radiation exposure: natural (50%) and artificial/man-made (50%).

- Ionization is caused by high-energy, short-wavelength electromagnetic radiations that break apart electrically neutral atoms.

- Two types of x-radiation are produced at the anode through energy conversion processes: bremsstrahlung radiation and characteristic radiation; bremsstrahlung radiation predominates.

- X-rays can interact with tissue cells and cause ionization; the interactions between x-rays and tissue cells that occur most often are Compton scatter and the photoelectric effect.

- Characteristics of photoelectric effect:
  - Low-energy x-ray photon gives up all of its energy ejecting an inner-shell electron.
  - It produces a characteristic ray.
  - It is a major contributor to patient dose.
  - It occurs in absorbers having a high atomic number.
  - It produces short-scale contrast (in analog imaging).

- Characteristics of Compton scatter:
  - It is the interaction that predominates in the diagnostic x-ray range.
  - A high-energy x-ray photon uses a portion of its energy to eject an outer shell electron.
  - It is responsible for scattered radiation fog to the image.
  - It poses radiation hazard to personnel.

- Exposure dose depends on beam attenuation and on the type of interaction that occurs between x-ray photons and tissue. Exposure dose is, therefore, affected by radiation quality (kV) and the subject being irradiated (i.e., thickness and nature of part; atomic number of part).

DOSE–RESPONSE RELATIONSHIPS

Dose–Response Curves

The association between a dose of ionizing radiation and the magnitude of the resulting response or effect is called a *dose–response, or dose–effect, relationship.* Dose–response curves are used to illustrate the relationship between exposure to ionizing radiation and possible resultant biologic responses (Fig. 8-8).

Linear (straight-line) relationships are those in which the response is directly proportional to the dose received; if the dose is increased, the biologic response is increased. In *nonlinear* relationships, the effects are not proportional to the dose. The term *threshold* refers to the dose below which no harmful effects are likely to occur, or the point/dose at which a response first begins. The two most frequently used dose–response curves in radiation protection are the *linear, nonthreshold* and the *nonlinear, threshold.* The Committee on the BEIR reports about the most current and comprehensive risk estimates for cancer and other health effects from exposure to low-level ionizing radiation (e.g., x-rays). Not only does the BEIR VII report support previously reported risk estimates for cancer and leukemia but newer and broader data also have *reinforced* confidence in these risk estimates. The BEIR VII report states that "a comprehensive review of available biologic and biophysical data supports a 'linear-no-threshold' (LNT) risk model—that the risk of cancer proceeds in a linear fashion at lower doses without a threshold and that the smallest dose has the potential to cause a small increase in risk to humans."

Most sources of ionizing radiation have a mixture of high- and low-linear energy transfer (LET) radiations. Low-LET radiations deposit less energy in cells/tissues along their path than high-LET radiations and are considered less destructive as they traverse tissues. The BEIR VII report identifies *low dose* as near zero to approximately 100 mSv (0.1 Sv) of low-LET radiation. The US population is exposed to average annual background radiation levels of approximately 6 mSv; exposure from a chest x-ray is approximately 0.10 mSv and exposure from a whole-body computerized tomography (CT) scan is approximately 10.0 mSv. The greatest portion of the public's annual exposure is from radon and thoron gases and medical procedures.

Linear: Threshold and Nonthreshold

The *linear, threshold* curve is shown in Figure 8-8D and illustrates responses that are proportional to the radiation dose received only after a particular dose is received—below this "threshold" dose, no response–effect is likely to occur. The *linear, nonthreshold* curve (Fig. 8-8A) is used to illustrate responses such as radiation-induced leukemia, cancer, and genetic effects. These are sometimes called *stochastic* or *probabilistic effects.* Stochastic effects occur randomly and are "all or nothing"–type effects, that is, they do not occur with degrees of severity. It must be noted that *in a nonthreshold curve there is no safe dose,* that is, no dose below which there will definitely be no biologic response—any dose can cause a biologic effect. Theoretically, even one x-ray photon can cause a biologic response. This is the curve of choice

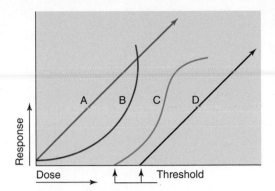

Figure 8-8. Dose–effect curves: (A) linear, nonthreshold; (B) nonlinear, nonthreshold; (C) nonlinear, threshold; (D) linear, threshold.

Average US Doses

- Annual background dose = approximately 6.2 mSv (620 mrem)
- Average chest x-ray = approximately 0.10 mSv (10 mrem)
- Average whole-body CT = approximately 10.0 mSv (1000 mrem)

Dose–Response Terminology

- *Linear:*
  Response is proportional to dose.
- *Nonlinear:*
  Response is not proportional to dose.
- *Threshold:*
  A dose must be received before a response can occur.
- *Nonthreshold:*
  No safe dose—even one photon can cause a response.

to predict effects of low-level (e.g., medical and occupational) exposure to ionizing radiation.

Nonlinear: Threshold and Nonthreshold

In *nonlinear* curves, the effects of radiation are not proportional to the dose received. Figure 8-8B and C illustrate nonlinear dose–response curves. In nonlinear curves, a considerable dose could be required before effects occur, after which effects might increase significantly with only a little more increase in the dose. Response could level off at some point and further doses might have much less effect, thus the term *nonlinear*. Nonlinear curves can be threshold or nonthreshold. A familiar nonlinear curve is the *S*, or *sigmoid*, type seen in Figure 8-8C. The *nonlinear (sigmoid), threshold* curve is used to illustrate certain radiation-induced somatic conditions such as skin *erythema*. These responses are *predictable* and often called *deterministic or nonstochastic effects*.

Late Effects

The Committee on the BEIR in 1990 reported in their revised risk estimates that effects of ionizing radiation exposure are approximately *3–4 times more than those reported in the previous statement*. The more recent (2005) BEIR VII report supports previously reported risk estimates for cancer and leukemia, and newer, broader data have *reinforced* confidence in these risk estimates.

Occupationally exposed individuals are concerned principally with *late* (i.e., *long-term* or *delayed*) effects of ionizing radiation such as radiation-induced *genetic effects, leukemia, cancers* (bone, lung, thyroid, breast), and *local effects* such as skin erythema, infertility, and cataracts—these can occur many years following initial exposure to low levels of ionizing radiation. These long-term/delayed effects are usually *chronic* and many are represented by the linear, nonthreshold dose–response curve.

History provides us with many examples of the delayed effects of ionizing radiation. Many of the early radiologists and radiation scientists, A-bomb survivors of Hiroshima and Nagasaki, and patients with ankylosing spondylitis in Great Britain in the 1940s developed leukemia and other *life-span–shortening* diseases as a result of exposure to varying quantities of ionizing radiation over a period of time. Some children irradiated in the 1940s for enlarged thymus glands developed thyroid cancer as adults 20 years later. Radium watch-dial painters in the 1920s developed a variety of bone cancers following a latent period of 20–30 years. These are all delayed effects of radiation and are represented by the linear, nonthreshold dose–response curve.

Cataractogenesis is another late effect of exposure to ionizing radiation, but it is represented by the *nonlinear, threshold* dose–response curve. An acute dose of approximately 200 rad is required to cause radiogenic cataracts. A far greater occupational or otherwise fractionated dose of approximately 1000 rad is required to induce cataracts.

Early, or short-term, effects of radiation are those responses that occur soon after exposure to ionizing radiation (within minutes, hours, days, or weeks). Short-term effects are usually *acute effects* and occur only after exposure to a very large amount of radiation all at one time (and

---

Early Effects

- Appear a short time after exposure
- Usually as a result of high dose in a short period of time
- Should not be seen in diagnostic radiology

Late Effects

Can appear years after exposure:
- Carcinogenesis
- Cataractogenesis
- Embryologic effect
- Life-span shortening

perhaps to the whole body) and therefore should not occur in diagnostic radiology.

Types of Risk

Risks associated with exposure to ionizing radiation can be divided into two categories: *nonstochastic/deterministic* and *stochastic/probabilistic*.

Deterministic risks are characterized by nonlinear dose responses and are associated with a threshold (safe) dose below which no effect is observed. Deterministic effects are believed to result from radiation-induced death of large groups of tissue cells, resulting in serious functional impairment. The severity of any injury increases with increasing ionizing radiation dose. Examples include radiation-induced skin injury, hypothyroidism, cataract formation, hair loss, temporary infertility, and sterility.

Although deterministic effects generally arise within days or weeks after exposure, some of the induced skin injuries, cataracts, and hypothyroidism have long latency periods.

"In recent years, there has been a marked increase in the number of patient skin injuries due to the increasing number and duration of fluoroscopically guided medical procedures" (*Shope T. Radiographics. 16;1996*). The Shope study and subsequent publication were the result of reports submitted to the FDA describing radiation-induced skin injuries from fluoroscopy. At present, there is heightened awareness of radiation skin dose, particularly in interventional fluoroscopic procedures. It is recommended that maximum radiation skin dose is better estimated using a dose-area product (DAP) meter. DAP meters measure the product of in-air radiation and the area of the x-ray field. This is generally thought to provide more useful information in potential high-dose procedures than simply recording the fluoroscopic time.

Stochastic effects include heritable genetic effects and some somatic effects. They are the foremost late effects that are expected to occur in populations exposed to ionizing radiation; somatic effects (i.e., radiation-induced cancer) are the leading health detriment.

For both somatic and genetic effects, the probability of their occurrence—but not their severity—is dependent on the radiation dose. However, for most stochastic effects, it is generally accepted that there is *no threshold*, that is, *no safe dose*. Radiation-induced cancers and genetic effects cannot be distinguished from those that appear spontaneously.

Types of Risks

Nonstochastic/deterministic:
- Threshold
- Nonlinear
- Includes all early effects
- Includes some later effects

Stochastic/probabilistic:
- No threshold
- Linear
- Genetic effects
- Cancer
- Includes most late effects

Summary

- Ionization of living tissue can cause chemical and biologic damage to somatic and/or genetic cells.

- A nonthreshold dose–response relationship indicates that there is no safe dose of radiation; any dose can cause a biologic effect.

- A linear dose–response indicates that the response is directly proportional to the dose.

- The linear, nonthreshold dose–response relationship illustrates stochastic (probabilistic) responses (cancer, genetic effects) and is the curve of choice used for occupational exposure.

- Occupationally exposed workers are concerned with late (i.e., long-term or delayed) effects of ionizing radiation such as radiation-induced genetic effects, leukemia, and cancers (bone, lung, thyroid, breast).

- Risks associated with exposure to ionizing radiation can be divided into two categories: *deterministic (nonstochastic)* and *probabilistic (stochastic)*.

BIOLOGIC EFFECTS OF IONIZING RADIATION

Law of Bergonié and Tribondeau

Before beginning our review of somatic and genetic effects of ionizing radiation, a brief review of *radiobiology* is in order. Radiobiology is the study of the effects of ionizing radiation on biologic material at the cellular level.

In 1906, two scientists, Bergonié and Tribondeau, proposed that certain cellular qualities made tissues more or less radiosensitive. The Law of Bergonié and Tribondeau addresses relative tissue sensitivity and states that the following are particularly radiosensitive:

1. Stem (undifferentiated, or precursor) cells

2. Young, immature tissues

3. Highly mitotic cells

Thus, very young cells, undifferentiated cells (nonspecialized in structure and function), and cells having the most reproductive activity are highly *radiosensitive*. Examples of highly radiosensitive tissues are intestinal epithelial cells and cells of the rapidly developing embryo and fetus.

Radiation Weighting and Tissue Weighting Factors

Ionization causes the removal of electrons from some atoms and the addition of electrons to other atoms. Thus, the stage is set for biologic effects; as a result of the ionization, appropriate chemical bonds cannot be maintained.

Similar absorbed doses of *different kinds* of radiation can cause different biologic effects to *tissues of differing radiosensitivity*. A *radiation weighting factor* (W_r) is a number assigned to different types of ionizing radiations so that their effect(s) may be better determined (e.g., x-rays vs. alpha particles). The W_r of different ionizing radiations is dependent on the LET of that particular radiation. A *tissue weighting factor* (W_t) represents the relative tissue radiosensitivity of the irradiated material (e.g., muscle vs. intestinal epithelium vs. bone).

The term *equivalent dose* (EqD) simply refers to the product of the absorbed dose (rad/Gy) and its radiation weighting factor (W_r).

The term *effective dose equivalent* refers to the dose from radiation sources internal and/or external to the body and is expressed in units of Sievert or rem. The factors used to determine effective dose (*EfD*) are as follows:

$$EfD = \text{radiation weighting factor } (W_r)$$
$$\times \text{ tissue weighting factor } (W_t)$$
$$\times \text{ absorbed dose } (D)$$

Radiation Type/Energy	W_r
X or gamma	1
Protons	2
Neutrons: 10–100 keV	10
Neutrons: 100 keV to 2 MeV	20
Alpha particles	20

Linear Energy Transfer and Relative Biologic Effectiveness Versus Biologic Damage

Radiation deposits energy as it passes through tissue. The rate at which this occurs is described as *LET*. LET is another means of expressing radiation quality and determining the W_r and expresses the ability of radiation to do tissue damage. As the LET of radiation increases, the radiation's ability to produce biologic damage also increases. This is described quantitatively by *relative biologic effectiveness (RBE)*; LET and RBE are directly related.

Because of the relative high effective atomic number (Z_{eff}) and mass density of biologic material, low-energy x-ray photons are more readily absorbed in biologic material than high-energy photons.

Diagnostic x-rays are considered low-LET radiation; the approximate LET of diagnostic x-rays is expressed as keV/μm. Energy transferred to tissue can cause molecular damage. Any manifestation of that damage will depend on the extent of molecular disruption and the type of tissue affected.

Organ/Tissue	W_t
Skin	0.01
Thyroid	0.05
Breast	0.05
Red bone marrow	0.12
Lung	0.12
Stomach	0.12
Gonads	0.20

Molecular Effects of Ionizing Radiation

The principal interactions that occur between x-ray photons and body tissues in the diagnostic x-ray range, the *photoelectric effect* and *Compton scatter,* are ionization processes producing photoelectrons and recoil electrons that traverse tissue and subsequently ionize molecules. These interactions occur randomly but can lead to molecular damage in the form of *impaired function* or *cell death*. The *target theory* specifies that deoxyribonucleic acid (DNA) molecules are the targets of greatest importance and sensitive to ionizing damage. However, because 65%–80% of the body is composed of water, most interactions between ionizing radiation and body cells will involve radiolysis of water rather than direct interaction with DNA. The two major types of ionizing effects that occur are the *direct effect* and the *indirect effect*.

Direct Effect. The direct effect occurs when the ionizing particle (e.g., an electron) interacts directly with the *key molecule* (DNA) or another critical enzyme or protein (i.e., RNA). Chemical damage can occur as chemical bonds are broken and the chemical structure is changed. This can result in impaired function or cell death. Direct effect usually occurs with high-LET radiations (e.g., alpha particles and neutrons) and when ionization occurs at the DNA molecule itself.

Indirect Effect. The *more frequently* occurring indirect effect happens when ionization takes place away from the DNA molecule, in cellular water. Ionization of water molecules in the body (i.e., *radiolysis of cellular water*) breaks water molecules into smaller molecules, often producing one or more atoms having unpaired electrons (*free radicals*). A free radical is very short lived but highly reactive; it can break chemical bonds in an effort to pair with another electron, and can even travel a considerable distance from its source. The indirect effect is predominant with low-LET radiations such as x-rays.

DNA is the primary target (key molecule) for cell damage from ionizing radiation. Possible types of damage to the DNA molecule are

Types of DNA Damage

- Main-chain, double–side rail break
- Main-chain, single–side rail break
- Main-chain breakage, cross-linking
- Base damage, point mutations

diverse. A single main-chain/side-rail scission (break) on the DNA molecule is *repairable.* A double main-chain/side-rail scission may repair with difficulty or may result in *cell death.* A double main-chain/side-rail scission on the same "rung" of the DNA ladder results in *irreparable* damage or *cell death.* Faulty repair of main-chain breakage can result in "cross-linking."

Damage to the nitrogenous bases, that is, damage to the base itself or to the rungs connecting the main chains, can result in alteration of base sequences causing a *molecular lesion/point mutation.* Any subsequent divisions result in daughter cells with incorrect genetic information.

Approximately 90% of cell damage is repairable. However, subsequent or multiple "hits" to the same cell are more likely to leave permanent damage.

Cellular and Relative Tissue Radiosensitivity

These types of molecular damage can occur to any of the somatic cells or to genetic cells. For example, high levels of radiation exposure to the bone marrow (where blood cells are produced) can cause a decrease in the number of circulating blood cells.

Tissue radiosensitivity is closely related to the cell (life and division) cycle. Cells divide for the purposes of reproduction, repair, and growth, and the cell cycle is an orderly arrangement of events. The cell cycle can be divided into two parts: interphase and *mitosis.* Interphase is further divided into three steps: gap 1 (G_1), synthesis (S), and gap 2 (G_2). Important, radiologically, is the fact that cells are *particularly radiosensitive* during late G_2 and mitosis (M). DNA replication occurs during the S phase, which is the *least radiosensitive* stage of the cell cycle (Fig. 8-9).

Lymphocytes, a type of white blood cell that plays an important role in the immune system, are particularly radiosensitive. If lymphocytes suffer radiation damage, the body loses its ability to fight infection and becomes more susceptible to disease.

Epithelial tissue, which lines the respiratory system and intestines, is also a highly radiosensitive tissue. In contrast, *muscle* and *nervous* tissues are comparatively insensitive to radiation. Because nerve cells in the adult do not undergo mitosis, they comprise the most *radioresistant* somatic tissue. However, nervous tissue *in the fetus* (particularly the 2nd to 8th weeks) is highly mitotic and, hence, highly *radiosensitive.*

The *genetic cells* of the gonads are considered especially radiosensitive tissues. Exposure to ionizing radiation can cause temporary infertility, permanent sterility, or mutations in succeeding generations. In

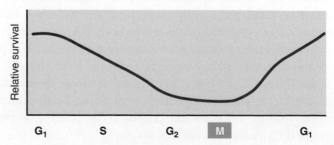

Figure 8-9. Cell radiosensitivity during cell cycle. Cells in late G_2 and in mitosis are most radiosensitive.

particular, the reproductive cells of the fetus and young children are exceptionally radiosensitive. Other factors that determine tissue response, and can modify radiation injury, include the following:

1. *Fractionation and protraction:* Small doses delivered over a long period of time produce a lesser effect. (The greatest effect of irradiation will be observed if a *large quantity* of radiation is delivered in a *short time* to the *whole body*.)

2. *Oxygen:* The greater the oxygen content of tissues, the greater is their radiosensitivity. Dissolved oxygen in tissues increases stability and toxicity of free radicals. The oxygen enhancement ratio (OER) can be determined by dividing the dose required to cause an effect *without* oxygen *by* the dose required to cause that effect *with* oxygen.

3. *Temperature:* Tissues are more radiosensitive at higher temperatures; chromosome aberrations are more likely to occur at lower temperatures because repair processes are inhibited.

4. *Age:* Fetal tissue is most radiosensitive. As the individual ages, tissue sensitivity decreases. Radiosensitivity increases again in old age, but only slightly.

5. *LET:* Radiation deposits energy as it passes through tissue. The rate at which this occurs is described as *LET*. As the LET of radiation increases, the radiation's ability to produce biologic damage also increases.

6. *RBE:* LET is described quantitatively by *RBE*; LET and RBE are directly related.

It is well established that sufficient quantities of ionizing radiation can cause a number of serious *somatic* and/or *genetic* effects. What is not clear, however, are the long-term effects of low-level (diagnostic and occupational) x-radiation.

Health care professionals involved in prescribing and delivering radiologic examinations have an obligation to keep nonproductive radiation exposure to all individuals as low as possible (the ALARA principle [keeping exposure *as low as reasonably achievable*]). Possible abusive overuse of radiologic (and other diagnostic) examinations is currently being scrutinized by many health care facilities as part of a continuous quality improvement program. Some formerly routine examinations are now considered excessive and unnecessary, for example, routine chest x-ray on admission to the hospital is no longer performed unless the patient is admitted to the pulmonary medicine or surgical service; preemployment chest and/or lumbar spine examinations are frequently considered to have little benefit.

Physicians and hospitals often assume the responsibility of hiring only credentialed radiographers in states having no *licensure* requirements for radiographers. Participation in *quality assurance* (QA) ensures that imaging equipment is functioning optimally, and that image quality is up to the expected standards.

Radiographers must consider patient dose when selecting exposure factors. One component of a radiographer's professionalism, as stated in the principles of the *ARRT® Code of Ethics,* is to consistently use every means possible to decrease radiation exposure to the population.

Radiographers must follow the *ALARA* principle as they carry out their tasks. The radiologic facility must undergo appropriate radiation surveys. Staff must be properly oriented, and regular in-service reviews of radiation safety must take place. Proper radiation monitoring and review of monthly radiation reports is essential.

Summary

- The Law of Bergonié and Tribondeau states that the most radiosensitive cells are young, undifferentiated, and highly mitotic.
- LET is another means of expressing radiation quality and determining the radiation weighting factor.
- W_r and W_t make a necessary distinction because identical doses of different kinds of radiation to different tissues will cause different biologic effects.
- EqD = absorbed dose $\times W_r$.
- EfD = $W_r \times W_t \times$ absorbed dose (D).
- Diagnostic x-radiation is low-energy, low-LET radiation.
- Ionizing radiation effect on cells is named according to the interaction site, namely, direct effect and indirect effect (on the key molecule: DNA).
- The most radiosensitive cell is the lymphocyte.
- As radiation professionals, we are obligated to keep radiation exposure to our patients and ourselves ALARA.

GENETIC EFFECTS

Pregnancy

There are a number of situations that require the radiographer's special attention. Irradiation during *pregnancy,* especially in early pregnancy, must be avoided. The fetus is particularly radiosensitive during the first trimester, during the time that pregnancy may not even be suspected. *Especially high-risk examinations* include pelvis, hip, femur, lumbar spine, cystograms and urograms, upper gastrointestinal (GI) series, and barium enema examinations.

During the first trimester, specifically the 2nd to 10th weeks of pregnancy (i.e., during major organogenesis), if the radiation dose is sufficient, fetal anomalies can be produced. *Skeletal and/or organ anomalies* can appear if irradiation occurs in the early part of this period, and *neurologic anomalies* can be formed in the latter part; *intellectual disability development* childhood *malignant diseases,* such as cancers or leukemia, and retarded growth/development can also result from irradiation during the first trimester.

Fetal irradiation during the second and third trimesters is not likely to produce anomalies, but with sufficient dose can contribute to development of various childhood malignant diseases. Fetal irradiation during the first 2 weeks of gestation (at least 250 mGy/25 rad) can result in *embryonic resorption or spontaneous abortion.*

It must be emphasized, however, that the likelihood of producing fetal anomalies at doses below 0.05–0.15 Gy (5–15 rad) is exceedingly small and that most general diagnostic examinations are likely to deliver fetal doses of less than 0.01–0.02 Gy (1–2 rad).

Females

Elective Scheduling/10-Day Rule. In consideration of the potential risk, female patients of childbearing age should be questioned regarding their last menstrual period (LMP) and the possibility of their being pregnant. Figure 8-10 is an example algorithm for questioning female patients having reproductive potential. Facilities offering radiologic services should make inquiries of their female patients regarding LMP and advise them about the risks associated with radiation exposure during pregnancy. The *10-day rule* identifies the first 10 days following onset of the menses as the safest time to schedule elective procedures of the abdomen/pelvis.

Patient Questionnaire. In addition to supporting the ALARA concept, many institutions also use a patient questionnaire as a guide for scheduling elective abdominal x-ray examinations on women of reproductive age. The patient completes a form that requests information concerning her LMP and the possibility of her being pregnant.

Posting. In place of either or both of the above-mentioned methods—or in addition to them—posters or signs can be displayed cautioning the patient to notify the radiologic technologist if she suspects that she might be pregnant. Most facilities will post these signs in waiting rooms, dressing rooms, and radiographic rooms.

Concern is occasionally expressed regarding dose received during diagnostic *mammography,* yet the risk associated with the x-ray dose received is minimal compared with the benefits of early detection of breast cancer. The use of dedicated mammography equipment with digital technique performed by credentialed radiographers delivers a very low skin and glandular dose.

> ### Ways to Reduce Risk to Recently Fertilized Ovum
>
> - Elective scheduling/10-day rule
> - Patient questionnaire
> - Posting

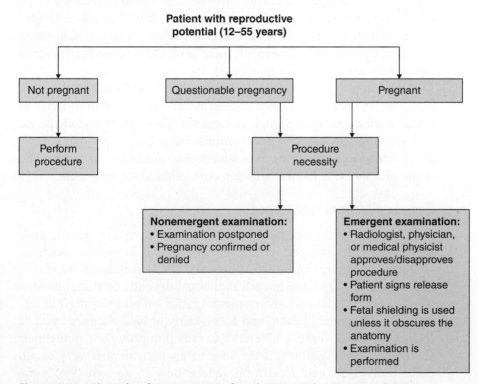

Figure 8-10. Algorithm for questioning female patients having reproductive potential. (Reproduced with permission from Tom Piccoli, DABR.)

Note: Starting in 2021, the National Council on Radiation Protection and Measurements (NCRP) advised against the use of gonadal shielding during pelvic and abdominal examinations. Reasons for the discontinuation of gonadal shielding during these examinations include the overall reduction in exposure factors used to acquire general x-ray examinations, unnecessary repeats due to improper shield placement, and the tendency for automatic exposure control (AEC) to administer more radiation than necessary when lead shields are in the collimated field.

Males

Because of the location of the gonads and *shielding* restrictions thus imposed in the female patient, the female gonads (ovaries) receive more radiation exposure than the male gonads (testes) undergoing similar examinations. The ovaries lie within the abdominal cavity and frequently cannot be effectively shielded during abdominal, pelvic, and lumbar spine radiography. Therefore, they can receive far more organ dose than the shielded testes (which are located outside the abdominal cavity) during diagnostic examinations of the abdominal region (e.g., lumbar spine, upper and lower GI, intravenous or retrograde pyelography).

It is important to note that the ovarian stem cells, the oogonia, reproduce only during fetal life. During childbearing years, there are only 400–500 mature ova accessible for fertilization, that is, 1 ovum per menstrual cycle for each of the fertile years. The male germ cells, spermatogonia, are produced continuously and longevity of fertility is quite different from that in the female.

Children

The female oogonia of fetal life and early childhood and male spermatogonia are especially radiosensitive because of their immature stage of development. Consequently, particular care should be taken to adequately shield the reproductive organs of pediatric patients. Children's reproductive lives are ahead of them and their reproductive cells particularly are radiosensitive.

Very sizable doses of radiation to children are also thought to be associated with increased incidence of leukemia and other radiation-induced malignancies. Examples of high-risk examinations might include pelvic and abdominal radiography and examinations requiring periodic follow-ups, such as scoliosis series. It is advisable to shield the hematopoietic bones of children to reduce radiation dose to blood-forming cells.

Genetically Significant Dose

Each member of the world's population bears a particular genetic dose of radiation. Its sources include environmental exposure, radiation received for medical and dental purposes, and occupational exposure. The quantity of exposure to each individual depends on that individual's geographic location (environmental radiation and elevation of terrain), overall general health, and accessibility of health care, as well as the occupational worker's adherence to radiation protection guidelines. Generally speaking, the genetic dose to an *individual* is very small. Some individuals may receive no genetic dose in a given year, some individuals are past their reproductive years, and some individuals will not or cannot bear children. Even if some individuals receive larger quantities of radiation exposure, its impact is "diluted" by the total population number. This concept is called *genetically significant dose (GSD)*, defined as the average annual gonadal dose to the population of child-bearing age and estimated to be 0.2 mSv (20 mrem).

An important part of radiation protection is care and attention to detail to avoid *repeated radiographic images*. Poor images resulting from technical error (e.g., incorrect positioning, improper selection of technical factors) or equipment malfunction must be repeated, thereby subjecting the patient to twice the necessary exposure dose. An exceedingly important feature of x-ray equipment, having potentially the most significant impact on patient dose, is appropriate *beam restriction/collimation*.

Another component of radiation protection is a QA program (through an ongoing preventive maintenance program and appropriate in-service education) that assures proper equipment function and compliance with established standards.

SOMATIC EFFECTS

Somatic effects of radiation are those that affect the irradiated body itself. Somatic effects are described as being *early* or *late*, depending on the length of time between irradiation and manifestation of effects.

Early somatic effects are manifested within minutes, hours, days, or weeks of irradiation, and occur only after a very large dose of ionizing radiation. It must be emphasized that doses received from diagnostic radiologic procedures are not sufficient to produce these early effects. An exceedingly *high dose of radiation delivered to the whole body in a short period of time* is required to produce *early* somatic effects.

Carcinogenesis

Late somatic effects are those that can occur years after initial exposure and are caused by low, chronic exposures. Occupationally exposed personnel are concerned with the late effects of radiation exposure. Some somatic effects such as *carcinogenesis* have been mentioned earlier: the *bone malignancies* developed by the radium watch-dial painters as a result of radiation exposure to bone marrow, the *thyroid* cancers of the individuals irradiated as children for thymus enlargement, the leukemia eventually developed by patients whose pain from ankylosing spondylitis was relieved by irradiation, and the *skin cancers* developed by early radiology pioneers working so closely with the "unknown ray." These malignancies are examples of somatic effects of radiation.

Cataractogenesis

Another example of somatic effects of radiation is *cataract* formation in the lenses of eyes of those individuals who are accidentally exposed to sufficient quantities of radiation (e.g., early cyclotron experimenters).

Life-Span Shortening

The lives of many of the early radiation workers were several years shorter than the lives of the general population. Statistics revealed that radiologists, for example, had a shorter life span than physicians of other specialties. *Life-span shortening,* then, *was* another somatic effect of radiation. Certainly, these effects should *never be experienced today.* Much has been learned about the biologic effects of radiation since its discovery, and a part of what we have learned has, sadly, been as a result of the experiences of the radiology pioneers.

Reproductive Risks

The human reproductive organs are particularly radiosensitive. *Fertility* and *heredity* are greatly affected by the *germ cells* produced within the testes (*spermatogonia*) and ovaries (*oogonia*). Excessive radiation exposure to the gonads can cause *temporary or permanent sterility,* and/or *genetic mutations.*

Embryologic/Fetal Effects

Embryologic/fetal effects are those experienced by the body of the developing embryo or fetus. Spontaneous abortion, skeletal or neurologic anomalies (intellectual disability development and microcephaly), and leukemia are examples of embryologic or fetal somatic effects.

Skin Effects

Acute Radiation Syndrome. After a large dose (at least 2 Gy/200 rad) of radiation to the *skin,* a mild *erythema* will result in 1 or 2 days. With a large enough dose, in approximately 2 weeks, a moist *desquamation* can occur followed by a dry desquamation. It takes approximately 5 Gy or 500 rad to produce skin erythema (*skin erythema dose [SED]*) in 50% of a population so exposed. This is termed SED_{50}. Another skin response is *epilation,* that is, hair loss as a result of damage to hair follicles and associated structures.

Blood Cell Effects

Most blood cells in circulation are manufactured by the bone marrow. The most radiosensitive of these cells are the *lymphocytes*—cells involved in immune response. They are the first to demonstrate depletion after a large enough exposure (0.25 Gy or 25 rad threshold), although all cells will decrease in number following a large dose of ionizing radiation.

Acute Radiation Syndrome. *Acute radiation syndrome* (ARS), sometimes called radiation sickness, is an acute condition caused by a large external penetrating exposure of ionizing radiation (at least 0.5–1.0 Gy/ 50–100 rad), all at one time or in a very short period of time, and to all or most of the body.

There are three types of ARS. *Hematopoietic* (or bone marrow) syndrome occurs at doses between 1 and 10 Gy (100–1000 rad) and can cause nausea, vomiting, diarrhea, decreased blood count, infection, and hemorrhage. *GI* syndrome generally occurs at doses between 6 and 10 Gy (600–1000 rad). It causes severe damage to the (stem) cells lining the GI, resulting in nausea, vomiting, diarrhea, blood changes, and hemorrhage; death usually occurs within 2 weeks. *Central nervous system* (CNS) or *cerebrovascular* (CV) syndrome usually occurs at doses greater than 50 Gy (5000 rad). The normally radioresilient central nervous and/or CV systems are affected very quickly. There is collapse of the circulatory system,

---

Acute Radiation Syndromes

- Hematopoietic
- Gastrointestinal
- Central nervous system

as well as increased pressure in the cranial vault, vasculitis, meningitis, ataxia, and shock. Death occurs in 3 days. Certainly, these syndromes are most likely to occur as a result of a nuclear accident or attack, atomic bomb fallout—and should never be a concern in diagnostic radiology.

ARS has four stages:

- *Prodromal stage:* Symptoms are nausea, vomiting, and diarrhea that occur 1 h to 2 days following exposure.
- *Latent stage:* Symptoms disappear; the exposed individual seems generally healthy for up to a few weeks. The length of the latent stage depends on the amount of exposure received (inversely related).
- *Manifest illness stage:* Symptoms depend on the specific syndrome and last up to several months, depending on severity. Medical attention is required.
- *Recovery or death:* Individuals who do not recover will die within weeks or months of exposure; recovery process can take from several weeks to 2 years. Those who recover must be concerned about long-term effects.

The whole-body dose of ionizing radiation that can be lethal to 50% of the exposed population within 30 days is called LD50/30. The LD50/30 for adult humans, without medical support, is estimated to be 3.02–4.0 Gy_t.

> ### Stages of Acute Radiation Syndrome
>
> - Prodromal
> - Latent
> - Manifest illness
> - Recovery or death

Summary

- Delivery of ionizing radiation during early pregnancy is potentially hazardous.
- Possible responses to irradiation in utero include spontaneous abortion, congenital anomalies, mental retardation, microcephaly, and leukemia or other childhood malignancies.
- Elective scheduling, patient questionnaire, and posting are suggested ways to avoid irradiation of a new embryo/fetus.
- Gonadal shielding is easier in the male patient because the reproductive organs are located externally.
- All children should be shielded whenever possible.
- Genetic effects refer to damage to reproductive cells, affecting the reproductive capacity of the individual, or creating mutations that will be passed on to future generations.
- The genetic dose of radiation borne by each member of the reproductive population is called the genetically significant dose.
- Somatic effects include those manifesting themselves in the exposed individual and can be described as early or late effects.
- Early somatic effects can occur only after a very large single exposure of radiation to the whole body (ARS).
- Late somatic effects include carcinogenesis, cataractogenesis, embryologic effect, life-span shortening, reproductive risks, and systemic effects.
- Occupationally exposed personnel are concerned with the late effects of radiation exposure.

COMPREHENSION CHECK

Congratulations! You have completed this chapter. If you are able to answer the following group of very comprehensive questions, you should feel confident that you have really mastered this section. You are then ready to go on to the "registry-type" questions that follow. For greatest success, do not go to the multiple-choice questions without first completing the following short-answer questions:

1. List various kinds of electromagnetic radiation; describe the electromagnetic spectrum in terms of energy, frequency, or wavelength (p. 250, 251).

2. Identify the way in which all electromagnetic radiations are similar and in what respects they differ (p. 249, 250).

3. Define the terms *wavelength* and *frequency* (p. 249).

4. Explain how wavelength and energy, and how frequency and energy, are related (p. 250).

5. Describe what is meant by the term *ionizing* radiation and how it differs from other electromagnetic radiations (p. 250).

6. Give examples of natural and artificial/man-made background radiations and identify the percentage each contributes to the population's annual radiation dose (p. 250, 251).

7. Which two sources of radiation exposure are the major contributors to the public annual dose (p. 251)?

8. What are the two ways in which x-ray photons are produced at the tungsten anode? Describe each. Which occurs more often (p. 252, 253)?

9. Describe photoelectric effect and Compton scatter. The following should be included in your description (p. 253, 254):

   A. energy required for production of each

   B. electron shell involved

   C. any electron shell vacancy or occupancy changes

   D. type of absorber (atomic number) most likely involved

   E. retention or loss of energy of incoming photon

   F. interaction associated with a recoil electron

   G. effect on image contrast

   H. impact on patient dose

10. Describe the purpose of dose–response (dose–effect) curves (p. 255).

11. Describe the difference between linear and nonlinear dose–response curves (p. 255, 256).

12. Describe the difference between threshold and nonthreshold dose–response curves (p. 256).

13. Differentiate between probabilistic/stochastic and deterministic/nonstochastic effects (p. 255, 257).

14. Name the type of dose–response curve that identifies *no* safe dose (p. 255).

15. Explain why occupationally exposed individuals are mainly concerned with the late, or long-term, effects of radiation exposure (p. 256).

16. List possible long-term effects of radiation exposure (p. 256).

17. List the three types of cells described by Bergonié and Tribondeau in 1906 as being the most radiosensitive (p. 258).

18. Discuss deterministic versus probabilistic risks; give examples of each (p. 257).

19. Discuss some reasons why the incidence of ionizing radiation–related skin injuries has increased, the kinds of medical imaging procedures in which skin injuries are most likely, and the ways in which radiation dose can be monitored during these procedures (p. 257).

20. What is described as the rate at which radiation deposits energy in tissue (p. 259)?

21. Why is a W_r assigned to different types of radiation, and a W_t assigned to different tissue types (p. 258)?

22. How can effective dose (*EfD*) be determined? How are LET and RBE related (p. 258, 259)?

23. With respect to the molecular effects of radiation, describe the difference between the direct and indirect effects; identify the one that occurs more frequently in the diagnostic range (p. 259).

24. What type(s) of DNA damage is/are repairable; which of these can result in cell death and mutation (p. 260)?

25. Identify each of the following as either radiosensitive or radioresistant: muscle, nerve (fetal and adult), and epithelial tissue; lymphocytes; and reproductive cells (p. 260).

26. How does each of the following affect the response of tissue to irradiation: tissue age, oxygen content, and fractionation/protraction of radiation delivery (p. 261)?

27. Identify the meaning of the acronym ALARA and how it relates to the radiographer; describe some ways in which the radiographer can use the ALARA principle (p. 261).

28. What is the most radiosensitive portion of the human gestational period? List four possible results of excessive radiation exposure during this period (p. 262).

29. What can result from excessive radiation exposure during the second and third trimesters of pregnancy (p. 262, 263)?

30. How much radiation exposure is necessary to produce fetal anomalies? Approximately how much fetal radiation do most diagnostic examinations deliver (p. 263)?

31. List three methods the radiology department can use to avoid irradiating a newly fertilized ovum (p. 263).

32. Explain the value of determining the LMP for female patients of childbearing age (p. 263).

33. What is the current NCRP advice and rationale regarding the use of gonadal shielding (p. 264)?

34. Describe the effectiveness of gonadal shielding in the male versus female patient; discuss the importance of shielding children (p. 264).

35. Describe the concept of GSD (p. 264, 265).

36. Why are we concerned with genetic dose? When do genetic effects manifest themselves (p. 264, 265)?

37. Distinguish between early and late somatic effects. When does each occur with respect to initial exposure? Can you give historic examples of each (p. 265, 266)?

38. What kind of radiation exposure would be required to cause early somatic effects? Give examples of early somatic effects (p. 265).

39. What kind of radiation exposure is characteristic of late somatic effects? Give examples of late somatic effects (p. 265).

40. Explain what is meant by LD50/30. What is the estimated LD50/30 for adults (p. 267)?

CHAPTER REVIEW QUESTIONS

1. Which dose–response curve would be used to illustrate the occurrence of skin erythema?
   (A) Nonlinear, nonthreshold
   (B) Nonlinear, threshold
   (C) Linear, nonthreshold
   (D) Linear, threshold

2. The most likely risk of a dose of 15 rad to the fetus during the latter part of the third trimester of pregnancy is
   (A) childhood malignant disease
   (B) skeletal anomalies
   (C) neurologic anomalies
   (D) spontaneous abortion

3. Linear energy transfer (LET) is
   1. a method of expressing radiation quality
   2. a measure of the rate at which radiation energy is transferred to soft tissue
   3. absorption of polyenergetic radiation
   (A) 1 only
   (B) 1 and 2 only
   (C) 1 and 3 only
   (D) 1, 2, and 3

4. Which of the following is the recommended method of choice for determining radiation skin dose during medical imaging procedures?
   (A) R meter
   (B) DAP meter
   (C) Fluoroscopy-on time
   (D) Total procedure time

5. What is the effect on relative biologic effectiveness (RBE) as linear energy transfer (LET) increases?
   (A) As LET increases, RBE increases
   (B) As LET increases, RBE decreases
   (C) As LET increases, RBE stabilizes
   (D) LET has no effect on RBE

6. The effects of radiation to biologic material are dependent on several factors. If a quantity of radiation is delivered to a body over a long period of time, the effect
   (A) will be greater than if it were delivered all at one time
   (B) will be less than if it were delivered all at one time
   (C) has no relation to how it is delivered in time
   (D) is solely dependent on the radiation quality

7. Which of the following account(s) for x-ray beam heterogeneity?
   1. Incident electrons interacting with several layers of tungsten target atoms
   2. Electrons moving to fill different shell vacancies
   3. Its nuclear origin
   (A) 1 only
   (B) 1 and 2 only
   (C) 1 and 3 only
   (D) 1, 2, and 3

8. What is used to account for the relative radiosensitivity of various tissues and organs?
   1. Tissue weighting factors (W_t)
   2. Radiation weighting factors (W_r)
   3. Absorbed dose
   (A) 1 only
   (B) 1 and 2 only
   (C) 2 and 3 only
   (D) 1, 2, and 3

9. How are wavelength and energy related?
   (A) Directly
   (B) Inversely
   (C) Chemically
   (D) Empirically

10. Deterministic effects of radiation include
    1. infertility
    2. cancer
    3. acute radiation syndrome
    (A) 1 only
    (B) 2 only
    (C) 1 and 3 only
    (D) 1, 2, and 3

Answers and Explanations

1. (B) The nonlinear, threshold curve is used to illustrate deterministic or nonstochastic effects after a certain dose is received. Skin erythema, or reddening of the skin, is shown to occur 24–48 h after a whole-body dose of 2.0 Sv. Compared with the linear, threshold dose, which shows a proportional relationship between a radiation dose and its biological effects, while a specific dose is required to initiate the biological effect, the relationship between the two does not follow a specific pattern. While a certain dose could be needed to cause the effect, an increase in severity or occurrence of the effect is not proportional to dose.

2. (A) Fetal irradiation during the first 2 weeks of gestation can result in *spontaneous abortion*. During the first trimester, specifically the 2nd to 8th weeks of pregnancy (during major organogenesis), if the radiation dose is at least 0.2 Gy or 20 rad, fetal anomalies can be produced. *Skeletal anomalies* usually appear if irradiation occurs in the early part of this period, and *neurologic anomalies* are formed in the latter part; mental retardation and childhood malignant diseases, such as cancers or leukemia, can also result from irradiation during the first trimester. Fetal irradiation during the second and third trimesters is not likely to produce anomalies, but rather, with sufficient dose (5–15 rad), some type of childhood malignant disease.

It must be emphasized, however, that the likelihood of producing fetal anomalies at doses less than 0.05–0.15 Gy (5–15 rad) is exceedingly small and that most general diagnostic examinations are likely to deliver fetal doses of less than 0.01–0.02 Gy (1–2 rad).

3. (B) When biologic material is irradiated, there are a number of modifying factors that determine what kind and how much response will occur in the biologic material. One of these factors is LET, which expresses the rate at which particulate or photon energy is transferred to the absorber. Because different kinds of radiations have different degrees of penetration in different materials, it is also a useful way of expressing the quality of the radiation.

4. (B) The Shope study (*Radiographics. 16;1996*) and subsequent publications were the result of reports submitted to the FDA describing radiation-induced skin injuries from fluoroscopy. There is heightened awareness of radiation skin dose, particularly in interventional fluoroscopic procedures. It is recommended that maximum radiation skin dose is better estimated using a dose-area product (DAP) meter. DAP meters measure the product of in-air radiation and the area of the x-ray field. This is generally thought to provide more useful information in potential high-dose procedures than simply recording the fluoroscopic time.

5. (A) LET expresses the rate at which photon or particulate energy is transferred to (absorbed by) biologic material (through ionization processes) and is dependent on radiation type and tissue absorption characteristics. RBE describes the degree of response or amount of biologic change we can expect of the irradiated material and is *directly related to LET*. As the amount of transferred energy (LET) *increases* (from interactions occurring between radiation and biologic material), the amount of biologic effect or damage (RBE) will also *increase;* as the amount of LET *decreases,* the RBE will also *decrease*.

6. (B) The effect of a quantity of radiation delivered to a body is dependent on several factors, including the amount of radiation received, the size of the irradiated area, and how the radiation is delivered in time. If the radiation is delivered in portions over a period of time, it is said to be fractionated and has a less harmful effect than if the radiation was delivered all at once. Cells have an opportunity to repair and some recovery occurs between doses.

7. (B) The x-ray photons produced at the tungsten target comprise a heterogeneous beam, that is, a spectrum of photon energies. This is accounted for by the fact that the incident electrons have different energies. Also, the incident electrons travel through several layers of tungsten target material, lose energy with each interaction, and therefore produce increasingly weaker x-ray photons. During characteristic x-ray production, vacancies may be filled in the K, L, or M shells, differing with each other in binding energies, and, therefore, a variety of energy photons are emitted.

8. (A) The *tissue weighting factor* (W_t) represents the relative tissue radiosensitivity of irradiated material (e.g., muscle vs. intestinal epithelium vs. bone). The radiation weighting factor (W_r) is a number assigned to different types of ionizing radiations to better determine their effect on tissue (e.g., x-ray vs. alpha particles). The W_r of different ionizing radiations is dependent on the

LET of that particular radiation. The following formula is used to determine *effective dose* (*EfD*):

$$EfD = \text{radiation weighting factor } (W_r)$$
$$\times \text{ tissue weighting factor } (W_t)$$
$$\times \text{ absorbed dose } (D)$$

9. (B) Frequency and wavelength are closely associated with the relative energy of electromagnetic radiations. *More energetic radiations have shorter wavelengths and higher frequency;* thus, they are inversely related. The relationship between frequency, wavelength, and energy is illustrated in the electromagnetic spectrum (see Fig. 8-1). Some radiations are energetic enough to rearrange atoms in materials through which they pass, and can therefore be hazardous to living tissue.

10. (C) Deterministic or nonstochastic effects of radiation are those that will occur after a specific radiation dose is received. Examples of deterministic effects include sterility/infertility, cataractogenesis, acute radiation syndrome, and skin erythema. These types of effects follow a threshold dose–response curve. Probabilistic or stochastic effects of radiation occur randomly and are therefore not predictable following a specific radiation dose. Probabilistic effects include radiation-induced cancer and some hereditary genetic effects and follow a nonthreshold dose–response curve.

Patient Protection

OBJECTIVES

At the conclusion of this chapter, the student will be able to:

- Explain the benefits of beam restriction.
- Describe how x-ray/light field congruence is achieved.
- Identify the factors that determine beam quantity and quality.
- Describe beam filtration purpose and requirements.
- Identify the various types and uses of protective shielding.
- Discuss the ways in which positioning, communication, and equipment can be used to reduce patient exposure.
- Discuss the effect(s) of grids on required exposure, patient dose, and image quality.
- List ways to decrease patient dose during fluoroscopic examinations.
- Identify NCRP recommendations for reducing patient exposure.

Medical imaging has demonstrated itself to be an invaluable diagnostic tool and its use has grown dramatically in recent years. However, the benefits of imaging technology must be carefully balanced with the risks associated with ionizing radiation exposure. We must remember that the risks are *invisible, long term,* and *cumulative. Ionizing radiation dose is directly and linearly related to risk.*

Statistics indicate that the number of radiologic imaging examinations performed annually is steadily increasing. The number of individuals receiving ionizing radiation doses, multiplied by extensive testing (more than 70 million CTs performed annually in the United States), involves a significant population risk. The ascribed cancer risk will rise correspondingly—at least 5% of cancers could result from diagnostic radiation.

The risk model of Biological Effects of Ionizing Radiation (BEIR) Committee VII for exposure to low-level radiation predicts that approximately 1 in 100 people is likely to develop solid cancer or leukemia from an exposure of 100 mSv above background dose.

All radiologic imaging professionals have the ethical responsibility to keep radiation exposure to patients (and themselves) to an absolute

Entrance Skin Exposure (ESD) per Examination

Conventional and fluoroscopy:	
Chest	0.1 mGy$_t$
C spine	1.5 mGy$_t$
L spine	3.0 mGy$_t$
Pelvis	1.5 mGy$_t$
Extremity	0.5 mGy$_t$
Skull	2.0 mGy$_t$
Abdomen	4.0 mGy$_t$
CT:	
Head	40 mGy$_t$
Abdomen/pelvis	20 mGy$_t$

minimum. One exceedingly important consideration in reducing patient exposure is *good patient communication*. Explaining the examination and answering the patient's questions will better ensure understanding and cooperation and reduce the chance for retakes. *Quality assurance (QA) programs* are in place to ensure that retakes will not be required as a result of equipment malfunction. *QA programs* cover all components of the entire system. Employees receive orientation on new equipment to ensure that it is used to best advantage and to reduce retakes as a result of unfamiliarity with equipment operation.

The concern about the risk of possible long-term effects of x-ray exposure obliges us to practice the *as low as reasonably achievable (ALARA)* principle. This chapter reviews the means of achieving this goal.

BEAM RESTRICTION

Purpose

Beam restriction, that is, limitation of irradiated field size, is probably the single most important factor in keeping patient dose to a minimum. The primary beam must be confined to the area of interest, so that only tissues of diagnostic interest should be irradiated.

Another benefit of beam restriction is that, because a smaller quantity of tissue is irradiated, less scattered radiation will be produced. Remember, scattered radiation does not carry useful information; it degrades the radiographic image by adding a layer of fog that impairs detail visibility.

There are three basic types of *beam restrictors:* aperture diaphragms, cones, and collimators.

Types

Aperture Diaphragms. The *aperture diaphragm* is the most elementary of the three types and is occasionally used in dedicated chest units, dental x-ray units, and trauma imaging equipment. It is simply a flat piece of lead (Pb) having a central opening that determines the size and shape of the x-ray beam. Regardless of the type, the aperture diaphragm should demonstrate adequate beam restriction by providing an unexposed border around the edge of the x-ray image.

Cones and Cylinders. *Cones* are circular, lead-lined devices that slide into place on the collimator housing. They may be the straight *cylinder* type, with proximal and distal diameters that are identical, or the infrequently used *flare type,* with a distal diameter that is greater than its proximal diameter. Cylinder cones are frequently able to extend, like a telescope, by means of a simple thumbscrew adjustment (Fig. 9-1). Although their use is limited, cylinder cones are most efficient because they provide beam restriction *closer to* the anatomic part being imaged.

A disadvantage of both the aperture and the cone is their fixed opening size, which will provide only one field size at a given distance. To

---

Beam Restriction

- Reduces patient dose
- Reduces production of scattered radiation
- Improves image quality

Beam Restrictor Types

- Aperture diaphragm
- Cone/cylinder
- Collimator

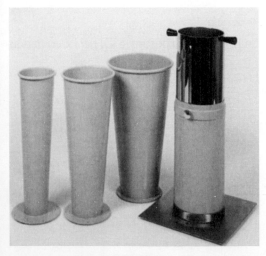

Figure 9-1. Cones and cylinders (Photo contributor: Burkhart Roentgen, Inc.)

change the size of the irradiated field, the radiographer must change to a different-sized aperture or cone. In addition, the cylinder cone can be used only for relatively small field sizes, such as the paranasal sinuses, L5–S1, or other small areas of interest.

Collimators. The *collimator* is the most practical and efficient beam-restricting device. The collimator box is attached to the tube head. Its uppermost aperture, the first set of shutters, is placed as close as possible to the x-ray tube port window (Fig. 9-2). This is done to control the amount of image-degrading extrafocal ("off-focus" or "stem") radiation leaving the x-ray tube (i.e., radiation produced when electrons strike surfaces other than the focal track). The next set/stage of *lead shutters* actually consists of two pairs of adjustable shutters—one pair for field length and another pair for field width. These lead shutters are used to regulate the length and width of the irradiated field.

Light-Localization Apparatus

Another important part of the collimator assembly is the *light-localization apparatus.* It consists of a small light bulb (to illuminate the field) and a 45° angle mirror to deflect the light. For the light field and x-ray field to correspond accurately, *the x-ray tube focal spot and the light bulb must be exactly the same distance from the center of the mirror* (Fig. 9-2). If the light and x-ray fields are not congruent, the part and image receptor will be misaligned. The misalignment could be enough to require repeat examination.

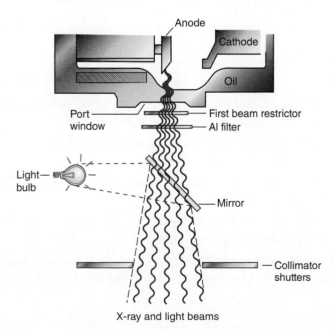

Figure 9-2. X-ray tube, filters, and collimator. The position of the collimator shutters can be seen. Note the position of the first beam restrictor, located at the x-ray tube port window. The oil coolant surrounding the x-ray tube contributes to inherent filtration. Added filtration includes the aluminum filter, the mirror, and collimator. (Reproduced with permission from Saia DA. *Lange Q&A Radiography Examination.* 7th ed. New York, NY: McGraw-Hill; 2009.)

Collimator accuracy should be regularly checked as part of the QA program. National Council on Radiation Protection and Measurements (NCRP) guidelines state that collimators must be accurate to within 2% of the source-to-image-receptor distance (SID).

Accuracy

Cylinder cones are sometimes attached to the tube housing and used in conjunction with collimators. It is important to collimate to the approximate cone diameter size; wide-open collimator shutters can lead to excessive scattered radiation production and can degrade the resulting radiographic image.

As a backup to the illuminated light field, should the light bulb burn out, there is a calibrated scale on the front of the collimator that indicates the x-ray field size at various SIDs.

An important safety feature of both radiographic and fluoroscopic collimators is *positive beam limitation (PBL)*. Sensors located in the Bucky tray, or other IR holder, signal the collimator to open or close according to the IR size being used in the Bucky tray. A properly calibrated PBL system will provide a small unexposed border on all sides of the finished image and is required by NCRP guidelines to be accurate to within 3% of the SID for a single side, and within 4% of the SID total for all sides. For example, if PBL is inaccurate by 2.75% in one direction, it is acceptable as long as any inaccuracy is less than 1.25% in other directions. The NCRP guideline for *manual* collimation is to be within 2% of the SID. The FDA regulation requiring PBL for all x-ray equipment was removed in 1994; therefore, many new x-ray units no longer have the PBL feature.

Summary

- Beam restriction is the most important way to reduce patient dose.
- Beam restrictors limit the volume of tissue being exposed, thereby reducing the production of scattered radiation.
- Beam restriction improves visibility of image details because less scattered radiation fog affects the IR.
- Types of beam restrictors include aperture diaphragms, cones and cylinders, and collimators.
- A properly calibrated PBL device will provide an unexposed border on all sides of the finished radiograph.
- For the light and x-ray field to correspond accurately, the focal spot and light bulb must be exactly the same distance from the mirror.

TECHNICAL FACTORS

Milliampere Seconds (mAs) and Kilovoltage (kV)

Selection of technical factors has a significant impact on patient dose. Remember that the exposure unit mAs is used to control the *quantity* of ionizing radiation delivered to the patient, and kilovoltage determines the *penetrability* of the x-ray beam. As kilovoltage is increased, more high-energy photons are produced, and the overall average energy of the beam is increased. An increase in mAs increases the *number* of photons produced at the target, but milliampere second is unrelated to photon *energy*.

Generally speaking, in an effort to keep radiation dose to a minimum, it makes sense to use the lowest mAs and the highest kV that will produce the desired radiographic results. An added benefit is that at high kilovoltage and low milliampere second values, the heat delivered to the x-ray tube is lower and tube life is extended.

Generator Type

Currently, three-phase and high-frequency generators predominate in radiologic equipment. They produce a nearly constant potential waveform, thereby offering the advantage of somewhat *reduced patient dose*. If voltage never drops to zero, more high-energy photons are produced—which have less likelihood of being absorbed by the patient. High-frequency generators are often smaller, more efficient, and less costly than high-voltage generators.

FILTRATION

X-ray photons emanating from the target/focal spot comprise a *polyenergetic* primary beam. There are many low-energy (or "soft") x-rays that, if not removed, would contribute significantly to patient *skin dose*. These low-energy photons are diagnostically useless; they do not have enough energy to penetrate the part and expose the image receptor; they penetrate only a small thickness of tissue before being absorbed. Filters, usually made of aluminum, are used in radiography to reduce patient dose by removing these low-energy photons, thereby decreasing beam intensity as well. Beam filtration results in an x-ray beam of *higher average energy*. *Total filtration* is composed of *inherent filtration* plus *added filtration*. The purpose of filtration is to reduce patient skin dose; filtration has no effect on receptor exposure.

Inherent Filtration

Inherent filtration is "built-in" filtration. It is composed of materials that are a permanent part of the x-ray tube and its tube housing. Once x-rays are produced at/within the tungsten target, many low-energy photons are absorbed by the anode surface itself. Other low-energy photons are removed by the *window* of the *glass envelope* of the x-ray tube, which has approximately 0.5-mm aluminum equivalent (Al equivalent) filtration. Other low-energy photons will be removed by the thin layer of oil coolant/insulation surrounding the x-ray tube. The glass envelope window in *mammographic* x-ray tubes is often made of *beryllium*, a substance having a low atomic number ($Z = 4$) and an inherent filtration of approximately 0.1-mm Al equivalent.

Inherent filtration tends to increase as the x-ray tube ages. With use, tungsten evaporates and is deposited on the inner surface of the

Factor	Function
Milliampere seconds	Controls quantity—no effect on quality
Kilovoltage	Controls quality, affects quantity

Total Filtration Requirements Summary

<50 kV = 0.5-mm Al equivalent

50–70 kV = 1.5-mm Al equivalent

>70 kV = 2.5-mm Al equivalent

glass envelope, effectively acting as additional filtration and decreasing x-ray output.

Added Filtration

Added filtration refers to the *thin sheets of aluminum* that are added to make the necessary total thickness of Al equivalent filtration (Fig. 9-2). For equipment operated above 70 kV, the total filtration requirement is 2.5-mm Al equivalent. Included in added filtration are the *collimator* and its *mirror,* having approximately 1.0-mm Al equivalent filtration.

The effect of total aluminum filtration is to remove the low-energy photons, thereby *decreasing patient skin dose* and resulting in an x-ray beam having *higher average energy.*

NCRP Guidelines

NCRP guidelines state that equipment operating above 70 kV must have a minimum *total* (inherent plus added) filtration of 2.5-*mm Al equivalent.* Equipment operating between 50 and 70 kV must have at least 1.5-mm Al equivalent filtration. X-ray tubes operating below 50 kV must have at least 0.5-mm Al equivalent filtration. Mammography equipment with a molybdenum target will have 0.025–0.03 mm molybdenum filtration. For magnification studies, a fractional tungsten target tube having at least 0.5-mm Al equivalent total filtration may be used.

Summary

- Low mAs and high kV factors help keep patient dose to a minimum.
- Proper calibration of equipment is essential for predictable results and patient safety.
- Proper selection of technical factors and an effective QA system help reduce radiation exposure.
- Filtration removes low-energy x-rays from primary beam, thereby
  - reducing patient skin dose
  - increasing the average energy of the beam
- Filtration is usually expressed in millimeter of Al equivalent.
- Inherent + added filtration = total filtration.
- Inherent filtration includes the glass envelope and oil coolant/ insulation.
- Added filtration consists of thin layers of Al, and includes the collimator and its mirror.
- Equipment operated above 70 kV must have at least 2.5-mm Al equivalent filtration.
- Inherent filtration increases with tube age, thereby decreasing tube output.

SHIELDING

Rationale for Use

Protective shielding has been used to reduce unnecessary radiation exposure especially to radiosensitive organs (i.e., gonads, blood-forming organs) and may still be provided to patients at their request or the request of the referring physician during radiographic and fluoroscopic examinations (Figs. 9-3–9-5; see also Figs. 9-6 and 9-7).

When requested or indicated, there are three indications for the effective use of gonadal shields: if the gonads lie in or within 5 cm of a well-collimated field*; if the patient has reasonable reproductive potential (a generally accepted procedure is to include all women younger than 55 years and all men younger than 65 years); and if diagnostic objectives permit gonadal shielding, that is, as long as the shield does not obscure diagnostic information.

Reasons for the discontinuation of gonadal shielding during these examinations include the overall reduction in exposure factors used to acquire digital x-ray examinations, unnecessary repeats due to improper shield placement, and the tendency for automatic exposure control (AEC) to administer more radiation than necessary when lead shields are incorrectly placed within the collimated field.

Protective shields must be carefully placed; superimposition on diagnostically important anatomic structures can cause retakes and exposure to unnecessary radiation. In addition, if gonadal shields are used during pelvic and abdominal examinations, it is crucial that the technologist manually selects their technique factors; AEC will attempt to penetrate the lead shield if it is within the collimated field, causing overexposure. By practicing manual technique selection, overirradiation will be avoided. Accurate positioning and beam restriction must always accompany gonadal shielding. When positioning body parts such as the extremities or the breast, the radiographer must be certain that the unshielded gonads do not intercept any of the primary/useful x-ray beams.

Gonadal shielding is far more effective in the male patient because the reproductive organs lie outside the body. Male patients are therefore more easily shielded, and shielding is much less likely to interfere with the diagnostic objectives of the examination. Female reproductive organs are located within the abdominal cavity, where shielding becomes a much less feasible option.

The use of requested protective shielding during *mobile radiography* must not be neglected.

Types and Placement of Shields

There are three types of gonadal shields available: flat contact shields, shadow shields, and contour (shaped) contact shields.

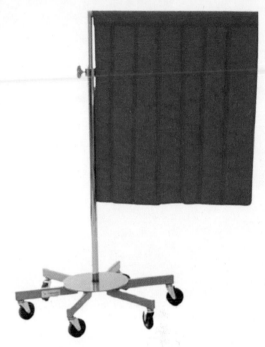

Figure 9-3. Portable lead shielding is useful for patient protection during diagnostic procedures. It is adaptable for fluoroscopic procedures. It can be moved easily and features adjustable height. (Photo contributor: Shielding International.)

Rationale for Gonadal Shielding

- The gonads lie in, or within 5 cm of, the collimated field.*
- The patient has reasonable reproductive potential.
- Diagnostic objectives permit.

---

*Starting in 2021, the NCRP advises against the use of gonadal shielding during pelvic and abdominal examinations.

Flat Contact. The simplest types are flat *contact shields,* such as pieces of lead-impregnated vinyl that are placed over the patient's gonads. Because these are difficult to secure in place, flat contact shields are useful primarily for anteroposterior (AP) or posteroanterior (PA) recumbent projections. Some flat contact shields are now equipped with straps for easy adjustment and a comfortable fit; without this feature, flat contact shields cannot be secured adequately for oblique, lateral decubitus, erect, or fluoroscopic procedures.

Shadow. *Shadow shields* attach to the x-ray tube head. These consist of a piece of leaded material attached to an arm extending from the tube head (see Fig. 9-4). The leaded material casts a shadow within the illuminated field that corresponds to the shielded area. Although shadow shields are initially more expensive, they are likely to be a one-time expense. Shadow shields can be used for more projections than flat contact shields and may also be used without contaminating a sterile field. These cannot be used for fluoroscopic procedures.

Contour (Shaped) Contact Shields. *Contour* (shaped) *contact shields* are very effective gonadal shields. When requested or indicated, ovarian shields can be used to protect the female ovaries from unnecessary radiation exposure (see Fig. 9-5). The ovarian shields are available with optional ties or other types of closure. Shields are also available to enclose and protect the male reproductive organs; the shield is held in place by disposable briefs. These are effective for a variety of projections, including oblique, erect, and fluoroscopic procedures.

Breast Shields. *Breast shields* are a type of flat, contact shield and should be used for female patients during scoliosis series. Scoliosis series are typically performed at ages when developing breast tissue is particularly radiosensitive. Breast shields are available incorporated in vertebral column compensating filters (Fig. 9-6), and as leaded vinyl vests ("spinal stoles"; Fig. 9-6C) that can be used in upright or recumbent projections. In addition, when performed *PA,* radiation dose to the breast can be reduced to *0.1%* of that received in the AP projection; magnification considerations are minimal.

Pediatric Shields. Pediatric shields are another type of flat, contact shield (Fig. 9-7). Body tissues are actively developing in children, and children have their reproductive futures ahead of them. Children should be shielded from all unnecessary radiation whenever possible. Child-friendly pediatric shields are available to protect pediatric patients and their appearance is more appealing and likely more tolerable.

Some companies have environment-friendly recycle/renew programs. They will recycle frontal or full protection aprons into smaller/half aprons, thyroid shields, gonad shields, and so on, for up to half the price of a new shield. Some companies will safely dispose of old lead aprons for a small fee.

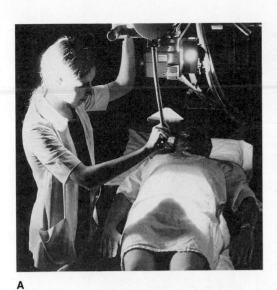
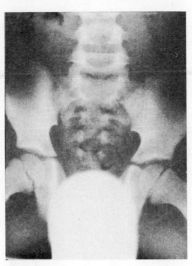

A

B

Figure 9-4. **(A)** A shadow single ("leaf shield") is attached to the collimator housing. It has a movable arm that allows a shield of the desired size and shape to be placed in the radiation field over the gonadal area. It is manually operated and swings away when not in use. (Photo contributor: Nuclear Associates.) **(B)** Correct placement of shadow shield. (Photo contributor: C.B. Radiology Design, Jamestown, New York.)

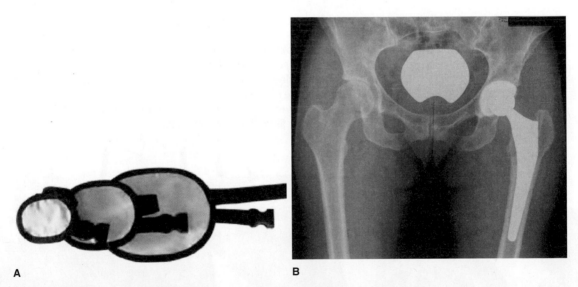

A

B

Figure 9-5 **(A)** When requested or indicated, ovarian shields can be used to protect the female ovaries from unnecessary radiation exposure. (Photo contributor: Shielding International.) **(B)** Excellent shielding of an AP female pelvis for hips. (Photo contributor: Department of Radiology & Imaging, Hospital for Special Surgery, New York, NY.)

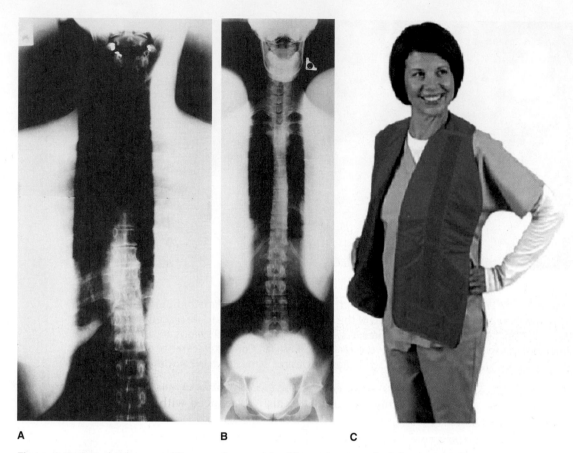

A　　　　　　　　　**B**　　　　　　　　　**C**

Figure 9-6. Spinal column studies are often required for evaluation of adolescent scoliosis, thus presenting a twofold problem: radiation exposure to youthful gonadal and breast tissues and significantly differing tissue densities and thicknesses. Both problems can be resolved with the use of a compensating filter (for uniform IR exposure) that incorporates lead shielding for the breasts and gonads. **(A)** Performed without the filter/shield. **(B)** Performed with the filter/shield. Note the improved visualization of the entire vertebral column and appropriate protection of the breasts and gonads. (Photo contributor: Nuclear Associates.) **(C)** Breast shields are available as leaded vinyl vests, "spinal stoles," which can be used in upright or recumbent positions. (Photo contributor: Shielding International.)

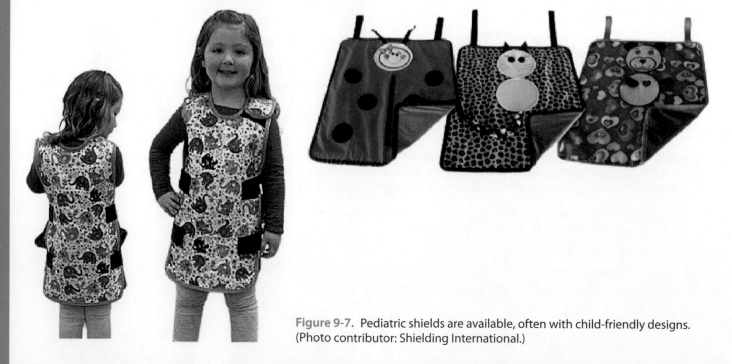

Figure 9-7. Pediatric shields are available, often with child-friendly designs. (Photo contributor: Shielding International.)

In addition, there are some new types of "lead" shields that are completely lead-free, environment friendly, and very light weight, and provide 0.5-mm lead equivalency.

Patient Position

Because the primary x-ray beam has a *polyenergetic* nature, the entrance/skin dose is significantly greater than the exit dose. This principle may be used in radiation protection by placing particularly radiosensitive organs away from the points of primary beam entry.

To place the gonads further from the primary beam and reduce gonadal dose, abdominal radiography should be performed as a PA projection whenever possible. Dose to the lens is significantly decreased when skull images are performed as a PA projection. Lens shields are available for use by personnel during fluoroscopy and/or other procedures that might increase exposure to the lens.

The same principle applies when performing scoliosis series on children/young adults. It is preferable to perform the examination in the PA projections in an effort to reduce gonadal dose and to decrease dose to breast tissue in young girls. The PA projection does not generally cause a significant adverse effect on recorded detail and is advocated to decrease dose to the reproductive organs and other radiosensitive areas. Dose to breast tissue during scoliosis survey can also be reduced with the use of breast shields (see Fig. 9-6).

Lead aprons can also be placed over chest/abdomen during radiography of various body parts to protect radiosensitive organs from unnecessary exposure to scattered radiation. Half aprons, or portable mobile shielding, can be used to protect the gonads from scattered radiation in chest radiography. Lead aprons/shielding can be placed *under* the patient during fluoroscopic procedures if they do not interfere with the objectives of the examination.

Summary

- Radiosensitive organs include the gonads and blood-forming organs.
- Rationale for gonadal shielding:
  - the gonads lie in or within 5 cm of *collimated* beam.
  - the patient has reproductive potential.
  - diagnostic objectives permit.
- Three types of gonadal shields are
  - flat contact
  - shadow
  - contour contact
- Male gonads are more easily and effectively shielded.
- Breast shields should be used as needed.
- To reduce exposure to reproductive organs and/or breasts, it is helpful to perform abdominal radiography and scoliosis series in the PA projection whenever possible.

REDUCING PATIENT EXPOSURE

Patient Communication

Gaining the patient's confidence and trust through effective communication is an essential part of the radiographic examination. Some patients will require a greater use of the radiographer's communication skills—patients who are seriously ill or injured; traumatized patients; patients who have impaired vision, hearing, or speech; pediatric patients; non–English-speaking patients; the elderly and infirm; the physically or mentally impaired; and alcohol and drug abusers. The radiographer must adapt his or her communication skills to meet the needs of many types of individuals and their condition/affliction. It is imperative that the radiographer takes adequate time to thoroughly explain the procedure or examination to the patient.

The radiographer requires the cooperation of the patient throughout the course of the examination. A thorough explanation will alleviate the patient's anxieties and permit fuller cooperation. Better understanding and cooperation will yield a good radiographic image and reduce the likelihood of repeat exposures. *Repeat exposures contribute to a significant increase in unnecessary patient exposure.*

Positioning of Patient

Another means of reducing patient exposure is by careful and accurate positioning. As already mentioned, repeat exposures/examinations contribute to a significant increase in unnecessary patient exposure, as well as increased facility expense.

Exact positioning and centering are particularly critical when using AEC. The anatomic part of interest must be positioned and centered accurately with respect to the AEC's sensors; otherwise, the resulting image can be overexposed or underexposed.

Automatic Exposure Control

An *AEC* is used to automatically regulate the amount of ionizing radiation delivered to the patient and image receptor, thereby serving to produce consistent and comparable radiographic results time after time. When an AEC is installed in the x-ray circuit, it is calibrated to produce radiographic receptor exposure as required by the radiologist for optimal diagnostic quality. AECs have sensors that signal to terminate the exposure once a predetermined, known-correct exposure has been reached.

Whether using analog or computerized/digital imaging equipment, *exact positioning and centering* are particularly critical when using equipment with AECs. The anatomic part of interest must be positioned and centered accurately with respect to the AEC's sensors; otherwise, the resulting image can demonstrate insufficient or excessive exposure.

There are two types of AECs: *ionization chambers* and *phototimers*.

Ionization Chamber. A parallel-plate *ionization chamber* consists of a radiolucent chamber just beneath the tabletop above the IR and grid (Fig. 9-8). As x-ray photons emerge from the patient, they enter the

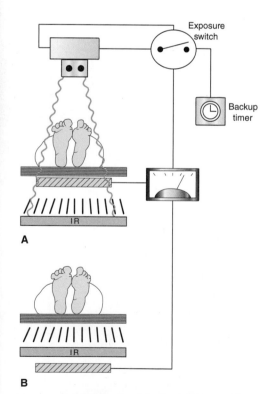

Figure 9-8. Two types of AECs. **(A)** The ionization chamber is positioned between the tabletop and the IR. **(B)** The phototimer is located below the IR. Note that a backup timer, which serves to terminate the exposure in the event of AEC failure, is used in conjunction with both AECs. (Reproduced with permission from Saia DA. *Lange Q&A Radiography Examination.* 7th ed. New York, NY: McGraw-Hill; 2009.)

chamber and ionize the air within. When a predetermined quantity of ionization has occurred (as determined by the selected technical factors), the exposure automatically terminates. The ionization chamber is the most commonly used AEC nowadays.

Phototimer. In the *phototimer,* a small fluorescent screen is positioned beneath the IR (Fig. 9-8). When remnant radiation emerging from the patient exits the IR, the fluorescent screen emits light. The fluorescent light charges a photomultiplier tube and, once a predetermined charge has been reached, the exposure is terminated.

Backup Timer. In either case, the manual timer should be used as *backup timer.* This ensures that in case of AEC malfunction, the exposure will terminate, and *patient overexposure and tube overload will be avoided.*

Minimum Response Time. Another important feature of the AEC to be familiar with is its *minimum response/reaction time.* This is the length of the *shortest exposure possible* with a particular AEC. If less than the minimum response time is required for a particular exposure, the image receptor will receive *greater* than required exposure. Decreasing the milliampere (preferable) or decreasing the kilovoltage will result in bringing the minimum response time within the established range of the AEC.

Summary

- Effective communication can increase patient cooperation and decrease repeats.
- Repeat exposures result in an increase in patient dose.
- When used properly, AECs ensure consistency of receptor exposure, patient dose, and image quality.
- There are two types of AECs: ionization chamber and phototimer.
- The ionization chamber type is located between the patient and the IR; the phototimer type is located beneath the IR.
- Every AEC has a minimum response time.
- AECs require accurate positioning and centering to produce predictable results.
- The manual timer must be used as backup timer to avoid patient overexposure and tube overload.

IMAGE RECEPTORS

An advantage of computerized radiography (CR), digital radiography (DR), and *digital fluoroscopy* (DF) is reduced patient dose—when used properly. CR and DR image receptors are far more sensitive to x-ray exposure than was film emulsion. The lower DF dose is possible because the DF x-ray beam is *pulsed,* rather than continuous. Static DF images are also lower dose because the TV camera tube or the charge-coupled device (CCD) also has greater sensitivity than spot film emulsion.

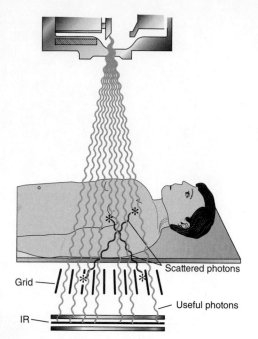

Figure 9-9. Scattered radiation generated within the patient can cause serious degradation of image quality. The improvement in image quality afforded by the use of grids more than makes up for the required increase in patient exposure.

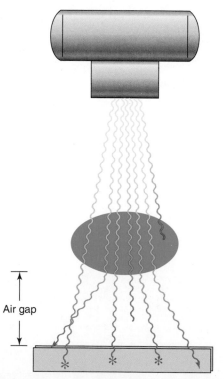

Figure 9-10. When an air gap is used, much of the scattered radiation generated within the patient never reaches the image receptor. An air gap may occasionally be used in place of a grid. (Reproduced with permission from Saia DA. *Lange Q&A Radiography Examination.* 7th ed. New York, NY: McGraw-Hill; 2009.)

GRIDS AND AIR-GAP TECHNIQUE

Grids, both stationary and moving, are used for parts measuring more than 10 cm and function to *remove a large percentage of scattered* (primarily Compton) radiation from the remnant beam before it reaches the image receptor, thereby improving radiographic contrast.

Because scattered radiation can contribute to overall receptor exposure, the addition of a grid (or an increase in grid ratio) must be accompanied by an appropriate *increase in technical factors* (usually mAs) to maintain the expected/required receptor exposure. The improvement in image quality is usually more significant than the *increased exposure to the patient* (Fig. 9-9).

However, the use of high-ratio grids at low kilovoltage levels is discouraged because of the unnecessary patient exposure required. Higher ratio grids are more effective in reducing the amount of scattered radiation reaching the IR, but their use requires more mAs (therefore, higher doses also result in higher x-ray tube heat production) and decreases positioning latitude of the x-ray tube. Lower ratio grids, such as 5:1 and 6:1, are often used in mobile imaging because they offer more (grid) positioning latitude.

An 8:1 grid is satisfactory for radiography up to 90 kV. A 16:1 grid ratio is frequently recommended for examinations using more than 100 kV. General radiographic fixed equipment commonly has a 10:1 or 12:1 grid.

It is interesting to note that, to produce a given receptor exposure, a moving grid generally requires more exposure than a stationary grid of the same ratio. As the lead strips continually change position while they move back and forth, some of the perpendicular rays will unavoidably be "caught" by the lead strips moving into their path.

An *air-gap* technique can function similar to, or in place of, a low-ratio grid. A distance is introduced between the anatomic part and the image receptor. Scattered photons emerging from the patient will continue to diverge and never reach the image receptor.

A "natural" air gap exists in the *lateral* projection of the cervical spine, and a 72-inch SID can be used *without* a grid (Fig. 9-10). *Transmitted* photons reach the IR, but *scattered* photons diverge and never reach the IR. Because no air gap is introduced in the *AP* projection of the cervical spine, it is usually radiographed at 40-inch SID *with* the use of a grid.

The object-to-image-receptor distance (OID) required in *magnification radiography* is an air gap and therefore grids are rarely needed when this special imaging technique is performed.

Air-gap technique may also be used in place of a grid in chest radiography. However, to maintain optimum recorded detail and avoid excessive magnification, the SID must be increased considerably (usually a 6-inch OID and a 7-foot SID), compensated for by an appropriate increase in mAs. Air-gap technique is limited to imaging of fairly thin parts, as more thick and dense tissues would require excessive and impractical radiation exposures.

In addition, equipment must be properly calibrated to produce consistently predictable results; specifically, the equipment must have *linearity* and *reproducibility.* When adjacent milliampere stations are tested, for example, 100 and 200 mA, and the exposure time is kept constant, the

200-mA station should produce twice the exposure rate of the 100-mA station—this is *linearity. Reproducibility* refers to consistency in exposure output during repeated exposures at a particular setting.

FLUOROSCOPY

Fluoroscopy is a potentially higher patient dose procedure. The principal reason for this is that the source of x-ray photons is in closer proximity to the patient than in overhead imaging. On September 30, 1994, the FDA issued the following advisory: "The FDA has received reports of occasional but at times severe radiation-induced burns to patients resulting from prolonged fluoroscopically-guided, invasive procedures." This is probably owing to the increasing number and duration of fluoroscopically guided medical procedures.

There are NCRP recommendations that provide guidelines for minimum source-to-skin distance (SSD), maximum tube output, collimation, timer and exposure switch specifications, and so on. Many of these important guidelines are listed in the following section.

An advantage of DF is reduced patient dose. The principal reason for lower patient dose in DF is that DF x-ray beams are *pulsed,* rather than continuous. In addition, the TV camera tube or CCD has greater sensitivity than did the film emulsion used in analog (film/screen) imaging.

Remember that the entrance/skin dose is significantly greater than the exit dose; this holds true in fluoroscopy as well as radiography. This principle may be used in radiation protection by placing particularly radiosensitive organs away from the primary beam. Moreover, lead aprons or half aprons can be placed *under* particularly radiosensitive areas (when using under-table fluoroscopy), as long as those areas are not of clinical significance.

High-kilovoltage technical factors are preferred to reduce patient dose in fluoroscopy as well as radiography. A 5-min cumulative timer must monitor the length of the fluoroscopic examination.

NCRP RECOMMENDATIONS FOR PATIENT PROTECTION

Note: Many of the means of patient protection serve to protect the operator as well.

- Equipment operating above 70 kV must have a minimum total (inherent plus added) *filtration* of 2.5-mm Al equivalent.
- *Reproducibility:* For a given group of technical factors, output intensity must be consistent from one exposure to the next; any variation in output intensity must not exceed 5%.
- *Linearity:* Output intensity must be constant when adjacent milliampere stations are used, with exposure times adjusted to maintain the same mAs; any variation in output intensity must not exceed 10%.
- X-ray tube *housing* must keep leakage radiation to less than 1 mGy$_a$/h (100 mR/h) when measured 1 m from the tube.
- A device (*centering light*) must be provided to align the center of the x-ray beam with the center of the image receptor.

- *Beam-limiting devices* must be provided; the *collimated* x-ray field must correspond with the visible light field within 2% of the SID in manual collimation and within 4% in PBL.

- The x-ray timer must be accurate. Single-phase equipment can be tested with a simple *spinning-top* test tool. Three-phase equipment is tested with a *synchronous spinning top* or an oscilloscope.

- *SSD* must not be less than 30 cm (12 inches) for all radiographic procedures other than dental radiography.

- The SSD must be at least 38 cm (15 inches) in stationary (fixed) fluoroscopic equipment, and at least 30 cm (12 inches) for mobile fluoroscopic equipment.

- The tabletop intensity/ESD of the *fluoroscopic* beam must be less than 100 mGy$_t$/min (10 R/min).

- The tabletop intensity/ESD of *interventional/high-level control* fluoroscopy must not exceed 200 mGy$_t$/min (20 R/min).

- A *cumulative timing device* must be available to signal the fluoroscopist (audibly, visibly, or both) when a maximum of 5 min of fluoroscopy time has elapsed.

- The *SID indicator* must be accurate to within 2% of the indicated SID.

- When more than one x-ray tube can be energized from a single control panel, there must be an obvious indicator on the control panel and on or near each tube housing that indicates which tube is being operated.

- The location of the *focal spot* must be indicated on the outside of the tube housing.

- Radiographic equipment should undergo regular QA testing.

- The radiographer must be able to see and communicate with the patient *at all times*.

- The exposure switches must be the *dead-man* type.

Summary

- When used correctly, digital imaging can significantly reduce patient dose.

- Grids improve the radiographic image by reducing the amount of scattered radiation fog, but necessitate an increase in exposure.

- An air gap can have the same effect as a low-ratio grid in decreasing the amount of scattered radiation reaching the image receptor; however, SID must be increased to decrease magnification and preserve recorded detail.

- Fluoroscopy delivers a higher patient dose than radiography because of decreased SSD.

- There are several important NCRP recommendations governing patient protection with which the radiographer should be familiar.

COMPREHENSION CHECK

Congratulations! You have completed your review of this chapter. If you are able to answer the following group of very comprehensive questions, you should feel confident that you have really mastered this section. You are then ready to go on to the "registry-type" questions that follow. For greatest success, do not go to the multiple-choice questions without first completing the following short-answer questions:

1. List some methods of achieving the ALARA goal (p. 273, 274).

2. What is the most important factor in minimizing patient exposure? Give an example of how it affects patient dose (p. 274).

3. List the three types of beam restrictors; describe the particular use(s) and efficiency of each (p. 274, 275).

4. What effect does beam restriction have on the production of scattered radiation (p. 274)?

5. To what degree of accuracy must beam restrictors be maintained (both manual and PBL) (p. 276)?

6. How is "off-focus" radiation minimized (p. 275, 276)?

7. Describe the relationship between the focal spot and collimator light bulb with respect to IR alignment (p. 276).

8. Explain the importance of an AEC's backup timer (p. 284, 285).

9. What is meant by the minimum response time of an AEC (p. 285)?

10. Why is positioning and centering so critical when using AECs (p. 288, 289)?

11. What combination of technical factors should be used, in general, to keep patient dose to a minimum (p. 277)?

12. How does filtration affect patient dose? How does filtration affect receptor exposure (p. 277, 278)?

13. Describe the two types of filtration that comprise total filtration (p. 277).

14. What are the NCRP filtration requirements (p. 278)?

15. How and why does inherent filtration change as the x-ray tube ages; how does it affect tube output (p. 279, 280, 281)?

16. List the three criteria for determining use of gonadal shielding (p. 282, 283).

17. Describe the three types of gonadal shielding (p. 281).

18. When might a breast or lens shield be used (p. 281, 282, 283)?

19. Explain the value of performing scoliosis series, abdominal, and skull radiography in the PA projection (p. 281, 283).

20. The NCRP makes several recommendations that can impact patient dose. Briefly describe the recommendations for each of the following (p. 287, 288):

    A. patient visibility during examination

    B. QA testing

    C. speed and care of intensifying screens

    D. external indication of focal spot

    E. energizing multiple x-ray tubes from one control panel

    F. minimum SSD in fluoroscopy units

    G. x-ray timer testing and accuracy

    H. beam limitation accuracy (manual and PBL) required

    I. beam alignment

    J. leakage radiation

    K. quantity of filtration

    L. linearity and reproducibility

CHAPTER REVIEW QUESTIONS

1. Which of the following is/are a feature(s) of x-ray equipment, designed especially to eliminate unnecessary radiation to the patient?

   1. Filtration
   2. Minimum SSD of 15 cm
   3. Collimator accuracy

   (A) 1 only
   (B) 1 and 2 only
   (C) 1 and 3 only
   (D) 1, 2, and 3

2. The quality assurance term used to describe consistency in exposure at adjacent milliampere stations is

   (A) reproducibility
   (B) linearity
   (C) beam limitation accuracy
   (D) automatic exposure consistency

3. How does filtration affect the primary beam?

   (A) Filtration decreases the average energy of the primary beam
   (B) Filtration increases the average energy of the primary beam
   (C) Filtration results in an increased patient dose
   (D) Filtration increases the intensity of the primary beam

4. Methods of decreasing patient exposure during fluoroscopic procedures include

   1. positioning the image intensifier as close to the patient as possible
   2. using the last image hold feature
   3. using the largest FOV

   (A) 1 only
   (B) 1 and 2 only
   (C) 2 and 3 only
   (D) 1, 2, and 3

5. Patient dose is affected by

   1. inherent filtration
   2. added filtration
   3. source–image distance

   (A) 1 only
   (B) 1 and 2 only
   (C) 1 and 3 only
   (D) 1, 2, and 3

6. Which of the following groups of technical factors will deliver the *least* amount of exposure to the patient?

   (A) 20 mAs, 100 kV
   (B) 40 mAs, 90 kV
   (C) 80 mAs, 80 kV
   (D) 160 mAs, 70 kV

7. The principal function of x-ray beam filtration is to

   (A) reduce operator skin dose
   (B) reduce patient skin dose
   (C) reduce image noise
   (D) reduce scattered radiation

8. Which of the following are types of gonadal shielding?

   1. Aluminum step wedge
   2. Shaped (contour) contact
   3. Shadow

   (A) 1 only
   (B) 1 and 2 only
   (C) 2 and 3 only
   (D) 1, 2, and 3

9. The advantages of beam restriction include

   1. production of less scattered radiation
   2. irradiation of less biologic material
   3. patient shielding will not be required

   (A) 1 only
   (B) 1 and 2 only
   (C) 2 and 3 only
   (D) 1, 2, and 3

10. Methods of decreasing patient exposure during fluoroscopic procedures include

    1. using a high pulse rate
    2. maximizing the use of boost mode
    3. using high kilovoltage/low milliampere combination

    (A) 1 only
    (B) 1 and 2 only
    (C) 3 only
    (D) 1, 2, and 3

Answers and Explanations

1. (C) According to NCRP regulations, radiographic and fluoroscopic equipment must have a total *filtration* of at least 2.5-mm Al equivalent whenever the equipment is operated at 70 kV or higher, to reduce excessive exposure to low-energy radiation. *Collimator* and beam alignment must be accurate to within 2% for manual, and 4% for PBL. The *SSD* must not be less than 30 cm (12 inches) for all procedures other than dental radiography. Distance is the single best protection from radiation. Excessively short SIDs/SSDs cause a significant increase in patient skin dose.

2. (B) Equipment must be properly calibrated to produce consistently predictable results; specifically, the equipment must have *linearity* and *reproducibility*. When adjacent milliampere stations are tested, for example, 100 and 200 mA, and the exposure time is kept constant, the 200-mA station should produce twice the exposure rate of the 100-mA station—this is *linearity*. *Reproducibility* refers to consistency in exposure output during repeated exposures at a particular setting.

3. (B) X-rays produced at the target comprise a heterogeneous primary beam. Filtration serves to eliminate the softer, less-penetrating photons leaving an x-ray beam of higher average energy. It is important in patient protection because unfiltered, low-energy photons not energetic enough to reach the image receptor are absorbed by the body and contribute to total patient dose.

4. (B) Fluoroscopic examinations have the potential to deliver significant patient dose, but there are a number of ways to keep that dose as low as possible: keeping the length of the fluoroscopic exposure/procedure to a minimum, using the last image hold feature, keeping the image intensifier as close to the patient as possible, using ABC settings with highest kilovoltage and lowest milliampere combinations, keeping the use of "boost" and magnification modes to a minimum, using the smallest practical FOV, using the lowest practical pulse rate, and adjusting tube angle/patient position to spread exposure dose over a larger area.

5. (D) *Inherent* filtration is composed of materials that are a permanent part of the tube housing, that is, the glass envelope of the x-ray tube and the oil coolant. *Added* filtration, usually thin sheets of aluminum, is present to make a total of 2.5-mm Al equivalent filtration for equipment operated above 70 kV. Filtration is used to

decrease patient dose by removing the weak x-rays having no value but contributing to skin dose. According to the inverse square law of radiation, exposure dose increases as *distance* from the source decreases, and vice versa.

6. (A) The selected mAs regulates the quantity of radiation delivered to the patient. Kilovoltage regulates the quality (penetration) of the ionizing radiation delivered to the patient. The higher the mAs, the greater is the patient dose. Higher energy (more penetrating) radiation—which is more likely to *exit* the patient—accompanied by a lower mAs is the safest combination for the patient.

7. (B) It is our ethical responsibility to minimize radiation dose to our patients. X-rays produced at the target comprise a heterogeneous primary beam. There are many "soft" (low-energy) photons that, if not removed, would contribute to only greater patient dose. They are too weak to penetrate the patient and expose the image receptor; they just penetrate a small thickness of tissue and are absorbed. Filters, usually made of aluminum, are used in *radiography to reduce patient dose by removing this low-energy radiation,* resulting in an x-ray beam of higher average energy. Total filtration is composed of inherent filtration plus added filtration.

8. (C) Gonadal shielding should be used whenever appropriate and possible during radiographic and fluoroscopic examinations. *Shaped contact (contour)* shields are best because they enclose the male reproductive organs, remaining in oblique, lateral, and erect positions—but they can be used only for male patients. *Shadow* shields that attach to the tube head are particularly useful for surgical sterile fields. *Flat contact* shields (flat sheets of flexible leaded vinyl) are useful for recumbent studies, but when the examination necessitates that oblique, lateral, or erect projections be obtained, they become less efficient. *Aluminum step wedges* are quality control (QC) tools used to determine the amount of radiation reaching the IR, they are not a variety of shielding.

9. (B) With greater beam restriction (i.e., smaller field size), less biologic material is irradiated, thereby reducing the possibility of harmful effects. If less tissue is irradiated, less scattered radiation is produced, resulting in improved image contrast. Protective shielding is used to reduce unnecessary radiation exposure to especially radiosensitive organs (i.e., gonads, lens, blood-forming organs) and should be provided to patients *whenever possible* during radiographic and fluoroscopic examinations. Beam restriction and shielding are essential components of patient protection.

10. (C) Fluoroscopic examinations have the potential to deliver significant patient dose, but there are a number of ways to keep that dose as low as possible: keeping the length of the fluoroscopic exposure/procedure to a minimum, using the last image hold feature, keeping the image intensifier as close to the patient as possible, using ABC settings with highest kilovoltage and lowest milliampere combinations, keeping the use of "boost" and magnification modes to a ***minimum***, using the smallest practical FOV, using the ***lowest*** practical pulse rate, and adjusting tube angle/patient position to spread exposure dose over a larger area.

Personnel Protection

OBJECTIVES

At the conclusion of this chapter, the student will be able to:

- List the cardinal principles of radiation protection.
- Identify the principal sources of personnel exposure.
- Explain how the cardinal principles of radiation protection are used to decrease occupational exposure.
- Discuss importance of the *as low as reasonably achievable* (ALARA) principle.
- List some National Council on Radiation Protection and Measurements (NCRP) guidelines related to occupational exposure in mobile and fluoroscopic procedures.
- Cite examples of primary and secondary radiation barriers.
- Identify factors considered when determining barrier thickness.
- Identify NCRP-recommended dose limits.

GENERAL CONSIDERATIONS

Occupational Exposure

Radiographers avoid unnecessary radiation exposure to themselves, and strive to keep patient dose to an absolute minimum. The sources of radiation exposure are the primary beam and the secondary radiation (scattered and leakage). *Radiographers must never be exposed to the primary, or useful, x-ray beam.*

The *patient* is the principal source of scattered radiation; protection guidelines address secondary radiation exposure. The National Council on Radiation Protection and Measurements (NCRP) recommends *personal monitoring* for individuals who may receive 5 mSv/year (0.50 rem/year), that is, 10% of the annual occupational dose-equivalent limit. Although the annual occupational dose-equivalent limit is 50 mSv/year (5 rem/year), the occupational dose to those performing general radiography most often does not exceed 1 mSv/year (100 mrem/year).

Time, distance, and *shielding* are the cardinal principles of radiation protection; dosimeter *monitoring* evaluates their effectiveness. Minimizing the length of a fluoroscopic procedure uses the principle of *time.* Increasing the distance between the x-ray source and the technologist, as in mobile radiography or in fluoroscopy, uses the principle of *distance.* Wearing a lead apron during fluoroscopy and providing the patient with gonadal shielding are examples of using the principle of *shielding.* The principles of time, distance, and shielding apply to both patient exposure and occupational exposure.

ALARA Principle

The use of radiation-monitoring devices helps us evaluate the *effectiveness* of radiation protection practices. Anyone who might receive 0.1 of the annual dose limit (i.e., 5 mSv/0.5 rem) must be provided a personal dosimeter. Effective dose limits take into account the weighted average to the tissues and organs. Reports received— monthly or quarterly—from dosimeter laboratories are official legal documents. They are reviewed, and attempts should be made to reduce *any* exposure no matter how small. Radiographers follow the *as low as reasonably achievable (ALARA)* principle as they carry out their tasks. Radiologic facilities undergo regular radiation surveys. New radiologic staff participate in radiation safety orientation, and regular radiation safety in-service education is conducted annually. Proper radiation monitoring and regular official review of radiation dosimeter reports are essential.

OCCUPATIONAL RADIATION SOURCES

Scattered Radiation

When primary x-ray photons intercept an object and undergo a change in direction, *scattered radiation* results.

The most significant occupational radiation hazard in diagnostic radiology is scattered radiation from the *patient,* particularly in *fluoroscopy,* where use of high kilovoltage results in energetic Compton scatter emerging from the patient. This poses a real occupational hazard to the radiologist and the radiographer.

The intensity of scattered radiation 1 m from the patient is approximately 0.1% of the intensity of the primary beam. Therefore, in terms of radiation protection, *the patient is considered the most important source of scattered radiation exposure.* Other scattering objects include the x-ray table, Bucky slot cover/closer, and control booth wall.

Leakage Radiation

Leakage radiation is that emitted from the x-ray tube housing in directions *other* than that of the primary beam. NCRP guidelines state that any leakage radiation from lead-lined x-ray tubes must not exceed

1 mGy$_a$/h (100 mR/h) when measured at a distance of 1 m from the x-ray tube.

NCRP Guidelines

NCRP guidelines regulate equipment design, among other things, in an effort to reduce exposure to personnel and patients. The following guidelines serve to reduce exposure to personnel:

- The control panel must somehow indicate when the x-ray tube is energized (i.e., "exposure-on" time) by means of an audible or visible signal.
- The x-ray exposure switch must be a "dead-man" switch and situated such that it cannot be operated outside the shielded area of the control booth.

Some patients, such as infants and children, are unable to maintain the required radiographic position. Mechanical immobilizing and restraining devices, carefully and intelligently used, serve to prevent motion on the resulting image. Additional help with immobilization, though infrequently required, can be a nonpregnant relative or friend (older than 18 years) or, as a last recourse, another hospital employee. The services of radiology personnel must *never* be used to help immobilize patients for x-ray procedures.

NCRP guidelines regarding protection of the *patient* and/or *personnel* during *fluoroscopic* procedures include the following:

- During fluoroscopic procedures, the *image intensifier* serves as a protective barrier from the primary beam and must be the equivalent of 2.0 mm Pb.
- The exposure switch must be the "dead-man" type.
- With under-table fluoroscopic tubes, a Bucky slot cover having at least the equivalent of 0.25 mm Pb must be available to attenuate scattered radiation (which is about at the fluoroscopist's gonad level).
- A cumulative timing device must be available to signal the fluoroscopist (audibly, visibly, or both) when a maximum of 5 min of fluoroscopy time has elapsed.
- A leaded screen drape and tableside shield, having at least the equivalent of 0.25 mm Pb, to reduce scattered radiation to the operator must be available.
- The tabletop intensity of the fluoroscopic beam must be less than 100 mGy$_a$/min (10 R/min).
- Protective *lead aprons* must be *at least 0.25-mm Pb* equivalent and must be worn by the workers in the fluoroscopy suite. *NCRP recommends a 0.5-mm Pb equivalent.*
- Protective *lead gloves* must be at least 0.25-mm Pb equivalent. The unshielded hand must not be placed in the unattenuated or useful beam.
- When fluoroscopy is performed with an *under-table* image intensifier, palpation must be performed mechanically.

> ### Rules for Selecting Someone to Assist the Patient in the Radiographic Department
>
> - A male (older than 18 years) is preferred; however, a female who is older than 18 years and not pregnant may also assist.
> - The individual must be provided with protective apparel.
> - The individual must not stand in the path of the useful beam.
> - The individual must be as far as possible from the useful beam.

Summary

- Time, distance, and shielding are the principal guidelines for reducing radiographic exposure; monitoring evaluates their effectiveness.

- Radiology professionals must practice the ALARA principle, that is, keeping exposure to ionizing radiation *as low as reasonably achievable.*

- The principal scattering object is the patient; others include the x-ray table, Bucky slot cover, and control booth walls.

- It is important to be familiar with pertinent guidelines established by NCRP reports: medical x-ray, electron beam, and gamma-ray protection for energies up to 50 MeV (Equipment Design, Performance and Use [1989; NCRP Report No. 102]; Radiation Protection for Medical and Allied Health Personnel [1989; NCRP Report No. 105]; Limitation of Exposure to Ionizing Radiation [1993; NCRP Report No. 116]; and Ionizing Radiation Exposure of the Population of the United States [2009; NCRP Report No. 160]).

- Mechanical restraining devices can be used to immobilize the patient/part as necessary during radiographic examinations.

- Persons occupationally exposed to radiation must never assist (hold) patients during radiographic/fluoroscopic exposures.

- If someone is required to assist a patient during radiographic/fluoroscopic exposures, it is essential that radiation safety guidelines are adhered.

- There are several NCRP guidelines regarding protection during fluoroscopic procedures with which the radiographer should be familiar.

FUNDAMENTAL METHODS OF PROTECTION

Cardinal Rules

The practice of effective radiation safety chiefly depends on common sense; that is, to safeguard yourself from something harmful, you generally remove yourself from it as soon as possible, stay as far away from it as possible, and keep a barrier between it and yourself—hence, the cardinal principles of *time, distance,* and *shielding.*

The greatest amount of occupational exposure is received in *fluoroscopic* procedures and *mobile* radiography. It is here that the radiographer must place special emphasis on the cardinal rules of radiation protection: time, distance, and shielding. Federal government controls also regulate manufacturing standards for the protection of both personnel and patients.

Inverse Square Law

Reducing the length of time exposed to ionizing radiation, as in reducing fluoroscopy time, results in a reduction of occupational exposure. Increasing the distance from the source of radiation results in a

---

Radiation Protection Rules

- Time
- Distance
- Shielding

reduction of occupational exposure, as illustrated by the *inverse square law*. Placing a barrier, such as a lead wall or lead apron, between you and the source of radiation results in a reduction of occupational exposure. Review the following examples:

- *Time:* If 0.1 mSv is received in 30 min of fluoroscopic procedure, how much dose will be received if the fluoroscopic time is reduced to 15 min? (If the fluoroscopic exposure time is cut in half, from 30 to 15 min, the exposure dose received would be correspondingly one-half of the original, or 0.05 mSv.)
- *Distance:* If 0.4 mSv is received at a distance of 40 inches from the x-ray source, what dose will be received at a distance of 80 inches from the source? (According to the inverse square law, if the distance from the radiation source is doubled, exposure dose will be one-fourth of the original quantity, or 0.1 mSv.)

To reduce exposure dose to health care professionals, patients, and the general population, we must minimize the *time* of exposure to the source of radiation, provide effective *shielding* from the radiation source, and, most importantly, maximize the *distance* from the source of radiation.

Primary Barriers

- Protect from the useful beam

Secondary Barriers

- Protect from scattered and leakage radiation

PRIMARY AND SECONDARY BARRIERS

NCRP Guidelines

Primary radiation barriers protect against direct exposure from the primary (useful) x-ray beam and have much greater attenuation capability than *secondary barriers*, which protect only from leakage and scattered radiation. An area occupied principally by radiology personnel and patients is referred to as a *controlled area*. Barriers must reduce controlled area exposure to less than 1 mSv (100 mrem) per week. Areas occupied by anyone are referred to as uncontrolled areas; barriers must reduce uncontrolled area exposure to 21 mSv/year, or 20 μSv/week. The three factors that determine the required thickness of primary barriers are *occupancy* factor, *workload,* and *use* factor.

Primary barriers are any surface that could be struck by the useful beam, such as the lead walls and doors of a radiographic room. Primary protective barriers of typical installations generally consist of walls with 1.5 mm (1⁄16-inch) lead thickness and 7 feet height.

Secondary radiation is defined as leakage and/or scattered radiation. As stated earlier, the x-ray tube housing protects from leakage radiation. The patient is the source of most scattered radiation.

Secondary radiation barriers include the portion of the walls above 7 feet in height; this area requires only 0.75 mm (1⁄32 inch) lead. The control booth is also a secondary barrier, toward which the primary beam must never be directed (Fig. 10-1). The radiographer must be protected by the control booth shielding during exposures, and the exposure switch or cord must be positioned and attached so that the exposure can be made only *within* the control booth. Leaded glass, usually 1.5-mm Pb equivalent, should be available for patient observation.

Factors Affecting Barrier Thickness

Occupancy factor

Refers to the amount of time the space beyond the barrier is occupied

Workload

Expressed in units of milliampere seconds per week or milliampere minutes per week

Use factor

The percentage of time the primary beam is directed at a particular barrier

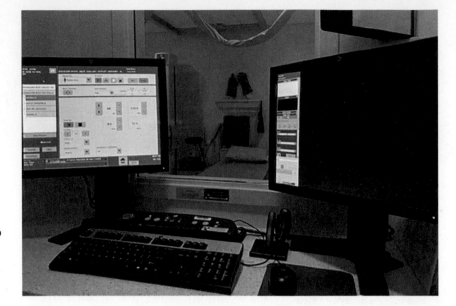

Figure 10-1. The control booth permits the operator to view the patient. The leaded booth and glass protect the operator from exposure to scattered radiation. The control booth is a secondary barrier toward which the primary beam must never be directed. (Photo contributor: Richard M. Kovatch R.T.(R).)

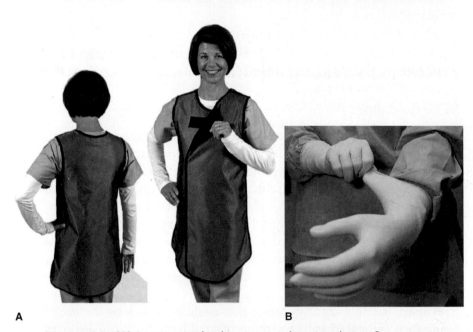

A   B

Figure 10-2. **(A)** A protective lead apron must be worn during fluoroscopic procedures. Various types/styles of lead aprons are available. The figure shows a wraparound-type protective apron. (Photo contributor: Shielding International.) **(B)** Attenuating sterile gloves are available for interventional procedures, diagnostic heart catheterization, coronary angioplasty, angiocardiography, pain management, orthopedics, and other fluoroscopic procedures. (Photo contributor: Shielding International.)

Attenuation Characteristics of Lead Aprons

X-ray attenuation at:

Pb equivalent thickness	75 kV	100 kV
0.25 mm	66%	51%
0.50 mm	88%	75%
1.0 mm	99%	94%

Protective Apparel and Its Care

During fluoroscopic procedures requiring the radiographer's presence in the radiographic department, the radiographer must wear protective apparel, including a lead apron (Fig. 10-2A). Lead aprons are secondary radiation barriers and *must* contain *at least* 0.25-mm Pb equivalent (as published in Title 10 of the CFR, Part 20), usually in the form of

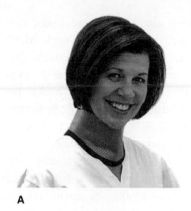

A

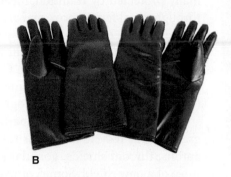

B

Figure 10-3. Other protective apparel available for fluoroscopic procedures include leaded eyewear, thyroid shield **(A)**, and leaded gloves **(B)**. (Photo contributor: Shielding International.)

lead-impregnated vinyl. Many radiology departments routinely use lead aprons containing 0.5 mm Pb (NCRP recommends minimum 0.5-mm Pb equivalent). These aprons are heavier, but they attenuate a higher percentage of scattered radiation (see the table "Attenuation Characteristics of Lead Aprons"). The fit of the apron is even more important than its thickness. It should not be drooping at the neckline or under the arms. Because the femur contains significant red bone marrow, it must be of appropriate length.

Other traditional useful protective apparel includes sterile attenuating gloves (Fig. 10-2B), thyroid shields, and leaded eyewear (Fig. 10-3). Lead aprons, lead gloves, and other apparel are secondary barriers; *they do not provide protection from the useful beam.*

Particularly useful for fluoroscopy in interventional and orthopedic procedures are the weightless/suspended "zero-gravity" protection systems (Fig. 10-4A and B). Traditional lead aprons are heavy; increased workloads for interventionalists and orthopedic surgeons using traditional lead aprons can result in extreme fatigue and even injury. The weightless/suspended "zero-gravity" protection systems offer superior radiation protection, eliminate body strain, and permit ease and freedom of movement within the sterile environment. Literature states that the 1.0-mm Pb equivalent body protection and 0.5-mm Pb/acrylic head shield reduce occupational exposure by at least 87%, compared with

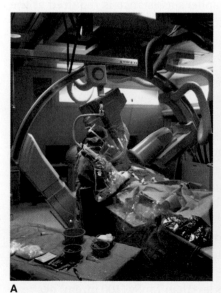

A

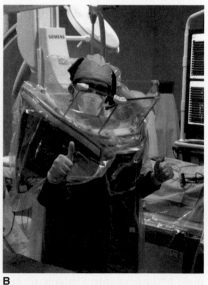

B

Figure 10-4 **(A)** Particularly useful for interventional and orthopedic fluoroscopic procedures are weightless/suspended "zero-gravity" protection systems. **(B)** The suspended "zero-gravity" protection systems offer superior radiation protection, eliminate body strain, and permit freedom of movement within the sterile environment. The systems also shield areas not normally protected by traditional lead aprons; they are extra long and shield through distal femur, proximal arm and axilla, and head and neck. (Photo contributor: Tidi Products, LLC.)

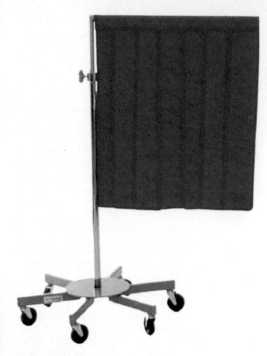

Figure 10-5. Movable leaded barriers can provide full or partial body protection for individuals required to remain in the room during the radiographic or fluoroscopic examination. Mobile barriers provide protection from secondary radiation and are available in a variety of sizes and lead equivalents. (Photo contributor: Shielding International.)

Pb Glove Protection Data

Kilovoltage level	60 kV	80 kV	100 kV
Percent attenuation	59%	49%	42%

traditional shielding systems. The system also shields areas not normally protected by traditional lead aprons; it is extra long and shields through distal femur, proximal arm and axilla, and head and neck.

Proper care of protective apparel is essential to ensure effectiveness. Lead aprons and gloves should be hung on appropriate racks, not dropped on the floor or folded. Careless handling can result in formation of cracks. Lead aprons and gloves should be imaged annually (either fluoroscopically or radiographically) to check for cracks.

Some companies have environment-friendly recycle/renew programs. They recycle frontal or full-protection aprons into smaller/half aprons, thyroid shields, gonadal shields, and so on, for up to half the price of a new shield. Some companies safely dispose of old lead aprons for a small fee.

In addition, there are some new types of protective "lead" shields that are completely lead-free, environmentally friendly, and very light weight, and provide 0.5-mm Pb equivalency.

Protective Accessories

Attenuating sterile gloves are also available for the interventional fluoroscopist. They are thin enough to permit good tactile sensitivity, yet effectively attenuate a good portion of x-ray exposure to the hands (see Fig. 10-2B and its table "Pb Glove Protection Data"). The gloves are nonlatex and are lead- and powder-free. They are useful for interventional procedures, diagnostic heart catheterization, coronary angioplasty, angiocardiography, pain management, orthopedics, and other fluoroscopic procedures. It is important to note that attenuating sterile gloves are meant *only* as a secondary barrier to scatter radiation and should never be used as protection from the primary beam.

Another device available for individuals required to remain in the fluoroscopy department is a mobile lead barrier (Fig. 10-5). These barriers feature optically clear and shatter-resistant lead acrylic windows and provide full-body protection from scattered radiation. They are usually available in a variety of lead equivalents.

Lead aprons can be placed under the patient's pillow during GI and BE examinations when the radiographer's assistance is required at the head end of the table during fluoroscopy.

SPECIAL CONSIDERATIONS

Pregnancy

A *pregnant radiographer* deserves special consideration in protection from occupational exposure. As soon as the radiographer knows that she is pregnant, it is advisable that she declares her pregnancy, in writing, to the health physicist. At that time, her occupational radiation history will be reviewed. She must be provided with a second (fetal) monitor. Modifications can be made to the pregnant radiographer's work assignments (e.g., no fluoroscopic assignments), but this is unnecessary if routine radiation safety guidelines are followed.

A radiographer who wears his or her radiation monitor on the collar outside the lead apron usually receives less than 1 mSv (100 mrem) per year.

If a *fetal monitor* is worn *under* the lead apron at waist level, the radiographer would receive 10% of that dose, or less than 0.1 mSv (10 mrem). Because the *gestational dose limit* to the fetus during the gestation period must not exceed *5 mSv* (500 mrem), under typical conditions, when sufficient protection measures are taken, modification of work assignments is not usually necessary. If a fetal, or "baby," monitor is worn, it must be clearly identified and not confused with the radiographer's regular monitor.

Radiation protection standards should be reviewed during pregnancy and dosimeter reports closely monitored. Many facilities document the counseling received by the pregnant radiographer from the time she apprises her supervisor of her pregnancy and makes the signed documents part of the employee's records.

Mobile Units

The potential for occupational exposure is greatest in interventional, fluoroscopic procedures and mobile imaging (Fig 10-6). In mobile imaging, it is essential to use two of the cardinal principles of radiation protection: shielding and distance. Each *mobile x-ray unit* should have a *lead apron* assigned to it. The radiographer should wear the apron while making the exposure at the furthest distance possible from the x ray tube. The mobile unit's exposure cord must permit the radiographer to stand at least *6 feet* from the x-ray tube and the patient.

Fluoroscopic Units and Procedures

Many of the fluoroscopic guidelines/rules serve to protect both the patient and the radiation worker. All *fluoroscopic* equipment must provide a gap of at least 30 cm (12 inches), and preferably 38 cm (15 inches), between the x-ray source (focal spot) and the x-ray tabletop (patient), according to NCRP Report No. 102. The *tabletop intensity/ entrance skin exposure* of the fluoroscopic beam must not exceed 100 mGy_a/min (10 R/min) or 21 mGy_a/min/mA (2.1 R/min/mA). With under-table fluoroscopic tubes, a Bucky slot cover having at least the equivalent of 0.25 mm Pb must be available to attenuate scattered radiation. Fluoroscopic milliamperes must not exceed 5 mA, although image-intensified fluoroscopy usually operates between 1 and 3 mA.

Because the fluoroscopic image receptor assembly functions as a primary barrier, it must have a lead equivalent of at least 2.0 mm. A cumulative timing device must be available to signal the fluoroscopist (audibly, visibly, or both) when a maximum of 5 min of fluoroscopy time has elapsed. Beam collimation must be apparent through visualization of unexposed borders on the TV monitor, and *total filtration* must be at least *2.5-mm Al* equivalent. Because occupational exposure to scattered radiation is of considerable importance in fluoroscopy, a *protective curtain/drape* of at least *0.25-mm Pb* equivalent must be placed between the patient and the fluoroscopist.

The effect of kilovoltage and milliampere adjustment on fluoroscopic images is similar to that on radiographic images. The automatic exposure control automatically varies the exposure required when viewing body tissues of widely differing tissue densities (e.g., between the abdomen and the chest). *As in radiography, high kilovoltage and low milliampere second values are preferred in an effort to reduce dose.*

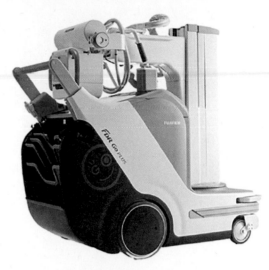

Figure 10-6. FUJIFILM Healthcare Americas Corp.

Summary

- The cardinal principles of radiation protection are time, distance, and shielding.
- Primary barriers protect from the useful (primary) beam, for example, the walls and doors of the radiographic department.
- Secondary barriers protect from sources of leakage and scattered radiation, for example, x-ray tube housing and the patient.
- Secondary barriers (e.g., control panel wall and lead apron) do not afford protection from the primary beam.
- There are several NCRP guidelines with which the radiographer should be familiar regarding required thickness and uses of protective shielding (see p. 295).
- A pregnant radiographer should apprise her supervisor of her condition as soon as possible.
- A pregnant radiographer wears a special second radiation monitor at waist level under her lead apron.
- Most occupational exposure is received in fluoroscopy and mobile radiography (especially C arm).

COMPREHENSION CHECK

Congratulations! You have completed your review of this chapter. If you are able to answer the following group of very comprehensive questions, you should feel confident that you have really mastered this section. You are then ready to go on to the "registry-type" questions that follow. For greatest success, do not go to the multiple-choice questions without first completing the following short-answer questions:

1. What are the three cardinal rules, or principal guidelines, for radiation protection (p. 294)?

2. When is personal radiation monitoring required (p. 293)?

3. What is the most significant scattering object in fluoroscopy and why? List the other scattering objects (p. 293).

4. What are the NCRP guidelines on leakage radiation, exposure switches, and exposure indicators (p. 294, 295)?

5. What resources should be used to assist and immobilize patients during radiographic examinations (p. 295)?

6. What rules apply if an individual is required in the radiographic department for assistance during a procedure (p. 295)?

7. Describe the NCRP guidelines that are in place for the patient and personnel protection during fluoroscopic procedures with respect to (p. 295):

    A. image intensifier lead equivalent

    B. exposure switch

    C. Bucky slot cover

    D. cumulative timer

    E. lead drape or curtain

    F. tabletop intensity maximum

    G. apron and glove lead equivalency

    H. palpation with remote fluoroscopy units

8. Distinguish between, and give examples of, primary and secondary barriers (p. 297).

9. What is the usual recommended thickness and recommended height of radiographic/fluoroscopic room walls (p. 297)?

10. What is leakage radiation? What protects from leakage radiation (p. 294, 295)?

11. Identify each of the following as primary or secondary barriers: x-ray room walls, control panel, lead aprons, and gloves (pp. 297–300).

12. How should lead aprons and gloves be cared for (p. 300)?

13. Describe how a pregnant radiographer may use a second personal monitor (p. 300, 301).

14. What is the gestational fetal dose limit (p. 301)?

15. What kinds of counseling and documentation are recommended for a pregnant radiographer (p. 300)?

16. Which areas of an x-ray facility generally have the highest occupational exposure (p. 301)?

17. Which NCRP guidelines govern mobile radiography with respect to availability of lead aprons, exposure cord, and fluoroscope source-to-skin distance (SSD) (p. 301)?

18. Which NCRP guidelines govern fluoroscopy equipment with respect to SSD, tabletop intensity, maximum milliampere, image intensifier lead equivalent, and fluoroscopy exposure switch (p. 295, 301)?

19. Which NCRP guidelines govern fluoroscopy equipment with respect to collimation, total filtration, protective curtain, Bucky slot cover, and cumulative timer (p. 295)?

20. Discuss differences/details with respect to mobile, fixed, and high-level control fluoroscopic equipment (p. 301).

CHAPTER REVIEW QUESTIONS

1. Any surface that can be struck by the useful x-ray beam is termed

   (A) primary barrier

   (B) secondary barrier

   (C) useful beam barrier

   (D) remnant radiation barrier

2. If an infant/child is unable to maintain the necessary radiographic position and mechanical restraining devices cannot be used, required assistance is most suitably obtained from

   (A) floor nurse

   (B) lead radiographer

   (C) friend or relative

   (D) student radiographer

3. How much protection is provided from a 100-kV x-ray beam when using a 0.50-mm Pb equivalent apron?

   (A) 65%

   (B) 75%

   (C) 88%

   (D) 99%

4. Features of fluoroscopic equipment designed specially to eliminate unnecessary radiation to the patient and personnel include

   1. protective curtain

   2. lead gloves

   3. collimation

   (A) 1 only

   (B) 1 and 2 only

   (C) 1 and 3 only

   (D) 1, 2, and 3

5. Which of the following groups of technical factors will deliver the *most* exposure to the patient?

   (A) 5 mAs, 90 kV

   (B) 10 mAs, 80 kV

   (C) 20 mAs, 68 kV

   (D) 40 mAs, 66 kV

6. If an individual received 0.45 mGy_a while standing at 4 feet from a source of radiation for 2 min, which of the following options will *most* effectively reduce his or her radiation exposure?

   (A) Standing 6 feet from the source for 2 min

   (B) Standing 5 feet from the source for 1 min

   (C) Standing 4 feet from the source for 3 min

   (D) Standing 3 feet from the source for 2 min

7. Guidelines used to reduce personnel and/or patient dose in fluoroscopy include

   1. maximum tabletop intensity of 200 mGy_a/min

   2. minimum SSD of 30 cm

   3. minimum filtration of 2.5-mm Al equivalent

   (A) 1 only

   (B) 1 and 2 only

   (C) 2 and 3 only

   (D) 1, 2, and 3

8. Occupational exposure to ionizing radiation is reduced by the following exposure cord guidelines:

   1. exposure cords on mobile equipment must allow the operator to be at a maximum of 6 feet from the x-ray tube

   2. exposure cords on fixed equipment must prevent the operator from leaving the control booth during an exposure

   3. exposure cords on fixed and mobile equipment should be the coiled expandable type

   (A) 1 only

   (B) 2 only

   (C) 1 and 3 only

   (D) 1, 2, and 3

9. The height of primary radiation barriers must be at least

   (A) 5 feet

   (B) 6 feet

   (C) 7 feet

   (D) 8 feet

10. Every time an x-ray photon scatters, its intensity at 1 m from the scattering object is what fraction of its original intensity?

    (A) $1/10$

    (B) $1/100$

    (C) $1/500$

    (D) $1/1000$

Answers and Explanations

1. (A) *Primary barriers* protect us from the primary or useful beam. They have much greater attenuation capability than secondary barriers that protect only from leakage and scattered radiation. The radiographic room walls are considered primary barriers because the primary beam is often directed toward them, as in chest radiography. *Secondary barriers* are surfaces that protect against scattered radiation. Most control booth barriers are *secondary barriers*. They are usually constructed of four thicknesses of gypsum board and/or 0.5–1 inch of plate glass. Remnant radiation penetrates the patient and forms the latent image on the image receptor. The primary x-ray beam must never be directed toward the control booth/secondary barrier.

2. (C) If mechanical restraint is not possible, a friend or relative accompanying the patient should be requested to hold the patient. If a friend or relative is not available, a nurse or transporter may be asked for help. Protective apparel, such as lead apron and gloves, should be provided to the person(s) holding the patient. *Radiology personnel must never assist in holding patients, and the individual assisting should* never *be in the path of the primary beam.*

3. (B) Lead aprons are worn by occupationally exposed individuals using fluoroscopic procedures. They are available with various lead equivalents; 0.25, 0.5, and 1.0 mm are the most common. The *1.0-mm* Pb equivalent apron will provide close to 100% protection at most kilovoltage levels, but it is rarely used because it weighs anywhere between 12 and 24 pounds. A *0.5 mm* apron will attenuate approximately 99% of a 50-kV beam, 88% of a 75-kV beam, and 75% of a 100-kV beam. A *0.25-mm* Pb equivalent apron will attenuate approximately 97% of a 50-kV x-ray beam, 66% of a 75-kV beam, and 51% of a 100-kV beam.

4. (C) The *protective* curtain is usually made of leaded vinyl with at least 0.25-mm Pb equivalent. It must be positioned between the patient and the fluoroscopist, and it greatly reduces exposure of the fluoroscopist to energetic scatter from the patient. Collimator or beam alignment must be accurate to within 2%. Just as overhead radiation barrier equipment, fluoroscopic total *filtration* must be at least 2.5-mm Al equivalent to reduce excessive exposure to low-energy radiation. Lead gloves serve only to protect the radiologist.

5. (D) Milliampere seconds regulate the *quantity* of radiation delivered to the patient. Kilovoltage regulates the *quality* (penetration) of the radiation delivered to the patient. Therefore, lower energy (less penetrating) radiation—which is less likely to exit the patient—accompanied by higher milliampere seconds would deliver the highest dose to the patient. *Lower* milliampere seconds at higher kilovoltage values *decreases* patient dose.

6. (B) A quick survey of the distractors reveals that options C and D will *increase* exposure dose; thus, they are eliminated as possible correct answers. Both A and B will serve to reduce radiation exposure, as distance is increased and exposure time is decreased in each case. It remains to be seen then which is more effective. Using the inverse square law of radiation, it is found that the individual would receive *0.2 mGy$_a$ at 6 feet in 2 min* and would receive *0.144 mGy$_a$ at 5 feet In 1 min*:

$$\frac{I_1}{I_2} = \frac{D_2^2}{D_1^2}$$

Substituting known values from distractor **A**, we get:

$$\frac{0.45\ \text{mGy}_a}{x} = \frac{6\ \text{feet}^2}{4\ \text{feet}^2}$$

$$\frac{0.45}{x} = \frac{36}{16}$$

$$36x = 7.2$$

$$x = 0.2\ \text{mGy}_a \text{ at 6 feet for 2 min}$$

Substituting known values from distractor **B**, we get:

$$\frac{0.45\ \text{mGy}_a}{x} = \frac{5\ \text{feet}^2}{6\ \text{feet}^2}$$

$$\frac{0.45}{x} = \frac{25}{16}$$

$$25x = 7.2$$

$$x = 0.228\ \text{mGy}_a \text{ at 5 feet for 2 min,}$$
$$\text{therefore 0.144 in 1 min}$$

Distractor **C** is the same distance, 4 feet, and the time is increased to 3 min, thereby delivering a greater exposure.

Substituting known values from distractor **D**, we get:

$$\frac{0.45\ mGy_a}{x} = \frac{3\ feet^2}{4\ feet^2}$$

$$\frac{0.45}{x} = \frac{9}{16}$$

$$9x = 7.2$$

$$x = 0.8\ mGy_a\ at\ 3\ feet\ in\ 2\ min$$

Therefore, **B** is most effective in reducing radiation exposure.

Note the inverse relationship between the distance and the dose. As distance from the source of radiation increases, dose rate significantly decreases.

7. (C) All *fluoroscopic* equipment (both stationary and mobile) must provide at *least* 30 cm (12 inches), and preferably 38 cm (15 inches), between the x-ray source (focal spot) and the x-ray tabletop, according to NCRP Report No. 102. Required filtration must be at least the equivalent of 2.5 mm Al. The tabletop *intensity* of the fluoroscopic beam must not exceed *100 mGy$_a$/min* (10 R/min), or *21 mGy$_a$/min/mA* (2.1 R/min/mA). Fluoroscopic milliampere must not exceed 5, although image-intensified fluoroscopy usually operates between 1 and 3 mA. The image intensifier functions as a primary barrier and has a lead equivalent of 2.0 mm.

8. (B) Radiographic and fluoroscopic equipment is designed to help decrease the exposure dose to the patient and the operator. One of the design features is the exposure cord. Exposure cords on *fixed* equipment must be short enough to prevent the exposure from being made outside the control booth. Exposure cords on *mobile* equipment must be long enough to permit the operator to stand *at least* 6 feet from the x-ray tube.

9. (C) Radiation protection guidelines have established that *primary radiation barriers* must be at least 7 feet high. Primary radiation barriers are walls toward which the primary beam might be directed. They usually contain 1.5 mm Pb, but this can vary depending on the *use factor* and other factors.

10. (D) One of the radiation protection guidelines for the occupationally exposed is that the x-ray beam must scatter twice before reaching the operator. Every time the x-ray beam scatters, its intensity at 1 m from the scattering object is approximately 0.1% of the intensity of the primary beam, that is, $^1/_{1000}$ of its original intensity. That is why, in terms of radiation protection, the patient is considered the most important source of scatter. Of course, the operator should be behind a shielded booth while making the exposure, but multiple scatterings further reduce danger of exposure from scattered radiation. Other scattering objects include the x-ray table, Bucky slot cover, and control booth wall.

Radiation Exposure and Monitoring

OBJECTIVES

At the conclusion of this chapter, the student will be able to:

- Name the traditional units of measure and their corresponding SI units.
- Describe the use of each unit of measure.
- Explain when a personnel monitor is required and the types of personnel monitors available.
- Describe the operation of each type of personnel monitor.
- Identify occupational dose limits.
- Differentiate between equivalent dose and effective dose.

UNITS OF MEASUREMENT

W.C. Röntgen's paper *On a New Kind of Rays* described the ionizing effect of x-rays on air, their penetrating effects on all forms of matter, and their effect on photographic emulsion. Röntgen's work was so thorough and complete that we know little more these days than was originally presented in his paper. We still use these principles today to detect and quantify radiation exposure.

The traditional/conventional radiation units of measurement are roentgen, rad, and rem. The Standard International (SI) units of measure have gained in usage in the United States and must be understood by the radiographer. The American Registry of Radiologic Technologists (ARRT®) Content Specifications for the Examination in Radiography indicate that the certification examination primarily uses the SI units of measurement.

Gray in Air (Gy$_a$)

The unit *kerma* expresses *kinetic energy released in matter*. X-rays expend kinetic energy as they ionize the air. Joule/kilogram is used to measure air kerma and 1 J/kg = 1 Gy$_a$. mGy$_a$ is the SI unit of measure of radiation exposure/intensity; the subscript *a* represents *air* as the absorber.

Air Kerma (*Kinetic Energy Released in Matter*)

- It measures energy transferred from x-ray photons to electrons during ionization.
- Symbol is Gy$_a$.
- 1 J/kg equals 1 Gy$_a$.

Roentgen

- It measures ionization in air (negative *or* positive ions counted).
- Symbol is R; measures x- and gamma radiation only.
- It is valid up to 3 MeV.

When used to express *rate*, roentgen is abbreviated as R/min or R/h. The roentgen expresses air ionization. Because x-rays ionize air, all ions of *either* sign (positive *or* negative) formed in a particular quantity of air are counted and equated to a quantity of radiation expressed in the unit roentgen. When used as a unit of measure, the roentgen is valid for x- and gamma radiations at energies up to 3 MeV (million/megaelectron volts).

SI Units	Traditional Units
Air kerma (Gy_a)	Roentgen
Gray (Gy_t)	rad
Sievert (Sv)	rem

Gray (Gy_t)

As ionizing radiation passes through matter, a certain amount of its energy is deposited in that matter, representing an absorbed dose. Note that we are again referring to energy released in matter, that is, *kerma.* The SI unit used to describe *absorbed dose* is *Gray* (Gy_t)—the subscript *t* representing *tissue.* It describes *tissue in general;* various organs and tissue types require assigned specific weighting factors in order to describe the *effective dose.* Absorbed dose and energy deposited are strongly related to chemical change and biologic damage. The amount of energy deposited in tissue and possible biologic damage are dependent on the following:

- Type of ionizing radiation
- Atomic number of the tissue
- Mass density of the tissue
- Energy of the radiation

1 Gray = 100 rad. *Rad* is an acronym for *radiation-absorbed dose.* It has been described as equivalent to *100 ergs* of energy deposited *per gram* of irradiated material. Because rad does not take into account the biologic effect of various *tissue types* and their *radiosensitivity,* it cannot be used to express effective dose or occupational exposure.

Sievert

The SI unit of measurement to describe effective dose to biologic material is the *Sievert (Sv).* Sievert is the unit of occupational radiation exposure.

Similar absorbed doses of *different kinds* of radiation can cause different biologic effects to *tissues of differing radiosensitivity.* A *radiation weighting factor* (W_r) is a number assigned to different types of ionizing radiations so that their effect(s) may be better determined (e.g., x-ray vs. alpha particles). The W_r of different ionizing radiations is dependent on the linear energy transfer (LET) of that particular radiation. The *average* absorbed dose multiplied by the radiation weighting factor equals *equivalent dose.*

TABLE 11-1. Quality Factor for Different Types of Radiation

Ionizing Radiation Type	Quality Factor
Gamma rays	1
X-ray photons	1
Alpha particles	20
Beta particles	1
Fast neutrons	20

A *tissue weighting factor* (W_t) represents the relative tissue radiosensitivity of the irradiated material (e.g., muscle vs. intestinal epithelium vs. bone). The weighting factor is like the *SI* equivalent of the formerly used quality factor (QF). For example, where rad × QF = *rem,* the SI expression is $Gy_t \times W_r = Sv$. The term *effective dose* is used to describe the product of the average absorbed dose, the type of radiation delivered, and the radiosensitivity of the exposed tissue.

The former unit of measure for dose to biologic material was *rem.* Rem is an acronym for *radiation equivalent man.* It uses the information collected for rad, but it also uses a QF to predict biologic effects from different types of radiation (Table 11-1). Thus, we have the following equation: rad × QF = rem. Radiations having a high QF have a higher LET and a greater potential to produce biologic damage. Rem is still often used as the unit of dose equivalency (DE) to express occupational exposure. 100 rem = 1 Sv.

Particulate Radiation

Particulate radiation (alpha, beta, etc.) is highly ionizing. As an *internal* source of radiation, it increases LET, and a significant biologic effect can result. As an *external* source of radiation, most is virtually innocuous. However, some beta particles (e.g., Mo-99 and Co-60 beta) are very energetic and can cause serious external damage.

As the *atomic number* of the irradiated tissue increases, a greater number of x-ray photons are absorbed by the tissue (i.e., the photoelectric interaction increases), and LET increases. As the *energy* of the ionizing radiation increases, it becomes more penetrating and LET decreases, thereby decreasing the likelihood of biologic effects.

MONITORING DEVICES

National Council on Radiation Protection and Measurements (NCRP) Guidelines for Use

Radiation monitoring is used to evaluate the effectiveness of the radiation safety policies and practices in place. Area dosimeters monitor radiation levels in a particular environment or area. Typical *personnel* dosimeters measure whole-body radiation exposure. They are worn at the collar/shoulder level; when using a lead apron, they are worn outside the lead apron. A fetal monitor is worn under a lead apron. Extremity dosimeters are worn on the finger, and dosimeters for the lens of the eye are usually worn behind eyeglasses. A *control dosimeter* accompanies every shipment of personnel monitors and used to monitor/ measure environmental radiation exposure received in transit and/or during storage in the radiology facility. It must be returned with the used personnel monitors. The radiation received by the control monitor is subtracted from radiation dose received by personnel monitors so that they reflect only the occupational dose.

The Code of Federal Regulations (CFR) states that monitoring should be provided for occupationally exposed individuals in a controlled area who are likely to receive more than ¹⁄₁₀th of *the dose-equivalent limit.*

Optically Stimulated Luminescent Dosimeter

Optically stimulated luminescence (OSL) dosimeters are gradually replacing the long-used film badges. They contain a thin layer of *aluminum oxide* (Al_2O_3). Aluminum oxide absorbs and stores the energy associated with exposure to ionizing radiation. OSL dosimeters are available with various combinations of filter packs (Fig. 11-1). Some contain a filter pack of tin, copper, and an open window. Others are available with aluminum oxide copper/aluminum, plastic, and an open window. These various *filters* serve to identify the type and energy of

---

Personnel Radiation Monitors

- Optically stimulated luminescence
- Thermoluminescent dosimeter
- Film badge
- Pocket dosimeter
- Ion storage device

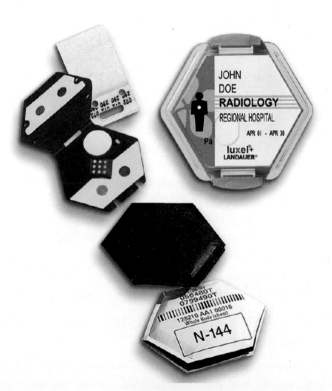

Figure 11-1. OSL dosimeters are available with various combinations of filters. Some contain a filter pack of tin, copper, and an open window. Others are available with aluminum, copper/aluminum, plastic, and an open window. Still others contain lead, copper/aluminum, plastic, and an open window. These various filters serve to identify the type and energy of radiation. (Photo contributor: Landauer Inc., Glenwood, IL.)

ionizing radiation that interacted with the dosimeter. For example, photons that penetrate the copper to interact with the dosimeter are more energetic than those that might have only enough energy to pass through the plastic filter.

When the OSL dosimeter is returned to the laboratory for processing, the Al_2O_3 chips are stimulated with green light from either a laser or a light-emitting diode source. The resulting blue light emitted from Al_2O_3 is proportional to the amount of radiation exposure. The quantity of light emitted is equated to a radiation quantity expressed in mrem on the written report returned to the user. Both high- and low-energy photons and beta particles can be measured with this technique.

The OSL dosimeter allows for multiple readouts and can be used to reconfirm reported radiation doses. This is because only a fraction of the radiation exposure signal contained in the Al_2O_3 material is used up on stimulation with the green light. Other advantages of the OSL dosimeter include the ability to measure radiation doses as low as 1 mrem (with a precision of ±1 mrem) and to be reanalyzed, if necessary. Its tamper-proof plastic package is unaffected by heat, moisture, and pressure. Although many facilities prefer monthly radiation reports, OSL dosimeters being so accurate and stable can be used for longer periods and "read" quarterly.

Film Badge Dosimeter

The ionizing radiation monitor used for many years was the *film badge*. The film badge consists of special radiation dosimetry film packaged like dental film and is enclosed in a special plastic holder. The plastic holder features an open window (through which the user's name appears) and various *filters* (which serve to identify the *type* and *energy of ionizing radiation* received by the user; Fig. 11-2).

Radiation that exposes the film behind an aluminum filter is more energetic than a radiation that passes through only the open window and less energetic than a radiation penetrating a copper filter. Film

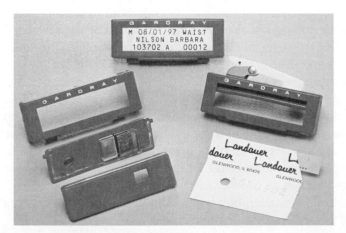

Figure 11-2. The radiation monitor used for many years was the *film badge,* consisting of special film packages such as dental film and enclosed in a special plastic holder. The plastic holder has an open window and various filters, which serve to identify the type and energy of radiation. (Photo contributor: Landauer Inc., Glenwood, IL.)

badges are used for *1 month,* collected, and sent to a special laboratory for processing. The degree of exposure is carefully evaluated and equated to a dose usually expressed in *mrem;* the film badge can measure doses as low as 10 mrem.

Film badges had once been the most widely used personnel radiation monitors but are frequently replaced by an OSL or a DIS dosimeter.

Thermoluminescent Dosimeter

The thermoluminescent dosimeter (TLD) (Fig. 11-3) contains crystalline chips of *lithium fluoride* (LiF). LiF absorbs and stores the energy associated with exposure to ionizing radiation. When the TLD is returned to the laboratory for processing, the LiF chips are heated. This process causes a release of visible light from the chips in proportion to the amount of ionizing radiation absorbed. The quantity of light emitted is equated to a radiation quantity expressed in mrem on the written report returned to the user.

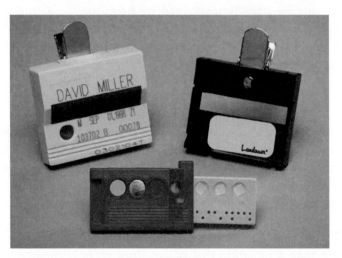

Figure 11-3. The TLD contains crystalline chips of LiF, which absorb and store the energy associated with exposure to ionizing radiation. (Photo contributor: Landauer Inc., Glenwood, IL.)

Similar to the film badges and OSLs, TLDs use various filters to determine the types and energy of exposure received. The TLD is more sensitive and precise than the film badge because it can measure doses as low as 5 mrem. The TLD is unaffected by heat or humidity, is reusable, and can be worn up to 3 months before processing. However, in the unlikely event that the user had unknowingly received excessive radiation exposure, the user should be made aware of it as soon as possible, and the event should be recent enough to be able to recall. The only disadvantage of the TLD is the inability to provide real-time dosage readings.

The OSL dosimeter, film badge, and TLD measure a variety of energies of x-, beta, and gamma radiations.

Pocket Dosimeter

The use of a *pocket dosimeter* (Fig. 11-4) is indicated when working with high exposures or large quantities of radiation for a short period of

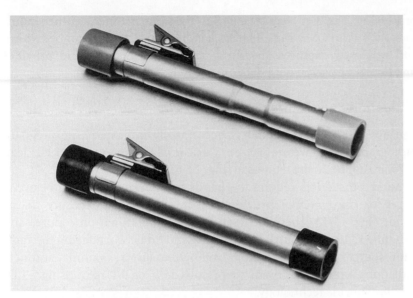

Figure 11-4. The pocket dosimeter contains a small ionization chamber that counts charges in proportion to the exposure received. (Photo contributor: Nuclear Associates.)

time, so that an immediate reading is available to the user. The pocket dosimeter is sensitive and accurate, but has limited application in diagnostic radiography.

The pocket dosimeter, or *pocket isolation chamber*, resembles a penlight. Within the dosimeter is a thimble ionization chamber. In the presence of x- or gamma radiations, a particular quantity of air is ionized and causes the fiber indicator to register radiation quantity in milliroentgen (mR). The self-reading type may be "read" by holding the dosimeter up to the light and, looking through the eyepiece, observing the fiber indicator. The pocket dosimeter can measure exposure quantities of 0–200 mR. Owing to its composition, the pocket dosimeter is a delicate instrument requiring careful handling. Sharp trauma, such as dropping the instrument, can result in inaccurate reading. The pocket dosimeter does not provide a permanent legal record of exposure.

Direct Ion Storage Dosimeter

One of the newest types of personnel monitoring devices is the revolutionary direct ion storage dosimeter (DIS). The DIS (Fig. 11-5) eliminates the need to collect and send dosimeters for monthly or quarterly

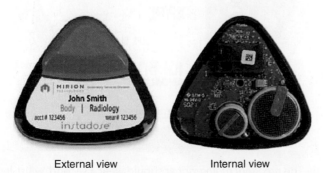

External view   Internal view

Figure 11-5. Direct ion storage dosimeter—external and internal views. (Photo contributor: Mirion Technologies, Inc.)

processing. The user wears the DIS in the same manner as other monitors, such as an OSL. The DIS has a gas-filled ionization chamber within and wirelessly captures, measures, analyzes, transmits, and provides immediate display of dose data on smart device or PC.

Evaluation and Maintenance of Records

The use of a *second monitor* is occasionally indicated. The pregnant radiographer may wear a second, waist-level dosimeter under her lead apron to approximate fetal dose (Fig. 11-6).

Some procedures require the hands to be near the useful beam. A *finger, or ring, monitor* provides information about exposure to the hands (Fig. 11-7). These are useful for interventional procedures and handling radioactive nuclides. The ring should be worn facing the radiation source. The ring monitors usually measure x-, gamma, and beta radiations with a minimum reportable dose of 0.1 mSv using TLD/lithium fluoride technology.

Personnel monitors should be worn consistently in the same place and facing forward (i.e., with the open window and user's identification visible). If the badge is correctly worn at the collar outside the lead apron, it will approximate dose to the head and neck and will provide an overestimation of dose to the shielded organs.

The radiographer is occupationally exposed to *low-energy, low-LET* radiation. Monitoring devices are worn *only for occupational purposes* and never if the individual is exposed for medical or dental reasons. The radiographer should review his or her record monthly (or quarterly, if a quarterly system is used) as the report is received by the institution. The RSO (radiation safety officer) is responsible for reviewing all dosimeter reports (Fig. 11-8) and being certain that the staff is monitored, educated, and regularly updated.

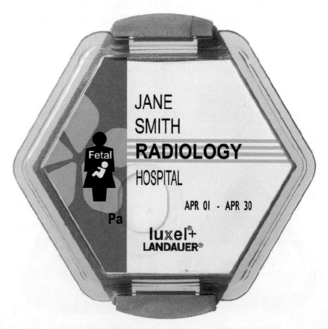

Figure 11-6. The *pregnant radiographer* should wear a second, waist-level, dosimeter under her lead apron that will measure the approximate fetal dose. (Photo contributor: Landauer Inc., Glenwood, IL.)

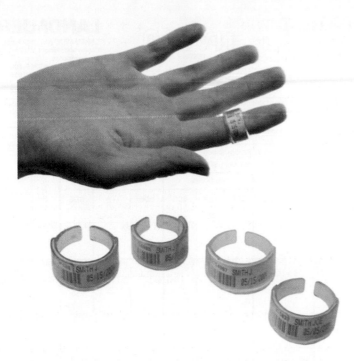

Figure 11-7. Finger/ring monitors are useful for interventional procedures and handling radioactive nuclides. (Photo contributor: Mirion Technologies, Inc.)

An *official written report* is sent to the sponsoring institution to document doses received from the OSL dosimeter, TLD, or film badge. A number of columns of specific data are reported. Exposure data that are *required* to appear are the current period exposure, the annual cumulative exposure, and separate readings for special dosimeters, such as fetal or extremity dosimeters.

NCRP RECOMMENDATIONS

A part of the professional radiographer's responsibility lies in keeping occupational exposure to a minimum. The use of radiation-monitoring devices helps evaluate the effectiveness of radiation protection practices. The periodic reports received from OSL dosimeter, film badge, or TLD laboratories are official legal documents that must be reviewed, and an attempt should be made to reduce *any* exposure no matter how small (i.e., the ALARA principle).

NCRP Report No. 116 and the CFR (10 CFR §20) require that occupationally exposed individuals aged 18 years and older do not receive exposures in excess of 50 mSv (5 rem) per year. A radiography student participating in clinical education before the age of 18 years must not receive an annual dose of more than 1 mSv/0.001 Sv (100 mrem/0.1 rem). Because the general population is not in the vicinity of man-made ionizing radiation on a daily basis, their annual dose limit is ¹⁄₁₀th that of a radiographer: 5 mSv (0.5 rem) per year.

The *cumulative* exposure for the occupationally exposed individual is determined using the following formula: age × 10 mSv. Thus, a 26-year-old radiographer's cumulative occupational exposure must not exceed 260 mSv (26 rem). The pregnant radiographer's *gestational* exposure to

---

NCRP-Recommended Occupational Dose Limits

Cumulative: age × 10 mSv

Annual: 50 mSv

Students younger than 18 years: 1 mSv

Skin, hands, feet: 500 mSv

Lens of eye: 150 mSv

Embryo/fetus: 0.5 mSv (month); 5.0 mSv (entire gestation)

140803 1
T
STILLED
TABULABLE
JACKSONVILLE,
India

Received Date / Reported Date	2021-03-25 / 2021-03-31
Page	1 of 3
Analytical Work Order / QC Release	2108400196 / LAH
Copy / Version	3 / 2

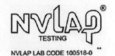
NVLAP TESTING
NVLAP LAB CODE 100518-0 **

LANDAUER®
LANDAUER, Inc., 2 Science Road
Glenwood, Illinois 60425-1586
landauer.com
Telephone: (708) 755-7000
Facsimile: (708) 755-7016
Customer Service: (800) 323-8830
Technical: (800) 438-3241

Radiation Dosimetry Report

**No NVLAP accreditation is available from NVLAP for thermal neutron or X type dosimeters. When exposure results are reported for thermal neutrons or X type dosimeters, this report contains data that are not covered by the NVLAP accreditation.

Account: 109907   Subaccount: 1289225   Series: ARA
Corrected

Copy 3 : Original sent to 140803 1, T, STILLED, TABULABLE, JACKSONVILLE, India

Dose Equivalent (mrem) for Periods Shown Below
DDE-Deep Dose Equivalent LDE-Lens Dose Equivalent SDE-Shallow Dose Equivalent

Participant Number / ID Number / Birth Date	Name	Dosimeter	Use	Rad. Type	Rad. Quality	Period Shown Below 2021-01-01 to 2021-03-31 DDE	LDE	SDE	Quarter to Date QUARTER 1 DDE	LDE	SDE	Year to Date 2021 DDE	LDE	SDE	Lifetime to Date LIFETIME DDE	LDE	SDE	Inception Date	Serial Number
00007	NEUTRON ELEKTA 1 CON NE	Ta	AREA	P / P / N / N	/ / T / F	3/3/M/M	3/3/M/M	3/3/M/M	3	3	3	3	3	3	64	60	64	2009/06	7311946K
00051	Flotsam, Stipes Vertigi 2000-01-31	Pa	AREA	P		M	2	2	M	2	2	M	2	2	143	150	181	1990/08	7311937K
00111	NEUTRON ELEKTA 1 DOOR N	Ta	AREA	P / P / N / N	/ / T / F	3/3/M/M	3/3/M/M	3/3/M/M	3	3	3	3	3	3	63	62	63	2009/06	7311947K
00112	Resultant, Ibices Caske 1982-03-07	Pa	CHEST			M	M	M	M	M	M	M	M	M	26	26	38	2010/05	7311945K
00149	Chemists, Redetermine E 1956-12-06	Pa	AREA			M	M	M	M	M	M	M	M	M	136	141	167	2008/05	7311941K
00205	AGILITY OFFICE	Ta	AREA	P / P / N / N	/ / T / F	2/2/M/M	2/2/M/M	2/2/M/M	2	2	2	2	2	2	158	157	169	2002/10	7311935K
00259	Carnauba, Leavers Everg 1951-11-23	Pa	AREA			M	M	M	M	M	M	M	M	M	474	472	507	2004/12	7311962K
00378	Appal, Aperient Continu 1996-05-23	Pa	AREA			M	M	M	M	M	M	M	M	M	1037	1039	1046	2004/12	7311961K
00411	Fescues, Brethren Carob 2002-08-29	Pa	AREA			M	M	M	M	M	M	M	M	M	424	436	471	2004/12	7311959K
00522	Amputated, Daimons Ener 1970-04-09	Pa	AREA			M	M	M	M	M	M	M	M	M	565	573	627	2004/12	7311960K

This report must not be used to claim product certification, approval, or endorsement by NVLAP, NIST, or any agency of the federal government.

Figure 11-8. An *official written report* documents doses received from the OSL dosimeter, TLD, or film badge. Columns of specific data are reported, including the current period exposure, annual cumulative exposure, and separate readings for special dosimeters, such as fetal or extremity dosimeters. (Photo contributor: Landauer Inc., Glenwood, IL.)

the embryo/fetus must not exceed 5 mSv (0.5 rem/500 mrem); the *monthly* embryo/fetal dose must not exceed 0.5 mSv (0.05 rem).

These are the recommended maximum dose-equivalent limits. The *actual* mean annual exposure to occupationally exposed medical personnel is 1–1.4 mSv (100–140 mrem), well below the recommended limit. However, the International Commission on Radiological Protection, in accordance with the ALARA concept, has *recommended* that the annual whole-body dose limit be reduced to 20 mSv (2 rem/2000 mrem).

Summary

- The unit *kerma* is used to express *k*inetic *e*nergy *r*eleased in *ma*tter, and is the SI unit of exposure replacing Roentgen (R unit).
- The SI unit used to describe absorbed dose is *Gray* (Gy_t).
- The SI unit of measure to describe effective dose is *Sievert* (*Sv*).
- Rad is an acronym for radiation-absorbed dose; the unit of absorbed dose is Gy_t.

- Rem describes effective dose and is often used as the unit of measure for personnel dosimeter results.
- The OSL dosimeter is the newest, most accurate personnel dosimeter; it can be processed monthly or quarterly. It uses a thin layer of Al_2O_3 to store information.
- Film badges are convenient, low-cost radiation monitors that are processed monthly.
- TLDs use LiF crystals to store exposure information. They are more precise and more expensive than film badges and may be processed quarterly.
- Film badges and TLDs measure exposure to x-, beta, and gamma radiations.
- Pocket dosimeters are thimble ionization chambers used to monitor larger quantities of radiation exposure, up to 200 mR.
- Radiographers strive to keep their occupational dose ALARA.
- NCRP Report No. 116 and the CFR (10 CFR §20) establish limits for exposure to ionizing radiation with which radiographers should be familiar.

COMPREHENSION CHECK

Congratulations! You have completed your review of this chapter. If you are able to answer the following group of very comprehensive questions, you should feel confident that you have really mastered this section. You are then ready to go on to the "registry-type" questions that follow. For greatest success, do not go to the multiple-choice questions without first completing the following short-answer questions:

1. Discuss R as a unit of measurement, including what it measures, the radiation(s) it measures, and up to what energy (p. 308).

2. What does the term *kerma* express? What is the SI unit of measure of radiation intensity (p. 307)?

3. What does the acronym rad mean? Define rad. Discuss/convert rad to SI unit (p. 308).

4. What is the SI unit of measure of energy deposited per gram of irradiated material (p. 308)?

5. Name the three factors influencing the amount of energy deposited (rad) in tissue (p. 308, 309).

6. Relate particulate radiation to degree of ionization in tissue, LET, and possible biologic effects (p. 309).

7. Discuss the function of weighting factors and quality factors (p. 308, 309).

8. What does the acronym rem mean? Discuss/convert rem to SI unit (p. 309).

9. Why could rem be accurately used to describe occupational DE, whereas rad could not (p. 308, 309)?

10. Describe the film badge. Include the following in your description (p. 311):
    (A) construction
    (B) purpose of filters
    (C) length of time used
    (D) type(s) of radiation detected
    (E) how it is "read" and in what unit
    (F) any advantages or disadvantages

11. Describe the TLD. Include the following in your description (p. 311, 312):
    (A) construction
    (B) type of crystals used and their unique characteristics
    (C) length of time used
    (D) type(s) of radiation detected
    (E) how it is "read" and in what unit
    (F) any advantages or disadvantages

12. Describe the pocket dosimeter. Include the following in your description (p. 312, 313):
    (A) construction
    (B) indications for use
    (C) how it is "read," in what unit, and up to what maximum limit
    (D) any advantages or disadvantages

13. Describe the OSL dosimeter to include (p. 310, 311):
    (A) component parts
    (B) type of crystal used, and how it reacts to radiation exposure
    (C) types and purpose of filters
    (D) how the OSL dosimeter is "read"
    (E) degree of accuracy
    (F) how it is affected by environmental condition

14. Describe the operation and advantages of the DIS dosimeter (p. 313).

15. What is the NCRP-recommended dose limit for occupational exposure in individuals younger than 18 years and older than 18 years (p. 315, 316)?

16. How is lifetime cumulative occupational exposure determined (p. 316)?

17. What is the NCRP-recommended dose limit for gestational fetal exposure (p. 316)?

CHAPTER REVIEW QUESTIONS

1. Which of the following units of measure is used to represent absorbed dose?

   (A) Air kerma

   (B) Gray

   (C) Sv

   (D) Relative biologic effectiveness (RBE)

2. What is the gestational dose limit for a pregnant radiographer?

   (A) 1 mSv

   (B) 5 mSv

   (C) 50 mSv

   (D) 100 mSv

3. The purpose of filters in personnel radiation monitors is to

   (A) eliminate harmful rays

   (B) measure radiation quality

   (C) prevent exposure from alpha particles

   (D) support the film contained within

4. The dose limits established for the OSL dosimeter, TLD, and film badge are valid for

   (A) alpha, beta, and x-radiations

   (B) x- and gamma radiations only

   (C) beta, x-, and gamma radiations

   (D) all ionizing radiations

5. The operation of personnel radiation-monitoring devices can depend on

   1. ionization

   2. thermoluminescence

   3. resonance

   (A) 1 only

   (B) 1 and 2 only

   (C) 2 and 3 only

   (D) 1, 2, and 3

6. What is the established monthly fetal dose-limit guideline for pregnant radiographers?

   (A) 0.5 mSv

   (B) 5 mSv

   (C) 50 mSv

   (D) 100 mSv

7. Which of the following crystals is used in a thermoluminescent dosimetry system?

   (A) Silver bromide

   (B) Aluminum oxide

   (C) Lithium fluoride

   (D) Ferrous sulfate

8. Potential ionizing radiation damage to tissue is dependent on the

   1. Z number of the tissue

   2. type of ionizing radiation

   3. mass density of the tissue

   (A) 1 only

   (B) 1 and 2 only

   (C) 2 and 3 only

   (D) 1, 2, and 3

9. The unit of measurement used to describe effective dose to biologic material is

   (A) Roentgen

   (B) Gray

   (C) Sievert

   (D) RBE

10. The NCRP recommends an annual effective occupational dose-equivalent limit of

    (A) 25 mSv

    (B) 50 mSv

    (C) 100 mSv

    (D) 200 mSv

Answers and Explanations

1. (B) The SI unit *kerma* is used to express *k*inetic *e*nergy *r*eleased in *ma*tter. The SI unit used to describe absorbed dose is *Gray* (Gy$_t$). The SI unit of measurement to describe effective dose is the Sievert (Sv). RBE is specific to the irradiated tissue, thereby being a valid unit of measurement of dose to biologic material.

2. (B) The pregnant radiographer's gestational exposure to the embryo/fetus must not exceed 5 mSv (0.5 rem/500 mrem); the monthly embryo/fetal dose must not exceed 0.5 mSv (0.05 rem).

3. (B) Film badge and OSL filters (usually aluminum and copper) serve to help measure radiation quality (energy). Only the most energetic radiation will penetrate the copper; radiation of lower levels will penetrate the aluminum, and the lowest energy radiation will pass readily through the unfiltered area. Thus, radiation of different energy levels can be recorded, measured, and reported.

4. (C) The occupational dose limit is valid for x-, beta, and gamma radiations. Traditional personnel monitors will not record alpha radiation because alpha particles are rapidly ionizing and capable of penetrating only a few centimeters of air. They are practically harmless as an external source of radiation but, potentially, the most harmful as an *internal* source. Pocket dosimeters measure x- and gamma radiations only; alpha and beta particles are not energetic enough to penetrate the device and enter the ionization chamber.

5. (B) Ionization is the fundamental principle of operation of both the film badge and the pocket dosimeter. In the film badge, the film's silver halide emulsion is ionized by x-ray photons. The pocket dosimeter contains an ionization chamber, and the number of ionizations taking place may be equated to exposure dose. Resonance refers to motion and has no application to personnel radiation monitoring.

6. (A) The declared pregnant radiographer poses a special radiation protection consideration, for the safety of the unborn individual must be considered. It must be remembered that the developing fetus is particularly sensitive to radiation exposure. Therefore, established guidelines state that the occupational radiation exposure to the fetus must not exceed 5 mSv (0.5 rem/500 mrem) during the entire gestation period; the *monthly* fetal dose must not exceed 0.5 mSv (0.05 rem).

7. (C) The thermoluminescent dosimeter (TLD) is a personnel radiation monitor that contains crystalline chips of lithium fluoride (LiF). LiF absorbs and stores the energy associated with exposure to ionizing radiation. During processing, the LiF chips are exposed to heat causing a release of visible light from the chips in proportion to the amount of ionizing radiation absorbed. The quantity of light emitted is equated to a radiation quantity expressed in mrem. OSL dosimeters use aluminum oxide crystals.

8. (D) Absorbed dose refers to the amount of energy deposited per unit mass and is strongly related to chemical change and biologic damage. The amount of energy deposited and, thus, the amount of possible biologic damage are dependent on the *type of ionizing radiation,* the *atomic (Z) number of the tissue,* the *mass density of the tissue,* and the *energy of the radiation.*

A radiation weighting factor (W_r) is a number assigned to different types of ionizing radiations so that their effect(s) may be better determined. The W_r of different ionizing radiations is dependent on the LET of that particular radiation. A tissue weighting factor (W_t) represents the relative tissue radiosensitivity of the irradiated material.

LET is another means of expressing radiation quality and determining the W_r. As the LET of radiation increases, the radiation's ability to produce biologic damage also increases. This is described quantitatively by RBE; LET and RBE are directly related.

Most sources of ionizing radiation have a mixture of high- and low-LET radiations. Low-LET radiations deposit less energy in cells/tissues along their path than high-LET radiations, and are considered less destructive as they traverse tissues.

9. (C) *Roentgen* is a unit of exposure; it was formerly used to measure the quantity of ionizations in air. The SI unit *air kerma* is used to express *k*inetic *e*nergy *r*eleased in *ma*tter, and its symbol is Gy$_a$. The SI unit used to describe absorbed dose is *Gray* (Gy$_t$). The SI unit of measurement to describe dose to biologic material is Sievert (Sv). RBE is specific to the irradiated tissue, thereby being a valid unit of measurement of dose to biologic material.

10. (B) A 1984 review of radiation exposure data revealed that the average annual dose equivalent for monitored radiation workers was approximately 2.3 mSv (0.23 rem). The fact that this is approximately 1/10th of the recommended limit indicates that the limit is adequate for radiation protection purposes. Consequently, the NCRP reiterates its 1971 recommended annual limit of 50 mSv (5 rem) (*NCRP Report No. 105, pp. 14–15*).

PART IV

Image Production

CHAPTER 12
Image Acquisition and Technical Evaluation
Introduction: Image Characteristics and Technical Factors
Image Quality
Digital Imaging
A. Image Qualities: Receptor Exposure and Contrast
Milliampere Seconds
Source-to-Image-Receptor Distance
Kilovoltage
Scattered Radiation
Grids
Filtration
Patient Factors
Beam Restriction
Anode Heel Effect
Generator Type
Computer Terminology
Terms
Postprocessing
Resolution and Visibility
Automatic Rescaling
Automatic Exposure Control
Types
Positioning Accuracy
Pathology
Technique Charts
Anatomically Programmed Technique
Exposure Indication
B. Image Qualities: Resolution and Distortion
Spatial Resolution
Contrast Resolution
Detective Quantum Efficiency
Noise

Resolution and Geometric Distortion
Terms and Factors
Distance
Patient Factors
Focal Spot Size
Motion

CHAPTER 13
Equipment Operation and Quality Assurance
Image Processing and Display
Image Identification
Imaging Plates and Photostimulable Phosphors
Image Processing
Exposure/Image Data Recognition
Histograms and Lookup Tables
Automatic Rescaling
Postprocessing/Image Manipulation
Digital Radiography
Image Communication and Interpretation
Radiographic and Fluoroscopic Equipment
Principles of Radiation Physics: X-ray Production
X-ray Beam
Photon Interactions With Matter
Types of Equipment
Fixed
Mobile
Dedicated
Electricity, X-ray Transformers, and Rectifiers
Alternating Current
High-Voltage Transformers
Autotransformers
Rectification
High-Frequency Generators

The X-ray Tube
Component Parts
X-ray Tube Characteristics
Filtration and Collimators
Safe Operation and Care
The Radiographic Circuit
Primary Circuit Components
Filament Circuit Components
Secondary Circuit Components
Circuitry Overview of a Single Exposure
Components of Digital Imaging
Anatomically Programmed Radiography
The Image Plate
The Photostimulable Phosphor
X-ray Absorption by PSP
Reading the PSP
PSP Sensitivity
Dynamic Range and Postprocessing
Exposure Indication
Indirect and Direct Digital Imaging
CR/DR Differences
Flat-Panel Detectors
Monitor Display
The Fluoroscopic System
Equipment
The Image Intensifier
Viewing Systems
Recording and Storage Systems

Computed Tomography
Component Parts
Couch/Table
Gantry
Computer
Operating Consoles
Generations of Computed Tomography
Standards of Performance and Equipment Evaluation
Regulations and Rationale
Equipment Calibration
Kilovoltage
Milliamperage
Timer
Beam Restriction
X-ray Tube Overload Protection
Reproducibility
Half-Value Layer
Focal Spot Size
Radiographic and Fluoroscopic Accessories
Imaging Plates and Photostimulable Phosphors
Grids
Fluoroscopic Exposure Rates
Lead Aprons and Gloves
Additional Digital Imaging Considerations

Image Acquisition and Technical Evaluation

OBJECTIVES

At the conclusion of this chapter, the student will be able to:

- Identify and discuss factors affecting image quality; distinguish between geometric and visibility factors.
- List the four x-ray exposure/technical factors and discuss the impact each can have on image quality and patient dose.
- Identify and discuss the factors that influence resolution and distortion.
- Calculate new image receptor exposure required with changes in SID.
- Discuss scattered radiation—its production, effect, and control.
- Discuss the types and function of grids; calculate required technical factor changes by using various ratio grids.
- Identify types of filtration and their purpose.
- Discuss various patient factors and their impact on technical factor selection and image quality.
- Describe AEC: types, purpose, correct use, and potential errors.
- Discuss the function and importance of the exposure indicator/index in digital imaging.
- List pixel and matrix qualities that improve image resolution.
- Describe DQE and relate it to various digital imaging components and their impact on spatial resolution.
- Discuss the effect of OID, SID, focal spot size, and motion on detail and distortion.

INTRODUCTION: IMAGE CHARACTERISTICS AND TECHNICAL FACTORS

The last several years have seen the process of x-ray image production undergo the most amazing changes since the discovery of x-ray itself in 1895. The majority of x-ray images produced nowadays are produced *electronically* (*digitally*), by using computed radiography (CR) or digital radiography (DR). We still have many new technologies being operated by a generational mix of imaging professionals. Seasoned radiographers who used analog imaging for years are now using digital imaging. Students who work side by side with them have learned much digital imaging in the classroom, but, in clinical settings, the students might still be putting "cassettes" into Bucky trays, reviewing their "films," and perhaps even getting "wet readings." Experienced radiographers who may have developed their own technique charts at one time are now using anatomically preprogrammed radiography (APR) technical factors.

There is also much that remains *unchanged* in the x-ray imaging chain and that remains dependent on the knowledge and skill of the radiographer—in order to obtain quality images, under ALARA conditions.

It is true that there are more variables than there are constants in x-ray imaging. How can one comprehend all the variables and control image quality when the equipment *seems* to make all the decisions? The most obvious variable, in which the least modification is possible, is the *patient*. Body habitus, muscle tone, pathology, trauma, and age all require accurate assessment prior to the intelligent selection of technical factors and/or preprogrammed exposure algorithms.

Body parts undergoing additive or destructive *pathologic changes* can require exposure modification to obtain the IR exposure and image quality.

To illustrate, a chest properly exposed on *inspiration* using a 14 × 17-inch IR cannot be duplicated, without a change in factors, when the exposure is made on *expiration*, or the field size is *collimated* to an 8 × 10-inch anatomic area.

Different exposures will be required for extremities with and without *casts*.

Body position plays an important role in obtaining the expected radiographic results. For example, a well-exposed image of a normal adult abdomen measuring 24 cm in the recumbent anteroposterior (AP) position cannot be duplicated by using the same factors in the prone, decubitus, or erect position. A *plain* image of a particular abdomen requires technical factors that are different from those of the same abdomen having a *barium*-filled stomach.

AECs will compensate for thickness and tissue density differences (including those caused by position and respiration), pathologic changes, and beam restriction. However, it should be emphasized that the radiographer's skill and accuracy in *positioning* and *photocell (ionization chamber) selection* play an important role in the proper function of AECs. An error in either of these factors could lead to the production of a subpar radiographic image.

What about circumstances that require deviation from the normal SID or the introduction of OID? What if the patient is unable to move from the stretcher or wheelchair, is unable to maintain the required position or suspend respiration, is in pain or semiconscious? How does beam restriction affect the radiographic image? How does scattered radiation affect a photostimulable phosphor (PSP)? Does kilovoltage (kV) affect receptor exposure and/or radiographic contrast? What is meant by the terms *contrast resolution, spatial resolution, and APR?* How do all these variables affect the image, and how can we use them to achieve optimal image quality? We are concerned with producing high-quality x-ray images—so how is image quality defined? Of what does it consist?

Image Quality

Image quality is evaluated according to image *brightness, gray scale, spatial resolution,* and *distortion.* The *visibility* factors are brightness and gray scale, whereas the *geometric* factors are spatial resolution and distortion.

The *exposure/technical factors* we use to create the image are milliamperage (*mA*), exposure time (*s*), kilovoltage (*kV*), and *SID.* Many other factors impact the image including beam restriction, grid selection, motion, and focal spot.

Patient variables that have significant impact on factor selection and the radiologic image include tissue density, tissue thickness, any pathology, and ability to communicate.

Digital Imaging

Computer hardware and software are required in both CR and DR. In digital imaging, x-ray detection, image display, and image storage are each carried out by a separate component of the digital system. Digital imaging is similar to analog imaging with respect to the production of x-rays, x-ray interaction and production of scatter, x-ray beam geometry, and factors affecting resolution/detail and distortion. However, the method of acquisition in digital imaging is either a one-step (*direct conversion*) or two-step (*indirect conversion*) process, as remnant x-ray photons are converted into an electric charge image.

In *digital* imaging, *brightness* and *contrast* are determined by computer software and monitor controls, but the principal factor in good digital image visibility and patient dose is still the result of proper IR exposure. If egregious errors are made in selection of technical exposure factors, the system will not be able to compensate and will produce an image of subpar diagnostic quality.

Diagnostic radiography is undergoing its most significant changes since the discovery of x-rays. Sonography and nuclear medicine made the change to digital; CT and MRI are intrinsically digital. Radiography was the last imaging modality to make the transition to digital.

Incentive for the transition was initially low because analog systems are reliable and produce excellent image quality. In addition, radiography's high spatial resolution and field of view (FOV) demand that electronic images carry a large amount of digital data. To illustrate: A typical postero-anterior (PA) chest image carries between 4 and 32 MB of digital data, whereas a single CT image holds approximately 0.5 MB of digital data. Therefore, radiographic images require a lot of digital storage space, a high bandwidth in *picture archiving and communication systems/medical image management and processing systems* (PACS/MIMPS), and require costly high-resolution monitors for diagnostic display. The language of DR includes, but is far from limited to, terms such as CR, DR, PSPs, *storage phosphor screens, charge-coupled devices* (CCDs), thin-film transistors (TFTs), flat-panel detectors (FPDs), and PACS/MIMPS. Tools available to us in digital imaging permit visualization of structures not demonstrated in analog imaging. IRs used in digital imaging respond to a wide range of exposures, providing outstanding dynamic range. Digital images can be shared and/or sent to distant locations via PACS/MIMPS.

Image Quality

- Brightness
- Gray scale/contrast
- Spatial resolution
- Distortion

The Prime Factors

- mAs (mA and time)
- kV
- Distance (SID)

- Digital image visibility and patient dose are dependent on correct IR exposure.
- Correct selection of kV and mAs is important in digital imaging.
- kV affects penetration but not contrast.
- mAs determines dose/receptor exposure but not brightness.

Digital Radiographic Images Require

- Large amount of digital storage space
- High bandwidth in PACS/MIMPS
- High-resolution display monitors

Advantages of Digital Imaging

- Image manipulation permits visualization of structures not seen in analog imaging.
- Digital IRs respond to a wide range of exposures; they provide a wide dynamic range.
- Digital images can be shared and/or sent to distant locations.

Summary

- There are many variables in x-ray imaging; the most important is the patient.
- Radiography's prime factors are mAs, kV, and SID.
- Image quality is evaluated according to image *brightness, gray scale, spatial resolution,* and *distortion.*
- The *visibility* factors are brightness and gray scale; *geometric* factors are spatial resolution and distortion. Motion is also a geometric factor.
- Patient variables have significant impact on factor selection and the radiologic image.
- Brightness and contrast are determined by computer software and monitor controls in digital imaging.
- Digital imaging can be a one-step direct conversion process or a two-step indirect conversion process.

There are *four qualities* by which every radiographic image is evaluated: brightness, contrast/gray scale, spatial resolution, and distortion.

There are a number of *technical factors* that affect one or more of these image qualities. These four radiographic qualities, and the factors that affect them, are discussed in the following text.

A. IMAGE QUALITIES: RECEPTOR EXPOSURE AND CONTRAST

The *visibility* factors are receptor/detector exposure and contrast. The term "detector exposure" specifically refers to digital imaging. However, the term "receptor exposure" is commonly used to identify the device that captures/records the x-ray image.

In digital imaging, *brightness* and *contrast* are determined by computer software and monitor controls—but the principal factor in good image quality and patient dose is still the result of proper receptor/detector exposure, as indicated by *exposure indicator/index* (EI) or *dose area product* (DAP) meter. Because EI often differed from one manufacturer to another, the American Association of Physicists in Medicine recommended a standardized indicator that would be consistent from one manufacturer to the next. This is the generic *deviation index* (DI) used on new equipment by all manufacturers. The DI is displayed to the operator immediately after every exposure.

Brightness refers principally to the amount of light transmitted by the display monitor, although ambient light and reflected light also contribute. Every effort is made to reduce glare. Monitor/image *brightness* can be adjusted by adjusting the *window level.*

Contrast exists whenever two or more differing brightness levels are present in a radiographic image. It allows the viewer to distinguish the subtle differences in density between adjacent structures. These differences exhibit a particular *gray scale.* The function of contrast is *to make details visible.*

Characteristics Determining Image Quality

Brightness	} *Visibility factors*
Gray scale/contrast	
Spatial resolution	} *Geometric factors*
Distortion	

- The function of contrast is to make details visible.

Contrast Terminology

High Contrast Is	Low Contrast Is
• short-scale contrast	• long-scale contrast
It Displays	**It Displays**
• few, very different, image/tissue densities	• many similar image/tissue densities

Subject contrast refers to the various body tissue densities and thicknesses, which results in *differential absorption* of the x-ray beam and *signal differences* within the remnant beam. X-ray photons undergo attenuation by various body tissues to differing degrees—with *less* exit radiation from more dense structures (i.e., structures having higher *attenuation coefficients*), and *more* exit radiation from less dense structures (i.e., structures having lower *attenuation coefficients*).

Milliampere Seconds

Milliampere seconds (*mAs*) is the *product* of milliamperes (mA) and exposure time (s). Technical factors are usually expressed in terms of mAs because there are many possible combinations of mA and time that will produce the desired mAs.

For example, if 10 mAs is required to produce a given receptor exposure, each of the following combinations should produce identical results: 100 mA and 100 ms, 200 mA and 50 ms, 300 mA and 33 ms, 400 mA and 25 ms, and so on. Any combination of mA and time that will produce a given mAs (i.e., a particular *quantity* of x-ray photons) will produce identical receptor exposure. This is called the *reciprocity law*.

mAs is a *quantitative* factor regulating the number of x-ray photons produced. mAs is *directly proportional* to x-ray beam *intensity, exposure rate, quantity—and therefore, patient dose.*

Summary

- The four critical image qualities are brightness, gray scale, spatial resolution, and distortion.
- There are a number of technical factors that affect one or more of these image qualities.
- Brightness and contrast are determined by computer software and monitor controls.
- The function of contrast is to make details visible.
- Subject contrast refers to body tissue densities and their differential absorption of the x-ray beam.
- mAs is the product of mA and exposure time in second(s).
- Any combination of mA and time that will produce a given mAs will produce identical receptor exposure according to the *reciprocity law*.
- mAs is a quantitative factor and is *directly proportional* to the number of photons delivered to the *IR* and the number of photons delivered to the *patient*.

Source-to-Image-Receptor Distance

As a child, you may have been told to "read your book next to the lamp, where you will have more light." Perhaps, your youthful eyes could see just fine where you were, but in fact your advisor was correct in saying that more light was available closer to its source (the lamp).

As distance from a light source increases, the light diverges and covers a larger area; the quantity of light available per unit area becomes

> **Reciprocity Law**
>
> Any combination of mA and exposure time that will produce a particular "mAs" will produce identical receptor exposure.

> mAs is directly proportional to receptor exposure.
>
> mAs has no impact on contrast.

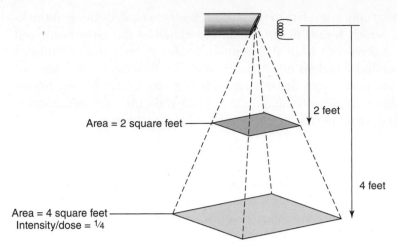

Figure 12-1. *The inverse square law.* Because x-ray beam coverage (area) increases with the square of the distance, the number of x-ray photons per unit area decreases by the same amount.

> SID is inversely proportional to receptor exposure.
>
> SID has no impact on contrast.

Use the Inverse Square Law to Determine the New Exposure Rate at a New Distance

$$\frac{I_1}{I_2} = \frac{D_2^2}{D_1^2}$$

---

less and less as the distance increases. The intensity (quantity) of light decreases according to the *inverse square law,* that is, the intensity of light at a particular distance from its source is inversely proportional to the square of the distance (Fig. 12-1). For example, if you decreased the distance between your book and the lamp from 6 to 3 feet, you would have 4 times as much light available.

Similarly, source-to-image-receptor distance (SID) has a significant impact on x-ray beam intensity/receptor exposure and patient dose. *As the distance between the x-ray tube and the IR increases, exposure rate decreases according to the inverse square law.* Therefore, as SID increases, the number of photons reaching the patient and IR decreases. Hence, SID is another important factor to determine IR exposure and patient dose.

Notice that according to the *inverse square law formula,* the exposure rate is *inversely* proportional to the square of the distance. This formula is used to calculate the resulting beam intensity as SID is changed. The *exposure maintenance formula* is a *direct* relationship and is used to calculate the new mAs required to keep the *same receptor exposure* as SID changes.

The two equations are as follows:

$$\frac{I_1}{I_2} = \frac{D_2^2}{D_1^2} \quad \text{Inverse square law}$$

$$\frac{\text{mAs}_1}{\text{mAs}_2} = \frac{D_1^2}{D_2^2} \quad \text{Exposure maintenance formula}$$

In the inverse square law equation, *I* represents intensity (a quantitative term referring to exposure rate; expressed as Gy_a/time or mGy_a/time) and *D* represents distance (SID). The original intensity is represented by I_1, the original distance squared is represented by D_1^2, and the new distance squared is represented by D_2^2. I_2 represents the new intensity (i.e., the new exposure rate). Note that the relationship is *inversely* proportional. Also note that the *opposite* is true in the exposure maintenance formula, that is, the relationship is *directly* proportional.

Example:
An x-ray image made using 12 mAs and 82 kV at 52-inch SID resulted in an exposure rate of 40 mR/min. Another image of the same part will be made at 44-inch SID. What is the exposure rate at the new distance?

Using the inverse square law and substituting known factors,

$$\frac{40}{x} = \frac{1936 \ (44^2)}{2704 \ (52^2)}$$

$$1936x = 108,160$$
$$x = 55.86 \ \text{mR/min at 44-inch SID}$$

This illustrates the relationship between distance and x-ray intensity. As the *distance* is *decreased*, the *intensity* of the x-ray beam *increases* according to the inverse square law. The resulting *increase* in *receptor exposure* will require an adjustment of mAs (according to the exposure maintenance formula) to reproduce the original receptor exposure.

Example:
In the aforementioned example, what new mAs value will be required at the new distance (44 inches) to maintain the original receptor exposure?

Using the exposure maintenance formula and substituting known factors,

$$\frac{\text{mAs}_1}{\text{mAs}_2} = \frac{D_1^2}{D_2^2}$$

$$\frac{12}{x} = \frac{2704 \ (52^2)}{1936 \ (44^2)}$$

$$2704x = 23,232$$
$$x = 8.59 \ \text{mAs at 44-inch SID}$$

At 44-inch SID, 8.59 mAs will be required to produce the same receptor exposure that was produced at 52-inch SID using 12 mAs.

> **Use the Exposure Maintenance Formula to Determine the New mAs at a New Distance**
>
> $$\frac{\text{mAs}_1}{\text{mAs}_2} = \frac{D_1^2}{D_2^2}$$

Summary

- Relatively small changes in SID can have a significant effect on receptor exposure.
- As the SID increases, the exposure rate and receptor exposure decrease.
- With changes in SID, the inverse square law is used to calculate the *new exposure rate*.
- With changes in SID, the exposure maintenance formula is used to calculate the *new mAs*.

Kilovoltage

As kV is increased, *more* electrons are driven to the anode with greater speed and energy. More high-energy electrons result in the production of *a greater number of high-energy x-rays*. Thus, kV affects both *quality* (energy/wavelength) and *quantity* of the x-ray beam. However, although

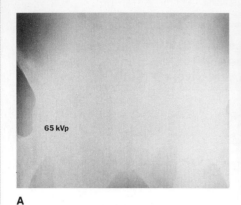

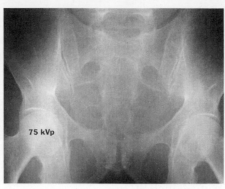

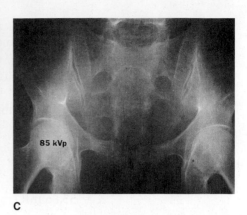

A　　　　　　　　　　　　　　　　**B**　　　　　　　　　　　　　　　　**C**

Figure 12-2. *Illustration of the 15% rule.* **(B)** Image was made using 15% more kV than image in **(A)** and demonstrates twice the exposure of image given in **(A)**. **(C)** Image was made using 15% more kV than the image in **(B)** and demonstrates twice the exposure of image given in **(B)**. (From the American College of Radiology Learning File. Photo contributor: The American College of Radiology.)

15% Rule

A 15% increase in kVp, no change to mAs = Double the IR exposure

A 15% decrease in kVp, no change to mAs = Half the IR exposure

---

kV has an impact on receptor exposure.

kV regulates beam quality/penetration and has a significant impact on image contrast in *analog* imaging.

---

kV and receptor exposure are directly *related,* they are not directly proportional. The effect of kV on quantity is not proportional because an increase in kV produces an increase in photons of *all energies.*

With respect to the effect of kV on receptor exposure, the *15% rule* can be used. If it is desired to double the receptor exposure, without adjusting the mAs, a similar effect can be achieved by *increasing the kV by 15%.* Conversely, the receptor exposure may be reduced to half by decreasing the kV by 15% (Fig. 12-2). Using the 15% rule to decrease mAs can play a significant role in decreasing patient absorbed dose because increased kV provides a *more penetrating* beam.

Example:
An x-ray image was obtained by using the following technical factors: 400 mA, 25 m, and 84 kV. It is necessary to produce another image with twice the receptor exposure. The maximum mA available is 400 and the exposure time cannot be increased because of involuntary motion. What alternate kV can be used to produce a radiograph with the desired receptor exposure?

If twice the original receptor exposure is needed, the kV may be increased 15% to produce the desired effect. Fifteen percent of 84 is 12.6. Therefore, using the same mAs and increasing the kV to 97 should produce an image with twice the original receptor exposure. *Note:* Increasing the kV can reduce patient dose (owing to decreased mAs) but can produce more scattered radiation. The production of scattered radiation increases with an increase in *kV,* an increase in *field size,* and an increase in part *thickness/density.*

Summary

- Increased kV produces *more* high-energy x-ray photons.
- An increase in kV will result in an increase in receptor exposure; a decrease in kV will result in a decrease in receptor exposure.
- When mAs manipulation is not possible, receptor exposure can be doubled or halved by using the 15% rule.
- High-energy photons are more penetrating in tissue and can decrease absorbed dose.
- Increasing kV increases the production of scattered radiation.

Scattered Radiation

High kV is desirable in terms of patient dose and x-ray tube life, but use of kV that is higher than appropriate for the anatomic part results in the production of excessive amounts of scattered radiation that can create fog and result in diminished visibility of image details (Fig. 12-3).

Much of the scattered radiation produced is highly energetic and exits the patient along with the useful image-forming radiation. However, scattered radiation carries no useful information but adds *noise* in the form of fog, thereby impairing visibility of detail.

Because scattered radiation can have a devastating effect on image contrast, it is essential that radiographers are knowledgeable about methods of controlling its production. The three factors that have a significant effect on the *production of scattered radiation* are beam restriction, kV, and thickness (volume) and density of tissues.

Perhaps, the most important way to limit the production of scattered radiation and improve contrast is by *limiting the size of the irradiated field* through *beam restriction* (Fig. 12-4).

As the size of the x-ray field is reduced, there are less area and tissue volume for scattered radiation to be generated. As the volume and/or density of the irradiated tissues increase, so does the quantity of scattered radiation produced (Fig. 12-5). Thicker and more dense anatomic structures will generate more scattered radiation. *Compression* of certain parts can occasionally be used to minimize the effect of scatter, but "tighter" *collimation* can *always* be used effectively.

Introduction of an OID (*air gap*) can have an effect on image contrast. An air gap introduced between the object and the IR has an effect similar to that of a grid. A 6-inch air gap is equivalent to the effectiveness of an 8:1 grid; a 10-inch air gap is equivalent to the effectiveness of a 16:1 grid. As energetic scattered radiation emerges from the body, it

> **Factors That Determine Production of Scattered Radiation**
>
> - Field size/beam restriction
> - Kilovoltage
> - Thickness/volume and density of tissues

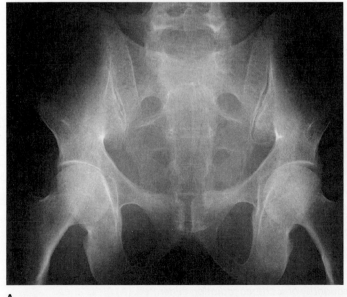
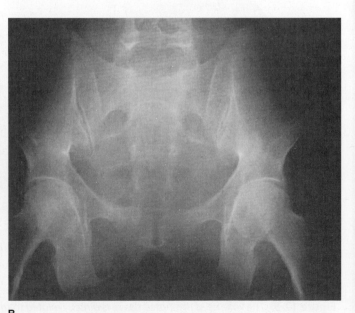

A   **B**

Figure 12-3. *Kilovoltage is directly related to the production of scattered radiation.* **(A)** Image made using 80 kV and 75 mAs. **(B)** Image made using 100 kV and 18 mAs, all other factors remaining the same. As kV is increased, the percentage of scattered radiation relative to primary radiation increases. Use of optimum kV for each anatomic part is helpful in keeping scatter to a minimum. (From the American College of Radiology Learning File. Photo contributor: The American College of Radiology.)

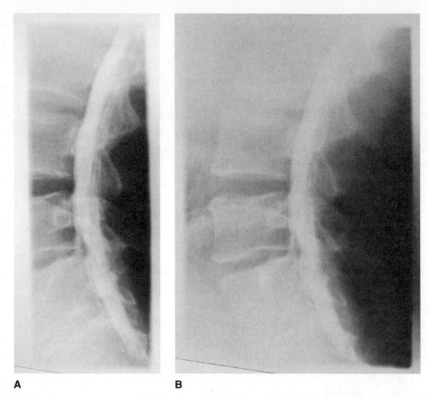

A   **B**

Figure 12-4. (A) Image demonstrates less scattered radiation fog than image given in **(B)**. Note the striking improvement in radiographic quality in image given in **(A)** as beam restriction is increased in this lateral lumbar myelogram. Although a 50% increase in technical factors was required to maintain appropriate receptor exposure in image given in **(A)** (to compensate for less scattered radiation reaching the IR), radiation protection is maintained because the volume of irradiated tissue is decreased. (From the American College of Radiology Learning File. Photo contributor: The American College of Radiology.)

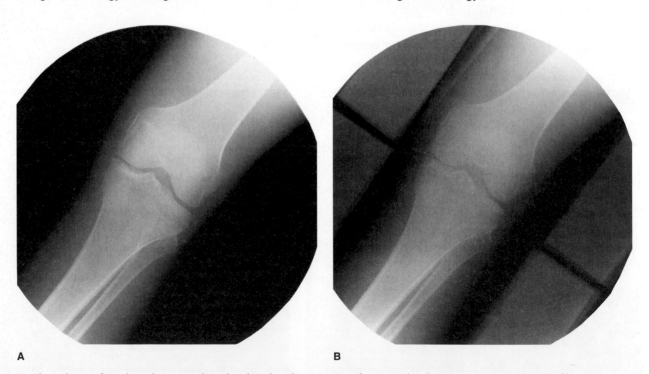

A   **B**

Figure 12-5. *The volume of irradiated tissue is directly related to the quantity of scattered radiation generated.* **(A)** AP of knee. **(B)** AP with paraffin absorbers *around* the knee. The loss of contrast exhibited in image given in **(B)** is caused by increased *volume* of irradiated material within the beam, resulting in increased scattered radiation fog. Note that the part need not be *thicker* to generate significant scatter, just that the total *irradiated volume* be greater. (From the American College of Radiology Learning File. Photo contributor: The American College of Radiology.)

continues to travel in its divergent fashion and, much of the time, will bypass the IR (see Fig. 12-15).

Summary

- Scattered radiation has an impact on receptor exposure.
- Scattered radiation can have a significant impact on contrast in analog imaging.
- kV selection determines the energy of x-ray photons and therefore the degree of penetration of various tissues.
- Scattered radiation is a result of x-ray photon interaction with tissue atoms via Compton scattering processes and adds quality-degrading fog to the radiographic image.
- The use of high kV reduces patient dose and reduces the production of x-ray tube heat but *increases* the production of scattered radiation fog.
- Scattered radiation carries no useful information but, rather, adds noise that impairs visibility of image details. Production of scattered radiation can be minimized by using optimum kV techniques and by restricting the size of the x-ray beam as much as possible.
- As the thickness and density of tissues increase, so does the production of scattered radiation; tissue thickness can sometimes be minimized with compression.
- As normal tissues undergo pathologic change, their penetrability frequently also changes in ways characteristic of the disease process (i.e., additive vs. destructive disease processes).

Grids

Use of Grids. As x-ray photons travel through a part, they either pass all the way through the IR or undergo interaction(s) that results in the photons either being absorbed by the part or being deviated in direction. Photons that change direction (scattered radiation) undermine and degrade the image.

The Part III, Safety section of this text discusses the origin of most scattered radiation, that is, Compton interactions. With respect to radiographic image quality, Compton interaction is responsible for most of the scattered radiation that reaches the IR. *Scattered radiation* adds image-degrading *fog* to the diagnostic image.

The single most important way to reduce the production of scattered radiation is to restrict the size of the x-ray field. Although *collimation*, optimum *kV*, and *compression* can be used (Fig. 12-6), a significant amount of scattered radiation is still generated within the part being imaged and can have a severely detrimental effect on image quality, as illustrated in the pelvis images shown in Figure 12-7.

A *grid* is a device interposed between the part and IR that functions to absorb a large percentage of scattered radiation before it reaches the IR. It is composed of alternating strips of lead foil and radiolucent filler material. X-ray photons traveling in the same direction as the primary

X-ray Photons Can

- *Penetrate* through the part
- *Scatter* within the part
- Be *absorbed* by the part

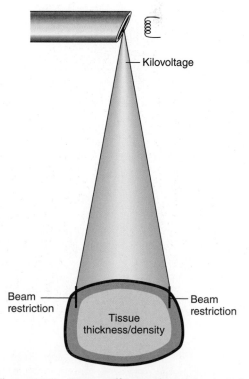

Figure 12-6. *Factors affecting the production of scattered radiation:* kilovoltage, beam restriction, and thickness and density of tissues.

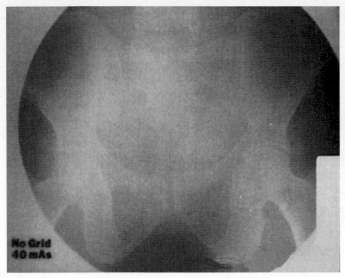
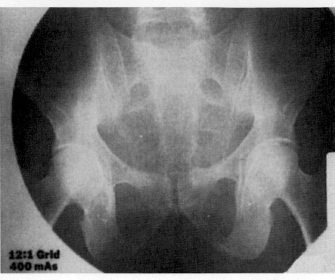

A   B

Figure 12-7. (A) Image made at 40 mAs without a grid. Because of the thickness and nature of the part imaged, a significant amount of scattered radiation was generated and exposed the (undiagnostic) image. **(B)** Image made using a 12:1 grid. Although an exposure increase to 400 mAs was required, a large percentage of the scattered radiation generated was removed before it reached the IR. (From the American College of Radiology Learning File. Photo contributor: The American College of Radiology.)

> Grids have a significant impact on receptor exposure.
>
> Grids have a significant impact on contrast in *analog* imaging.

beam pass between the lead strips. X-ray photons, having undergone interactions within the body and deviated in various directions, are absorbed by the lead strips; this is called "cleanup" of scattered radiation (Fig. 12-8).

The use of grids is recommended for body parts measuring greater than 10 cm. The major exception to this rule is the chest, which can frequently be examined without a grid because its contents (mostly air) do

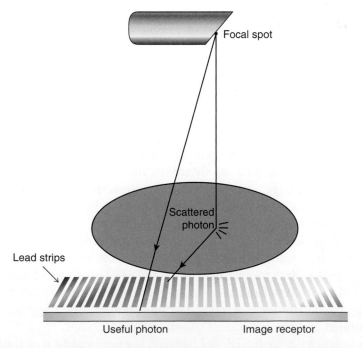

Figure 12-8. X-ray photons undergo interactions within the body and are deviated in various directions. Many of these scattered photons are absorbed by the lead strips. Useful photons travel between the lead strips and contribute to the diagnostic image.

not generate significant quantities of scattered radiation. Even so, many institutions perform most chest examinations by using a grid and high kV factors.

When imaging large body parts without the use of a grid, scattered radiation contributes to more than 50% of the total IR exposure. If a grid is introduced, there will be significantly *fewer* photons reaching the IR, hence a very significant decrease in receptor exposure. To maintain appropriate receptor exposure then, the addition of a grid must be accompanied by an appropriate increase in *mAs*. Before beginning a discussion of the impact of grids on technical factors, a more complete study of them is in order.

Types of Grids. A grid may be *stationary* or *moving*. Stationary grids are the simplest type and consist of alternating *vertical* lead strips (i.e., a *parallel* grid) and radiolucent interspace filler material. A "slip-on," or "wafer," grid is an example of stationary grids. *Stationary grids* are useful in mobile radiography and horizontal beam (cross-table) radiography; they are usually low ratio. A potential disadvantage of stationary grids is visibility of grid lines.

A *moving grid* is in motion during the exposure, and grid lines are effectively blurred out of the radiographic image. The lead strips and interspace material of a moving grid are slightly *angled* so that, at a given distance from the focal spot, the angle of the lead strips will conform with the divergence of the x-ray beam. A grid with lead strips angled thus is called a *focused grid*; if an imaginary line is extended up from each lead strip, the point of intersection is called the *convergence line,* and the distance from the convergence line to the surface of the grid is the *focusing distance* (Fig. 12-9). That focusing distance is the ideal SID, although grids usually specify a *focal range* in which they can be safely used.

A focused grid must be used with the correct side facing the x-ray beam. Figure 12-11 illustrates a grid error caused by using a

Origin of Scattered Radiation and Methods for Controlling Its Production

- The larger the x-ray field size, the more SR produced. *Solution:* Collimate!
- The higher the kV, the greater the production of SR (a result of the higher incidence of Compton scatter interactions). *Solution:* Use optimum kV.
- The thicker and denser the body tissues, the greater the amount of SR produced. *Solution:* When possible, use part compression/prone position to decrease effect of fatty abdominal tissue.

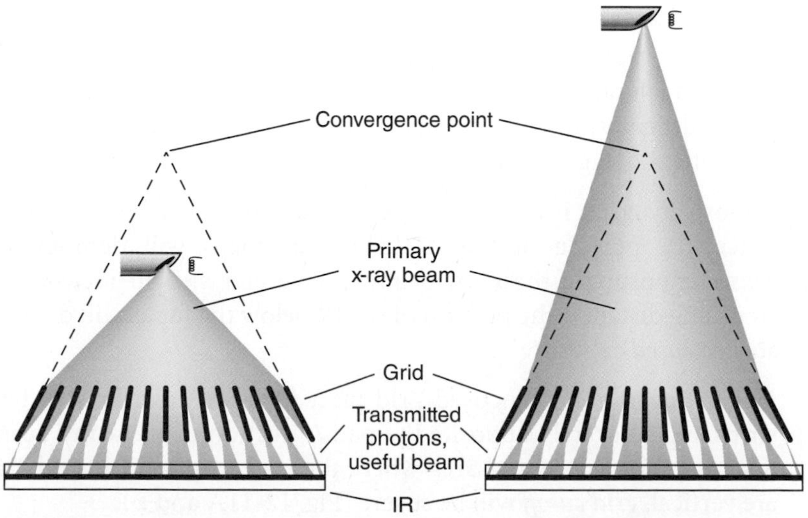

Figure 12-9. Grid cutoff will be apparent if the SID is above or below the specified focal range limits and will be characterized by receptor exposure loss at the periphery of the image. This is described as an *off-focus error* or *focus–grid distance decentering.*

focused grid upside down. If a focused grid is placed upside down, the divergent x-ray beam will be absorbed by the grid's lead strips everywhere but the grid's central portion—where lead strips are vertical.

Another type of grid is the *crossed grid;* it has a second series of lead strips aligned perpendicular to the first. Crossed grids may be parallel or focused and are extremely efficient in absorbing scattered radiation; however, their use prohibits *any* x-ray tube angulation and requires that the x-ray tube be *exactly* in the center of the grid. Any misalignment or tube angulation can result in severe *grid cutoff* (absorption of the useful beam). Crossed grids are not frequently used in general radiography.

Grid Errors. Care must be taken to avoid errors common in the use of focused grids, including angulation errors, off-level errors, off-focus errors, off-center errors, and upside-down grid placement.

- *Angulation errors:* The x-ray tube may be safely angled in the direction of the lead strips; angulation "against" the lead strips causes *grid cutoff,* that is, absorption of the useful beam with resulting loss of exposure across the IR.

- *Off-level errors:* If the planes of the x-ray tube and grid surface are not parallel, *grid cutoff* will occur. This can happen if the x-ray tube is angled "against" the lead strips or if the grid is tilted under the patient during mobile radiography. To avoid cutoff, the grid surface must be perpendicular to the central ray and, if CR angulation is required, the tube angle must be parallel with the direction of the lead strips.

- *Off-focus errors:* If the SID is below the lower limits or above the upper limits of the specified focal range, *grid cutoff* will occur. This type of error is also called *focus–grid distance decentering.* Off-focus errors are usually characterized by loss of exposure at the *periphery* of the IR. An example of an off-focus and lateral decentering error is seen in Figure 12-9.

- *Off-center errors:* If the x-ray beam is not centered to the grid (i.e., if it is shifted laterally), *grid cutoff* will occur. This type of error is called lateral decentering and characterized by a *uniform loss of exposure* across the IR (Fig. 12-10).

If the x-ray beam is both off-center *and* off-focus *below* the focusing distance, the portion of the IR below the focus will demonstrate *increased* exposure; if the x-ray beam is off-center *and* off-focus *above* the focusing distance, the portion of the IR below the focus will demonstrate *decreased* exposure.

- *Upside-down grid:* A focused grid placed upside down has its lead strips angled exactly opposite the path/direction of the x-ray beam. So, except for the central area where the lead strips and x-ray beam are vertical, *grid cutoff* will be severe (Fig. 12-11A and B).

Grid Characteristics. Two of a grid's *physical characteristics* that determine its degree of efficiency in the removal of scattered radiation are grid ratio and the number of lead strips per inch.

> **Grids Can Be**
>
> - Parallel or focused
> - Stationary or moving

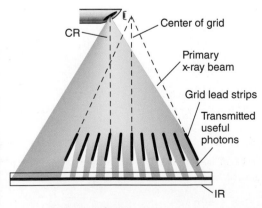

Figure 12-10. *A uniform loss of exposure* across the IR will occur if the x-ray beam is off-center laterally.

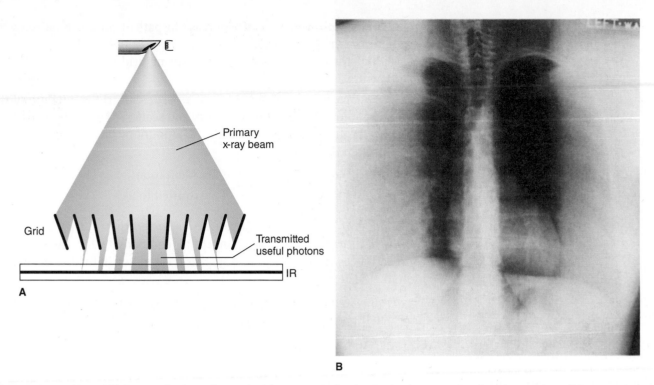

B

Figure 12-11. (A and B) An *upside-down focused grid* presents its lead strips in the opposite direction to that of the x-ray beam. This results in severe grid cutoff everywhere except in the central portion of the radiographic image.

- *Grid ratio: Grid ratio* is defined as the height of the lead strips compared with the distance between them (Fig. 12-12):

$$\text{Grid ratio} = \frac{\text{Height of Pb strip (H)}}{\text{Width of interspace material (D)}}$$

For example, a grid having lead strips 1.5 mm tall separated by interspace material 0.15 mm wide has a grid ratio of 10:1.

As the lead strips are made taller, or the distance between them decreases, scattered radiation is more likely to be trapped before reaching the IR. A 12:1 ratio grid will absorb more scattered radiation than an 8:1 ratio grid.

- *Grid frequency: It describes the number of lead strips per inch within the grid.* The advantage of many lead strips per inch is that there is less *visibility* of the lead strips. As the number of lead foil strips per inch increases, the lead foil strips must become *thinner* and therefore *less visible*. There is, of course, a disadvantage here. If the lead strips get thinner, more energetic scattered radiation can pass through them and reach the *IR*. So, to maintain the efficiency of a grid having many lead strips per inch, its grid *ratio* is often increased as well, that is, the lead strips are made taller to increase the likelihood of their trapping scattered radiation before it reaches the IR.

The radiolucent interspace material is most frequently made of plastic or fiber, particularly in pediatric imaging and mammography; some grids use aluminum as the interspace material. Aluminum is sturdier; it gives the image a smoother appearance free of objectionable *grid lines* and can perhaps have an additional filtering effect on scattered

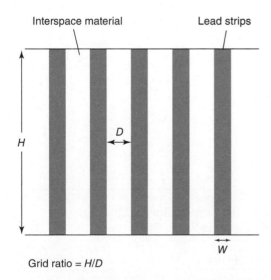

Figure 12-12. Cross-section of a grid. *Grid ratio* is defined as the height of the lead strips (*H*) to width of the interspace material (*D*). Grid ratio = *H/D*. The width of the lead strip is *W*. (Reproduced with permission from Saia DA. *Lange Q&A Radiography Examination*. 7th ed. New York, NY: McGraw-Hill; 2009.)

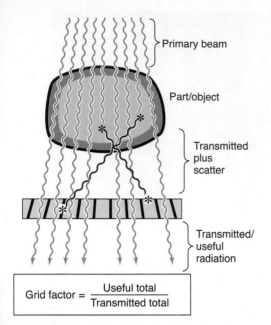

$$\text{Grid factor} = \frac{\text{Useful total}}{\text{Transmitted total}}$$

Figure 12-13. The grid factor (G) is the *grid conversion factor* and expresses the x-ray quantity/exposure at the grid surface compared to the quantity of x-ray transmitted through the grid.

Grid Conversion Factors for Various Ratio Grids

Grid Ratio	Conversion Factor
No grid	1
5:1	2
6:1	3
8:1	4
10 or 12:1	5
16:1	6

radiation. However, a greater increase in patient dose is required with aluminum interspace grids.

Other ways of expressing and measuring grid efficiency include the following:

- *Grid factor:* The *grid factor* (G) of a particular grid is the ratio of the total amount of radiation (primary and scattered) incident on the surface of the grid compared with the amount of radiation transmitted through the grid:

$$G = \frac{\text{Incident total}}{\text{Transmitted total}}$$

The grid factor is the grid conversion factor, that is, that amount by which the mAs must be changed to compensate for the radiation absorbed by the grid (Fig. 12-13). This is discussed in further detail later in this section.

- *Contrast improvement factor (CIF):* The ratio of radiographic contrast obtained with a grid to the contrast obtained without a grid is called the CIF. Grids have a major impact on contrast resolution:

$$\text{CIF} = \frac{\text{Contrast with grid}}{\text{Contrast without grid}}$$

- *Selectivity:* The ratio between the quantity of *useful photons transmitted* through the grid and the quantity of *scattered photons transmitted* is called the selectivity (S) of the grid:

$$S = \frac{\text{Useful photon transmission}}{\text{Scattered photon transmission}}$$

An undesirable but unavoidable characteristic of grids is that they do absorb some useful photons as well as scattered photons. The higher the grid ratio, the more pronounced this will be. The higher the ratio of *useful* photon to *scattered* photon transmission, the more desirable the grid.

- *Lead content:* This is perhaps least familiar to the radiographer because it applies little to the practical use of the grid. Although the definitions of *grid ratio* and *grid frequency* do not take into account the thickness of the lead strip, the term *lead content* does express this. Lead content is measured in g/cm^2 and expresses the amount of lead contained within a particular grid.

How must technical factors be adjusted to maintain appropriate receptor exposure when changing from nongrid to grid? How can technical factors be changed to preserve the IR exposure when changing from one ratio grid to another?

In actual practice, the grid conversion factor varies slightly according to the kV range used. The ARRT recognizes that different textbooks cite slightly different grid conversion factors and states that the distractors in calculation problems will not be so close as to cause conflict with the keyed correct answer. The conversion factors listed in the accompanying table are probably the most commonly used factors and can be used to calculate grid conversions in technical factor problems.

Example:

A particular examination was performed at the tabletop/nongrid at 40-inch SID using 7 mAs and 90 kV. To reduce the amount of image-degrading scattered radiation, another image will be made by using a 12.1 ratio grid. What new mAs factor will be required to maintain the original receptor exposure?

The grid conversion formula is

$$\frac{mAs_1}{mAs_2} = \frac{Grid\ factor_1}{Grid\ factor_2}$$

Substituting known quantities

$$\frac{7}{x} = \frac{1}{5}$$

$$x = 35\ mAs\ required\ with\ 12{:}1\ grid$$

Example:

A lumbar spine was imaged laterally at 40-inch SID using 40 mAs and 95 kV and an 8:1 ratio grid. To improve scattered radiation cleanup, another image will be made by using a 12:1 grid. What new mAs factor will be required to maintain the original level of receptor exposure?

By using the grid conversion formula shown earlier and substituting known quantities,

$$\frac{400}{x} = \frac{4}{5}$$

$$4x = 200$$

$$x = 50\ mAs\ required\ with\ 12{:}1\ grid$$

In general, an 8:1 grid is satisfactory for radiography up to 90 kV. A 16:1 grid ratio is frequently advocated for radiography greater than 100 kV. General radiographic fixed equipment usually has a 10:1 or 12:1 grid.

The use of high ratio grids at low kV levels is discouraged because of the unnecessary patient exposure required. Higher ratio grids are more effective in reducing the amount of scattered radiation reaching the IR; however, their use requires more mAs and decreases the positioning latitude (of the x-ray tube). Lower ratio grids (5:1, 6:1) are often used in mobile imaging because they offer more (grid) positioning latitude.

Remember, to avoid detrimental changes in receptor exposure, mAs adjustments are essential when changing grid ratios.

Development of Virtual Grid technology demonstrates ability to obtain quality images without the use of traditional grids. This technology reduces patient dose and can be particularly useful in emergency and mobile imaging (Fig. 12-14).

An *air gap* introduced between the object and the IR can have an effect similar to that of a grid. As energetic scattered radiation emerges from the body, it continues to travel in its divergent fashion and, much of the time, will bypass the IR (Fig. 12-15). A 6-inch air gap produces an effect similar to an 8:1 grid, whereas a 10-inch air gap is equivalent to a 16:1 grid. It is necessary to increase the SID to reduce the magnification caused by the air gap/OID.

Similar to the use of grids, employment of the air-gap technique causes a decrease in the number of photons that will be incident on the image receptor. Therefore, to maintain proper exposure, it is necessary to increase

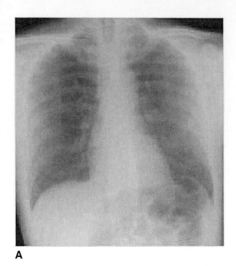

A

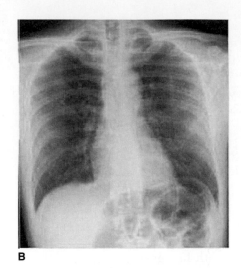

B

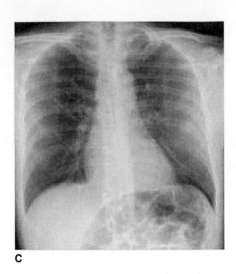

C

Figure 12-14. Illustration of chest without use of a grid (**A**), use of virtual grid (**B**), and using a traditional grid (**C**). (FUJIFILM Healthcare Americas Corp.)

the mAs to compensate for this loss. To calculate this increase, the grid conversion formula and the 8:1 ratio conversion factor can be used.

Summary

- The amount of scattered radiation reaching the IR is decreased through the combined use of collimators and grids.
- Receptor exposure is significantly impacted with the use of grids.
- Grids are made of alternating strips of lead and radiolucent material; they are placed between the patient and the IR to absorb scattered radiation exiting from the part.
- Grids may be stationary or moving, parallel, or focused.
- Focused grids require that the
  - correct surface should face the x-ray tube (i.e., not upside down).
  - tube angulation parallels the lead strips.
  - long axes of the x-ray tube and grid surface are parallel.
  - SID should be within the stated focusing distance/range.
  - x-ray beam should not be off-center (laterally) with the center of the grid.
- If focused grid requirements are not met, the resulting image will demonstrate a loss of receptor exposure as a consequence of grid cutoff (i.e., absorption of the useful beam).
- The most common way of expressing grid efficiency is by grid ratio and the number of lead strips per inch.
- Because grids remove many x-ray photons that would have contributed to receptor exposure, the addition of a grid requires a significant increase in mAs.
- When implementing a grid or changing grid ratio, a grid conversion factor must be used to determine required mAs change to avoid undesirable changes in receptor exposure.

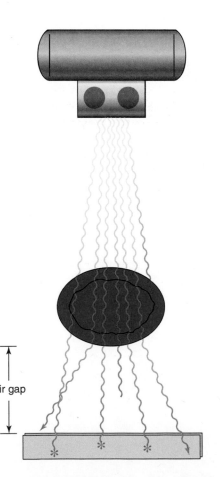

Air gap

Figure 12-15. Air-gap technique. As scattered radiation emerges from the part, it continues to travel in its divergent fashion, bypassing the IR.

Filtration

The primary beam generally has a total filtration of 2.5-mm Al equivalent for patient protection purposes. In general-purpose radiographic tubes, the glass envelope usually accounts for approximately 0.5-mm Al equivalent and the collimator provides approximately 1.0-mm Al equivalent. These are considered *inherent filtration*. The manufacturer adds another 1.0-mm Al (*added filtration*) to meet the minimum requirements of 2.5-mm Al equivalent total filtration for radiographic tubes operated above 70 kV.

This type of filter serves to remove the diagnostically useless x-ray photons that contribute only to patient skin dose. These x-ray photons are low energy (soft) and do not reach the IR; thus, x-ray tube total *protective* filtration *has no effect on receptor exposure*. Filtration increases the *overall average energy* of the x-ray beam, often called "hardening" the beam.

Compensating filters can be used to provide more uniform receptor exposure when imaging structures having widely different *attenuation coefficients* (x-ray absorbing properties) because of thickness or tissue composition. Usually made of aluminum or clear plastic, they slide into tracks in the collimator housing similar to a cylinder cone or attach magnetically to the undersurface of the collimator housing.

If an x-ray image of a foot demonstrates well-exposed tarsals, the toes might appear overexposed (Fig. 12-16A). Because the foot varies in thickness and tissue density along its long axis, it can be difficult to achieve uniform image quality. A *wedge*-shaped compensating filter can remedy the situation (Fig. 12-16B). The filter is placed so that the thin portion is over the tarsals and the thick portion over the toes. Technical factors appropriate for tarsals are used, and the thick portion of the filter removes enough of the primary beam to prevent overexposure of the toes. Thus, a foot image having uniform quality is achieved. A wedge filter can be useful for femur examinations and decubitus abdomen images (Fig. 12-16C and D).

Another type of compensating filter is the *trough* filter (Fig. 12-17A), so named because its central portion is thin and its lateral portions are thicker, thus forming a central trough. A trough filter can be used in chest radiography to permit visualization of the denser mediastinal structures without overexposing the more radiolucent lungs and pulmonary vascular markings.

Balancing uneven tissue densities is less problematic in digital imaging. Probably, the greatest advantage of digital imaging is its dynamic range and contrast resolution.

Patient Factors

Normal tissue variants and pathologic processes that alter tissue thickness and composition can have a significant effect on differential absorption, the amount of SR generated, and the number of photons reaching the IR. It is helpful for the radiographer to recognize the specific pathologic conditions/processes that will impact the number of x-ray photons likely to reach the IR and conditions/processes that are likely to generate more SR. Exit beam quantity and characteristics will

Filtration (Protective)

- Reduces patient skin dose
- Minimum 2.5-mm Al equivalent
- Inherent + added = total filtration
- Increases overall average energy of the x-ray beam

Protective filtration has *no* impact on receptor exposure.

Protective filtration has *no* impact on contrast.

Filtration (Compensating)

- Used for anatomic parts having very different thickness/absorption properties
- Used to "balance" tissue densities; improves visualization of all tissues

Compensating filtration can be used to impact receptor exposure.

Compensating filtration has an effect on contrast in *analog* imaging.

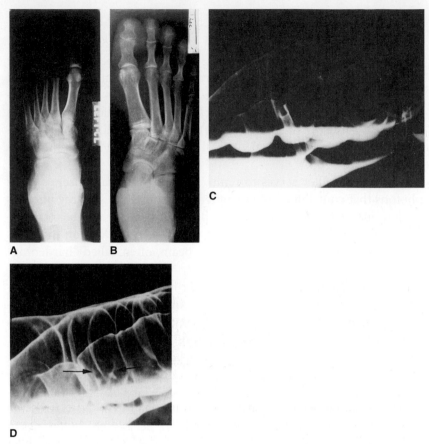

Figure 12-16. **(A)** Typical foot imaged without the use of a *compensating filter;* although the tarsals and metatarsals are well demonstrated, the phalanges are significantly overexposed. **(B)** Image made using a compensating filter whose thicker portion was placed over the phalanges to balance receptor exposure. **(C)** Lateral decubitus image of an air- and barium-filled colon. Abdominal tissues often shift to the dependent side in the decubitus position, making the "down" side thicker than the "up" side. Excessive exposure of the air-filled structures can obliterate pathology. **(D)** Use of a wedge-shaped compensating filter can equalize tissue density differences, thus providing more uniform receptor exposure and improved visualization of any pathology (a polypoid lesion is demonstrated).

vary—depending on whether the condition is additive or destructive. If AEC is used correctly, the required exposure change will be automatic. If AEC is not used, it is the radiographer's responsibility to recognize and adapt the correct exposure modification.

In 1916, R. Walter Mills presented an article at the American Roentgen Ray Society meeting in Chicago (published in *American Journal of Roentgenology,* April 1917), describing "The Relation of Bodily Habitus to Visceral Form, Position, Tonus and Motility." In his article, he coined the terms *hypersthenic, sthenic, hyposthenic,* and *asthenic* (defined in Chapter 6) to describe the various body types. He noted that most physicians came into the field prejudiced by their early anatomic teachings and had fixed conceptions, "which the revelations of the roentgen ray ruthlessly outraged."

Radiographers still use these terms nowadays to describe *body habitus* and its normal variants. Knowledge of each of the body types and its associated tissue characteristics, position and tonus of associated

Examples of *Additive* Pathologic Conditions

- Ascites
- Rheumatoid arthritis
- Paget's disease
- Pneumonia
- Atelectasis
- Congestive heart failure
- Edematous tissue

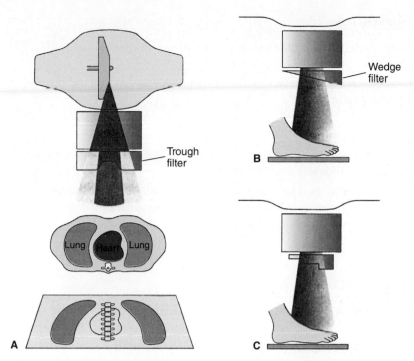

Figure 12-17. (A) *Trough filter* in place for chest radiography. The thicker lateral portions of the trough reduce the intensity of the beam directed toward the lungs, whereas the thinner central portion does not attenuate the beam directed to the denser mediastinal structures. **(B and C)** Two types of *wedge filters* used to "graduate" the x-ray beam intensity, with a greater number of photons directed to the thicker tarsal area and fewer photons toward the thinner areas of metatarsals and phalanges. (Reproduced with permission from Shephard CT. *Radiographic Image Production and Manipulation*. New York, NY: McGraw-Hill; 2003.)

organs, and so on, helps us position more accurately and use the control panel exposure options to best advantage.

For example, the same body part, such as the stomach, in two different individuals will require very different central ray points of entry if one individual is hypersthenic and the other asthenic (see Figs. 6-4 and 6-5). A particular body part, such as the shoulder, might measure the same on two different individuals; yet, it may not be appropriate to select identical technical factors for each if one is a muscular sthenic build and the other a hyposthenic type with little muscle tone.

Other factors that influence receptor exposure are age, gender, and pathology. Various abnormal pathologic conditions, disease processes, and trauma can affect tissue density and, consequently, receptor exposure. Normal variants of muscle development result from different lifestyles, occupations, and age and will affect receptor exposure.

Some pathologic conditions are called *destructive,* such as osteoporosis and conditions involving necrosis or atrophy. These conditions can cause an undesirable increase in receptor exposure unless they are recognized and appropriate changes are made in technical factors, either manually or via AEC. Other conditions such as ascites, rheumatoid arthritis, and Paget's disease are *additive,* and an increase in technical factors is required to maintain adequate receptor exposure.

Patient factors can have a significant impact on receptor exposure.

Patient factors can have a significant effect on contrast in *analog* imaging.

Examples of *Destructive* Pathologic Conditions

- Osteoporosis
- Osteomalacia
- Pneumoperitoneum
- Emphysema
- Degenerative arthritis
- Atrophic and necrotic conditions

Summary

- Protective x-ray tube filtration of 2.5-mm Al has no effect on receptor exposure.
- In the absence of AEC, variations in tissue density will be noted in the image as variations in IR exposure.
- Normal tissue density differences occur as a result of body habitus, age, gender, and level of activity.
- Trauma and pathologic conditions can change normal tissue densities, thereby affecting a change in IR exposure.
- The radiographer must be knowledgeable about conditions affecting normal and abnormal changes in tissue density to make appropriate selection of technical factors, especially in the absence of AEC.

> Beam restriction has an impact on receptor exposure.
>
> Beam restriction has an impact on contrast in *analog* imaging.

Beam Restriction

A change in receptor exposure will occur with changes in the size of the irradiated field, all other factors remaining constant. *Beam restriction* (i.e., reducing the volume of tissue irradiated) reduces the production of scattered radiation and, consequently, decreases receptor exposure. The reverse is also true: As field size increases, receptor exposure increases as a result of increased production of scattered radiation.

Therefore, as changes are made in the size of the irradiated field, an accompanying change in mAs will occur (automatically) to maintain the same receptor exposure.

> ### Anode Heel Effect Conditions
>
> - At short SIDs
> - With large-size IRs
> - With small anode angle x-ray tubes

> Anode heel effect has minimal impact in digital imaging.
>
> Anode heel effect can have a significant impact on contrast and on receptor exposure in *analog* imaging.

Anode Heel Effect

Figures 12-18 and 12-19 illustrate how a portion of the divergent x-ray beam is absorbed by the anode, resulting in diminished receptor exposure at the anode end of the image.

When using general x-ray tubes at standard distances, the heel effect is noticeable only when imaging parts of uneven thickness such as the femur and thoracic spine. In these cases, the heel effect may be used to advantage by placing the thicker body portion under the cathode end of the x-ray beam, thus having the effect of "balancing/evening out" tissue densities. When parts having uneven thickness are positioned correctly under the x-ray tube, observation of the anode heel effect is minimal in digital imaging.

Generator Type

Conventional 60-Hz full-wave rectified power is converted to a higher frequency of 500–25,000 Hz in the most recent generator design—the *high-frequency generator*. Because high frequency generators produce higher average kV, improved penetration can result in a slightly lower subject contrast at the IR; since digital systems readily compensate for this, generator type has little/no impact on image contrast. The high-frequency generator is small in size, in addition to producing an almost

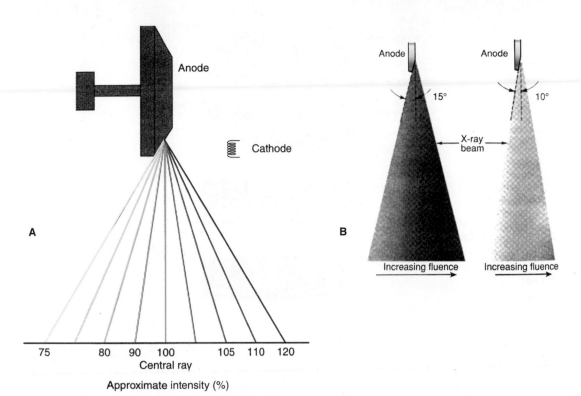

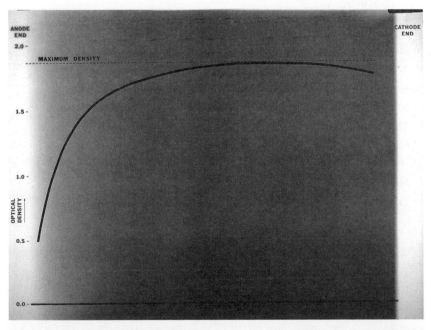

Figure 12-18. (A and **B)** *The anode heel effect*. As x-ray photons are produced within the anode, a portion of the divergent beam is absorbed by the anode's "heel." This represents a decrease in x-ray beam intensity at the anode end of the x-ray beam. (Reproduced with permission from Shephard CT. *Radiographic Image Production and Manipulation*. New York, NY: McGraw-Hill; 2003.)

Figure 12-19. *Radiographic illustration of the anode heel effect*. Note the gradual increase in radiographic receptor exposure toward the cathode end of the beam. (From the American College of Radiology Learning File. Photo contributor: The American College of Radiology.)

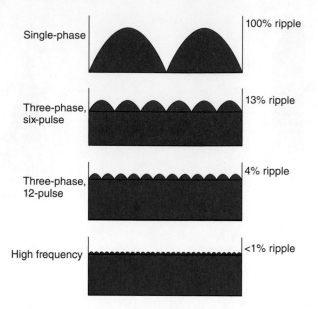

Figure 12-20. *Single-phase (1ø) and three-phase (3ø) waveforms.* Compared with the one useful impulse available per ¹⁄₆₀th s with alternating current, single-phase rectified current has two useful impulses, 3ø 6p rectified has 6 useful impulses, and 3ø 12p has 12.

Generator type has no impact on receptor exposure.

Generator type has no impact on contrast.

constant potential waveform (Fig. 12-20). High-frequency generators first appeared in mobile x-ray units and were then adopted by mammography and CT equipment.

More radiographic equipment use high-frequency generators nowadays. Their compact size makes them popular, and the fact that they produce nearly constant potential voltage helps improve image quality and decrease patient dose (fewer low-energy photons to contribute to skin dose).

Correction for generator type is unnecessary in digital imaging.

Summary

- Correction for generator type is unnecessary in digital imaging.
- High-frequency generators have the advantage of compact size and almost constant potential waveform.
- Changing of size of the irradiated field affects receptor exposure as a result of increased/decreased scattered radiation production.
- The anode heel effect is characterized by greater x-ray intensity (i.e., quantity) at the cathode end of the beam. The anode heel effect is most pronounced at short SIDs, with large IRs, and with x-ray tubes having small anode angles.
- The anode heel effect has little impact in digital imaging.

COMPUTER TERMINOLOGY

Terms

The computer hardware interprets all information as a simple "yes" or "no" decision. This is symbolically represented with digits 1 and 0. A *bit* in computer terminology refers to an individual 1 or 0 and is a single bit of information. Image storage is located in a *pixel* (Fig. 12-21), which is a two-dimensional "picture element." Pixels are measured in the "XY" direction. Bit *depth* refers to the number of *bits per pixel* and identifies

Bit

Binary digit

Smallest unit of computer data

Bit Depth

Number of bits per pixel

Determines gray scale

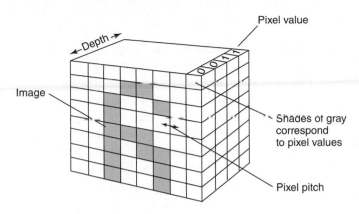

Figure 12-21. A digital image may be likened to a three-dimensional object made up of many small cubes, each containing a binary digit or bit. The image is seen on one surface of the block, whose depth is the number of bits required to describe each pixel's gray level.

the *values of gray/gray scale*. Gray scale is variations in brightness resulting from intensity variations. A *histogram* is a graphic representation of pixel value distribution (Fig. 12-22A and B) demonstrating the number of pixels and their value.

The third dimension in the *matrix* of pixels is the depth that, together with the pixel, is called the *voxel* (Fig. 12-23). Voxels are measured in the "Z" direction. Voxel is often defined as the volume of tissue that is represented in a pixel. The depth of the block, *bit depth*, is the number of bits required to describe the number of *gray levels* that each pixel can take on.

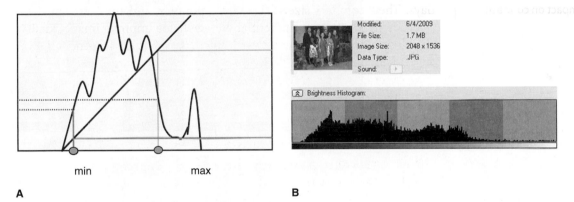

A

B

Figure 12-22. (A) A graphic representation illustrating the distribution of pixel values. (Photo contributor: Courtesy of FUJIFILM Medical System USA.) Nowadays, many digital cameras can also display the histogram distribution **(B)** of pixel values, for example, for a typical graduation photograph. (Photo contributor: Christina Cheong, RT(R)(M).)

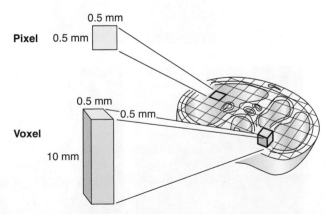

Figure 12-23. The third dimension in the matrix of pixels is the depth, which together with the pixel is called the voxel (volume element).

Postprocessing

Postprocessing is the ability to *manipulate the image after exposure.* Among other things, image manipulation postprocessing can be used for *grayscale/contrast* modification via *windowing.* The window *width* controls the shades of gray, whereas the window *level* corresponds to the *brightness* (Fig. 12-24). Narrower windows (i.e., decreased window width) result in higher (shorter scale) contrast. Pixel values *below* the window range will be displayed as *black,* whereas pixel values *above* the window range will be displayed as *white.* Pixel values between the two limits are spread over the full scale of gray. The second factor involved in grayscale adjustment is the lookup table (LUT), to be discussed later. Another type of postprocessing is *contrast enhancement* or contrast scaling. Image contrast is optimized to improve diagnostic interpretation. Rescaling of pixel values is achieved by using an LUT.

Dynamic range and *contrast resolution* are other terms commonly used to describe the range of grays a particular digital system is capable of resolving/demonstrating. The *higher* the contrast resolution, the

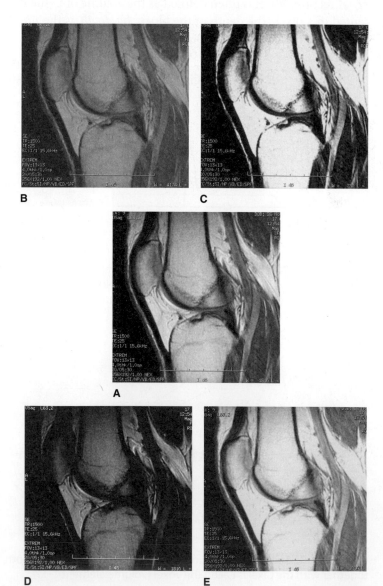

Figure 12-24. Changes in *window width* and *window level.* **(A)** Image *(center)* has a window width of 590 and window level of 270. **(B)** In this image, the window width is increased to 1340, and in **(C),** the window width is decreased to 302, leaving window level unchanged. The changes in image *contrast* are evident. Next, images given in **(D)** and **(E)** are compared with the image given in **(A). (D)** In this image, the window level is increased to 441, and in image given in **(E),** it is decreased to 45. This time the changes in image *brightness* are obvious.

better the ability to see similar adjacent gray shades. As mentioned earlier, the greater the number of bits per pixel (bit depth), the greater the capability of displaying many shades of gray.

Resolution and Visibility

Good resolution can be obscured by scattered radiation or incorrect brightness, thus impairing resolution *visibility*. The term *visibility* refers to how readily the anatomic details can be perceived; for example, excessive/incorrect brightness or scattered radiation fog impairs visibility because it obscures the image details. Brightness and fog have no effect on how sharply an image detail is rendered; they do, however, determine how easily we are able to recognize/perceive those details. This quality is *contrast resolution*.

Although mAs, kV, and so on, have little to no effect on brightness and contrast resolution characteristics of digital x-ray images, the IR must still receive the correct exposure in terms of quantity/mAs and quality/kV of x-ray photons to produce an optimal image free of graininess and scattered radiation fog and to keep patient dose to a minimum.

Software processing algorithms control digital image *brightness*. One way in which it does so is by determining the *number* of x-ray photons produced during an exposure. By using anatomically programmed radiography (APR), the digital system will provide predetermined exposure factors (mAs and kV) for the body part being imaged. In doing so it will directly impact the intensity, or number of photons present in the x-ray beam. This controls the amount of exposure incident on the image receptor, affecting image quality. APR is discussed in greater detail later in this section.

The total number of x-ray photons exiting the part is divided among all the pixels—and each pixel must have enough x-ray photons to provide a *grayscale* range. If there are insufficient x-ray photons for each pixel, noise (graininess) increases, that is, as signal-to-noise ratio (SNR) decreases, noise increases. *Graininess* of digital images can be caused by underexposure, incorrect processing, incorrect algorithm/LUT selection (from the anatomic menu), inadequate collimation, and grid cutoff.

> **Causes of Graininess**
>
> - Underexposure
> - Incorrect processing algorithm/LUT
> - Excess scattered radiation
> - Inadequate beam restriction
> - Grid misalignment; cutoff

Automatic Rescaling

Digital imaging exposure data/field recognition (*EDR/EFR*) and *automatic rescaling* offer wide latitude and automatic optimization of the radiologic image. EDR, by using the selected processing algorithm and its LUT, enables compensation for approximately 80% underexposure and 500% overexposure. Although automatic/computerized optimization of the radiologic image is a wonderful method, radiographers must be even more aware of their role in keeping patient dose to a minimum.

Summary

- Bit depth identifies grayscale values.
- A histogram is a graphic representation of pixel value distribution.
- The ability to manipulate the image after exposure is called postprocessing.

- Window width controls shades of gray; more narrow windows result in higher contrast.
- Window level corresponds to brightness.
- *Dynamic range* and *contrast resolution* are terms used to describe the gray scale.
- As SNR decreases, noise in the form of graininess increases.
- Although EDR and automatic rescaling optimize our images, imaging professionals must be aware of their responsibility to keep patient dose to a minimum.

AUTOMATIC EXPOSURE CONTROL

AEC is used to automatically regulate the amount of ionizing radiation delivered through the anatomic part to the IR, regardless of the IR type, thereby serving to produce consistent and comparable radiographic results with minimum patient exposure. When AEC is installed in the x-ray circuit, it is calibrated to terminate the exposure once the predetermined desirable exposure has been made.

Exact positioning and centering are particularly critical when using AEC. The anatomic part of interest must be aligned (centered) accurately with respect to the AEC sensors; otherwise, the result can be over- or underexposure. The correct AEC sensors must be selected; otherwise, the exposure will be optimized for the wrong tissue density. If the *volume of interest (VOI) is small,* AEC detectors not covered by anatomy are likely to cause premature termination of exposure, resulting in quantum noise. A large metal orthopedic prosthetic should not be positioned directly over an AEC sensor because an excessive exposure time can result, causing patient and image overexposure.

Types

In one type of AEC, there is a (radiolucent) parallel plate *ionization chamber* just beneath the tabletop, *above* the IR (Fig. 12-25). The part to be examined is centered to the sensor and imaged. As x-ray photons emerge from the patient, they enter the chamber and ionize the air within. When a predetermined quantity of ionization has occurred, indicating that correct exposure has been reached, the exposure automatically terminates.

The other type of AEC is the (radiopaque) *phototimer* type in which a small fluorescent screen is positioned *beneath* the IR. When the exit radiation emerging from the part interacts with and exits the IR, the fluorescent screen emits light and charges a photomultiplier tube. Once a predetermined charge has been reached, the exposure is automatically terminated.

In either case, the *manual* timer should always be used as a *backup timer*. In case of AEC malfunction, the backup timer would terminate the exposure, thus *avoiding patient overexposure and tube overload.*

Another important feature of the AEC is its *minimum response/reaction time.* This is the length of the *shortest exposure possible* with a particular AEC (10–30 ms). If less than the minimum response time is required for a particular exposure, the resulting image will exhibit

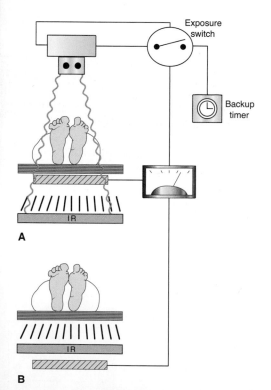

Two Types of AECs

- Phototimer
- Ionization chamber

Figure 12-25. The two types of *automatic exposure devices* are the *ionization chamber* (located just below the tabletop) **(A)** and the *phototimer* (located below the IR) **(B)**. Note the *backup timer* that functions to terminate the exposure should the AEC fail to operate properly. (Reproduced with permission from Saia DA. *Lange Q&A Radiography Examination.* 7th ed. New York, NY: McGraw-Hill; 2009.)

overexposure. The only way to remedy this is to either decrease the mA or decrease the kV. Each maneuver will result in increased exposure time to within the response time capabilities of the AEC.

Positioning Accuracy

To achieve the expected receptor exposure, the appropriate detector(s)/sensor(s) must be selected and the part of interest must be correctly positioned directly above the appropriate detector(s)/sensor(s).

If a structure having less tissue density than the part of interest is incorrectly positioned above the detector, or if the detector is incompletely covered, the detector will terminate the exposure more quickly and the area of interest will be *underexposed*. On the contrary, if the sensor is positioned under a structure having greater tissue density than the part of interest (e.g., if the center detector is used for a PA chest image), the exposure will be greater than required and an *overexposed* image can result and/or EI error will be noted.

Similarly, if the incorrect sensor for the anatomic part is selected, a receptor exposure error will result. If the sensor selected is under a tissue of higher density than the anatomy of interest, the image will be overexposed. Conversely, if the sensor selected is beneath a tissue of lower density than the anatomy of interest, the image will be underexposed. In each case, the error is likely to be reflected by the EI.

Consequently, although the exposure is "automatic," knowledge of anatomy, accurate positioning skills, and correct equipment use are essential to producing optimal image quality.

Pathology

The presence of pathology often modifies tissue composition. Changes that occur are generally spoken of as *additive* or *degenerative*. Additive pathology is that which increases tissue density, requiring an increase in technical factors (e.g., ascites, pulmonary edema). Degenerative pathology involves deterioration of the part (e.g., osteoporosis, emphysema) and requires a decrease in technical factors.

Because the function of an automatic exposure device is to "recognize" differences in tissue density and thickness, it will compensate for most pathologic changes by adjusting the mAs.

Technique Charts

Fixed Versus Variable kV Technique. In a *variable kV technique* chart, the mAs is fixed and the kV is increased as part thickness increases. For each centimeter increase in thickness, the kV is increased by two. For every 4–5 cm increase in thickness, the mAs is doubled. Accurate measurement with calipers is required. The variable kV technique chart is not frequently used in formulating manual techniques nowadays because it is associated with increased scattered radiation production and inconsistent contrast and receptor exposure.

A *fixed kV technique* chart specifies a particular kV for each body part or type of examination. A kV is selected that will provide adequate penetration; mAs is used to compensate for variation of patient size and condition.

Examples of Additive Pathologic Conditions

- Ascites
- Rheumatoid arthritis
- Paget's disease
- Pneumonia
- Atelectasis
- Congestive heart failure
- Edematous tissue

Examples of Destructive Pathologic Conditions

- Osteoporosis
- Osteomalacia
- Pneumoperitoneum
- Emphysema
- Degenerative arthritis
- Atrophic and necrotic conditions

Fixed kV Technique Chart

	Fixed kV	Grid
Extremities	55	No grid
Skull	75	Grid
Abdomen	75	Grid
Lateral lumbar	90	Grid
Barium studies	120	Grid
Chest examinations	120	Grid

Accurate caliper measurement of the part to be imaged is essential with the *variable* kV technique chart because the kV increases by two for every 1-cm increase in part thickness. *Fixed* kV charts may specify a specific kV for the "small," "medium," or "large" patient, which corresponds to measurements within a particular range (e.g., 10–12 cm = small; 13–15 cm = medium; and 16–18 cm = large). Accurate measurement may be essential for the correct application of each method. Structures imaged by using AECs do not require measurement because the AEC automatically adjusts the exposure for tissue variations.

AEC and Technique Charts. Fixed kV techniques are generally used with AECs. An optimum kV for each body part (femur, abdomen, hip, chest, etc.) is selected and the exposure is automatically terminated once the predetermined correct exposure (mAs) has been reached.

The AEC automatically adjusts the exposure required for body parts that have different thicknesses and tissue densities, regardless of the type of the IR. Proper functioning of the AEC depends on accurate positioning by the radiographer. The *correct photocell*(s) must be selected, and the anatomic part of interest must *completely* cover the photocell to achieve the desired image quality. If the *VOI is small,* as in pediatric cases, AEC detectors not covered by anatomy are likely to cause premature termination of exposure, resulting in quantum mottle/noise. If *collimation* is inadequate and a field size larger than the part is used, excessive scattered radiation from the body or tabletop can cause the AEC to terminate the exposure prematurely, resulting in an underexposed radiograph. In addition, a large metal orthopedic prosthetic should not be positioned directly over an AEC sensor because an excessive exposure time can result, causing patient and image overexposure. This is a result of the increased attenuation of the x-ray photons as they encounter the high-density metal prosthetic device, causing fewer photons to reach the sensor. The AEC system will seek additional photons for that exposure, leading to an increased exposure time.

Backup time always should be selected on the manual timer to prevent patient overexposure and to protect the x-ray tube from excessive heat production should the AEC malfunction. Selection of the optimal kV for the part being radiographed is essential—no practical amount of mAs can make up for inadequate penetration (kV). Excessive kV can cause the AEC to terminate the exposure prematurely.

A *technique chart,* therefore, is strongly recommended for use with AEC; it should indicate the optimal *kV* for the part, the *photocells* that should be selected, and the *backup time* that should be set.

ANATOMICALLY PROGRAMMED TECHNIQUE

By using automatically programmed technique, or APR, the radiographer uses console graphics or a touch screen to *select the anatomic part, the desired position/procedure, and the relative size* (S, M, L) of the part

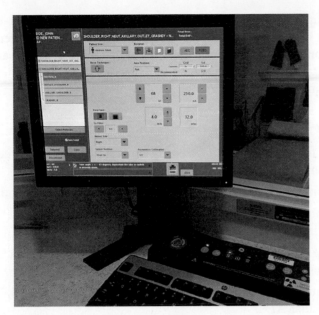

Figure 12-26. Acquisition workstation of APR unit. (Photo contributor: Richard Kovatch, RT(R).)

to be imaged (Fig. 12-26). The unit's microprocessor chooses the appropriate preprogrammed mAs and kV algorithm for that particular part and size—from the "internal technique chart" predetermined and stored on installation. Both AEC and manual exposure factors are typically recommended so that under nonroutine conditions, the radiographer can modify the preset/programmed factors.

APR is used in conjunction with AEC and is therefore still highly dependent on the skillfulness of its user. Accurate positioning, photocell selection, and control of scattered radiation are essential to the production of quality images.

Exposure Indication

Digital imaging offers *wide dynamic range* and *automatic optimization of the radiologic image.* Digital imaging can compensate for approximately 80% underexposure and 500% overexposure—this is termed *EDR.* This can be an important advantage particularly in trauma and mobile radiography. The radiographer must still be vigilant in patient dose considerations—overexposure, although correctable via EDR, results in *increased patient dose;* underexposure results in decreased image quality because of increased image *noise.*

Digital systems provide some type of *EI or DI* to serve as a quality control and radiation safety tool in an effort to avoid "dose creep." The EI name varies according to the manufacturer: an *S* (sensitivity) number, *EI* (exposure index), *REX* (reached exposure index), or other identifying EI depending on the manufacturer used. The manufacturer usually provides a chart identifying the acceptable *range* the EI numbers should be within for various examination types. This *range* represents the acceptable *exposure latitude.* Although in one manufacturer's system a high *S* number is related to *under*exposure, a high *EI* number in another manufacturer's system is related to *over*exposure—it is essential for radiographers to be knowledgeable about the various types of equipment they use.

Although EI or DI is useful in determining the amount of x-ray exposure incident on the image receptor, it is important to remember that it alone is not an accurate measure of patient dose. There are many other factors that would need to be considered to determine patient dose during an exposure.

Summary

- AECs function to produce consistent and comparable receptor exposures.
- There are two types of AECs: ionization chamber and phototimer.
- Ionization chambers are located between the x-ray table and the IR; phototimers are located beneath the IR.
- Backup timers are used in conjunction with AECs and function to terminate the exposure in case of AEC malfunction.
- Minimum reaction time is the shortest exposure time possible with a particular AEC.
- AECs will compensate for tissue thickness and density differences; they require accurate positioning and correct photocell selection.
- Pathologic conditions may be either additive or degenerative; correct use of the AEC will compensate for pathologic conditions and will be reflected in appropriate EI range.
- The fixed kV-type chart uses an optimal kV for each anatomic part; its advantage is consistency of image contrast.
- Calipers are used to measure anatomic part thickness.
- The variable kV-type chart increases/decreases the kV by two for each 1 cm increase/decrease in body thickness; thus, accurate part measurement is necessary.
- APR utilizes selection of anatomic part, rather than selection of specific technical factors.
- The image EI or DI assists in evaluating the image quality and patient exposure.
- The EI value must be within the range indicated as correct by the manufacturer for the particular examination.

COMPREHENSION CHECK

1. List the four image qualities used to evaluate x-ray images; list the four technical factors fundamental to every exposure (p. 325).

2. List at least three patient variables (p. 324).

3. Describe the process of automatic rescaling (p. 348, 349).

4. List three advantages of digital imaging (p. 324, 325).

5. How do the terms *receptor* and *detector* differ (p. 326)?

6. What is the reciprocity law? How does it apply to digital imaging (p. 327)?

7. How is mAs related to receptor exposure, beam intensity, and patient dose in digital imaging (p. 327)?

8. How is SID related to receptor exposure, beam intensity, and patient dose in digital imaging (p. 327, 328)?

9. Does the inverse square law illustrate a direct or indirect relationship (p. 328)?

10. How is kV related to photon energy, scattered radiation, receptor exposure, beam intensity, and patient dose in digital imaging (p. 329, 330)?

11. What is the 15% rule? How is it used (p. 330)?

12. What are the three ways to decrease the production of scattered radiation? Of the three, which is considered the most important (p. 331, 332)?

13. How does beam restriction impact detector/receptor exposure in digital imaging (p. 331, 332)?

14. What is a stationary grid? Give some examples of its use. What are its disadvantages (p. 335)?

15. What is a moving grid? How does its construction generally differ from the stationary grid? What is its advantage over a stationary grid (p. 335)?

16. Define convergence line, focusing distance, focal range, and crossed grid (p. 335).

17. Define grid cutoff, lateral decentering, and focus–grid distance decentering (p. 336).

18. Describe grid ratio, number of lead strips per inch, and lead content; describe their relationship to *cleanup* and receptor exposure (p. 336, 337).

19. Of what material(s) is grid interspace material usually made? How is each related to efficiency, patient dose, and sturdiness (p. 335)?

20. Describe contrast improvement factor and selectivity (p. 338).

21. Describe how grid conversion factors can be used to determine required mAs adjustment (p. 338, 339).

22. How can an air gap influence receptor exposure and what mAs adjustments are needed when it is employed (p. 339)?

23. What is inherent filtration? What is added filtration? What does each consist of (p. 341)?

24. What is the primary purpose of total filtration? What effect does it have on receptor exposure (p. 341)?

25. Describe how body position, condition, and pathology can affect receptor exposure (p. 341, 342, 343).

26. Differentiate between and give examples of destructive and additive pathologic conditions (p. 343).

27. How can beam restriction impact receptor exposure (p. 344)?

28. How can the anode heel effect impact receptor exposure? Under what conditions is the heel effect most noticeable (p. 344)?

29. How is SID related to receptor exposure, beam intensity, and patient dose in *digital* imaging (p. 328, 353)?

30. How is kV related to photon energy, scattered radiation, receptor exposure, beam intensity, and patient dose (p. 330, 331)?

31. How are grids related to scattered radiation, receptor exposure, and patient dose (p. 333, 334, 335)?

32. How is protective filtration related to photon energy, receptor exposure, and patient dose (p. 341)?

33. Define the following computer terms: bit, pixel, bit depth, gray scale, histogram, matrix, postprocessing, and dynamic range (p. 346, 347, 326).

34. What controls brightness and contrast in digital imaging (p. 325)?

35. List at least three causes of graininess in CR images (p. 363, 349).

36. Define image contrast; what is the function of image contrast (p. 326, 327)?

37. Describe the concept of differential absorption and its impact on image contrast (p. 326, 327).

38. List the three factors that determine the production of scattered radiation (p. 330, 331).

39. Describe the two types of AECs. Include in your description (p. 350, 351):

    i. the location of each, relative to the tabletop and the IR

    ii. operation of each, and how exposure is terminated

40. Explain the importance of the backup timer used in AEC (p. 350, 352).

41. Explain the importance of proper AEC sensor/photocell selection; describe typical errors in photocell selection and the subsequent radiographic results (p. 351).

42. Why are fixed kV technique charts preferred to variable kV technique charts (p. 351, 352)?

43. Discuss why positioning accuracy is essential to proper function of the AEC (p. 351).

44. Describe APR. How are appropriate technical factors selected by using APR (p. 352, 353)?

45. Discuss the function and importance of the EI in digital images (p. 353, 354).

CHAPTER REVIEW QUESTIONS

1. Which of the following systems uses a preprogrammed, internal technique chart to produce appropriate mAs and kV values for an exposure?

    (A) AEC

    (B) APR

    (C) TFT

    (D) CCD

2. In an AEC system, which component is responsible for avoiding overexposure of the patient and potential tube overload?

    (A) Minimum response timer

    (B) Ionization chamber

    (C) Backup timer

    (D) Phototimer

3. The effects of scattered radiation on the x-ray image include the following:

    1. it produces fog

    2. it decreases contrast resolution

    3. it increases grid cutoff

    (A) 1 only

    (B) 2 only

    (C) 1 and 2 only

    (D) 1, 2, and 3

4. Which of the following can impact receptor exposure?

    1. Tissue density

    2. Pathology

    3. Beam restriction

    (A) 1 and 2 only

    (B) 1 and 3 only

    (C) 2 and 3 only

    (D) 1, 2, and 3

5. If it is desired to reduce the receptor exposure by one-half, which of the following would best accomplish this?

    (A) Decrease the kV by 50%

    (B) Decrease the kV by 15%

    (C) Decrease the SID by 25%

    (D) Decrease the grid ratio

6. The use of optimum kV for small, medium, and large body parts is the premise of

    (A) fixed kV, variable mAs technique chart

    (B) variable kV, fixed mAs technique chart

    (C) fixed mAs, variable body part technique

    (D) fixed mAs, variable SID technique

7. An exposure was made using 200 mA, 50-ms exposure, and 75 kV. Each of the following changes will effectively double radiographic receptor exposure, except

    (A) change to 0.1-s exposure

    (B) change to 86 kV

    (C) change to 20 mAs

    (D) change to 100 mA

8. A radiographic procedure requires technical factors of 75 kV and 5 mAs for a nongrid exposure. If a 10-inch air-gap technique was to be employed, what mAs should be used to preserve IR exposure?

    (A) 5 mAs

    (B) 20 mAs

    (C) 25 mAs

    (D) 30 mAs

9. Of the following groups of technical factors, which will produce the greatest receptor exposure?

    (A) 200 mA, 50 ms, 36-inch SID

    (B) 400 mA, 0.05 s, 72-inch SID

    (c) 400 mA, 0.10 s, 72-inch SID

    (D) 200 mA, 100 ms, 36-inch SID

10. Which of the following pathologic conditions would require an increase in technical factors?

    (A) Pneumoperitoneum

    (B) Obstructed bowel

    (C) Renal colic

    (D) Ascites

11. The *term* used to describe the number of bits per pixel, which has a significant effect on gray scale, is

    (A) voxel

    (B) bit depth

    (C) histogram

    (D) TFT

12. All of the following statements regarding automatic exposure control are true, except

    (A) AECs function to produce consistent and comparable receptor exposures

    (B) ionization chambers are located between the x-ray table and the IR

    (C) AECs will compensate for tissue thickness and density differences

    (D) minimum reaction time is the longest exposure time possible with a particular AEC

13. Which of the following statement(s) regarding protective filtration is/are true?

    1. Protective filtration functions to reduce patient skin dose

    2. Protective filtration increases the overall average energy of the x-ray beam

    3. Protective filtration has no impact on receptor exposure

    (A) 1 only

    (B) 1 and 2 only

    (C) 1 and 3 only

    (D) 1, 2, and 3

14. A satisfactory receptor exposure was obtained by using 12 mAs and 400 mA. What exposure time would be required to produce the same receptor exposure by using 1200 mA?

    (A) 0.1 ms

    (B) 1.0 ms

    (C) 10 ms

    (D) 100 ms

15. Grid absorption of the useful beam is termed

    (A) cleanup

    (B) cutoff

    (C) focusing

    (D) compensation

Answers and Explanations

1. (B) By using APR, the radiographer uses console graphics or a touch screen to *select the anatomic part and its relative size* (S, M, L) to be imaged. The unit's microprocessor chooses the appropriate preprogrammed mAs and kV algorithm for that particular part and size—from the "internal technique chart" predetermined and stored on installation.

APR is used in conjunction with AEC and is therefore still highly dependent on the skillfulness of its user. Accurate positioning, photocell selection, and control of scattered radiation are essential to the production of quality images using APR and AEC.

2. (C) An AEC system can have one of two devices to modulate exposures: an ionization chamber or a phototimer. In *ionization chamber systems*, x-ray photons leave the patient's body and are collected in the chamber. The air inside will be ionized until a predetermined amount has been reached. In *phototimer* systems, x-ray photons will leave the patient and interact with a fluorescent screen. This screen will emit light in proportion to the exposure received and charge a photomultiplier tube until a predetermined amount has been reached. All AEC systems have a minimum response timer and a backup timer. The *minimum response timer* determines the shortest exposure possible, and the *backup timer* functions to terminate the exposure should a malfunction occur that causes the exposure to continue for longer than expected. This prevents both overexposure of the patient and tube overload.

3. (C) Scattered radiation is produced as x-ray photons travel through matter, interact with atoms, and are scattered (change direction). If these scattered rays are energetic enough to exit the body, they will strike the IR from all different angles. Because the scattered photons have lost energy during the interactions within the body, they will add excessive low density (gray) tones to the image. They therefore do not carry useful information—merely producing a *gray fog* over the image, adding noise, and producing *less contrast resolution*. Grid cutoff decreases receptor exposure, increases contrast in analog imaging, and is caused by improper relationship between the x-ray tube and the grid.

4. (D) The radiographic subject, that is, the patient, is composed of many different tissue types of varying densities, resulting in varying degrees of photon attenuation and absorption. This *differential absorption* impacts receptor exposure and contributes to contrast resolution. Normal tissue density can be significantly altered in the presence of pathology. For example, destructive bone disease can cause a dramatic decrease in tissue density. Abnormal accumulation of fluid (as in ascites) will cause a significant increase in tissue density. Muscle atrophy, or highly developed muscles, will similarly decrease, or increase, tissue density. Perhaps, the most important way to improve contrast resolution and limit the production of scattered radiation is by limiting the size of the irradiated field through *beam restriction*. As the size of the field is reduced, there is less tissue volume irradiated; therefore, less scattered radiation will be produced.

5. (B) Receptor exposure is proportional to mAs. However, other methods may be used to adjust receptor exposure. A decrease in kV by 15% will effectively halve the receptor exposure. SID adjustment is not recommended for making receptor exposure changes because image magnification and patient dose are affected as well. Decreasing the grid ratio will increase the receptor exposure.

6. (A) The optimum kV (or fixed kV) technique separates anatomic parts into small, medium, and large categories and assigns an optimum kV for that particular body part. Patient thickness (measurement in centimeters) determines mAs.

7. (D) Receptor exposure is directly proportional to mAs. If exposure time is doubled from 0.05 ($\frac{1}{20}$) s to 0.1 ($\frac{1}{10}$) s, receptor exposure will double. If the mAs is doubled from 10 to 20 mAs, receptor exposure will double. If the kV is increased by 15%, from 75 to 86 kV, receptor exposure will double according to the 15% rule. Changing to 100 mA will halve the mAs, effectively halving the receptor exposure.

8. (D) The air-gap technique can be used in place of a grid in some situations, but a subsequent increase in mAs is still needed to preserve IR exposure. A 10-inch air gap is the equivalent of a 16:1 grid. To change nongrid to grid exposure, you must multiply the original mAs by the appropriate grid ratio factor:

No grid = 1 × original mAs
5:1 grid = 2 × original mAs
6:1 grid = 3 × original mAs
8:1 grid = 4 × original mAs
12:1 grid = 5 × original mAs
16:1 grid = 6 × original mAs

Therefore, to change from nongrid to a 10-inch air gap, multiply the original mAs by a factor of 6. A corrected mAs of 30 is required.

9. (D) By using the formula mA × second = mAs, determine each mAs. The greatest receptor exposure will be produced by the combination of greatest mAs and shortest SID. Groups A and C should produce identical receptor exposure, according to the inverse square law, because group C is twice the distance and 4 times the mAs of group A. Group B has twice the distance of group A but only twice the mAs; it has, therefore, less receptor exposure than groups A and C. Group D has the same distance as group A and twice the mAs, making it the group of technical factors that will produce the greatest receptor exposure.

10. (D) Because pneumoperitoneum is an abnormal accumulation of air or gas in the peritoneal cavity, it would require a decrease in technical factors. Obstructed bowel usually involves distended, gas-filled bowel loops, again, requiring a decrease in technical factors. With ascites, there is an abnormal accumulation of fluid in the abdominal cavity, necessitating an increase in technical factors. Renal colic is the pain associated with the passage of renal calculi; usually no change from the normal technical factors is required.

11. (B) Image storage is located in a *pixel,* a two-dimensional "picture element," measured in the "XY" direction. Bit *depth* refers to the number of *bits per pixel* and identifies the *values of gray/gray scale.* Gray scale is variations in brightness resulting from intensity variations. A *histogram* is a graphic representation of pixel value distribution demonstrating the number of pixels and their value. The third dimension in the *matrix* of pixels is the "volume element"—the voxel, measured in the "Z" direction. A TFT, thin-film transistor, is associated with FPDs.

12. (D) AEC is used to automatically regulate the amount of ionizing radiation delivered through the anatomic part to the IR, regardless of the IR type, thereby serving to produce consistent and comparable radiographic results with minimum patient exposure. The two types of AECs are ionization chamber and phototimer. Ionization chambers are located between the x-ray table and the IR; phototimers are located beneath the IR. Backup time always should be selected on the manual timer to prevent patient overexposure and to protect the x-ray tube from excessive heat production should the AEC malfunction. Minimum reaction time is the *shortest* exposure time possible with a particular AEC. Pathologic conditions may be either additive or degenerative; correct use of the AEC will compensate for changes in tissue thickness, density, and/or pathologic conditions and will be reflected in appropriate EI range.

13. (D) The primary beam generally has a total filtration of 2.5-mm Al equivalent for patient protection purposes. Protective filtration serves to remove the diagnostically useless x-ray photons that contribute only to patient skin dose. These x-ray photons are low energy and would not reach the IR; thus, x-ray tube *protective* filtration *has no effect on receptor exposure.* Because low-energy photons are removed, filtration increases the *overall average energy* of the x-ray beam. In general-purpose radiographic tubes, the glass envelope usually accounts for approximately 0.5-mm Al equivalent and the collimator provides approximately 1.0-mm Al equivalent. These are considered *inherent filtration.* The manufacturer adds another 1.0-mm Al to meet the minimum requirements of 2.5-mm Al equivalent total filtration for radiographic tubes operated above 70 kV.

14. (C) Using 12 mAs and 400 mA, the exposure time was 30 ms. Because mA × time = mAs, then $1200x = 12$; $x = 0.01$ s (10 ms). Therefore, 10-ms exposure would be required with 1200 and may produce the same receptor exposure.

15. (B) X-ray photons scatter within the anatomic part and cause image-degrading fog. Grids are used to *cleanup* scattered radiation before it reaches the IR. Grids must be used correctly to avoid absorption of the useful beam, termed grid *cutoff.*

B. IMAGE QUALITIES: RESOLUTION AND DISTORTION

If tiny anatomic details of images made under different conditions are carefully inspected, it is noted that the anatomic details appear with varying degrees of resolution/clarity. Some details are clearly defined, whereas others exhibit degrees of unsharpness/blurriness. *Resolution* describes how closely fine details can be associated and still be recognized as separate details (Fig. 12-27A). Spatial resolution can be expressed in mathematical terms of modulation transfer function, or MTF, which describes the amount of blur and contrast of a system component or the entire imaging system.

Spatial Resolution

Spatial resolution is the term used to describe the IR's impact on image detail. Spatial resolution is receptor dependent. *Spatial resolution is measured in line pairs per millimeter (lp/mm). One line pair refers to one line and one space adjacent to it.* The spatial resolution of digital imaging is not as good as that of analog imaging. Although analog resolution is better, digital imaging's ability to perceive small differences in tissue densities (i.e., better contrast resolution) is often more valuable, particularly when viewing soft tissues. For example, analog imaging provides a spatial resolution of about 10 lp/mm, whereas digital ranges between 2.5 and 5 lp/mm! However, the wide dynamic range capabilities of digital imaging compensate for the loss of spatial resolution.

Because digital detectors have a lower spatial resolution than analog detectors, it is essential that radiographers control the other factors impacting resolution.

The IR's spatial resolution in *direct digital* systems is *fixed* and is related to the detector element (*DEL*) size of the *TFT*. The smaller the TFT DEL size, the better the spatial resolution. TFT DEL sizes range from approximately 140 to 200 μm.

Spatial resolution in *indirect* imaging improves with increased *sampling frequency* (pixels/mm or pixel density), smaller *pixel pitch*, smaller *pixel size*, and larger image matrix.

Digital Image Resolution Improves With

- Smaller pixel size
- Smaller pixel pitch
- Larger image matrix
- Greater pixel density

Spatial Resolution Factors

Direct Digital
- Pixel pitch
- DEL size of the TFT

Indirect Digital
- Pixel pitch
- Sampling frequency

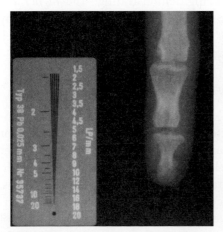
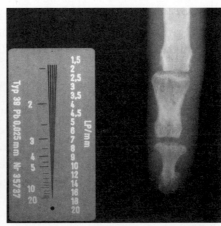
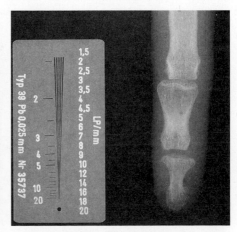

Figure 12-27. (A) *Magnified views of the second phalanx.* (*Left*) Significant blur/unsharpness of image details; resolution is approximately 6 lp/mm. (*Center*) Improved resolution of approximately 8 lp/mm. (*Right*) Best resolution of approximately 12 lp/mm. (From the American College of Radiology Learning File. Photo contributor: The American College of Radiology.) (*continued*)

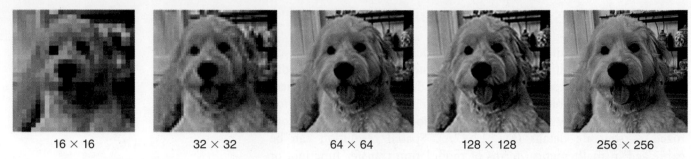

16 × 16   32 × 32   64 × 64   128 × 128   256 × 256

Figure 12-27. *(Continued)* **(B)** The matrix is the number of pixels in the *XY* direction. The larger the matrix size, the better the image resolution.

Spatial resolution is detector dependent.

Matrix Size, FOV, Pixel Size, and Spatial Resolution

As matrix size increases → pixel size decreases → spatial resolution increases

As matrix size decreases → pixel size increases → spatial resolution decreases

As FOV increases → matrix remains the same → pixel size increases → spatial resolution decreases

As FOV decreases → matrix remains the same → pixel size decreases → spatial resolution increases

---

- One outstanding quality of digital imaging is its exceptional *contrast resolution*.

A digital image is formed by a matrix of pixels in *rows and columns* (Fig. 12-27B). This allows for the organized placing of pixels within the image, providing an accurate representation of the anatomical structures that were radiographed. A matrix having 512 pixels in each row and column is a 512 × 512 matrix. The term *FOV* is used to describe how much anatomy (e.g., 150 mm diameter) is included in the image.

The matrix or FOV can be changed without one affecting the other, but changes in either will affect the pixel size. As matrix size is increased, there are more and smaller pixels in the matrix, therefore improving spatial resolution. As FOV is decreased, the matrix size will remain the same but must fit into a smaller area. This causes the pixels to become smaller, improving spatial resolution.

Other CR image processing factors contribute to image resolution and are addressed in the later section.

Contrast Resolution

What digital imaging might lack in spatial resolution, it more than makes up for in contrast resolution. The number of subtle grayscale differences able to be demonstrated is far greater, resulting in a significantly better contrast resolution. The terms *dynamic range* and *contrast resolution* are commonly used to describe the range of grays a particular digital system is capable of resolving/demonstrating. The *higher* the contrast resolution, the better the ability to see similar adjacent gray shades. As mentioned earlier, the greater the number of bits per pixel, the greater the capability of displaying many shades of gray.

Detective Quantum Efficiency

Detective quantum efficiency (DQE) describes the percentage of incoming x-ray photons that are detected and absorbed by the detector for transformation to the x-ray image. Detector systems having higher DQEs have the ability to produce high-quality images at lower doses. In CR, the receptor is the PSP. Digital detectors include TFTs and CCDs. DR can be either direct or indirect conversion. Systems without a scintillation/light conversion step have a higher DQE, with the exception of the new *complementary metal oxide semiconductor* capture systems. In general, amorphous selenium TFTs have the highest DQE. Details are addressed in Chapter 13.

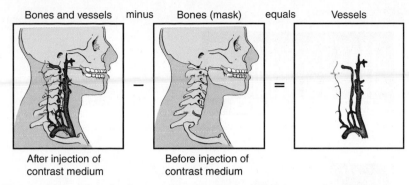

Figure 12-28. Digital subtraction angiography (DSA). Image details not required for diagnosis can be subtracted from an image. Only vessels containing contrast medium are visualized in the final image.

Noise

Noise is an electronic term for anything that interferes with visualization of the image we wish to see. The *SNR* is important in image quality. The signal is the x-ray photons. An insufficient number of x-ray photons (mAs) can result in image noise. Digital images are subject to noise; it can appear as *graininess* called *quantum mottle*. Noise cannot be removed in postprocessing.

As SNR increases, image quality increases but at the expense of exposure dose. Intelligent selection of technical factors is still required, and radiographers must be even more vigilant in minimizing patient exposure.

RESOLUTION AND GEOMETRIC DISTORTION

Terms and Factors

The degree of resolution, or detail, transferred to the IR is a function of the resolving power of each of the system components and can be expressed in mathematical terms as MTF, which describes the amount of blur and contrast of a system component or the entire imaging system.

Resolution can be expressed in line pairs per millimeter (Fig. 12-29) when measured by using a *resolution test pattern. One line pair refers to one line and the one space adjacent to it.* Resolution describes how closely fine details may be associated and still be recognized as separate details before seeming to blend into each other and appear "as one."

The term *distortion* refers to misrepresentation of the actual *size* (*magnification*) or *shape* (*foreshortening* or *elongation*) of the structures imaged, which may be partly or wholly caused by inherent object unsharpness.

All of the geometric factors—OID, SID, focal spot size, distortion, structural position and shape, and motion—impact resolution/detail.

Each of the factors having an effect on spatial resolution and geometric distortion is discussed in the following sections.

Typical Image Matrix Sizes Used in Medical Imaging Are

- Nuclear medicine   128 × 128
- Digital subtraction   1024 × 1024
  angiography (Fig. 12-28)
- CT   512 × 512
- Chest radiography   2048 × 2048

Factors Affecting Resolution

- OID (magnification distortion)
- SID (magnification distortion)
- Focal spot size (focal spot blur)
- Patient factors (structural shape/position)
- Motion (motion blur)

Distortion

- *Size* distortion (magnification)
- Shape distortion (elongation/foreshortening)

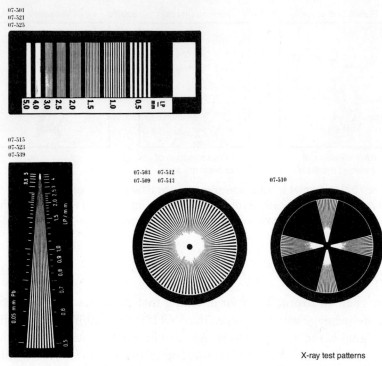

X-ray test patterns

Figure 12-29. Resolution is measured with a *resolution test pattern* and expressed in line pairs per millimeter. Resolution test tools are pictured. The *star pattern* is generally used for focal spot size evaluation. (Reproduced with permission from Nuclear Associates, Carle place, NY.)

Geometric Factors Affecting Distortion

- *Size* distortion (magnification):
  OID
  SID
- Shape distortion (elongation/foreshortening):
  Alignment of x-ray tube, anatomic part, and IR

Remember, *image quality* is evaluated according to image *brightness, gray scale, spatial resolution,* and *distortion.* The *visibility* factors are the previously discussed brightness and gray scale; the *geometric* factors are spatial resolution and distortion, discussed in the following sections.

Summary

- Spatial resolution refers to the sharpness of structural detail borders; it is affected by OID, SID, focal spot size, patient factors, and motion.
- Spatial resolution can be measured by using a resolution test pattern and expressed in line pairs per millimeter.
- MTF is a method of mathematically describing the blur and contrast of the system or one of its components.
- DQE describes a system's percentage of detected incoming x-ray photons.
- Systems having a higher DQE are able to produce quality images at lower doses.
- Distortion relates to the size and/or shape of the imaged part compared with the actual size and shape of the anatomic object.
- The terms *magnification, elongation,* and *foreshortening* are used when describing distortion.
- Visibility factors are brightness, contrast, and noise.

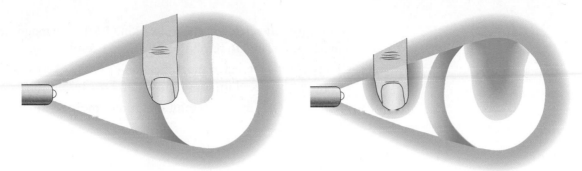

Figure 12-30. *Effect of OID on magnification and detail.* As the finger moves *away* from the surface (toward the light source), the shadow image becomes *magnified* and *blurry.*

Distance

If you place your hand between a flashlight and a wall, or any flat surface of a dimly lit room, the shadow of your hand will vary in *size and clarity* as it changes position with respect to the flashlight and the surface. As your hand moves farther from the surface, the shadow becomes larger and less distinct. As your hand is brought closer to the surface (and farther from the flashlight), the shadow becomes more like the actual size of your hand and appears with more clarity (Fig. 12-30).

OID. The aforementioned experiment and Figure 12-30 illustrate the effect of *OID* on spatial resolution and geometric distortion. Therefore, like visible light, the x-ray beam diverges as it leaves its source; an increase in OID will increase *magnification.* X-ray photons strike all parts of the object, continue traveling in a divergent fashion, and "deposit" the (now magnified and unsharp) image on the IR (Fig. 12-31). *Geometric resolution/detail is degraded as OID increases.*

OID has a much greater effect on magnification than SID. The significance of the effect can be realized when recalling that each 1 inch of OID is remedied by 7-inch increase in SID!

SID. A similar example can be used to show the effect of *SID* on image geometry and resolution. If your hand is placed at a given distance from the flat surface, any change in the *distance between the light source and the surface* will affect the magnification and clarity of the shadow image. As the flashlight moves closer to your hand, the shadow will become larger and less distinct. As the flashlight is moved farther from the surface, the shadow approaches the actual size of your hand and becomes sharper and more distinct (Fig. 12-32). Similarly, as the distance between the x-ray source and the IR increases, the x-ray image is less magnified and more distinct (Fig. 12-33). *Geometric resolution/detail improves as SID increases.*

Summary

- Resolution and magnification are *inversely* related, that is, resolution *increases* as magnification *decreases.*

- SID and OID regulate magnification and therefore influence the geometric properties, and hence resolution, of the radiographic image.

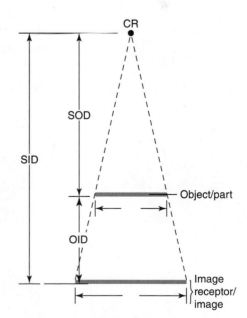

Figure 12-31. As distance from the object to the IR (OID) increases, the projected size of the image increases, that is, magnification increases. (Reproduced with permission from Saia DA. *Lange Q&A Radiography Examination.* 7th ed. New York, NY: McGraw-Hill; 2009.)

- SID is *inversely* related to magnification (↑ SID = ↓ magnification) and *directly* related to resolution (↑ SID = ↑ resolution).

- OID is *directly* related to magnification (↑ OID = ↑ magnification) and *inversely* related to resolution (↑ OID = ↓ resolution).

- Changes in OID impact resolution 7 times more significantly than similar changes in SID.

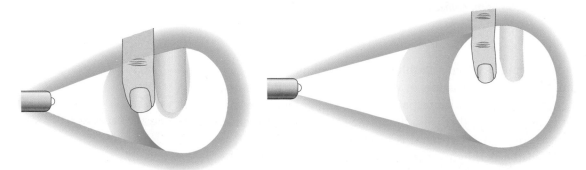

Figure 12-32. *Effect of SID on magnification and detail.* As the light source moves closer to the finger, the shadow image becomes magnified and blurry.

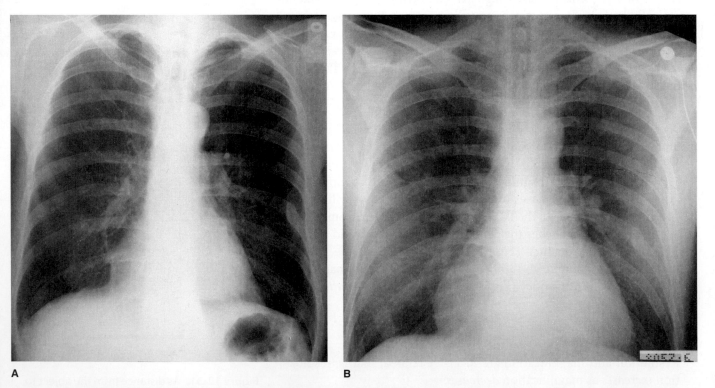

A   B

Figure 12-33. (A) PA erect chest taken at a distance of 6 feet demonstrates an accurate representation of the heart shadow and various parenchymal and bony structures. **(B)** AP erect at 50 inches of the same patient taken within 24 h and with no change in patient condition. The *heart appears markedly larger* (15.5 cm on PA and 20 cm on AP) for two *reasons:* (1) The heart is farther from the IR in the AP projection and (2) the SID is decreased; thus, the heart is magnified. (From the American College of Radiology Learning File. Photo contributor: The American College of Radiology.)

Patient Factors

A certain amount of object unsharpness is an inherent part of every radiographic image because *of the position and shape of anatomic structures within the body.*

Structure Position. Structures within the three-dimensional human body lie in different planes. For example, the frontal sinuses are more anterior than the sphenoids, the ureters are more anterior than the kidneys, the upper renal poles lie in a plane posterior to the lower renal poles, the fundus of the stomach is more posterior than its body and pylorus, and the posterior portions of the sacroiliac joints are more medial than their anterior portions.

Structural Shape. In addition, the three-dimensional shape of solid anatomic structures rarely coincides with the shape of the divergent beam. Consequently, some structures are imaged with more inherent distortion than others, and shapes of anatomic structures can be entirely misrepresented. Structures *farther* from the IR will be distorted (i.e., *magnified*) more than those *closer* to the IR.

For the *shape* of anatomic structures to be accurately recorded, the structures must be *parallel* to the x-ray tube and the IR and aligned with the central ray. The shape of anatomic structures lying at an angle within the body or placed away from the central ray will be misrepresented on the IR (Fig. 12-34).

There are two types of shape distortion. If a linear structure is angled within the body, that is, not parallel with the long axis of the part/body and not parallel to the IR, that anatomic structure will appear *smaller*—it will be *foreshortened.* A good example of foreshortening is demonstrated in the PA projection of the wrist. The curved carpal scaphoid appears smaller than its actual size because of foreshortening. On the contrary, *elongation* occurs when the x-ray tube is angled. This is often

> ### Subject/Object Unsharpness Results When
>
> - Object shape does not coincide with the shape of the x-ray beam
> - Object plane is not parallel with the x-ray tube and/or the IR
> - Anatomic object(s) of interest is not in the path of the CR
> - Anatomic object(s) of interest is at a distance from the IR

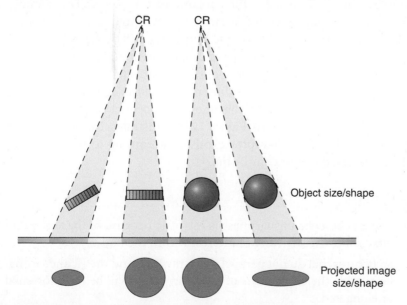

Figure 12-34. The shape of various structures can be radiographically misrepresented (i.e., *foreshortened or elongated*) as a result of their position in the body. That misrepresentation can be exaggerated when the part is away from the central axis of the x-ray beam. (Reproduced with permission from Saia DA. *Lange Q&A Radiography Examination.* 7th ed. New York, NY: McGraw-Hill; 2009.)

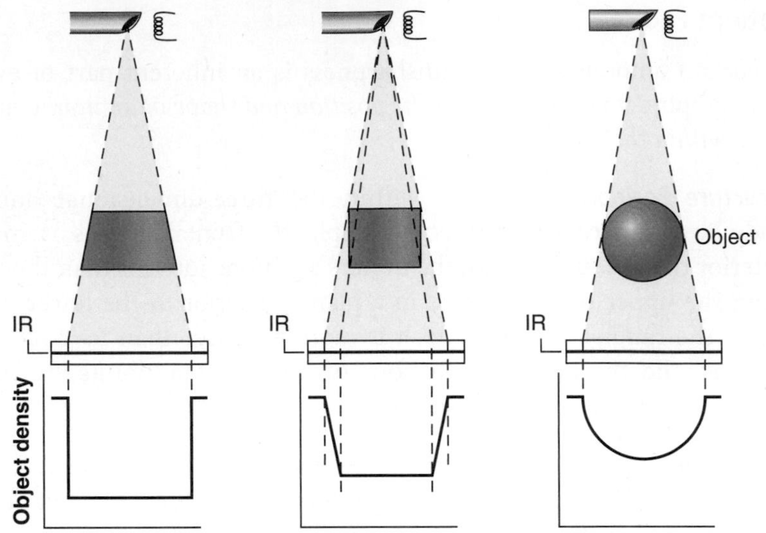

Figure 12-35. Blur or unsharpness results when the *shape* of a three-dimensional object does not coincide with that of the x-ray beam. Blur is accompanied by changes in receptor exposure as a result of differing thicknesses traversed by the x-ray beam.

used to advantage in radiography. In the Towne method of the skull, the occipital bone is better visualized when the central ray is angled 30° caudally because the facial bones are projected inferiorly and removed from superimposition on the occipital bone. Similarly, the tortuous sigmoid colon can be "opened up" in the AP axial projection by using a cephalad angle. Thus, intentional distortion can be used to improve visualization of some structures.

Image details placed away from the central ray will be exposed by more divergent rays, resulting in *rotation distortion*. This is why the central ray must be directed to the part of greatest interest. For example, if bilateral hands are requested, it might be better to image them individually; if imaged simultaneously, the central ray will be directed to no anatomic part (between the two hands) and rotation distortion will occur increasingly with the divergence of the x-ray beam.

Unless the edges of a three-dimensional *object* conform to the shape of the x-ray beam, blur or unsharpness will occur at the partially attenuating edge of the object. As Figure 12-35 illustrates, this will be accompanied by changes in receptor exposure according to the thickness of areas traversed by the x-ray beam.

Summary

- Some geometric unsharpness is intrinsic because of the shape and position of the structure of interest within the body.

- Structures that do not parallel the x-ray tube and the IR and/or that lie outside the central axis of the x-ray beam will be foreshortened or elongated.

- Structures within the body lie at varying distances from the x-ray IR, producing varying degrees of magnification.

Focal Spot Size

Another factor influencing the geometry of the image, and having a significant impact on spatial resolution, is focal spot size. If x-ray photons were emitted from a single-point source, structures would be recorded and resolved with great clarity. However, because x-ray photons emerge from a measurable focus, image details are represented with unsharp edges.

As shown in Figures 12-36 and 12-37, photons emerging from various points on a measurable focal spot are responsible for producing anatomic details having *blurred, unsharp edges.* The extent or size of the unsharp area is *directly* related to focal spot size and OID and *inversely* related to the SID, that is, unsharpness increases as focal spot size and OID increase and as the SID decreases.

This border of unsharpness around image details is geometric unsharpness often called *focal spot blur, edge gradient, or penumbra.* The *smaller* the focal spot size, the less blur and the *better the spatial resolution.*

A distinction is made between the *actual focal spot* (AFS) and the *effective* (or projected) *focal spot* (EFS). The AFS is the finite area on the tungsten target that is actually bombarded by electrons from the filament. The EFS is the foreshortened size of the focus as it is projected down toward the IR. This is called *line focusing* or the *line focus principle* (Fig. 12-38A–C). Radiographers generally speak in terms of the effective, or projected, focal spot, which is the focal spot size stated by x-ray tube manufacturers. The smaller the EFS, the better the image resolution.

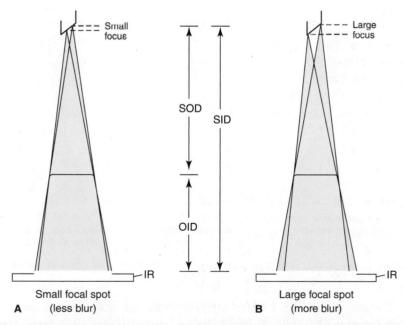

A Small focal spot (less blur)

B Large focal spot (more blur)

Figure 12-36. X-ray photons emitted from a small but measurable focal spot **(A)** will produce a small zone of blur or unsharpness around each image detail. X-ray photons emitted from a larger focal spot **(B)** will produce a larger degree of unsharpness/blur. The degree of blur is directly related to the *size of the focal spot.*

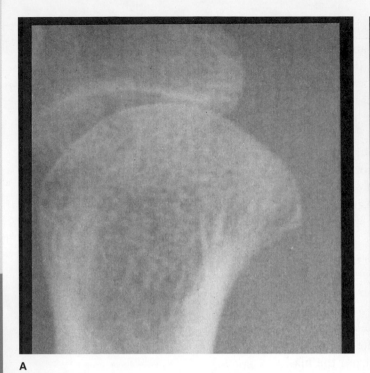

A

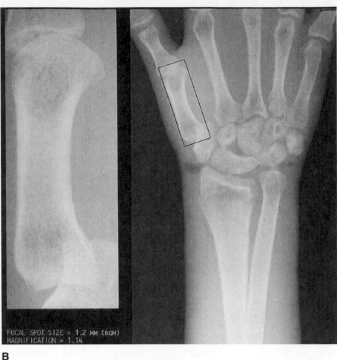

B

FOCAL SPOT SIZE = 1.2 MM (NOM)
MAGNIFICATION = 1.14

Figure 12-37. *Effect of focal spot on spatial resolution.* Both images were produced using direct exposure technique to better show the effect of focal spot size on resolution. **(A)** Magnified image of the first metacarpal, made with a 0.6-mm focal spot. Note the blur or unsharpness associated with bony trabeculae, especially noticeable on the magnified image. **(B)** Image made under identical conditions but using a 1.2-mm focal spot; more severe degradation of spatial resolution is demonstrated as a result of blur from the use of a larger focal spot. *Note:* Magnification views must be made with a 0.3-mm (*fractional*) focal spot, or smaller, to preserve spatial resolution. (From the American College of Radiology Learning File. Photo contributor: The American College of Radiology.)

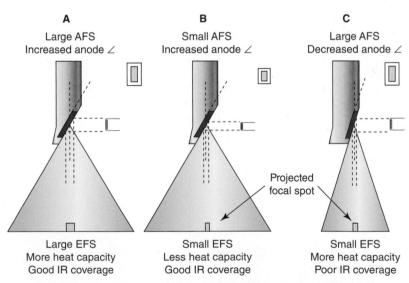

Figure 12-38. (A–C) The figures demonstrate how focal spot size and anode angle affect EFS, heat load capacity, and IR field coverage.

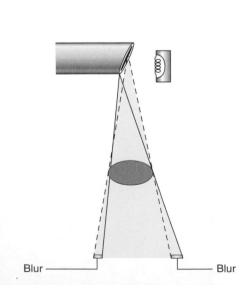

Figure 12-39. Because of the angle of the anode, unsharpness or blur is greatest at the cathode end of the IR. (Reproduced with permission from Saia DA. *Lange Q&A Radiography Examination.* 7th ed. New York, NY: McGraw-Hill; 2009.)

The size of the EFS, with its associated blur or unsharpness, actually *varies along the length of the IR,* being largest in size (and associated with most blur) at the cathode end of the IR and smallest at the anode end (Figs. 12-39 and 12-40).

The anode angle can also have a significant effect on image resolution. Differences in anode angle, all other factors remaining constant, will affect the size of the EFS, as illustrated in Figure 12-38.

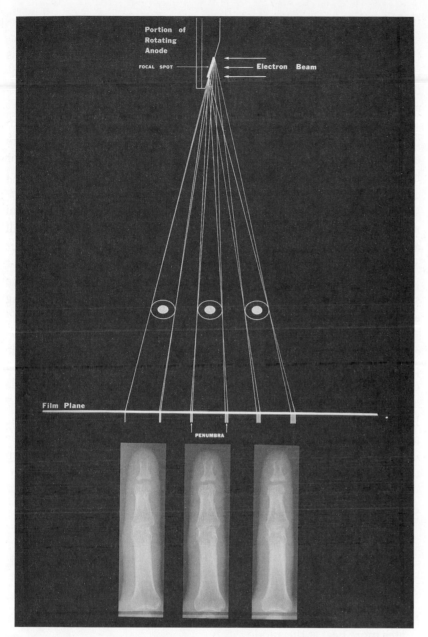

Figure 12-40. *Variation of effective focal spot size along the longitudinal tube axis.* Three images of the third phalanx are shown: one taken at the anode end of the x-ray beam, one at the central portion of the beam, and one at the cathode end. The images clearly illustrate gradual loss of resolution toward the cathode end of the x-ray beam. (From the American College of Radiology Learning File. Photo contributor: The American College of Radiology.)

If the use of a smaller focal spot size provides us with better resolution, why is the smallest available focal spot not always used? Simply because focal spot size is also associated with the buildup of *heat* within the x-ray tube. Large quantities of heat delivered to the x-ray tube, especially in a short period of time, can be very damaging to the tube and can shorten its life span.

The larger the surface area bombarded by electrons, the greater the heat load capacity of the x-ray tube. Heat load capacity is limited when using a small AFS. But notice in Figure 12-38C that a small EFS can be achieved by using a large AFS if anode angle is decreased. This will

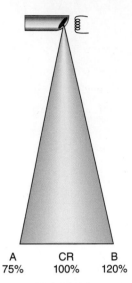

A
75%

CR
100%

B
120%

Figure 12-41. *The anode heel effect.* As x-ray photons are produced at the anode focus, a portion of the divergent beam nearest the anode end (A) is absorbed by the anode's "heel." This represents a decrease in x-ray beam intensity at the anode side of the x-ray beam. The smaller/steeper the anode angle/bevel, the more pronounced the heel effect.

Spatial Resolution Factors

- OID
- SID
- SOD
- Focal spot size
- Motion
- Distortion
- Structural position and shape

improve resolution and increase the heat load capacity, but IR field coverage is compromised because of heightened anode heel effect. A "fractional" (0.3 mm or smaller) EFS can be achieved, spatial resolution is improved, and anode heat load tolerance is not compromised. This feature is useful in magnification and visualization of small blood vessels and other tiny anatomic details.

If the AFS is small, heat is confined to a tiny area; localized melting of the target material and anode *pitting* and/or cracking can occur more easily. The larger the focal spot, the greater the surface area available for heat dispersion (via conduction, convection, and radiation). The perfect combination would, of course, be a large actual focus that could withstand heat and still provide a small effective focus for optimum spatial resolution. This can be achieved by using an x-ray tube with a small anode *angle* of approximately 7°–10°. As mentioned earlier, the smaller angle enables a larger "face" to be presented to the electron stream, that is, a larger surface area over which to disperse heat (Fig. 12-38). The slight anode angle causes significant foreshortening of the AFS, creating a very small *EFS*.

A difficulty associated with the use of a small anode angle, however, is maintaining a large (14 × 17) field size. The small anode angle produces a pronounced *anode heel effect* (Fig. 12-41) with resulting compromise in field coverage (Fig. 12-38). By using a small anode angle, a typical radiographic distance of 40-inch SID, and a 14 × 17 IR, there will be approximately 2 inches of unexposed area at the anode end of the image. This can be remedied with an increase in SID, which must be accompanied by an appropriate increase in technical factors.

Summary

- Focal spot size affects spatial resolution by influencing the degree of blur or unsharpness: ↑ focal spot size = ↑ blur = ↓ detail.
- Unsharpness/blur is *directly* related to focal spot size and OID and *inversely* related to SID.
- The use of a small focal spot improves spatial resolution but generates more heat at the anode.
- The effective or projected focal spot size is always smaller than the AFS according to the line focus principle.
- EFS size varies along the longitudinal axis of the IR, being largest at the cathode end and smallest at the anode end of the x-ray beam.
- Smaller anode angles can permit larger AFS sizes while maintaining small EFS sizes—at the expense of accentuating the *anode heel effect*.
- Use of a small anode angle can limit IR coverage at traditional and short SIDs.
- The anode heel effect is most pronounced using large IRs, short SIDs, and small anode angles.

Motion

Motion is probably the greatest challenge to good spatial resolution. Image blur or unsharpness, as a result of motion, can cause severe degradation of spatial resolution (see Fig. 12-9A and C). The best method of minimizing *voluntary motion* is through good *communication* and *suspended respiration.* A patient who understands what to expect and what is expected of him or her is better prepared and more likely to cooperate than a patient whose concerns have been inadequately addressed.

Involuntary motion, such as peristaltic activity, muscle spasms, and heart action, cannot be controlled by the patient. The best way to minimize involuntary motion is by using the shortest possible *exposure time.* Motion is often a problem in mobile radiography with machines of limited output (thereby prohibiting the use of short exposure times).

Special positioning devices (such as pediatric immobilizers), positioning sponges, and carefully placed sandbags are frequently used to assist the patient in maintaining the required position.

Equipment motion can cause an effect similar to that caused by patient motion. Bucky/grid motion can cause motion of the part during tabletop examinations; x-ray equipment sometimes has a switch to turn off the bucky/grid when doing tabletop work. Bumping an improperly balanced x-ray tube housing/collimator box just before making an exposure can result in motion blur or unsharpness if the exposure is made while the x-ray tube is still vibrating.

Motion blur is probably the greatest enemy of spatial resolution and is most obvious when the motion is close to the IR. Part motion is more damaging to spatial resolution than tube motion.

Deliberate motion is occasionally used to blur out unwanted structures so that the area of interest can be seen to better advantage. The "breathing techniques" of a transthoracic shoulder (Fig. 12-42A) and lateral thoracic spine (Fig. 12-42B) are typical examples. Another is the infrequently performed procedure of (conventional) *tomography,* in which a preselected structure plane will be clearly delineated whereas structures above and below that plane are blurred (Fig. 12-43).

> **To Minimize Voluntary Motion**
> - Good communication
> - Suspended respiration
>
> **To Minimize Involuntary Motion**
> - Short exposure time
> - Part support and stabilization
> - Special immobilization devices

Summary

- Motion is the greatest adversary of spatial resolution.
- Voluntary patient motion can be minimized through good communication.
- Involuntary patient motion is best minimized by using the shortest possible exposure time.
- Various radiographic accessories are available to help minimize both voluntary and involuntary patient motions.
- Equipment motion can also result in loss of spatial resolution in the form of image blur.
- Special techniques that introduce motion are sometimes used to see some structures particularly well.

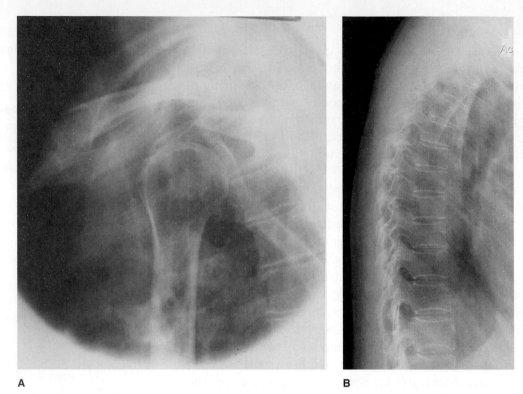

A   B

Figure 12-42. (A) Intentional motion, "breathing technique," to improve visualization of the transthoracic shoulder. Respiration motion blurs pulmonary vascular markings and superimposed bony structures. (Photo contributor: David Sack, BS, RT(R), CRA, FAHRA.) **(B)** Intentional motion, as a result of respiration during a long exposure, is used to blur ribs and pulmonary vascular markings, thereby promoting better visualization of thoracic vertebrae. (Photo contributor: Stamford Hospital, Department of Radiology.)

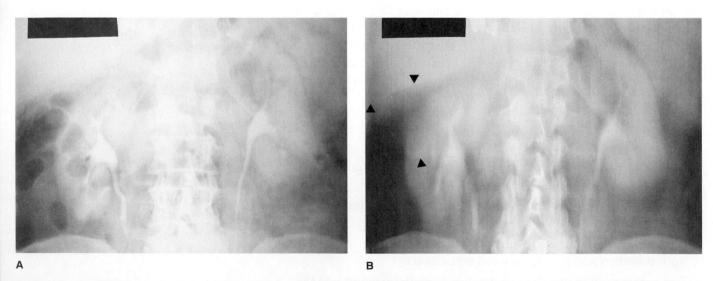

A   B

Figure 12-43. (A) Plain intravenous urogram with no visible abnormalities. **(B)** An 8-cm tomographic section of the same patient clearly depicting a 7-cm renal cyst overlying the right mid-renal cortex. (From the American College of Radiology Learning File. Photo contributor: The American College of Radiology.)

COMPREHENSION CHECK

1. To what does the term spatial resolution refer; how is it measured and expressed (p. 361)?

2. What is meant by FOV? How is it related to matrix size, pixel size, and spatial resolution (p. 325, 362)?

3. What do the terms *dynamic range* and *contrast resolution* describe (p. 325, 341, 348, 349, 361)?

4. Relate spatial resolution to pixel size, pixel pitch, and image matrix size (p. 361).

5. List the geometric factors affecting distortion (p. 363).

6. List the resolution factors that apply to digital imaging (pp. 363–372).

7. Compare the impact of OID versus SID on magnification distortion (p. 365).

8. What does one "line pair" consist of (p. 361)?

9. How are the terms *magnification, elongation,* and *foreshortening* related to *distortion* (p. 367, 368)?

10. What is the relationship between OID, spatial resolution, and magnification? What is the relationship between SID, spatial resolution, and magnification (p. 365)?

11. What are the two types of shape distortion? How can shape distortion be avoided (p. 367, 368)?

12. What causes object unsharpness and how is it, with respect to its three-dimensional shape and OID, an inherent part of every radiographic image (p. 368)?

13. Distinguish between actual and effective/projected/apparent focal spot size; what is the line focus principle (p. 369, 370)?

14. How is AFS size related to spatial resolution? How does the size of the projected focus vary along the length of the IR (p. 371, 372)?

15. How are focal spot size and anode angle related to x-ray tube heat load capacity (p. 371)?

16. Discuss the difference between voluntary and involuntary motions, and describe the most effective means of avoiding each (p. 373).

17. Why is motion intentionally introduced in some radiographic examinations? Give some examples (p. 373).

18. Define noise and its impact on SNR and image quality (p. 349, 363).

CHAPTER REVIEW QUESTIONS

1. Image detector spatial resolution in direct digital systems is
   1. fixed
   2. inversely related to the TFT DEL size
   3. always variable
   (A) 1 only
   (B) 1 and 2 only
   (C) 2 and 3 only
   (D) 1, 2, and 3

2. Factors impacting spatial resolution in indirect digital imaging include
   1. pixel pitch
   2. sampling frequency
   3. DEL size of the TFT
   (A) 1 only
   (B) 1 and 2 only
   (C) 2 and 3 only
   (D) 1, 2, and 3

3. Which of the following describes the percentage of incoming x-ray photons that are identified and absorbed by the detector?
   (A) Dynamic range
   (B) Field of view
   (C) Detective quantum efficiency
   (D) Contrast resolution

4. The electronic term used to describe anything that interferes with visualization of the x-ray image is
   (A) scintillation
   (B) MTF
   (C) postprocessing
   (D) noise

5. Factors that can impact image resolution include
   1. patient factors
   2. focal spot size
   3. SID
   (A) 1 only
   (B) 1 and 2 only
   (C) 2 and 3 only
   (D) 1, 2, and 3

6. Misalignment of the tube–part–IR relationship results in
   (A) shape distortion
   (B) size distortion
   (C) magnification
   (D) blur

7. An algorithm, as used in x-ray imaging,
   (A) is a geometric formula
   (B) produces specific exposure factors
   (C) is a series of variable instructions
   (D) produces predetermined exposure factors

8. Foreshortening of an anatomic structure means that
   (A) it is projected on the IR smaller than its actual size
   (B) its image is more lengthened than its actual size
   (C) it is accompanied by geometric blur
   (D) it is significantly magnified

9. In electronic imaging, as digital image matrix size increases,
   1. pixel size decreases
   2. resolution decreases
   3. FOV decreases
   (A) 1 only
   (B) 2 only
   (C) 1 and 2 only
   (D) 2 and 3 only

10. Focal spot blur is greatest
    (A) directly along the course of the central ray
    (B) toward the cathode end of the x-ray beam
    (C) toward the anode end of the x-ray beam
    (D) as the SID is increased

11. An increase in the size of the FOV would cause a
    1. decrease in spatial resolution
    2. increase in pixel size
    3. increase in matrix size
    (A) 1 only
    (B) 1 and 2 only
    (C) 2 and 3 only
    (D) 1, 2, and 3

12. What principle explains the difference in intensity at different ends of the x-ray beam?

(A) Anode heel effect

(B) Effective focal spot

(C) Penumbra

(D) Actual focal spot

13. A change in which of the following would have the greatest impact on image magnification?

(A) FOV

(B) SID

(C) Matrix size

(D) OID

Answers and Explanations

1. (B) *Spatial resolution* is the term used to describe the detector's impact on recorded detail in digital imaging. Spatial resolution is detector dependent. The detector's spatial resolution in direct digital systems is *fixed* and is inversely related to the *DEL* size of the *TFT*. The *smaller* the TFT DEL size, the greater the spatial resolution. TFT DEL sizes range from approximately 140 to 200 μm.

2. (B) Spatial resolution in *indirect* imaging improves with increased *sampling frequency* (pixels/mm or pixel density), smaller *pixel pitch,* smaller *pixel size,* and larger image matrix. The smaller the pixels and pixel pitch (i.e., distance between the center of one pixel to the center of adjacent pixel), the better the resolution.

DEL size of the TFT is related to *direct* digital imaging.

3. (C) DQE describes the percentage of incoming x-ray photons that are detected and absorbed by the detector for transformation to the x-ray image. Detector systems having higher DQEs have the ability to produce high-quality images at lower doses. DR can be either direct or indirect conversion. Systems without a scintillation/light conversion step generally have a higher DQE. Dynamic range and contrast resolution describe the range of grays that can be displayed by an imaging system. The field of view (FOV) describes how much anatomy is covered in the x-ray and included in the image matrix.

4. (D) *Noise* is an electronic term for anything that interferes with visualization of the image we wish to see. The *SNR* is important in image quality. The signal is the x-ray photons. An insufficient number of x-ray photons (mAs) can result in image noise. Digital images are subject to noise; it can appear as *graininess* called *quantum mottle,* as seen in Figure 12-4. Noise cannot be removed in postprocessing.

As SNR increases, image quality increases but at the expense of exposure dose. Intelligent selection of technical factors is still required, and radiographers must be even more vigilant in minimizing patient exposure.

5. (D) A certain amount of object unsharpness is an inherent part of every radiographic image because of the position and shape of *anatomic structures* within the body. Anatomic structures are frequently not parallel to, and at some distance from, the IR. Consequently, some structures are imaged with more inherent distortion than others, and shapes of anatomic structures can be entirely misrepresented. As OID increases, structures farther from the IR will be distorted (magnified), resulting in decreased resolution. *SID* is directly related to resolution/detail and inversely related to magnification. As SID increases, magnification decreases and detail increases.

Photons emerging from various points on a measurable *focal spot* are responsible for producing anatomic details having blurred, unsharp edges. The extent or size of the unsharp area is *directly* related to focal spot size and OID and *inversely* related to the SID, that is, unsharpness increases as focal spot size and OID increase and as the SID decreases.

6. (A) Shape distortion (e.g., foreshortening or elongation) is caused by improper alignment of the tube, part, and IR. Size distortion, or magnification, is caused by too great an OID or too short an SID. Focal spot blur is caused by the use of a large focal spot.

7. (C) An algorithm is a series of computerized step-by-step instructions used to solve a problem. The instructions are flexible, that is, variable, and various options are checked to produce the best possible results from the range of available options.

Radiographically speaking, the algorithm will test a range of variations to produce the best possible group of exposure factors for the particular anatomic part and circumstances.

8. (A) If a structure of a given length is not positioned parallel to the IR, it will be projected smaller than its actual size (foreshortened). An example of this can be a lateral projection of the third digit. If the finger is positioned so as to be parallel to the IR, no distortion will occur. If, however, the finger is positioned so that its distal portion rests on the IR whereas its proximal portion remains at a distance from the IR, foreshortening will occur.

9. (A) A digital image is formed by a matrix of pixels (picture elements) in rows and columns. A matrix that has 512 pixels in each row and column is a 512 × 512 matrix. The term *FOV* is used to describe how much anatomy (e.g., 150 mm diameter) is included in the matrix. The matrix and the FOV can be changed independently without one affecting the other, but changes in either will change pixel size. Spatial resolution is measured in line pairs per millimeter. As matrix size is increased (e.g., from 512 × 512 to 1024 × 1024), there are more and smaller pixels in the matrix and therefore improved resolution. Fewer and larger pixels result in poor resolution, a "pixelly" image, that is, one in which you can actually see the individual pixel boxes. Spatial resolution is measured in line pairs per millimeter. One line pair refers to one line and one space adjacent to it.

10. (B) Focal spot blur, or geometric blur, is caused by photons emerging from a large focal spot. The AFS is always larger than the effective (or projected) focal spot, as illustrated by the line focus principle. In addition, the effective focal spot size varies along the longitudinal tube axis, being greatest in size at the cathode end of the beam and smallest at the anode end of the beam. Because the projected focal spot is greatest at the cathode end of the x-ray tube, geometric blur is also greatest at the corresponding part (cathode end) of the x-ray image.

11. (B) FOV has a direct relationship with pixel size, and an indirect relationship with resolution. In other words, as the field of view increases, or gets larger, the size of the pixels will increase. Larger pixels result in a lower spatial resolution. FOV does not affect matrix size.

12. (A) The anode heel effect states that as x-rays are created, a portion of the beam closer to the anode side of the tube will be absorbed by the angled portion of the anode, or its heel. This causes a decrease in intensity at that end of the exposure. Penumbra, or focal spot blur, refers to the border of unsharpness surrounding a radiographic image. The effective focal spot is the actual location on the anode that is bombarded by electrons during the x-ray production process. The effective focal spot is the foreshortened focus that projects from the angled anode disk, down toward the patient.

13. (D) Changes in both SID and OID will influence the magnification of a radiographic image. SID is inversely related to magnification. This means that when SID is increased, magnification will decrease. OID is directly related to magnification, meaning that when OID is increased, magnification is also increased. Changes in OID impact resolution 7 times more significantly than similar changes in SID.

FOV and matrix size do not have an impact on image magnification.

Equipment Operation and Quality Assurance

OBJECTIVES

At the conclusion of this chapter, the student will be able to:

- List the patient information that is required to be on every x-ray image.
- Describe the structure and function of imaging plates and photostimulable phosphors (PSPs).
- Explain the process of PSP image formation and processing through a computed radiography reader.
- Explain the function of histograms and lookup tables.
- Discuss the importance of accurate exposure field recognition.
- List and describe the effects of various types of postprocessing functions on the radiographic image.
- Identify various image artifacts.
- Discuss the process of x-ray beam production and its characteristics.
- List the various types and features of x-ray equipment found in radiology.
- Explain the function and operation of transformers.
- Describe the structure and function of the x-ray tube.
- Identify the portions of the x-ray circuit and their component parts.
- Describe the fundamentals of anatomically programmed radiography.
- Define relevant terms for digital imaging.
- Describe both computed radiography and digital radiography (DR) systems.
- Differentiate between indirect and direct conversion DR systems.
- Discuss the purpose and use of exposure index systems.
- Discuss the rationale and elements of a quality control program.
- Identify various calibration tests performed on radiographic equipment and their acceptable standards.
- Describe the care and maintenance of imaging accessories.
- Describe the care and maintenance of protective apparel.

- Explain the specific information found about the different informatics systems used in radiography, such as HIS, RIS and EMR.
- Explain the basics of computer networking in relation to the imaging department (PACS/MIMPS and DICOM).

IMAGE PROCESSING AND DISPLAY

Image Identification

All essential medicolegal information must be visible on each x-ray image: patient name or identification number, side marker, date, and institution. Much of the demographic information is entered in the console computer. Accurate markers are essential for every image. This includes a left or right marker, properly placed and not superimposed on essential anatomy. Often special additional markers will be necessary to indicate that the examination was performed in the upright position, in the decubitus position, as a comparison image, and so on.

A type of exposure index (EI) (i.e., exposure dose) value should be identifiable and evaluated for appropriateness on each image. EI values often differed considerably among equipment manufacturers. The American Association of Physicists in Medicine proposed the term deviation index (DI) to be standardized among manufacturers. The DI should be visible to the operator on the control panel immediately following every exposure.

The radiograph must include the anatomic *areas of interest* in the desired position and projection. To ensure patient radiation safety, there must be visible evidence of *beam restriction/collimation. Protective shielding* has been used to reduce unnecessary radiation exposure to especially radiosensitive organs (i.e., gonads, blood-forming organs) and may still be provided to patients at their request or the request of the referring physician during radiographic and fluoroscopic examinations (see new shielding recommendations in Chapter 9).

> **Information Required on Each X-ray Image**
> - Patient name/identification number
> - Side marker, right or left
> - Examination date
> - Institution's name
>
> **Optional Information on Each X-ray Image**
> - Patient age or date of birth (DOB)
> - Attending physician
> - Time of day
> - Radiographer identification

Summary

- Medicolegal implications require that every image includes the patient's name or identification number, left- or right-side marker, examination date, and name of institution.
- When multiple images are taken of a patient the same day, the time of day should be indicated on each image.
- Image ID systems are electronic or radiographic.

Imaging Plates and Photostimulable Phosphors

The imaging plates (IPs) have a protective function (for the flexible photostimulable phosphor [PSP] within), are used in the Bucky tray or under the anatomic part, and come in a variety of sizes (Fig. 13-1A). The IPs need not be light-tight because the PSP inside is not light sensitive. One corner of the IP's rear panel has a memory chip for patient information; the IP also has a thin lead foil backing to absorb any backscatter.

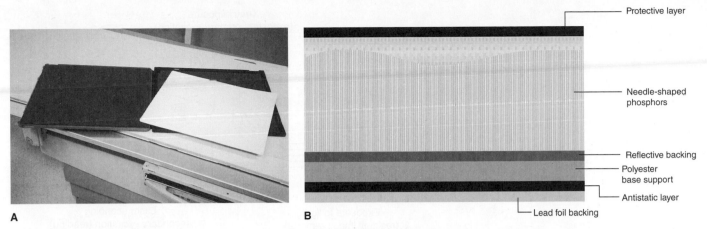

Figure 13-1. **(A)** An IP holds the PSP between its front and rear panels. **(B)** Barium fluorohalide is either granular or "needle shaped." The "needlelike" phosphors have the advantage of *better x-ray absorption and less light diffusion*. (Reproduced with permission from Shephard CT. *Radiographic Image Production and Manipulation*. New York, NY: McGraw-Hill; 2003.)

The PSP is composed of europium-doped barium fluorohalide (mixed with a binder) coated on a storage plate. The $BaF:Eu^{2+}$ crystal is usually in the form of *granular* or *turbid* phosphors. Other examples of turbid phosphors are gadolinium oxysulfide (Gd_2O_2S) and rubidium chloride. *Needle*-shaped (Fig. 13-1B) or *columnar* phosphors (usually cesium iodide [CsI]) have the advantage of *better x-ray absorption* and *less light diffusion.*

Just under the barium fluorohalide layer is a *reflective layer* that helps direct emitted light toward the computed radiography (CR) reader. Below the reflective layer is the base, behind that is an *antistatic layer*, and then the *lead foil* to absorb backscatter. There is a *protective layer* over the top of the barium fluorohalide.

On exposure, the x-ray photons interact with the $BaF:Eu^{2+}$ crystals. As a result of this interaction, a small amount of visible light is emitted, but most of the x-ray energy is stored (hence the term *storage plate*). This stored energy represents the latent image.

When the barium fluorohalide absorbs x-ray energy, electrons are released and they divide into two groups. One electron group initiates the *immediate luminescence* (primary excitation) during the excited state of Eu^{2+}. The other electron group becomes trapped within the phosphor's halogen ions, forming a "color center" (also called "F center"). These are the phosphors that ultimately form the radiographic image because, when exposed to a *monochromatic* laser light source, these phosphors emit *polychromatic* light (secondary excitation), termed *photostimulated luminescence* (PSL).

After exposure, the IP is placed in the CR scanner/reader (see Fig. 13-2), where the PSP is automatically removed. A narrow monochromatic, high-intensity helium–neon laser or a solid-state laser beam scans back and forth across the PSP while it is being pulled under the laser to progressively read the entire PSP. The movement of the PSP under the laser can be called subscan motion.

The phosphors are activated by the monochromatic red laser light (≈ 400 nm); however, PSL is a different color (bluish purple, blue–green, ≈ 550 nm). These two lights (PSL and laser) must not interfere with each other. To improve the image signal-to-noise ratio (SNR), the

---

PSP Storage Plate: Three Stages

- X-ray exposure
- Scanning/reading
- Erasure

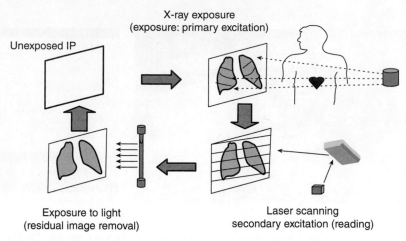

X-ray exposure
(exposure: primary excitation)

Unexposed IP

Exposure to light
(residual image removal)

Laser scanning
secondary excitation (reading)

Figure 13-2. The recording, reading, and erasure cycles. The PSP, within the IP, is exposed to x-ray photons, scanned/read, and then erased for reuse. (Photo contributor: Courtesy of FUJIFILM Medical System USA.)

image-carrying PSL must be of a different wavelength/color from, and physically separate from, that of the laser excitation light. An *optical filter* is used that permits transmission of the PSL but attenuates the laser light; this filter is mounted in front of a photomultiplier tube (PMT). The optical filter is generally a blue glass filter placed between the light guide and the PMT to filter out red laser light.

The PSL signal represents varying tissue densities and the latent image. The PMT or photodiode (PD) detects the PSL and converts it to electrical signals (Fig. 13-3), which are then transferred to an analog-to-digital converter (ADC)—converting the analog electrical signal to digital data. These digital data are then transferred to a digital-to-analog converter (DAC) to be converted to a perceptible analog image on the display monitor. The monitor image can be electronically transmitted, windowed, manipulated, postprocessed, and stored efficiently

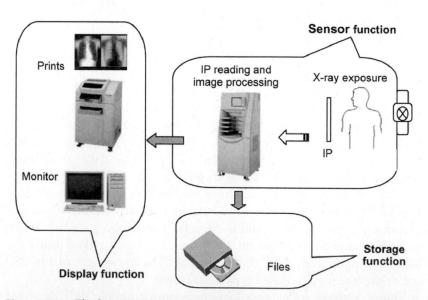

Sensor function

Prints

IP reading and
image processing

X-ray exposure

IP

Monitor

Display function

Files

Storage function

Figure 13-3. The latent image on the PSP is changed to a visible image as it is moved at a constant speed and scanned by a narrow, high-intensity helium–neon laser or a solid-state laser to obtain the pixel data. (Photo contributor: FUJIFILM Healthcare Americas Corp.)

(archived). Postprocessing functions can include edge enhancement; this technique can be used to improve the visibility of structures such as chest tubes by accentuating their edges.

The PSP layer can *store* its latent image for several hours; however, after approximately 8 h, significant image *fading* will occur as a result of "color center" electron signal loss. The europium activator is important for the *storage* characteristic of the PSPs; without europium, the image will not become visible.

Some PSP storage plates are manufactured specifically for better resolution (e.g., for mammography). Some higher resolution PSPs "read" the information from both sides of the PSP storage plates.

PSP storage plates must be maintained by regular inspection and cleaning. Dust and scratches cause image artifacts (Fig. 13-4).

IPs must be used with the correct side facing up. Figure 13-5 illustrates an image made with the IP inadvertently used upside down. Artifacts from the IP rear panel are imaged superimposed on the anatomic part. Care must be taken to keep the exposed IPs separate from the unexposed ones. Figure 13-6 is an example of double exposure. Notice that, although double exposed, the image does not look overexposed—as a result of *automatic rescaling*.

Once the PSP storage plate–reading process is completed, any remaining data stored on the PSP are erased by exposing it to high-intensity light (called "erasure"); the PSP storage plate is then ready for reuse. If the erasure process is incomplete, remnants of the previous image remain and degrade the new image. Figure 13-7 is an example of incomplete erasure.

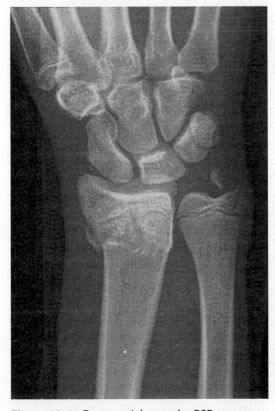

Figure 13-4. Dust particles on the PSP create exposure artifacts.

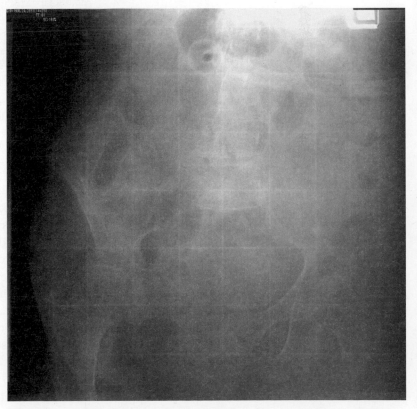

Figure 13-5. IP inadvertently used upside down. Artifacts from the IP rear panel are superimposed on the anatomic part.

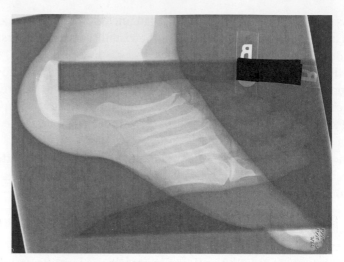

Figure 13-6. Double exposure. Care must be taken to keep exposed IPs separate from unexposed ones. (Photo contributor: Stamford Hospital, Department of Radiology.)

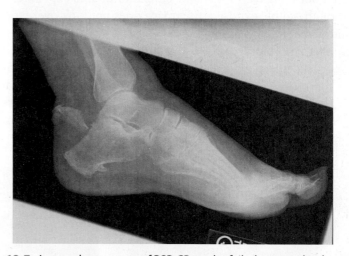

Figure 13-7. Incomplete erasure of PSP. CR reader failed to completely erase the previous image. Faint image of ribs can be seen outside the collimated area, above the foot. (Photo contributor: Stamford Hospital, Department of Radiology.)

Thus, the PSP undergoes three cycles: (i) x-ray exposure, (ii) reading, and (iii) erasure (see Fig. 13-2).

Figure 13-8 is an example of a double-exposed PSP. The same part was imaged twice by using the same PSP. Again, notice that automatic rescaling has corrected the appearance of the image—even though it received *twice* the correct exposure.

When two or more exposures are desired on one image receptor (IR), the *partition pattern* (or *exposure recognition*) process becomes essential for achieving good images. Unexposed portions of the IP must be well collimated and shielded to protect from exposure to scattered radiation (SR). X-ray fields must not overlap or be too close together without being shielded. Figure 13-9 illustrates the effect of improper partitioning of the IP.

An artifact associated with digital imaging and grids is *aliasing* (sometimes called "Moiré effect"). If the direction of the lead strips and the grid lines per inch (i.e., grid frequency) match the scan frequency of

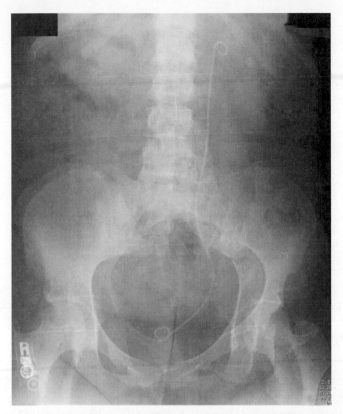

Figure 13-8. Double exposure. Note how CR will "correct" the exposure values; the image does not appear overexposed, but the second abdomen image is visible. (Photo contributor: Stamford Hospital, Department of Radiology.)

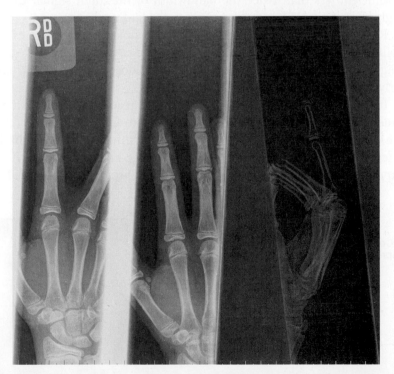

Figure 13-9. The "partition pattern recognition process" in CR will determine whether the image is divided, and if so, how it is divided. In the CR image above, one image was not recognized probably because the x-ray field was too close to the adjacent field. (Reproduced with permission from Shephard CT. *Radiographic Image Production and Manipulation*. New York, NY: McGraw-Hill; 2003.)

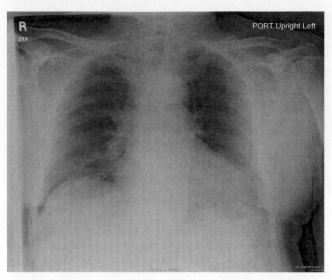

Figure 13-10. If the direction of the lead strips and the grid lines per inch/grid frequency matches the scan frequency of the scanner/reader, the "aliasing" artifact can occur. (Photo contributor: Stamford Hospital, Department of Radiology.)

the scanner/reader, this artifact can occur (Fig. 13-10). Aliasing appears as superimposed images slightly out of alignment, an image "wrapping" effect. This most commonly occurs in mobile radiography with stationary grids and can be a problem with digital radiography (DR) flat-panel detectors (FPDs). Aliasing can also occur when sampling frequency is insufficient/less than twice the bandwidth of the input signal. Use of high-frequency (HF) grids is recommended in digital imaging.

Recent development of Virtual Grid technology demonstrates the ability to obtain quality images without the use of traditional grids (Fig. 13-11). This technology reduces patient dose and can be particularly useful in emergency and mobile imaging.

Image *fading* occurs if there is a delay in reading the PSP. After a time, trapped photoelectrons are released from the "color center" and are therefore unable to participate in PSL. PSL intensity *decreases* in the interval between x-ray exposure and the image-reading process. If the exposed PSL is not delivered to the reader/processor for 8 h, PSL

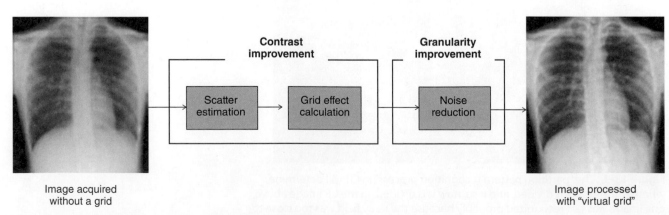

Image acquired without a grid

Contrast improvement

Scatter estimation → Grid effect calculation

Granularity improvement

Noise reduction

Image processed with "virtual grid"

Figure 13-11. Virtual Grid technology provides quality images without the use of traditional grids and with significant reduction in patient dose. (Photo contributor: FUJIFILM Healthcare Americas Corp.)

decreases by approximately 25%. Fading also increases as environmental temperature increases.

PSP storage plates are very sensitive (10× more than film emulsion) to not only x-rays but also ultraviolet, gamma, and particulate radiations. Environmental conditions are therefore an important consideration in their storage. Building materials such as concrete, marble, and others constantly emit natural radiation; bedrock in some geographic areas contributes significantly to background radiation. If PSPs are stored for extended periods of time, the possibility of artifacts must be considered. These artifacts typically appear as randomly placed small black spots. *If an IP and its PSP storage plate have been stored, unused, for 48 h or more, the PSP storage plate should be erased prior to use.*

The mechanical consistency and accuracy of the laser optics and transport systems of the CR scanner/reader are extremely important for image quality—inconsistent scanning motion can result in a wavy, or otherwise distorted, image. This is sometimes called *laser jitter* and should be evaluated monthly as part of the CR quality assurance (QA) monitoring.

Summary

- The IP functions to protect the PSP within.
- The active ingredient within the PSP is $BaF:Eu^{2+}$.
- X-ray photons interact with $BaF:Eu^{2+}$ crystals; a small amount of visible light is emitted, but most of the x-ray energy is stored as the latent image.
- PSL is released by phosphors on stimulation by monochromatic laser light.
- PSL is collected by the PMT or PD and converted to electrical signals.
- PSL is converted to an electrical signal and transferred to the ADC; digital data are then transferred to DAC.
- Image fading can occur if the PSP is not processed promptly.
- CR enables image manipulation after exposure (postprocessing).
- "Windowing" changes image contrast and/or brightness.

Image Processing

The polyenergetic x-ray beam is captured very efficiently by the digital receptors. However, the range of x-ray photons is so large that *raw images* are unclear and require digital processing to be of diagnostic quality. X-ray photons are converted to electrical signals, which are then available for processing and postprocessing. Digital processing permits visualization of an infinite number of tissue densities captured by the digital detector. According to the Nyquist theorem, when the electric signals are sampled for conversion to a digital image, the sampling frequency must be more than twice the frequency of the input signal to best duplicate that original signal. This assures that the image will be as close to the original signal as possible and that it will be of the highest quality, even if some data are lost along the image creation process. At least twice the number of pixels required to form the image must be sampled, or the resolution will be compromised.

Exposure/Image Data Recognition

The CR reader scans the entire PSP and identifies and analyzes the region(s) of interest (ROI). It can separately analyze ROIs when more than one exposure is made to a single PSP. This is most typical in extremity imaging, and the process is termed *exposure field recognition, partition pattern recognition, or segmentation*. The scanner/reader distinguishes the number and orientation of images by identifying their collimated borders and analyzing only that exposure within the borders. For the best results, collimated borders should be sharp and well defined. This ensures that unnecessary information outside the collimated edges, such as scatter, will be eliminated from the histogram analysis. If the PSP is analyzed incorrectly, the ensuing histogram would be skewed and the resulting image far from optimum.

Other common conditions that can cause failure of exposure field recognition are poor or overlapping collimation (Fig. 13-12), SR (especially from adjacent field), and metallic bodies such as prostheses.

Common Causes for Exposure Field Recognition Failure

Nondefined collimation borders

Overlapping collimation

Scatter radiation

Metallic bodies

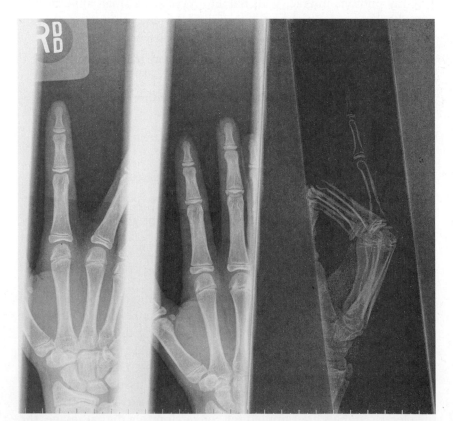

Figure 13-12. The "partition pattern recognition process" in CR will determine whether the image is divided, and if so, how it is divided. In the CR image above, one image was not recognized. (Reproduced with permission from Shephard CT. *Radiographic Image Production and Manipulation.* New York, NY: McGraw-Hill; 2003.)

Histograms and Lookup Tables

In digital imaging, there are numerous *brightness and tonal values* that represent various *tissue densities*, for example, bone, muscle, fat, blood-filled organs, air/gas, metal, contrast media, and pathologic processes. The CR scanner/reader recognizes all these values and constructs a representative grayscale *histogram* of them, corresponding to the anatomic characteristics of the programmed part. Thus, all posteroanterior (PA) chest histograms are similar, all lateral chest histograms are similar, all pelvis histograms are similar, and so on.

A histogram itself does not illustrate the anatomic part, if it is positioned correctly or if the image has good resolution. But it does provide information about the tonal values of the pixels within the image—blacks are to the left, whites are to the right. Think of it as being similar to a bar graph that plots the number of each pixel value for the radiographic image, allowing it to be displayed properly. In a *narrow* histogram, the blacks from the left and the whites from the right are squeezed to the center of the histogram, resulting in a very gray *low-contrast* image. In a *wide* histogram, the mid-histogram gray pixels have moved laterally toward the blacks and whites, resulting in a *higher contrast* image. In an image having *low brightness* (dark), the histogram pixels have shifted to the left and the histogram becomes somewhat narrower. In an image having *high brightness* (light), the histogram pixels have shifted to the right and the histogram becomes somewhat wider.

A histogram is a *graphic representation* of pixel value distribution (Fig. 13-13B and C). The histogram is an analysis and graphic representation of all the information from the PSP screen, demonstrating the quantity of exposure, the number of pixels, and their value. Histograms are unique to each body part imaged. Over time, if required diagnostic image characteristics change, the default histogram can be updated to reflect the latest required characteristics.

In anatomically programmed radiography (APR), the radiographer selects a *processing algorithm* by selecting the anatomic part and particular projection on the computer/control panel. After a part is exposed/imaged, its PSP is read/scanned and its own histogram is developed and analyzed. The resulting analysis, and histogram of the *actual* imaged part, is compared with the *programmed* representative histogram for that part.

If the incorrect anatomical part/menu is selected, histogram analysis will be faulty and the resulting image will be unsatisfactory. Figure 13-3 illustrates this effect. Often, an incorrectly applied part/menu can be switched to the correct part/menu during or after image preview. However, the results can vary depending on the equipment manufacturer. Sometimes, the selected new menu will be applied to the original raw data (best results); other manufacturers apply on top of the originally incorrect menu (less optimal results).

The CR unit then matches that information with a particular *lookup table* (LUT)—a "characteristic curve" that best matches the anatomic part being imaged; it identifies each of the tonal values and their distribution in the x-ray image. Permanent LUTs function to manipulate grayscale values to provide the appropriate grayscale rendition. The observer is able to review the image and, if desired, change its appearance (through "windowing"); postprocessing changes the variable LUT.

CR Resolution Increases As

- PSP size decreases
- Laser beam size decreases
- Monitor matrix size increases

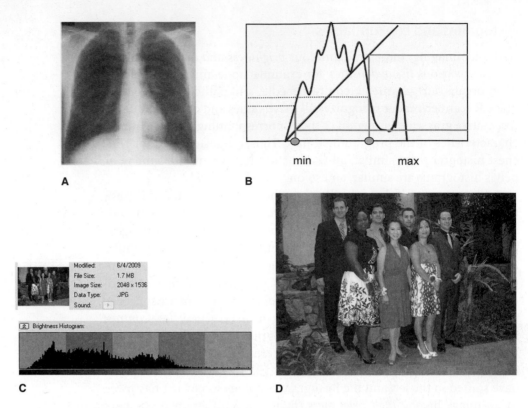

Figure 13-13. PA chest **(A)** and its histogram **(B)**; a graphic representation illustrating the distribution of pixel values. (Photo contributor: FUJIFILM Healthcare Americas Corp.) Many digital cameras nowadays can also display the histogram distribution **(C)** of pixel values, for example, for typical graduation photographs **(D)**. (Photo contributor: Christina Cheong, RT(R)(M).)

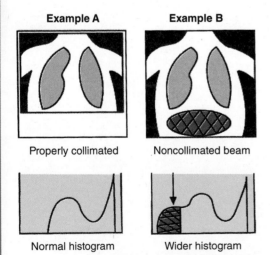

Figure 13-14. Average exposure level and exposure latitude in image B has changed as a result of poor collimation. This will be reflected in the image informational numbers (e.g., "S number," "EI"). Other factors affecting histogram appearance include selection of the processing algorithm, any changes in SR, SID, OID, in addition to beam restriction. (Photo contributor: Courtesy of FUJIFILM Medical System USA.)

Hence, *histogram analysis* and use of the appropriate *LUT* together function to produce predictable image quality in CR.

It is important to note that *histogram appearance* and *patient dose* can be affected by the radiographers' knowledge and skill by using digital imaging, in addition to their degree of accuracy in *positioning* and *centering*. Beam restriction is exceedingly important to avoid *histogram analysis errors*. Lack of adequate collimation can result in signals outside the anatomic area being included in the exposure data recognition (EDR)/histogram analysis. This can result in a variety of histogram analysis errors including excessively light, dark, or noisy images.

As seen in Figure 13-14, because of poor collimation, the average exposure level and exposure latitude have changed; these changes are reflected in the images' *exposure indicator* numbers ("S number," "EI," etc.). Other factors affecting histogram appearance, and therefore these exposure indicator factors, include selection of the *correct processing algorithm* (e.g., chest vs. femur vs. cervical spine), changes in *scatter*, *source-to-image-receptor distance* (SID), *object-to-image-receptor distance* (OID), and *collimation*—in short, anything that affects scatter and/or dose. One other factor is *delay in processing* from time of exposure. Delay in processing can result in *fading* of the image. Normal examination times and short delays between projections are generally not a problem.

The image seen on the monitor, then, is the "default" image—one that has been obtained by using parameters that have been prescribed consistent with department preferences.

Automatic Rescaling

Digital imaging *EDR* and *automatic rescaling* offer wide latitude and automatic optimization of the radiologic image. Automatic rescaling compensates for too little/too great an exposure. EDR, by using the selected processing algorithm and its LUT, enables compensation for approximately 80% underexposure and 500% overexposure. Although automatic/computerized optimization of the radiologic image is a wonderful tool, radiographers must be even more aware of their role in keeping the patient dose to a minimum.

Postprocessing/Image Manipulation

Postprocessing is the ability to *manipulate the image after exposure*. Among other things, image manipulation postprocessing can be used for *grayscale/contrast* modification via *windowing*. The window *width* controls the shades of gray, whereas the window *level* corresponds to the *brightness* (Fig. 13-15). Narrower windows result in higher (shorter

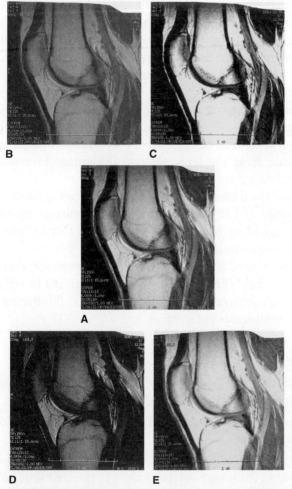

Figure 13-15. Changes in *window width* and *window level*. Image **A** (*center*) has a window width of 1810 and window level of 761. In image **B,** the window width is increased to 4174. In image **C,** the window width is decreased to 732, leaving the window level unchanged. The changes in image *gray scale* are evident. Next, images **D** and **E** are compared with image **A**. In image **D,** the window level is increased to 1497. In image **E,** it is decreased to 325. This time the changes in image *brightness* are obvious.

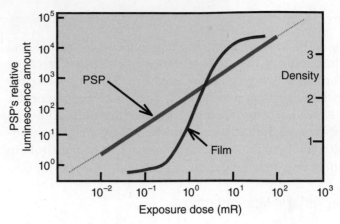

Figure 13-16. Illustration of *wide dynamic range* (scale of contrast) afforded by PSP (compared to film emulsion) enabling detection of slight differences in x-ray absorption characteristics among various tissue densities. (Courtesy of FUJIFILM Medical System USA.)

scale) contrast. Pixel values *below* the window range will be displayed as *black,* whereas pixel values *above* the window range will be displayed as *white.* Pixel values between the two limits are spread over the full scale of gray. The radiographer must keep dose reduction in mind. The *same* technical factors as those selected manually, *or less,* are generally recommended for CR/DR.

Therefore, windowing and other postprocessing mechanisms permit the radiographer to effect changes in the image and produce "special effects" such as *contrast enhancement, edge enhancement, image stitching* (for anatomic areas too large for one IR), image inversion, rotation, reversal, and image annotation.

Because of the digital system's automatic rescaling function and wide dynamic range of PSP (Fig. 13-16), overexposure of up to 500% and underexposure of up to 80% (due to technical factors) are reported as recoverable, thus eliminating most retakes.

Shuttering is used to remove the bright unexposed areas outside of the collimated field (Fig. 13-17A–D) that contribute to *veil glare.* Glare interferes with accurate perception of details. Shuttering is *never* a substitute for adequate collimation.

Digital Imaging

- Brightness changes with changes in window *level.*
- Contrast changes with changes in window *width.*
- It has wide dynamic range/latitude.
- Fading can occur with delayed CR processing.
- CR IPs are very sensitive to x-ray and background radiation fog.

Summary

- X-ray photons are converted to electrical signals and available for processing and postprocessing.
- To ensure correct PSP analysis, collimated borders should be sharp and well defined.
- A histogram provides information about the tonal values of the pixels within the image corresponding to the anatomic characteristics of the selected part.
- A histogram is a *graphic representation* defining all the grayscale values of a particular image.
- A *processing algorithm* is selected when the radiographer selects the part and projection on the computer.

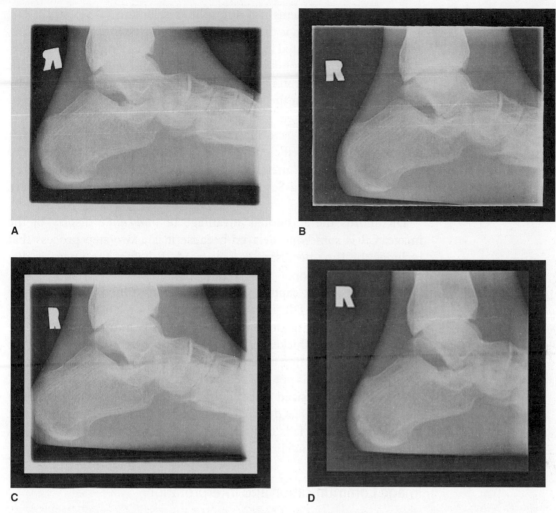

Figure 13-17. **(A)** A lateral calcaneus with collimation and no masking. **(B)** The use of automask feature. **(C)** The use of automask feature with added collimation to indicate its use. **(D)** The use of manual masking with no evidence of collimation.

- An LUT matches the anatomic part being imaged and functions to manipulate grayscale values to provide the appropriate grayscale rendition.
- *Histogram analysis* and the appropriate *LUT* together function to produce predictable image quality in CR.
- Windowing, edge enhancement, and other features are available as postprocessing functions.

Digital Radiography

The PSP is the x-ray photon receptor/detector in *CR* systems. *DR* systems do not use PSPs; DR systems are *direct-* or *indirect*-capture and conversion systems of x-ray imaging. DR uses solid-state detector plates (FPDs) as the x-ray image detector to intercept the x-ray beam.

Indirect-capture systems are FPDs that use thin-film transistors (TFTs) or charge couple devices (CCDs). Both indirect-capture systems involve *scintillation*. One type of indirect-capture FPD systems uses CsI or Gd_2O_2S as the *scintillator*. The scintillator captures x-ray photons and emits light. That light is then recorded via a CCD *or* TFT.

Direct-capture systems use amorphous selenium (a-Se) and TFTs. a-Se, a semiconductor, is the x-ray photon detector. On x-ray exposure, x-ray energy is converted to an electrical signal in a single layer of material such as the semiconductor a-Se. Electric voltage is applied to both surfaces of a-Se, electron hole pairs are created, and charges are read by TFT arrays located on the surfaces. The electrical signal is transferred directly to the ADC.

Systems *without* a scintillation/light conversion step have *higher* detective quantum efficiency (DQE), with the exception of the new complementary metal oxide semiconductor (*CMOS*) capture systems. In general, a-Se TFTs used in direct-capture systems have the highest DQE.

DR affords the additional advantage of *immediate* display of the image; CR is somewhat delayed because it is a two-step process that includes the time necessary to scan/read IP before the image is displayed on the monitor.

Thus, the direct-capture system *eliminates the scintillator step* required in indirect DR. Because selenium has a relatively low *Z* number (compared with gadolinium [*Z* = 64] or cesium [*Z* = 55]), a-Se detectors are made thicker to *improve detection,* thus compensating for the low x-ray absorption of selenium. There is no diffusion of electrons, so *spatial resolution* is not affected in this manner.

It must be emphasized that although the biggest advantage of digital/electronic imaging is its *dynamic range,* patient overexposure can result if the radiographer fails to keep technical factors within the system's recommended EI/guidelines.

Image Communication and Interpretation

The quantity of patient information and diagnostic image data stored by hospitals is ever increasing. It is essential that this information be stored, managed, and utilized efficiently. *Hospital information system* (HIS) networks allow the archiving and distribution of vast amounts of image information from all modalities, managing it all with a single system. *Radiology information system* (RIS) centrally processes and stores image data within a hospital, enabling image retrieval from the server by any department over the hospital network, and display image at the requesting department's *modality work list (MWL).* Using a *picture archiving and communications system* (PACS) and *teleradiology,* digital images can be sent anywhere there is an equipment to receive and display them. The FDA recently announced that PACS will now be calleds medical image management and processing systems (MIMPS); https://www.intelerad.com/en/2021/04/29/pacs-are-now-mimps-says-the-fda/. Effective operation of these systems requires designated standards for image and data communication exchange. These standards are provided by Digital Imaging and COmmunications in Medicine (DICOM) and Health Level 7 (HL7) to ensure compatibility and security.

DICOM is a universally accepted, standard network protocol that allows for the sharing of imaging data between different types of diagnostic machines. This is incredibly important in the health care setting where there are multiple modalities attempting to use the same

---

DR affords the advantage of *immediate* display of the image; CR is somewhat delayed because it is a two-step process.

- CR:

  Two-step process

  Delayed image display

- DR:

  One-step process

  Immediate image display

Information Found in the HIS and RIS

HIS: holds information related to the patient's all-around medical care

- Hospital billing
- Inpatient ordering system
- Treatment information

RIS: holds information related to the imaging department

- Imaging history
- Radiology scheduling information
- Radiologist's reports

PACS/MIMPS network. HL7 is a protocol that facilitates communication between both the HIS and RIS, defining what relevant patient information can be shared and used in the creation of digital images.

Interpretation of digital images can be made from the display monitor (softcopy display). In addition, "hardcopies" can be made on a film by using a laser printer. A *laser camera* records the displayed image by exposing a film with laser light; it can also record several images on one film. The laser printer is connected for immediate processing of the images.

Summary

- Digital FPD can be either a direct or indirect system.
- Indirect-capture FPDs use TFTs or CCDs and involve *scintillation*.
- Direct-capture systems use a-Se and TFTs; a-Se, a semiconductor, is the x-ray photon detector.
- Voltage is applied to the a-Se surfaces; the resulting charges are read by TFT arrays, and the electrical signal is transferred to the ADC.
- Systems without a scintillation/light conversion step have a higher DQE.
- By using PACS/MIMPS and *teleradiology,* digital images can be sent anywhere there is an equipment to receive and display them.
- "Hardcopies" can be made on (single emulsion) films by using a laser printer.
- Standards to ensure compatibility and security of image and data communication exchange are provided by DICOM and HL7.

COMPREHENSION CHECK

1. What is the function of the IP (p. 382)?

2. What phosphor is most often used for PSPs in computed radiography? What is the term used to describe the light released by these phosphors on x-ray absorption (p. 383)?

3. What is the difference between turbid and columnar phosphors? How is it related to resolution (p. 384)?

4. How is the exposed PSP "read" (p. 384)?

5. What kind of laser is used to stimulate the PSP (p. 383)?

6. What is the purpose of the optical filter (p. 384)?

7. What is the value of postprocessing (p. 385)?

8. What is image *fading*? How can it be avoided (p. 385, 389)?

9. Why should PSPs be erased prior to use if they have been unused for an extended period of time (p. 384, 385)?

10. Cite the differences between indirect and direct DR (p. 395).

11. What are the two indirect digital methods; describe each (p. 395).

12. Which device functions to transfer the x-ray image from the PSP screen to the display monitor (p. 384)?

13. What does a histogram represent in CR (p. 390, 391)?

14. What is the purpose of an LUT in CR (p. 391, 392)?

15. How does the radiographer select a processing algorithm (p. 391)?

16. What is windowing? What does a change in window width and/or window level affect (p. 393)?

17. What can change the appearance of the histogram and therefore affect its analysis (p. 390)?

18. In what two ways can a CR reader identify and analyze multiple images on one PSP (p. 390)?

19. What two systems currently provide standards that ensure compatibility and security of PACS/MIMPS and teleradiology systems (p. 396)?

20. What system is used to send digital images anywhere there is equipment available to receive and display them (p. 396)?

21. What device is used to make "hardcopies" of images seen on display monitors (p. 397)?

22. Describe the difference between primary and secondary excitation of barium fluorohalide phosphors (p. 383).

23. Identify the cause of PSP fading (p. 385, 388, 389).

24. List types of postprocessing functions (p. 384, 385, 394).

25. Describe the appearance and cause of aliasing artifact (p. 386, 388).

26. Differentiate between the various layers of the PSP based on function (p. 383, 384).

27. What are some common image artifacts encountered in PSP systems (p. 386, 388, 389)?

CHAPTER REVIEW QUESTIONS

1. For medicolegal reasons, radiographic images are required to include all the following information, *except*

   (A) the patient's name and/or identification number

   (B) the patient's birth date

   (C) a right- or left-side marker

   (D) the date of the examination

2. The component of a CR IP that records the radiologic image is the

   (A) emulsion

   (B) helium–neon laser

   (C) photostimulable phosphor

   (D) scanner–reader

3. If a PSP has been stored, unused, for 48 h or more, it should be erased prior to use to avoid

   (A) phantom image formation

   (B) image fog

   (C) aliasing artifact

   (D) image distortion

4. Factors that can affect histogram appearance include

   1. beam restriction

   2. centering errors

   3. incorrect SID

   (A) 1 only

   (B) 1 and 2 only

   (C) 2 and 3 only

   (D) 1, 2, and 3

5. By adjusting the window width of a digital image, the technologist would be changing

   (A) spatial resolution

   (B) contrast

   (C) pixel size

   (D) matrix size

6. The main difference between the *direct*-capture and *indirect*-capture DR is that

   (A) direct capture/conversion has no scintillator

   (B) direct capture/conversion uses a PSP

   (C) in direct capture/conversion, light is detected by CCDs

   (D) in direct capture/conversion, light is detected by TFTs

7. What feature is used to display RIS information about current patients?

   (A) HIS

   (B) MWL

   (C) PACS/MIMPS

   (D) DICOM

8. The x-ray photon detector in direct-capture systems is

   1. a semiconductor

   2. a-Se

   3. CsI

   (A) 1 only

   (B) 1 and 2 only

   (C) 2 and 3 only

   (D) 1, 2, and 3

9. The *processing algorithm* has its own predetermined histogram that is representative of the

   (A) pixel value distribution of the exposure

   (B) anatomic part and projection

   (C) image gray scale

   (D) pixel size

10. The function of *shuttering* is to

    (A) remove bright, unexposed areas outside collimated field

    (B) prevent overexposure

    (C) prevent underexposure

    (D) substitute for, or supplement, collimation

11. Which of the following are considered benefits of increased collimation, or beam restriction?

    1. Reduction in histogram analysis errors

    2. Reduction in image fog caused by scatter radiation

    3. Reduction in patient dose

    (A) 1 only

    (B) 2 only

    (C) 2 and 3 only

    (D) 1, 2, and 3

12. Which layer of the PSP is responsible for directing emitted light toward the CR reader?

    (A) Protective layer

    (B) Lead foil

    (C) Reflective layer

    (D) Antistatic layer

Answers and Explanations

1. (B) Every radiographic image *must* include (1) the patient's name or ID number; (2) the side marker, right or left; (3) the date of the examination; and (4) the identity of the institution or office. Additional information *may* be included: the patient's birth date or age, name of the attending physician, and the time of day. When multiple examinations (e.g., chest examinations or small bowel images) of a patient are carried out on the same day, it becomes crucial that the time the radiographs were taken be included on the image. This allows the physician to track the patient's progress.

2. (C) Inside the IP is the *photostimulable phosphor* (*PSP*). This PSP (or SPS—storage phosphor screen), with its layer of europium-activated barium fluorohalide, serves as the IR because it is exposed in the traditional manner and receives the latent image. The PSP can *store* the latent image for several hours; after about 8 h, noticeable image fading will occur. Once the IP is placed into the CR processor (*scanner* or *reader*), the PSP plate is removed automatically. The latent image on the PSP is changed to a manifest image as it is scanned by a narrow, high-intensity *helium–neon laser* to obtain the pixel data. As the PSP is scanned in the reader, it releases a violet light—a process called *PSL*.

3. (B) PSP storage plates are very sensitive to not only x-rays but also ultraviolet, gamma, and particulate radiations. Building materials such as concrete, marble, and others constantly emit natural radiation; bedrock in some geographic areas contributes significantly to background radiation. If PSPs are stored for extended periods of time, the possibility of artifacts must be considered. These artifacts typically appear as randomly placed small black spots. If an IP and its PSP storage plate have been stored, unused, for 48 h or more, the PSP should be erased prior to use.

Aliasing artifact can occur if a grid's lead strip pattern (i.e., frequency) matches the scanning (sampling) pattern of the scanner/reader. Phantom image artifacts are a result of incomplete erasure of a previous image on that PSP. Image fading occurs if an exposed PSP has been left several hours without processing and usually affects the entire image.

4. (D) Numerous *tonal values* represent various *tissue densities* (i.e., x-ray attenuation properties), for example, bone, muscle, fat, blood-filled organs, air/gas, metal, contrast media, and pathologic processes. The CR scanner/reader recognizes these values and constructs a representative *grayscale* histogram of them, corresponding to the *anatomic characteristics of the imaged part*.

A histogram is a *graphic representation* of *pixel value distribution*. The histogram is an analysis and graphic representation of all the PSP information, demonstrating the quantity of exposure, the number of pixels, and their value. Histograms are *unique to each body part* imaged.

Histogram appearance and *patient dose* can be affected by radiographers' knowledge and skill by using digital imaging, in addition to their degree of accuracy in *positioning* and *centering*. Collimation is exceedingly important to avoid *histogram analysis errors*. Lack of adequate collimation can result in signals outside the anatomic area being included in the EDR/histogram analysis.

Other factors affecting histogram appearance include selection of the *correct processing algorithm* (e.g., chest vs. femur vs. cervical spine), changes in *scatter, SID, OID*, and *collimation*—that is, anything that affects scatter and/or dose.

5. (B) The digital image's *scale of contrast* (*contrast resolution*) and brightness can be changed electronically through leveling and windowing of the image. The *level control* determines the *mid-brightness*, whereas the *window control* determines the *total number* of grays (to the right and left of the central/mid-brightness). Matrix and pixel sizes are related to (spatial) resolution of digital images.

6. (A) One type of *indirect*-capture FPD uses CsI or Gd_2O_2S as the *scintillator*, that is, which captures x-ray photons and emits light. That light is then transferred via a photodetector coupling agent—a CCD or TFT. In *direct*-capture FPD systems, x-ray energy is converted to an electrical signal in a single layer of material such as the semiconductor a-Se. Electric charges are applied to both surfaces of a-Se, electron–hole pairs are created, and charges are read by TFT arrays located on the surfaces. The electrical signal is transferred directly to the ADC. The number of TFTs is equal to the number of image pixels.

Thus, the direct-capture system *eliminates the scintillator* step required in indirect DR. Because selenium has a relatively low Z number (compared with gadolinium [Z = 64] or cesium [Z = 55]), a-Se detectors are made thicker to improve detection, thus compensating for the low x-ray absorption of selenium. There is no diffusion of electrons, so spatial resolution is not affected in this manner.

7. (B) Patient demographic and examination information originates from the hospital/facility HIS, where it is obtained when the patient is initially registered and accessible later as needed. Typical patient information includes name, DOB or age, sex, ID number, accession number, examination being performed, date, and time of examination.

A feature that is useful in sorting examinations and decreasing (but not eliminating) errors is the *modality work list* (*MWL*). The MWL "brings up" existing RIS information, that is, the examinations scheduled for each imaging modality. The technologist selects the correct patient, which includes that patient's particular demographics, from the particular MWL.

PACS/MIMPS is used by health care facilities to economically store, archive, exchange, transmit digital images from multiple imaging modalities; it replaces the need to manually file, retrieve, and transport film and film jackets.

RIS and HIS can be integrated with PACS/MIMPS for electronic health information storage. The purpose of HIS is to manage health care information and documents electronically and to ensure data security and availability. RIS is a system for tracking radiologic and imaging procedures. RIS is used for patient registration and scheduling, radiology workflow management, reporting and printout, manipulation and distribution and tracking of patient data, and billing. RIS complements HIS and is critical to competent workflow of radiologic facilities.

8. (B) One type of *indirect*-capture FPD uses CsI or Gd_2O_2S as the *scintillator,* that is, which captures x-ray photons and emits light. That light is then transferred via a photodetector coupling agent—a CCD or TFT. In *direct*-capture FPD systems, x-ray energy is converted to an electrical signal in a single layer of material such as the *semiconductor a-Se*. Electric charges are applied to both surfaces of a-Se and charges are read by TFT arrays. The electrical signal is transferred directly to the ADC. The direct-capture system *eliminates the scintillator* step required in indirect DR.

9. (B) The radiographer selects a *processing algorithm* by selecting the anatomic part and particular projection on the computer/control panel. The CR unit then matches that information with a particular LUT—a characteristic curve that best matches the anatomic part being imaged. This information is then compared to the values from the incoming exposure and the image is rescaled. The observer is able to review the image and, if desired, change its appearance (through "windowing"); doing so changes the LUT. Hence, histogram analysis and use of the appropriate LUT together function to produce predictable image quality in CR.

10. (A) *Shuttering* is used to remove the bright, unexposed areas outside of the collimated field that contribute to *veil glare*. Glare interferes with accurate perception of details. Shuttering is *never* a substitute for adequate collimation. Because it is occurring after an exposure has occurred, it will have no bearing on the patient dose.

11. (D) Collimation, or beam restriction, has many benefits to both the patient and the quality of a digital image. Increased collimation reduces exposure to the tissues surrounding the anatomical part of interest, thus reducing the number of opportunities for the radiographic beam to scatter. This means fewer of these low-energy scattered photons will be absorbed by the patient or reach the image receptor. Scattered photons add unwanted signals that are outside of the required range, causing histogram analysis errors and radiographic fog.

12. (C) Because visible light travels in many directions, it can be easy to lose valuable diagnostic information during the readout of a PSP. The reflective layer aids in the processing of the PSP by directing the emitted light from the emulsion layer toward the CR reader. The antistatic layer absorbs static discharge from adjacent CR reader components preventing unwanted artifact on the image. The lead foil absorbs backscatter photons from the incident x-ray beam that penetrate through the PSP and ricochet back toward the IP. The protective layer is a special coating that is placed over the barium fluorohalide to give it some rigidity and durability.

RADIOGRAPHIC AND FLUOROSCOPIC EQUIPMENT

Principles of Radiation Physics: X-ray Production

Diagnostic x-rays are produced within the x-ray tube when high-speed *electrons* are rapidly decelerated on encountering the tungsten atoms of the anode. The *source of electrons* is the heated cathode filament; when thousands of volts (kilovolts [kV]) are applied, a potential difference is created within the x-ray tube, driving the electrons across to the anode focal spot. When the high-speed electrons are suddenly stopped at the focal spot, their kinetic energy is converted to x-ray photon energy in one of two ways:

1. *Bremsstrahlung* (brems) or "braking" *radiation:* A high-speed electron, passing near or through a tungsten atom, is attracted and "braked" (i.e., slowed down) by the positively charged nucleus and deflected from its course with a loss of energy. *This energy loss is given up in the form of an x-ray photon* (Fig. 13-18). The electron might not give up all its kinetic energy in one interaction; it can go on to have several more interactions deeper in the anode, each time producing an x-ray photon having less and less energy. This is one reason the x-ray beam is *polyenergetic,* that is, has a *spectrum of energies.* Brems radiation *comprises 70%–90% of the x-ray beam.*

2. *Characteristic radiation:* In this case, a high-speed electron having an energy of at least 70 keV encounters a tungsten atom within the anode and *ejects* a K-shell electron (Fig. 13-19), leaving a vacancy in that shell. An electron from the adjacent L shell moves to the K shell

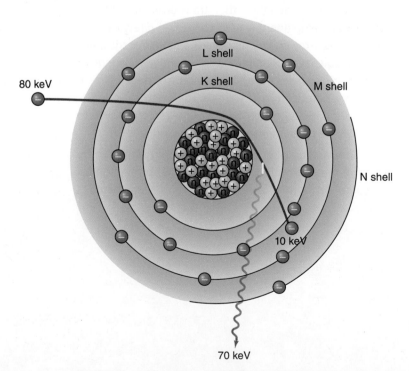

Figure 13-18. Production of bremsstrahlung (brems) radiation. A high-speed electron is deflected from its path, and the loss of kinetic energy is emitted in the form of an x-ray photon.

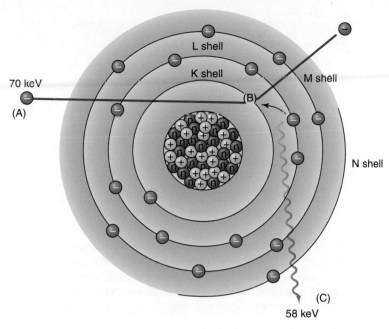

Figure 13-19. Production of characteristic radiation. A high-speed electron (A) ejects a tungsten K-shell electron, leaving a K-shell vacancy (B). An electron from the L shell fills the vacancy and emits a K-characteristic ray (C).

to fill its vacancy, and in doing so *emits a K-characteristic ray*. The *energy* of the characteristic ray is equal to the *difference in energy between the K- and L-shell energy levels.*

X-ray Beam

Frequency and Wavelength. All *electromagnetic radiations*, including x-rays, can be described as wave-like fluctuations of electric and magnetic fields (Fig. 13-20). Figure 13-20 illustrates that visible light, microwaves, and radio waves, as well as x-rays and gamma rays, are all part of the *electromagnetic spectrum*. All electromagnetic radiations have the same *velocity*, 186,000 miles per second (3×10^8 m/s); however, they differ greatly in *wavelength*.

> **X-ray Production**
>
> • Brems (70%–90%)
> • Characteristic (10%–30%)

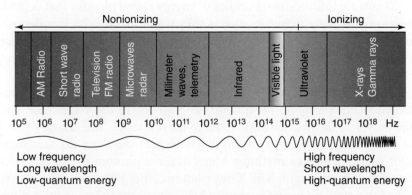

Figure 13-20. The electromagnetic spectrum. Frequency and photon energy are *directly* related; frequency and photon energy are *inversely* related to wavelength.

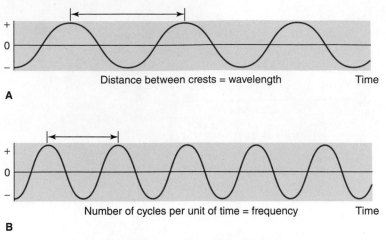

Figure 13-21. Wavelength **(A)** versus frequency **(B)**. *Wavelength* is described as the distance between successive crests. The shorter the wavelength, the more crests or cycles per unit of time (e.g., per second). Therefore, the shorter the wavelength, the greater the *frequency* (number of cycles per second). Wavelength and frequency are *inversely* related.

Wavelength refers to the distance between two consecutive wave crests (Fig. 13-21). *Frequency* refers to the number of cycles per second (cps); its unit of measurement is the *hertz* (Hz), which is equal to 1 cps. Frequency and wavelength are closely associated with the relative *energy* of electromagnetic radiation. More energetic radiations have *shorter wavelength* and *higher frequency*. The relationship among frequency, wavelength, and energy is graphically illustrated by the electromagnetic spectrum.

Beam Characteristics. Some radiations, such as x-rays, are energetic enough to rearrange atoms in materials through which they pass, and they can therefore be hazardous to living tissue. These radiations are called *ionizing* radiation because they have the energetic potential to break apart electrically neutral atoms, resulting in the production of negative and/or positive *ions*. X-ray photons, having the *dual nature* of both particles and electromagnetic waves, are highly energetic ionizing radiation. Diagnostic x-rays are extremely short, between 10^{-8} and 10^{-12} m in wavelength. The unit formerly used for such small dimensions is the angstrom (Å); 1 Å = 10^{-10} m.

X-rays are infinitesimal bundles of energy called *photons* that deposit some of their energy into matter as they travel through it. This deposition of energy, and subsequent *ionization,* has the potential to cause chemical and biological damage. Several of the outstanding properties of x-ray photons are listed in the *summary box*.

The possibility of tissue damage as a result of exposure to x-ray photons depends partly on the *quantity* and *quality* of the x-ray beam and the technical factors that contribute to these factors. The *primary beam* of x-rays refers to the x-ray beam that emerges from the x-ray tube focal spot, before it strikes anything. Many of these photons then encounter the part to be radiographed. X-ray photons emerging from the part are called the *remnant or exit beam* and help contribute in image formation. The principal factor affecting beam *quantity* is milliampere seconds (mAs), whereas the principal factor affecting beam *quality* is kilovoltage

Shorter Wavelength Is Associated With

- Higher frequency (cps)
- Higher energy
- Increased ionizing potential

(kV). Another x-ray beam characteristic is described by the *inverse square law* of radiation. The inverse square law is particularly important in radiation protection considerations and in the selection of technical factors. These factors and many others are thoroughly discussed in Part III, Chapter 12, Image Acquisition and Technical Evaluation and in Part IV, Safety.

Photon Interactions With Matter

The gradual decrease in exposure rate as radiation passes through tissues is called *attenuation*. Attenuation is principally attributable to the two major types of interactions that occur between x-ray photons and tissue in the diagnostic x-ray range of energies.

Photoelectric Effect. In the *photoelectric effect,* a relatively low-energy (low kV) x-ray photon uses all its energy (true/total absorption) to eject an inner shell electron, leaving an orbital vacancy. An electron from the shell above drops down to fill the vacancy and, in doing so, gives up energy in the form of a characteristic ray (Fig. 13-22A).

The photoelectric effect is more likely to occur in absorbers having *high atomic number* (e.g., bone and positive contrast media) and contributes significantly to patient dose, as all the photon energy is absorbed by the patient (and contributes to short-scale contrast in analog imaging).

Compton Scatter. In *Compton scatter,* a fairly *high*-energy (high kV) x-ray photon ejects an *outer shell* electron (Fig. 13-22B). Although the x-ray photon is deflected with somewhat reduced energy (modified scatter), it retains most of its original energy and exits the body as an energetic scattered photon.

Because the scattered photon exits the body, it poses little radiation hazard to the patient. Some internal scatter, however, can contribute to patient dose. Compton scatter contributes to *image fog* and poses *radiation hazards to personnel* (as in fluoroscopic procedures).

X-ray Quantity and Quality

Quantity, or intensity: the number of photons
 • Controlled by mAs

Quality: penetrating power of the photon
 • Controlled by kVp

Properties of X-ray Photons

• X-rays are not perceptible by the senses.
• X-rays travel in straight lines.
• X-rays travel at the speed of light.
• X-rays are electrically neutral.
• X-rays have a penetrating effect on all matter.
• X-rays have a physiological effect on living tissue.
• X-rays have an ionizing effect on air.
• X-rays have a photographic effect on film emulsion.
• X-rays produce fluorescence in certain phosphors.
• X-rays cannot be focused.
• X-rays have a spectrum of energies.

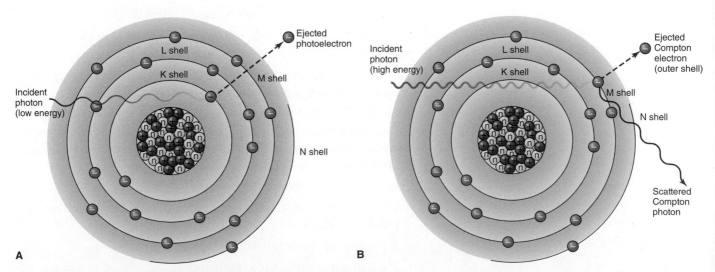

Figure 13-22. (A) In the photoelectric effect, all of the incoming (low-energy) photon's energy is absorbed as it ejects an inner shell electron from orbit. **(B)** In Compton scatter, the incoming (high-energy) photon uses *part* of its energy to eject an outer shell electron; in doing so, the photon changes direction (scatters) but retains much of its original energy.

Coherent (Classical) Scatter. The process of *coherent* scatter is also known as *classical, unmodified,* Rayleigh, or Thomson scatter. This interaction between x-rays and matter occurs with very low energy x-ray photons—energies rarely used in diagnostic radiology. When a very low energy x-ray photon interacts with a single atomic electron (Thomson) or several/all the electrons of a single atom (Rayleigh) of matter, the photon "disappears," as it is absorbed by the atom, and leaving the atom in an excited state. As the atom returns to its normal state, it releases an x-ray photon of *identical* wavelength but travels in a direction different from that of the incident photon (i.e., a *scattered photon*). It is important to note that this is the only interaction between x-ray photons and matter in which *no ionization occurs.*

Tissue Attenuation. The radiologic image is obtained as a result of the attenuation processes occurring in the body. Tissues that are very dense will allow little or no passage of x-rays—those tissues appear white or light on the image. Other tissues are easy for x-ray photons to penetrate—those tissues appear darker.

Sometimes, we use artificial contrast agents to better demonstrate certain parts; depending on the nature of the contrast agent, these parts will look lighter or darker. Some body parts are smaller, whereas others are larger. Various pathologic conditions can alter the nature of the tissues they affect; this can also influence how light or dark the image will be.

All this indicates that the *thickness* or size of body parts, as well as the *atomic number* of the tissue (e.g., bone vs. soft tissue), has a significant influence on photon interactions and therefore attenuation of the x-ray beam by various anatomic tissues.

Summary

- All radiations of the electromagnetic spectrum travel at the *same* velocity, 186,000 miles per second, but *differ* in wavelength.
- Wavelength is the distance between two consecutive wave crests.
- The number of cycles and crests per second is frequency; its unit of measure is Hz.
- Wavelength and frequency are inversely related.
- Ionization is caused by high-energy, short-wavelength electromagnetic radiation that breaks apart electrically neutral atoms.
- Two types of x-rays are produced at the anode through energy conversion processes: brems radiation and characteristic radiation; brems radiation predominates.
- X-rays can interact with tissue cells and cause ionization; interactions between x-rays and tissue cells are the photoelectric effect, Compton scatter, and coherent (classical) scatter.
- Characteristics of photoelectric effect:
  - Low-energy x-ray photon gives up all its energy, ejecting an inner shell electron.
  - It produces a characteristic ray (secondary radiation).
  - It is a major contributor to patient dose.
  - It occurs in absorbers having high atomic number and mass density.

- Characteristics of Compton scatter:
  - It predominates in the diagnostic x-ray range.
  - High-energy x-ray photon uses a portion of its energy to eject an outer shell electron.
  - It is responsible for SR fog to the image.
  - It poses radiation hazards to personnel and to patients as internal scatter.
- Characteristics of coherent scatter:
  - Very low energy x-ray photon interacts with the atom, disappears, and sets the atom into an excited state.
  - As the atom returns to a normal state, an identical photon is emitted but in a different direction.
  - This is the only interaction that does not cause ionization.
- Contributors to exposure dose are beam attenuation and the type of interaction. Exposure dose is, therefore, impacted by radiation quality (kV) and the subject being irradiated (i.e., thickness and nature of part; atomic number of part).

TYPES OF EQUIPMENT

The various kinds of x-ray machines are generally named according to the x-ray energy they produce or the specific purpose(s) for which they are designed, for example, mammographic unit, tomographic equipment, mobile unit, 150-kV chest unit, 1200-mA (milliampere) general diagnostic unit, digital fluoroscopy (DF), DR and fluoroscopy (R/F), or CR.

Fixed

Most x-ray equipment is *fixed* or stationary, that is, it is installed in a particular place and cannot be moved. Most general radiographic and fluoroscopic (RF) equipment in the radiology/imaging department is fixed. Fixed equipment will have an x-ray table that is either the *stationary*/pedestal type or the *floating* type. A tilting RF tabletop is necessary for many types of x-ray examinations, especially fluoroscopy. Typically, the tabletop will move 30° Trendelenburg and 90° vertically; footboard and shoulder support accessories are used with the tilting tabletop. Current tilting tabletops are also very useful for patients with limited mobility (Fig. 13-23). Adjustable height is an optional feature especially helpful for the patient and the radiographer. The x-ray tube support can be wall-mounted, floor-mounted, or suspended overhead. Fixed interventional equipment is conducive to C-arm configuration.

Mobile

Mobile x-ray equipment is designed to be transported to the patients who are unable to travel to the radiology/imaging department, for example, the very ill, incapacitated patients, and patients in surgery or

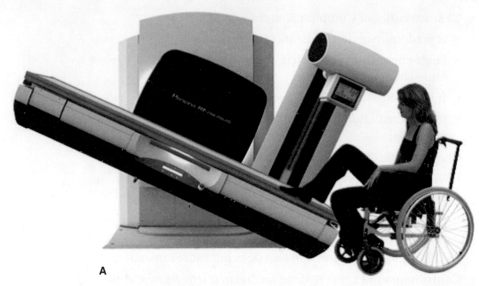

A

Figure 13-23. (A) A tilting tabletop is necessary for many types of x-ray examinations, especially fluoroscopy. RF tabletops typically move 30° Trendelenburg and 90° vertically. Tilting tabletops are also useful for patients with limited mobility. (FUJIFILM Healthcare Americas Corp.)

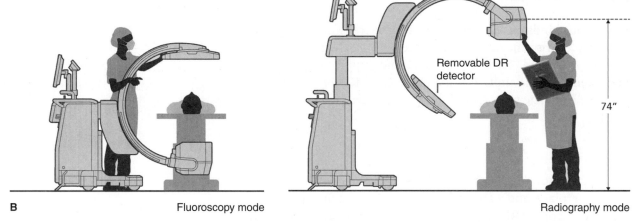

B   Fluoroscopy mode   Radiography mode

Removable DR detector

74"

Figure 13-23. (B) Some mobile equipment can function in radiographic and/or fluoroscopic mode. (FUJIFILM Healthcare Americas Corp.)

---

isolation. Mobile equipment is available for radiographic and/or fluoroscopic x-ray procedures (see Fig. 13-23B). Mobile equipment operates on rechargeable batteries with HF output. Immediate image display is possible via FPD systems and built-in monitors. Detectors can be either tethered or the wireless type.

Dedicated

X-ray equipment that is designed for a specific purpose or type of examination is called *dedicated equipment*. Examples of dedicated equipment are mammography equipment, chest units, bone densitometry equipment, and dental x-ray units.

Generators

- Change mechanical energy to electrical energy

Motors

- Change electrical energy to mechanical energy

ELECTRICITY, X-RAY TRANSFORMERS, AND RECTIFIERS

Alternating Current

A basic understanding of magnetism and electricity is fundamental to the study of x-ray equipment. The relationship between magnetism and electricity is central to the operation of many x-ray circuit components; therefore, it is important to review these concepts before reviewing x-ray circuit components.

Generators function to change mechanical energy to electrical energy (whereas *motors* convert electrical energy to mechanical energy). Electrical current flowing through a conductor in only one direction and with constant magnitude is called *direct current* (DC); a familiar source of DC is the *battery*.

Electricity is more efficiently transported over long distances at low-current and high-voltage values to avoid excessive power loss (according to the power, or heat loss formula: $P = I^2R$). Most applications of electricity require the use of *alternating current* (AC), in which the amplitude and polarity of the current vary periodically with time (Fig. 13-24).

The HF generator is small in size, in addition to producing an almost constant potential waveform. HF generators first appeared in mobile

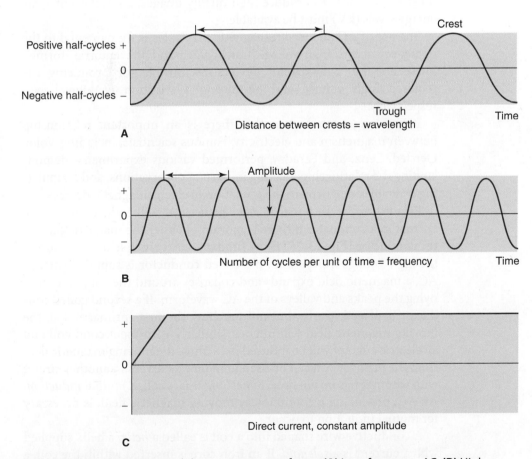

Figure 13-24. Alternating and direct current waveforms. **(A)** Low-frequency AC. **(B)** High-frequency AC. Compare the distance between crests and troughs in image **B** with those in image **A**. **(C)** Direct current, like that supplied by a battery, is characterized by constant amplitude (peak potential).

Alternating Current

- *Amplitude* and *polarity* vary periodically
- *Wavelength:* distance between two consecutive crests; one positive half-cycle and one negative half-cycle
- *Crest:* positive half-cycle peak
- *Trough:* negative half-cycle peak
- *Amplitude:* height of the wave
- *Frequency:* number of cps
- *Hertz:* unit of frequency

x-ray units and were then adopted by mammography and computed tomographic (CT) equipment.

HF generators are favored nowadays for a few reasons. Their compact size makes them popular and the fact that they produce nearly constant potential voltage helps improve image quality and decrease patient dose (fewer low-energy photons to contribute to skin dose).

AC consists of sinusoidal waves. One *wavelength* consists of two half-cycles: a *positive half-cycle* and a *negative half-cycle*. A *wavelength* is defined as the distance between two consecutive *crests*. A *crest* is the positive half-cycle peak, and a *trough* is the negative half-cycle peak. The maximum height of the wave/impulse is called its *amplitude* and represents electrical potential, that is, voltage. *AC is therefore characterized by varying amplitude and periodic reversal of polarity.* The number of cycles per unit of time is called *frequency* (Fig. 13-24), and its unit of measurement is the *hertz* (Hz). In the United States, AC is generated at 60 Hz or cps, that is, 60 cycles (60 positive half-cycles and 60 negative half-cycles) occur each second. One half second, therefore, would include 30 cycles; consequently, four cycles represent a $\frac{4}{60}$- or $\frac{1}{15}$-s time interval.

X-rays are produced when high-speed electrons are suddenly decelerated on encountering the tungsten atoms of the anode. To produce x-rays of diagnostic value, high voltage (thousands of volts, i.e., kV) must be available. To produce high-quality images, a selection of x-ray energy levels (kV) must be available.

The use of AC and electromagnetic principles is fundamental to the operation of the high-voltage transformer and the autotransformer. These are the x-ray circuit devices responsible for producing the required high voltage and permitting a selection of kilovoltages, respectively.

It has long been known that there is an important relationship between magnetism and electricity. Famous scientists, including Volta, Oersted, Lenz, and Faraday, performed various experiments demonstrating the relationship, making important observations, and formulating principles that explain the operation of electromagnetic devices.

Faraday's observation that a *magnetic field* will induce an electric current in a conductor if there is motion of either the magnetic field or the conductor (Fig. 13-25) is the fundamental principle of operation of the high-voltage *transformer*. If a coiled conductor is supplied with an AC, a magnetic field expands and collapses around the coil, accompanying the peaks and valleys of the AC waveform. If a second coiled conductor is placed nearby, but not touching the first (primary) coil, the moving magnetic field will interact similarly with the second coil and an electric current will be induced in it. Thus, the moving magnetic field from the primary coil can be used to induce a current in another circuit with whom it has *no physical connection;* this is called *mutual induction.* An AC, producing a continuously moving magnetic field, is necessary for mutual induction to occur.

A conductive wire shaped into a coil is called a *helix;* a helix supplied with a current is a *solenoid.* If an iron core is inserted within the coil, a simple *electromagnet* is formed and the magnetic lines of force are intensified. Thus, a transformer's conductor is frequently coiled around an iron core to increase its efficiency.

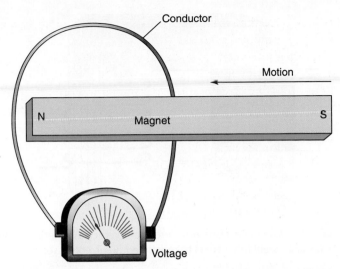

Figure 13-25. Electromagnetic induction. An electric current will be induced in a conductor whenever there is relative motion between a conductor and magnetic field; that is, if a conductor moves through a magnetic field, if a magnetic field moves across a conductor, or if the magnetic field is constantly changing (as in AC).

Summary

- X-ray equipment may be described as either fixed or mobile.

- Fixed equipment tabletops are either *pedestal* or *floating.*

- Tilting tabletops must move 90° vertically and 30° Trendelenburg.

- X-ray tube supports can be floor-mounted, wall-mounted, or suspended overhead.

- X-ray equipment designed for a particular purpose is termed *dedicated.*

- A generator converts mechanical energy to electrical energy; a motor converts electrical energy to mechanical energy.

- Electricity is transported over long distances at high-voltage and low-current values to minimize energy loss, according to the heat loss formula: $P = I^2R.$

- AC is characterized by constantly changing polarity and amplitude.

- A coil of wire is a helix; supplied with current, it is a solenoid; with an iron core, it is the simplest type of electromagnet.

- X-ray transformers operate on the principle of mutual induction.

High-Voltage Transformers

X-ray transformers are used to increase the incoming voltage to the more useful *kilovoltage* required for x-ray production. Transformers that increase the voltage are called *step-up transformers* or high-voltage transformers. The degree to which transformers increase the voltage is determined by their *turns ratio,* that is, the number of turns in the secondary (high-voltage) coil compared with the number of turns in the primary (low-voltage) coil; the higher the ratio, the greater the voltage

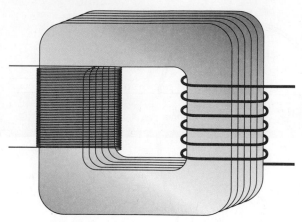

Figure 13-26. The *closed-core* transformer reduces loss of magnetic flux. Note the *laminated* silicon steel that serves to reduce *eddy current* losses.

increase; however, current decreases proportionally according to the (transformer law) equation that follow:

$$\frac{V_s}{V_p} = \frac{N_s}{N_p} \qquad \frac{N_s}{N_p} = \frac{I_p}{I_s}$$

Note that the relationship between the turns ratio and the *voltage* is a *direct one,* whereas there is an *inverse* relationship between the turns ratio and the *current.* So, as the voltage increases, the current decreases proportionally.

For example, if a particular x-ray transformer has a turns ratio of 500:1 and is supplied with 50 A and 220 V, *what is its kV and mA output?*

$$\frac{x}{220} = \frac{500}{1} \qquad\qquad \frac{500}{1} = \frac{50}{x}$$

$$x = 500 \times 220 \qquad\qquad 500x = 50$$
$$x = 110{,}000 \text{ volts} = 110 \text{ kV} \qquad x = 0.1A = 100 \text{ mA}$$

Transformers can also be the *step-down* type, such as that found in the x-ray filament circuit.

Although transformers operate at approximately 95% efficiency, energy loss varies according to transformer design. An *open-core* transformer consists of two parallel iron cores with conductive windings; however, a loss or leaking away of magnetic flux occurs at the ends of the iron cores. A *closed-core* transformer (Fig. 13-26) consists of a ring-shaped core of iron that serves to reduce leakage flux energy loss. A *shell*-type transformer has a central partition, effectively dividing it into two halves. The transformer primary and secondary coils are wound around the center bar (but not touching each other), and this arrangement serves to reduce energy loss still further.

Autotransformers

The x-ray circuit transformer is a *fixed*-ratio transformer, that is, the turns relationship is constant. How, then, are we able to have a selection of kilovoltages from which to choose? It is through the use of an *autotransformer,* which sends the correct amount of *voltage* to the primary

---

Types of Transformer Losses

- *Copper losses* are caused by the resistance to current flow that is characteristic of all conductors and are reduced by using larger *diameter* conductive wire.

- *Hysteresis losses* are a result of the continually changing magnetic domains of the core material (as a result of changing polarity of AC) and can be reduced by using core material of greater permeability (e.g., silicon).

- *Eddy current* losses are a result of small currents (eddy currents) built up in the core material as a result of the continually changing magnetic fields. Eddy current losses are reduced by laminating the core material; any current generated can travel only the small distance between laminations and therefore represents a smaller energy loss.

coil of the high-voltage transformer to be stepped up to the required *kilovoltage* level.

The autotransformer consists of an iron core with a single coil wrapped around it (that serves as its primary and secondary windings) and operates on the principle of *self-induction.* Each coil turn has a contact or tap. A movable contact (corresponding to the kV selector dial on the control panel) makes connection with the appropriate tap on the autotransformer. The voltage sent to the primary coil of the high-voltage transformer depends on the number of coils "tapped." For example, a particular autotransformer has 2000 windings and is supplied with 220 V. If 500 windings are tapped, *what voltage is sent to the primary of the step-up transformer?* The solution can be determined by using the *autotransformer law* (which is the same as the transformer law):

$$\frac{V_s}{V_p} = \frac{N_s}{N_p}$$

$$\frac{x}{220} = \frac{500}{2000}$$

$$2000x = (500)(220)$$
$$2000x = 110,000$$

$$x = 55 \text{ V sent to the primary coil of the step-up transformer}$$

Summary

- High-voltage (step-up) transformers function to provide the necessary kilovoltage for x-ray production.
- As the high-voltage transformer steps up voltage to kilovoltage, it proportionally steps down current according to the primary-to-secondary turns ratio and the transformer law.
- The transformer and autotransformer laws are expressed by the following equations:

$$\frac{V_s}{V_p} = \frac{N_s}{N_p} \qquad \frac{N_s}{N_p} = \frac{I_p}{I_s}$$

- Step-down transformers are also called filament transformers; they function on the same principles as step-up transformers and are placed in the filament circuit.
- Transformers can be designed as open core, closed core, or shell type; transformers are approximately 95% efficient.
- Types of transformer losses include copper losses, eddy current losses, and hysteresis losses.
- The autotransformer, operating on the principle of self-induction, functions to provide a selection of kilovoltages.
- Both the transformer and the autotransformer require AC for operation.

Rectification

Some x-ray circuit devices, such as the transformer and autotransformer, operate only on AC. The efficient operation of the x-ray tube, however, requires the use of *unidirectional* current, so current must be

Transformers
- Step-up transformers increase voltage (and decrease amperage proportionally)
- Step-down transformers decrease voltage (and increase amperage proportionally)
- Require AC for operation
- Operate on the principle of mutual induction

Autotransformers
- Select the amount of voltage sent to the transformer (kV selector)
- Operate on the principle of self-induction
- Require AC for operation

Comparison of Technical Factors Required

1φ	3φ 6p	3φ 12p
mAs	⅔ 1φ mAs	½ 1φ mAs

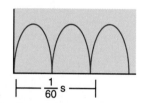

A Single-phase, full-wave rectified

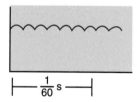

B Three-phase, six-pulse

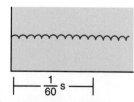

C Three-phase, 12-pulse

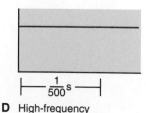

D High-frequency

Figure 13-27. (A-D) Waveforms.

rectified before it gets to the x-ray tube. The process of full-wave *rectification* changes the nonuseful negative half-cycle to a useful positive half-cycle.

An x-ray circuit rectification system is located between the secondary coil of the high-voltage transformer and the x-ray tube. Rectifiers are solid-state diodes made of *semiconductive materials* such as silicon, selenium, or germanium that conduct electricity *in only one direction*. Thus, a series of rectifiers placed between the transformer and the x-ray tube function to change AC to a more useful unidirectional current.

Although rectification remedies the changing polarity problem of single-phase AC, the problem of constantly varying *amplitude* remains. The continually changing voltage from zero to maximum potential and back to zero produces a pulsating beam of x-rays having a wide range of energies. *Three-phase (3φ) rectification* superimposes three AC waveforms, each separated from the other two by 120° and resulting in a pulsating waveform. Although *single-phase (1φ) rectification* produces a waveform having 100% "ripple" (i.e., 100% drop in potential between pulses), three-phase, six-pulse (3φ 6p) rectification presents a 13% ripple; three-phase, 12-pulse (3φ 12p) rectification presents a 4% ripple (Fig. 13-27).

High-Frequency Generators

Conventional 60-Hz full-wave rectified power is converted into a higher frequency of 500–25,000 Hz in most recent generator design—the *HF generator*. AC power is rectified and smoothed by a large capacitor, becoming a DC voltage supply. An HF *inverter* then converts the DC voltage back into an HF AC voltage of up to 100 kHz. This is then conducted to the primary winding of the high-voltage transformer. From the secondary side of the high-voltage transformer, full-wave rectification takes place, which doubles the *number* of x-ray pulses per second up to 175,000.

The HF generator is small in size, in addition to producing an almost constant potential waveform. HF generators first appeared in mobile x-ray units and were then adopted by mammography and CT equipment.

Nowadays, more general radiographic equipment use HF generators. Their compact size makes them popular and the fact that they produce nearly constant potential voltage (less than 1% ripple) helps improve image quality and decrease patient dose (fewer low-energy photons decrease skin dose) (see Fig. 13-27).

3φ 6p Rectification presents a 13% ripple; 3φ 12p rectification presents a 4% ripple, and HF presents less than 1% ripple. Therefore, the overall average energy of the x-ray beam increases. For example,

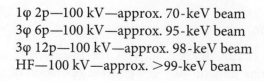

1φ 2p—100 kV—approx. 70-keV beam
3φ 6p—100 kV—approx. 95-keV beam
3φ 12p—100 kV—approx. 98-keV beam
HF—100 kV—approx. >99-keV beam

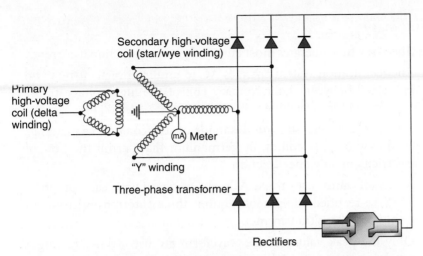

Figure 13-28. A simplified diagram of the secondary (high-voltage) side of a
3φ 6p–rectified x-ray circuit. 3φ Equipment requires the use of three autotransformers (not shown) and one transformer having three windings arranged
in *delta* and *star* (or wye) configuration. (Reproduced with permission from
Saia DA. *Lange Q&A Radiography Examination.* 7th ed. New York, NY:
McGraw-Hill; 2009.)

The quantity and quality of x-ray photon production increase from
1φ generators to 3φ 6p generators to 3φ 12p generators to HF generators, which produce the greatest quantity and quality of x-ray photons.
Because 3φ and HF x-ray generation provides a more uniform spectrum
of x-ray photon energies, the term kV has replaced kVp.

3φ Rectification requires the use of *three autotransformers* (one for
each incoming current) and *one transformer* having three windings.
A transformer winding can be arranged in either *star* (wye) or *delta*
configuration (Fig. 13-28).

Generator ratings are expressed in kilowatts (kW). The formula to
determine the power rating of a 3φ generator is as follows:

$$W = V \times A$$

or

$$W = kV \times mA \div 1000$$

For example, to determine the power rating for a 3φ generator that is
capable of delivering 150 kV at 1200 mA to the x-ray tube, first change
kV and mA to V and A and then use the equation

$$W = V \times A$$
$$W = 150,000 \times 1.2$$
$$W = 180,000 \ (180 \ kW)$$

or

$$W = kV \times mA \div 1000$$
$$W = 150 \times 1200 \div 1000$$
$$W = 180 \ kW$$

Summary

- The x-ray tube operates most efficiently on unidirectional current.
- The rectification system changes AC to unidirectional current and is located between the secondary coil of the high-voltage transformer and the x-ray tube.
- Rectifiers are solid-state diodes made of semiconductive materials such as silicon, selenium, or germanium that permit the flow of electricity in only one direction.
- 3φ Rectification uses three ACs out of phase with each other by $120°$; 3φ-rectified equipment requires three autotransformers and one high-voltage transformer.
- Only the peak values of the waveform are used, thus creating a nearly constant potential current.
- 3φ Rectification may be six pulse (13% ripple) or 12 pulse (4% ripple), depending on the number of rectifiers used.
- 3φ High-voltage transformer windings are arranged in either star (wye) or delta formation.
- HF generators use inverter circuits to change the supplied DC into pulsed voltage.
- X-ray photon quality and quantity increase from three-phase to HF generators.
- Generator ratings are expressed in kW; to determine the power rating of a 3φ generator, use $W = V \times A$ or $W = kV \times mA \div 1000$.

COMPREHENSION CHECK

1. Describe the two types of x-ray production and the contribution of each to the primary beam (p. 402, 403).

2. Discuss what is meant by the dual nature of the x-ray beam; list at least eight properties of x-ray photon (p. 404).

3. Describe the interactions between x-ray photons and the matter in the diagnostic x-ray range, their frequency of occurrence, the circumstances in which each is more likely to occur, and implication(s) of each for patients and the IR (p. 405, 406).

4. Discuss the differences between fixed and mobile equipment; give examples of typical/required features of each (p. 407, 408).

5. Define and give examples of dedicated x-ray equipment (p. 408).

6. Distinguish between AC and DC waveforms (p 409).

7. Discuss the following characteristics of AC: amplitude, polarity, wavelength, and frequency (p. 409, 410).

8. Define helix, solenoid, and electromagnet (p. 410).

9. Describe the function of the transformer, and identify the principle on which it operates (p. 410).

10. By using the transformer law, determine the voltage and current delivered to the x-ray tube (p. 412).

11. Identify four types of x-ray transformer construction (p. 412, 413).

12. Describe three types of transformer energy losses and methods by which they can be reduced (p. 412).

13. Describe the function of the autotransformer, and identify the principle on which it operates (p. 412, 413).

14. Using the autotransformer law, determine the voltage sent to the transformer primary coil (p. 413).

15. Identify the type of current required for operation of the transformer and autotransformer (p. 413).

16. Define the function of the generator and the motor (p. 408, 409).

17. Describe the rectification process (p. 413, 414).

18. Identify and give examples of the type of material of which solid-state diodes are made (p. 414).

19. Differentiate among single-phase; three-phase, six-pulse; and three-phase, 12-pulse waveforms (p. 414).

20. Identify the pulse ripple for single-phase; three-phase, six-pulse; and three-phase, 12-pulse rectification (p. 414).

21. Identify the number of autotransformers and transformers required for three-phase rectification (p. 415).

22. Identify the two types of transformer winding configurations (p. 415).

CHAPTER REVIEW QUESTIONS

1. Diagnostic x-rays are generally associated with
   (A) high frequency and long wavelength
   (B) high frequency and short wavelength
   (C) low frequency and long wavelength
   (D) low frequency and short wavelength

2. To eject a K-shell electron from a tungsten atom, the incoming electron must have an energy of *at least*
   (A) 60 keV
   (B) 70 keV
   (C) 80 keV
   (D) 90 keV

3. The advantages of HF generators over earlier types of generators include
   1. smaller size
   2. nearly constant potential
   3. lower patient dose
   (A) 1 only
   (B) 1 and 2 only
   (C) 1 and 3 only
   (D) 1, 2, and 3

4. Which of the following can be associated with mobile x-ray equipment?
   1. Wireless detector
   2. Rechargeable batteries
   3. HF output
   (A) 1 only
   (B) 1 and 2 only
   (C) 2 and 3 only
   (D) 1, 2, and 3

5. The device used to change AC to unidirectional current is
   (A) a capacitor
   (B) a solid-state diode
   (C) a transformer
   (D) a generator

6. Which of the following circuit devices operate(s) on the principle of self-induction?
   1. Autotransformer
   2. Choke coil
   3. High-voltage transformer
   (A) 1 only
   (B) 1 and 2 only
   (C) 2 and 3 only
   (D) 1, 2, and 3

7. The relationship between wavelength and energy is correctly described as
   (A) directly related
   (B) inversely related
   (C) directly proportional
   (D) inversely proportional

8. The primary coil of the high-voltage transformer receives
   (A) AC
   (B) direct current
   (C) pulsating direct current

9. The two main characteristics of AC are
   (A) constant amplitude and periodic change in flow
   (B) bidirectional amplitude and periodic flow
   (C) periodic amplitude and unidirectional flow
   (D) varying amplitude and periodic reversal of direction

10. The x-ray interaction with matter that is responsible for the majority of SR reaching the IR is
    (A) the photoelectric effect
    (B) Compton scatter
    (C) classical scatter
    (D) Thompson scatter

11. The relationship between frequency and energy is correctly described as
    (A) directly related
    (B) inversely proportional
    (C) directly proportional
    (D) inversely related

12. What type of x-ray generator will produce the greatest voltage ripple?
    (A) Single-phase, full-wave rectified
    (B) Three-phase, six-pulse
    (C) Three-phase, 12-pulse
    (D) High-frequency

Answers and Explanations

1. (B) Electromagnetic radiation can be described as wave-like fluctuations of the electric and magnetic fields. There are many kinds of electromagnetic radiation; visible light, microwaves, and radio waves, as well as x-rays and gamma rays, are all part of the electromagnetic spectrum. All the electromagnetic radiations have the same velocity, that is, 3×10^8 m/s (186,000 miles per second); however, they differ greatly in wavelength and frequency. Wavelength refers to the distance between two consecutive wave crests. Frequency refers to the number of cycles per second (cps); its unit of measurement is hertz (Hz), which is equal to 1 cps. Frequency and wavelength are closely associated with the relative energy of electromagnetic radiation. More energetic radiations have *shorter wavelength and higher frequency*. The relationship among frequency, wavelength, and energy is graphically illustrated in the electromagnetic spectrum.

Some radiations are energetic enough to rearrange atoms in materials through which they pass, and they can therefore be hazardous to living tissue. These radiations are called *ionizing radiation* because they have the energetic potential to break apart electrically neutral atoms, resulting in the production of negative and/or positive ions.

2. (B) X-ray photons are produced in two ways as high-speed electrons interact with target tungsten atoms. First, if the high-speed electron is attracted by the nucleus of a tungsten atom and changes its course, as the electron is "braked," energy is given up in the form of an x-ray photon. This is called *bremsstrahlung* (braking) *radiation,* and it is responsible for most of the x-ray photons produced at the conventional tungsten target. Second, a high-speed electron having an energy of at least 70 keV may eject a tungsten K-shell electron, leaving a vacancy in the shell. An electron from the next energy level, the L shell, drops down to fill the vacancy, emitting the difference in energy as a K-characteristic ray. Characteristic radiation makes up only about 15% of the primary beam.

3. (D) HF generators first appeared in mobile x-ray units and were then adopted by mammography and CT equipment. Nowadays, more and more radiographic equipment use HF generators. Their compact size makes them popular, and the fact that they produce nearly constant potential voltage helps improve image quality and decrease patient dose (fewer low-energy photons to contribute to skin dose).

4. (D) Mobile x-ray equipment is designed to be transported to the patients who are unable to travel to the radiology/imaging department—the very ill, incapacitated patients, and patients in surgery or isolation. Mobile equipment is available for radiographic and/or fluoroscopic x-ray procedures. Mobile equipment operates on rechargeable batteries with HF output. Immediate image display is possible via FPD systems and built-in monitors. Detectors can be either tethered or the wireless type.

5. (B) Some x-ray circuit devices, such as transformers and autotransformers, will operate only on AC. The efficient operation of the x-ray tube, however, requires the use of unidirectional current, so current must be *rectified* before it gets to the x-ray tube. The process of full-wave *rectification* changes the negative half-cycle to a useful positive half-cycle. An x-ray circuit rectification system is located between the secondary coil of the high-voltage transformer and the x-ray tube. Rectifiers are solid-state diodes made of *semiconductive materials* such as silicon, selenium, or germanium that conduct electricity *in only one direction*. Thus, a series of rectifiers placed between the transformer and the x-ray tube function to change AC to a more useful unidirectional current.

6. (B) The principle of self-induction is an example of the second law of electromagnetics (Lenz's law), which states that an induced current within a conductive coil will oppose the direction of the current that induced it. It is important to note that self-induction is a characteristic only of AC. The fact that AC is constantly changing direction accounts for the opposing current setup in the coil. Two x-ray circuit devices operate on the principle of self-induction. The autotransformer operates on the principle of self-induction and enables the radiographer to vary the kilovoltage. The choke coil also operates on the principle of self-induction; it is a type of variable resistor that may be used to regulate filament current. The high-voltage transformer operates on the principle of mutual induction.

7. (B) All electromagnetic radiations can be described as wave-like fluctuations of the electric and magnetic fields. All electromagnetic radiations have the same velocity, 186,000 miles per second (3×10^8 m/s); however, they differ greatly in wavelength.

Wavelength refers to the distance between two consecutive wave crests. *Frequency* refers to the number of cycles per second (cps); its unit of measurement is the hertz (Hz), which is equal to 1 cps. Frequency and wavelength are associated with the relative *energy* of electromagnetic radiation. Frequency is directly related to photon energy, whereas wavelength is inversely related. That is, photon energy increases as wavelength decreases and frequency increases. More *energetic* radiations have *shorter wavelength* and *higher frequency*.

8. (A) Faraday's observation that a *magnetic field* will induce an electric current in a conductor if there is motion of either the magnetic field or the conductor (see Fig. 13-25) is the fundamental principle of operation of the high-voltage *transformer*. If a coiled conductor is supplied with an AC, a magnetic field expands and collapses around the coil, accompanying the peaks and valleys of the AC waveform. If a second coiled conductor is placed nearby, but not touching the first (primary) coil, the moving magnetic field will interact similarly with the second coil and an electric current will be induced in it. Thus, the moving magnetic field from the primary coil can be used to induce a current in another circuit with whom it has *no physical connection;* this is called *mutual induction.* An AC, producing a continuously moving magnetic field, is necessary for mutual induction to occur.

9. (D) AC consists of sinusoidal waves. One *wavelength* consists of two half-cycles: a *positive half-cycle* and a *negative half-cycle.* A *wavelength* is defined as the distance between two consecutive *crests.* A *crest* is the positive half-cycle peak, and a *trough* is the negative half-cycle peak. The maximum height of the wave/impulse is called its *amplitude* and represents electrical potential, that is, voltage. *AC is therefore characterized by varying amplitude and periodic reversal of polarity.* The number of cycles per unit of time is called *frequency* (see Fig. 13-24), and its unit of measurement is the *hertz* (Hz). In the United States, AC is generated at 60 Hz or cps, that is, 60 cycles (60 positive half-cycles and 60 negative half-cycles) occur each second. One-half second, therefore, would include 30 cycles; consequently, four cycles represent a $^4/_{60}$- or $^1/_{15}$-s time interval.

10. (B) In the photoelectric effect, a relatively low-energy photon uses all its energy to eject an inner shell electron, leaving a vacancy. An electron from the shell above drops down to fill the vacancy and in so doing gives up a characteristic ray. This type of interaction is most harmful to the patient because all of the photon energy is transferred to tissue. In Compton scatter, a high-energy incident photon ejects an outer shell electron. In doing so, the incident photon is deflected with reduced energy, but it usually retains most of its energy and exits the body as an energetic scattered ray. This scattered ray will either contribute to image fog or pose a radiation hazard to personnel depending on its direction of exit. In classic scatter, a low-energy photon interacts with an atom but causes no ionization; the incident photon disappears into the atom and then is released immediately as a photon of identical energy but with changed direction. Thompson scatter is another name for classic scatter.

11. (A) All electromagnetic radiations can be described as wave-like fluctuations of the electric and magnetic fields. All electromagnetic radiations have the same velocity, 186,000 miles per second (3×10^8 m/s); however, they differ greatly in wavelength.

Wavelength refers to the distance between two consecutive wave crests. Frequency refers to the number of cycles per second (cps); its unit of measurement is the hertz (Hz), which is equal to 1 cps. Frequency and wavelength are associated with the relative energy of electromagnetic radiation. Frequency is directly related to photon energy, whereas wavelength is inversely related. That is, photon energy increases as wavelength decreases and frequency increases. More energetic radiations have shorter wavelength and higher frequency.

12. (A) The single-phase, full-wave rectified generator will produce the greatest voltage ripple at 100%. After rectification, the voltage will continually vary from maximum potential, back to zero, creating a pulsating beam of x-rays with a wide range of energies. This was improved on with three-phase rectification that superimposed three AC waveforms separated by 120°. Three-phase, six-pulse has a 13% ripple, whereas three-phase, 12-pulse has a 4% ripple. High-frequency generators offer the smallest voltage ripple at 1%, allowing for a nearly constant potential.

THE X-RAY TUBE

X-rays are produced when high-speed electrons emitted from the cathode filament are suddenly decelerated as they encounter tungsten atoms of the x-ray tube anode or target. This can happen in two ways; a review of the two processes is as follows:

1. *Bremsstrahlung* (brems) or "braking" *radiation:* A high-speed electron, passing through a tungsten atom, is attracted and "braked" by the positively charged nucleus and deflected from its course with a resulting loss of energy. *This energy loss is given up in the form of an x-ray photon* (see Fig. 13-18). Very often, the electron does not give up all its kinetic energy in one such interaction; it goes on to have several more interactions deeper in the target, each time giving up an x-ray photon having less and less energy—accounting for the polyenergetic nature of the x-ray beam. Brems radiation comprises 70%–90% of the x-ray beam.

2. *Characteristic radiation.* In this case, a high-speed electron encounters the tungsten atom and ejects a K-shell electron, leaving a vacancy in that shell. An electron from an adjacent shell (i.e., the L or M shell) fills the vacancy and in doing so *emits a K-characteristic ray* (see Fig. 13-19). The energy of the characteristic ray is equal to the difference in energy level between the K shell and the shell that gave up the electron to fill the K vacancy. The energy of L- and/or M-characteristic radiation will be less than the K-characteristic ray. The varying energies of characteristic radiation also account for the energy spectrum of the x-ray beam.

Component Parts

X-ray tubes are used for both radiographic and fluoroscopic purposes. Their basic components are the *anode* (positive electrode) and *cathode* assembly (negative electrode), enclosed within an evacuated (vacuum) *glass envelope* (Fig. 13-29).

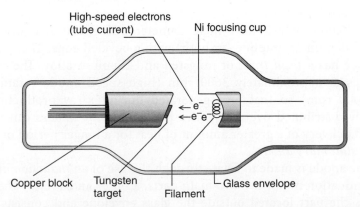

Figure 13-29. A simplified illustration of a *stationary* anode x-ray tube. The tungsten target is embedded in a solid block of copper that serves to conduct heat away from the tungsten and into the oil coolant that surrounds the glass envelope. Most x-ray tubes nowadays use *rotating* anodes as a means of more even heat distribution.

X-ray Tube

- Anode (positive electrode)
- Cathode (negative electrode)
- Glass envelope (vacuum)

Anode

- Graphite/molybdenum disk with beveled edge
- Tungsten/rhenium alloy focal track (0.6–1.2 mm)
- Molybdenum stem (support for anode disk)

Induction Motor

- Rotates anode
- Stator (outside glass envelope)
- Rotor (inside glass envelope)

Characteristics of Tungsten (W) as Target Material

- High atomic number ($Z = 74$) increases x-ray production
- High melting point (3410°C) to resist pitting and cracking
- Thermal conductivity for heat dissipation

The *glass envelope* enclosure creates a *diode* (two electrodes) tube somewhat reminiscent of early radio and television tubes. The x-ray tube glass enclosure, however, is made of glass that is extremely heat resistant to maintain the necessary *vacuum* for the production of x-rays. Should the vacuum begin to deteriorate, air molecules within the tube would collide with, and decelerate, the high-speed electrons traveling to the anode, thus diminishing the production of x-rays. The condition of air within the glass envelope is called a "gassy tube" and will eventually cause oxidation and burnout of the cathode filament.

The cathode assembly consists of one or more *filaments,* their supporting wires, and a *nickel focusing cup.* The filament is a fine (~0.2-mm diameter) 1- to 2-cm coil of tungsten wire that, when heated to incandescence by approximately 4 A of current, boils off/releases outer shell tungsten electrons. This event is called *thermionic emission.* Most x-ray tubes actually have two or more filaments and are called *double-focus tubes.* The typical x-ray tube has two filaments, one small and one large, to direct electrons to either the small or large anode focal spot. Each filament is closely embraced by a negatively charged focusing cup that serves to direct the electrons toward the anode. The two filaments are arranged in a three-wire/conductor system. A low-voltage conductor carries low voltage to heat the selected (large or small) filament. The third conductor is common to both filaments and carries the high voltage necessary to propel liberated electrons to the anode (see Fig. 13-31B).

As the filament releases electrons, small quantities of tungsten can be vaporized and deposited on the inner surface of the glass envelope. If tungsten is deposited on the port window, it acts as a filter and reduces the intensity of the x-ray beam; it can also affect the tube vacuum and ultimately leads to tube failure.

The filament is heated with the required 3–5 A and 10–12 V by the *filament circuit.* The filament current is kept at a standby quantity until the rotor is activated; at that time, the *filament booster circuit* brings it up to the level required for exposure. The rotor switch should not be activated for extended periods because the filament current is at maximum potential and tungsten vaporization can increase. Extended activation can also result in bearing damage and decreased tube life.

The anode is a 2- to 5-inch diameter disk made of lightweight molybdenum or graphite (or both) with a beveled edge. The beveled surface has a *focal track* of tungsten and rhenium alloy. The anode rotates at approximately 3600 rpm (high-speed anode rotation is ~10,000 rpm) so that heat generated during x-ray production is evenly distributed over the entire track. *Rotating anodes* can withstand delivery of a greater amount of heat for a longer period of time than *stationary anodes.*

The anode is made to rotate through the use of an *induction motor.* An induction motor has two main parts, a *stator* and a *rotor.* The stator is the part located outside the glass envelope and consists of a series of electromagnets occupying positions around the stem of the anode. The stator's electromagnets are supplied with current, and the associated magnetic fields function to exert a drag or pull on the rotor within (Fig. 13-30).

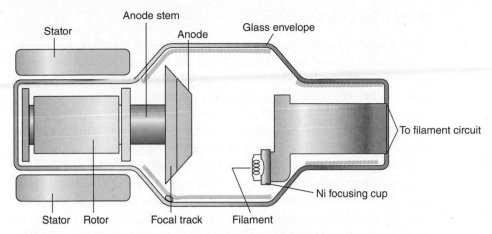

Figure 13-30. The component parts of a rotating anode x-ray tube. Note the position of the stator and the rotor. Note the beveled edge of the anode, forming the focal track, and the position of the filament directly across from the rotating focal track. (Reproduced with permission from Saia DA. *Lange Q&A Radiography Examination.* 7th ed. New York, NY: McGraw-Hill; 2009.)

Tungsten (W) is usually chosen as target material because of its *high atomic number* (Z = 74), *high melting point* (3410°C), and *thermal conductivity* (equal to that of copper). The high atomic number serves to increase the efficiency of x-ray production; its high melting point makes it resistant to pitting and cracking; its thermal conductivity helps dissipate the heat produced during x-ray production. Rhenium is added to further resist anode pitting at high temperatures (Fig. 13-31A).

Summary

- X-rays (brems and characteristic) are produced by the abrupt deceleration of high-speed electrons by tungsten atoms within the focal track.
- The x-ray tube is a diode, that is, it has a negative electrode (cathode) and a positive electrode (anode).
- The x-ray tube's electrodes are enclosed within a vacuum glass envelope; a "gassy" tube produces x-rays less efficiently and results in filament oxidation/burnout.
- The cathode assembly consists of tungsten filament(s) with supporting wires and a (negatively charged) nickel focusing cup.
- X-ray tubes have at least two filaments, one for each focal spot.
- Heating of the filament to incandescence (with 3–5 A, 10–12 V) and subsequent release of electrons is called thermionic emission.
- The anode is a 2- to 5-inch molybdenum or graphite disk with a peripheral focal track of tungsten and rhenium alloy.
- Tungsten is the target material of choice because of its high atomic number, high melting point, and thermal conductivity; rhenium helps prevent pitting.
- An induction motor, consisting of a stator and a rotor, rotates the anode at 3600–10,000 rpm.

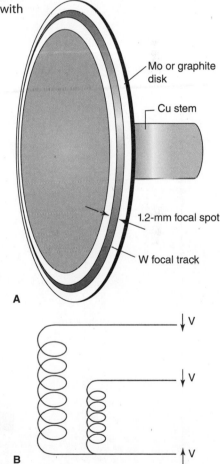

Figure 13-31. (A) A typical rotating anode. The anode disk is usually made of molybdenum and has a beveled edge containing a "band" of tungsten/rhenium alloy that forms the focal track. **(B)** Two filaments are arranged in a three-supporting wire/conductor system. A *low*-voltage conductor carries low voltage to heat the selected (large or small) filament. The third conductor is common to both filaments and carries the *high* voltage necessary to propel liberated electrons to the anode. The filament is supplied with 3–5 A and 10–12 V.

X-ray Tube Characteristics

The production of x-rays involves the generation of significant amounts of heat; *only 0.2% of the kinetic energy of the electron stream is converted to x-rays,* and the rest of the energy is converted to *heat.* Because heat can be very damaging to the x-ray tube and its efficient operation, several features are incorporated to expedite its dissipation. The *thermal conductivity* of tungsten is one feature; however, most cooling is a result of heat diffusion to the oil that surrounds the x-ray tube.

If large quantities of heat were continually directed to a single stationary small spot, that spot would be subjected to all the heat generated and would suffer more abuse and subsequent damage. Large quantities of heat delivered to the x-ray tube, especially in a short period of time, can be very damaging to the tube and can shorten its life span. The focal track of the *rotating* anode serves to *spread generated heat over a large area.* The width of the focal track on the anode's beveled edge is approximately 6 mm. Rotating anodes having a diameter of 2–5 inches will therefore provide significant surface area for the production and dissipation of heat.

The width of the beveled focal track is called the *actual* focal spot size. A distinction is made between the actual focal spot and the *effective,* projected, or apparent focal spot. The actual focal spot size is the width of the finite area on the tungsten target that is actually bombarded by electrons from the filament. The effective, projected, or apparent focal spot is the *foreshortened* size of the focus, as it is projected down toward the IR, that is, as it would be seen looking up into the x-ray tube (Fig. 13-32). This is called line focusing or the *line focus principle.* The effective focal spot size is also affected by the degree of focal track bevel, or anode angle. Anode angles are usually 5°–20°.

When using an x-ray tube with a small anode angle, a larger actual anode area (i.e., actual focal spot) can be bombarded and still maintain

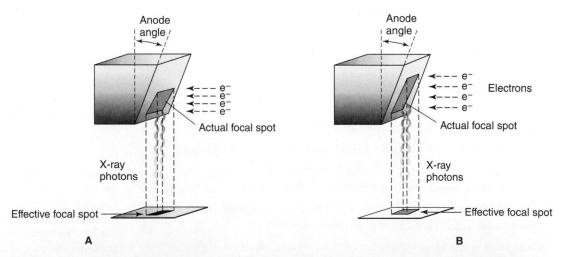

Figure 13-32. Line focus principle. Note how foreshortening of the actual focal spot impacts the effective (projected or apparent) focal spot. **(A)** A square actual focal spot produces a rectangular effective focal spot. **(B)** An elongated actual focal spot produces a square effective focal spot. As the anode *angle* is made smaller, the actual focal spot may be made larger while a small effective focal spot is still maintained. (Reproduced with permission from Saia DA. *Lange Q&A Radiography Examination.* 7th ed. New York, NY: McGraw-Hill; 2009.)

a small effective focal spot—anode heat load tolerance is not compromised and recorded detail is improved.

The size of the effective focal spot *varies along the length of the IR,* being largest in size (and associated with most blur) at the cathode end of the IR and smallest at the anode end (Fig. 13-33).

A phenomenon associated with the anode's focal spot is called focal spot *blooming.* With the use of high mA, the focal spot can become hot enough to temporarily grow in size, resulting in diminished resolution.

A difficulty associated with the use of a small anode angle, however, is a marked *anode heel effect* (Fig. 13-34). The anode heel effect results in a portion of the x-ray beam being absorbed by the anode, resulting in diminished beam intensity and receptor exposure at the anode end of the image.

Using a small anode angle, a typical radiographic distance of 40-inch SID, and a 14 × 17 IR, will result in approximately 2 inches of unexposed area at the anode end of the image. This can be remedied with an increase in SID, which must be accompanied by an appropriate increase in technical factors.

When using general x-ray tubes at standard distances, the heel effect is noticeable only when imaging parts of uneven thickness such as the femur and the thoracic spine. In these cases, the heel effect may be used to advantage by placing the thicker body portion under the cathode end of the x-ray beam, thus having the effect of "balancing/evening out" tissue densities.

The *line focus principle* and the *anode heel effect,* and their effects on radiographic quality, are discussed more fully in Chapter 12. When specifying focal spot size, it is the effective focal spot size that is quoted. We often speak of "double-focus" x-ray tubes, meaning that a small (e.g., 0.6 mm) and a large (1.2 mm) focal spots are available to choose from.

These x-ray tubes actually have only *one focal track;* a portion of it is used for the small focus setting. It is more accurate to say that these are *double filament* tubes, for there are two filaments: the smaller one is activated when the small focal spot is selected, and the larger one is activated for the large focal spot.

The amount of heat produced at the target is expressed in terms of *heat units* (HU). Exposure factor selection has a significant effect on the production of heat as expressed in the following equation:

$$HU = mA \times s \times kV \text{ (single phase)}$$

For example,

$$300 \text{ mA} \times 0.4 \text{ s} \times 80 \text{ kV} = 9600 \text{ HU}$$
$$300 \text{ mA} \times 0.2 \text{ s} \times 92 \text{ kV} = 5520 \text{ HU}$$

Thus, a greater number of HU are produced with higher mAs and lower kV technical factors. *A correction factor* is added to the equation when using 3φ equipment.

$$HU = mA \times s \times kV \text{ (1φ)}$$
$$HU = mA \times s \times kV \times 1.4 \text{ (3φ and HF)}$$

For example,

$$300 \text{ mA} \times 0.4 \text{ s} \times 80 \text{ kV} = 9600 \text{ HU (1φ)}$$
$$300 \text{ mA} \times 0.4 \text{ s} \times 80 \text{ kV} \times 1.4 = 13,440 \text{ HU (3φ/HF)}$$

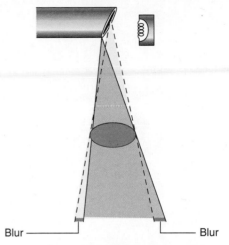

Figure 13-33. Because of the angle of the anode, unsharpness or blur is greatest at the cathode end of the image receptor. (Reproduced with permission from Saia DA. *Lange Q&A Radiography Examination.* 7th ed. New York, NY: McGraw-Hill; 2009.)

Line Focus Principle

The effective focal spot is always smaller than the actual focal spot.

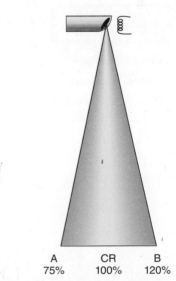

Figure 13-34. *The anode heel effect.* As x-ray photons are produced at the anode focus, a portion of the divergent beam nearest the anode end (A) is absorbed by the anode's "heel." This represents a decrease in x-ray beam intensity at the anode side of the x-ray beam. The smaller/steeper the anode angle/bevel, the more pronounced the heel effect.

Summary

- Most of the energy used to produce x-rays is converted to heat; only 0.2% is converted to x-rays.

- Heat is damaging to x-ray tubes; x-ray tubes are surrounded with oil to carry heat away from the anode (also for insulating purposes).

- The width of the focal track is identified as the actual focal spot; its bevel (angle) projects a smaller, effective focal spot to the IR according to the line focus principle.

- The degree of anode bevel (angle) influences the degree of heel effect; the smaller the angle, the more pronounced the heel effect.

- Blooming causes temporary enlargement of the focal spot and diminished resolution.

- HU are used to express the degree of accumulation of anode heat and determined by mA × time × kV; the correction factor for 3φ is 1.41.

Filtration and Collimators

X-ray photons produced at the focal spot are *polyenergetic,* and the low-energy x-ray photons, if not removed, would contribute significantly to patient *skin dose.* They do not have enough energy to reach the IR; they penetrate only a small thickness of tissue before being absorbed. Filters, usually made of aluminum, are used in radiography to reduce patient dose by removing low-energy photons. Filtration results in an x-ray beam of higher average energy. *Total filtration* is composed of *inherent filtration* plus *added filtration.*

Inherent, "built-in," filtration is composed of materials that are a permanent part of the x-ray tube and its housing (glass envelope, porch window, oil coolant). During the x-ray production process, many low-energy photons are absorbed by the anode surface itself. The window of the x-ray tube's glass envelope has approximately 0.5-mm Al equivalent and removes other low-energy photons. The thin layer of oil coolant/insulation surrounding the x-ray tube will remove more low-energy photons.

Inherent filtration tends to increase as the x-ray tube ages. With use, tungsten evaporates and is deposited on the inner surface of the glass envelope, effectively acting as additional filtration and decreasing the x-ray output.

Added filtration refers to the *thin sheets of aluminum* that are added to make the necessary total thickness of aluminum equivalent filtration. For equipment operated above 70 kV, the total filtration requirement is 2.5-mm Al equivalent. Added filtration includes the *collimator,* and its *mirror* having approximately 1.0-mm Al equivalent.

Adjustable lead shutter *collimators* are used to define the size and shape of the x-ray field that emerge from the x-ray tube port window. The fixed diaphragm located just outside the x-ray tube's port window functions to significantly reduce the effect of off-focus radiation.

Another important part of the collimator assembly is the *light localization apparatus.* It consists of a small light bulb (to illuminate the field) and a 45°-angle mirror to deflect the light. The x-ray tube focal spot and the light bulb must be exactly at the same distance from the

Filtration Summary

<50 kV = 0.5-mm Al equivalent

50–70 kV = 1.5-mm Al equivalent

>70 kV = 2.5-mm Al equivalent

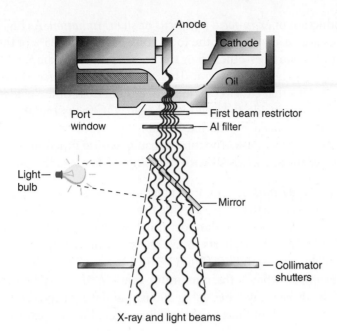

Figure 13-35. X-ray tube, filters, and collimator. The position of the collimator shutters can be seen. Note the position of the first beam restrictor, located at the x-ray tube port window. For light field and x-ray field congruence, the focal spot and the light bulb must be exactly at the same distance from the center of the mirror. The oil coolant surrounding the x-ray tube contributes to inherent filtration. Added filtration includes the aluminum filter, the mirror, and the collimator. (Reproduced with permission from Saia DA. *Lange Q&A Radiography Examination.* 7th ed. New York, NY: McGraw-Hill; 2009.)

center of the mirror for the light and x-ray fields to correspond accurately (Fig. 13-35). If the light and x-ray fields are not congruent, the anatomic part and the IR will be misaligned.

Collimator accuracy should be regularly checked as part of the QA program. National Council on Radiation Protection and Measurements (NCRP) guidelines state that collimators must be accurate to within 2% of the SID.

Safe Operation and Care

X-ray Tube Ratings. X-ray tubes are rated according to allowable *kilowatts* (kW) at an exposure time of 0.1 s (100 ms), and at the maximum amperage as determined by the *tube rating chart* and dependent on focal spot size.

$$\text{Power (in watts)} = 100 \text{ kV} \times \text{maximum A at } 0.1 \text{ s}$$
$$\text{(at a given focal spot size)}$$

Example:
If the maximum A at 0.1 s and 100 kV is 300, what is the x-ray tube power rating?

$$\text{Power} = 100 \text{ kV} \times 0.3 \text{ A} = 30 \text{ kW}$$

The typical x-ray tube kilowatt rating is usually rated between 20 and 80 kW.

As stated earlier, the use of very high mA can cause the focal spot to grow in size, a phenomenon called *blooming*, which has a degrading effect on image resolution. Another occurrence within the x-ray tube is

> **X-ray Tube Rating**
>
> - X-ray tubes are usually rated in kW
> - kW = 100 kV × maximum A at 100 ms

the production of *extra-focal (off-focus* or *stem) radiation*. As high-speed electrons are headed toward the focal spot, as many as 25% of them can interact with surfaces other than the focal spot, for example, the glass envelope and the anode stem. This interaction produces low-energy brems photons that either contribute to patient dose or are evidenced as exposed areas outside the collimated field. Off-focus radiation can be significantly reduced by the fixed diaphragm located just outside the x-ray tube's port window. The tube housing, whose function is to reduce leakage radiation, also assists with reducing off-focus radiation.

Safe X-ray Tube Limits. Each x-ray tube has its own *tube rating chart* and *anode cooling curve* that illustrate safe tube *heat limits* and the particular *cooling characteristics* of the anode. It is essential that the radiographer know how to use these charts to use the x-ray tube properly and safely and to prolong its useful life (Fig. 13-36).

For example, what is the maximum safe kV that may be used with each of the three x-ray tubes using 200 mA and 0.2-s exposure?

Do this for each of the x-ray tubes illustrated: Find the exposure time on the horizontal axis, follow it up until it meets the 200-mA line, and then follow that across to the vertical axis and read the kV.

> A = approximately 147 kV
> B = greater than 150 kV (off the chart)
> C = approximately 57 kV

Comparing these answers with the information provided in the legend for Figure 13-36, it can be seen that the *size of the focal spot* and the *type of rectification* significantly impact heat-loading characteristics of an x-ray tube.

Next, refer to the anode cooling curve. For example, if the x-ray tube were saturated with 1,300,000 HU, it would take 30 min to cool down to 300,000 HU. How long would it take to cool from 700,000 to 450,000 HU? (Answer: ~10 min.)

X-ray tubes are like incandescent light bulbs. Their useful life is dependent on proper use. X-ray tubes should be warmed prior to their first use in the morning. Exceeding tube exposure and/or heat limits will shorten a tube's life. System voltage fluctuations, drops or sags in incoming power, can decrease tube life. X-ray tubes should have appropriate preventive maintenances and calibrations. New x-ray tubes must be installed properly and should have had a minimum shelf/storage time before installation. Careless treatment or abuse of the x-ray tube, as well as normal wear and tear, will lead to its ultimate demise.

Some Causes of X-ray Tube Failure

Vaporized tungsten: As a result of thermionic emission, quantities of tungsten can be vaporized and deposited on the inner surface of the glass envelope. When deposited on the port window, tungsten acts as a filter and reduces the intensity of the beam; it can also alter the tube vacuum and finally leads to tube failure.

Pitted anode: Exposures made exceeding the tube rating create enough excessive heat to produce many small melts, or pits, over the surface of the focal track. X-ray photons are absorbed by these surface irregularities and, consequently, x-ray intensity is reduced. Extensive

---

Safe X-ray Tube Limits Illustrated In

- Tube rating charts
- Anode cooling curves

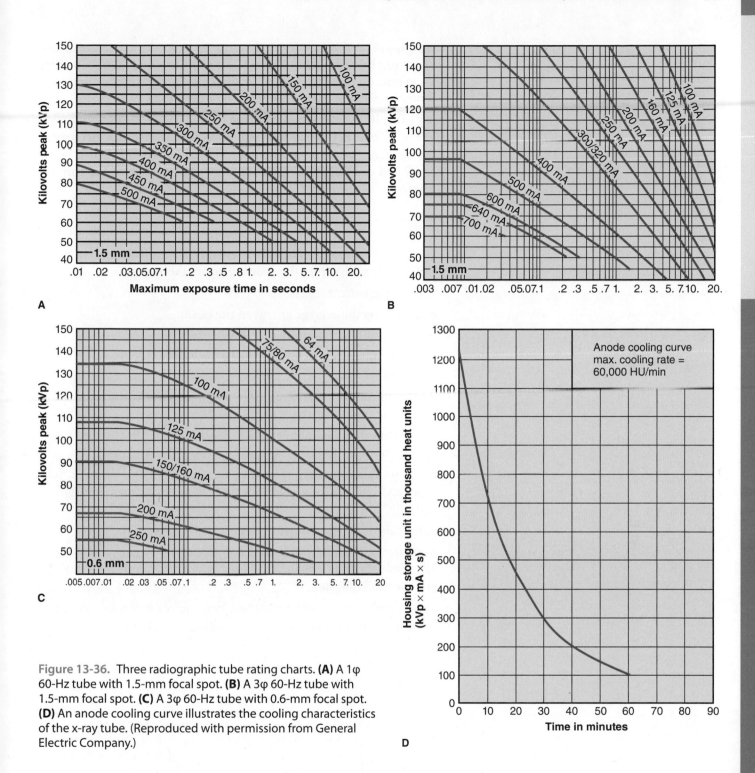

Figure 13-36. Three radiographic tube rating charts. **(A)** A 1φ 60-Hz tube with 1.5-mm focal spot. **(B)** A 3φ 60-Hz tube with 1.5-mm focal spot. **(C)** A 3φ 60-Hz tube with 0.6-mm focal spot. **(D)** An anode cooling curve illustrates the cooling characteristics of the x-ray tube. (Reproduced with permission from General Electric Company.)

pitting also results in *vaporized* tungsten deposited on the inner surface of the tube window that acts as an additional filter and further reduces beam intensity. Arcing can occur between the filament and tungsten deposit, resulting in a cracked glass envelope.

Cracked anode: A single, large, excessive exposure to a cold anode can be severe enough to crack the anode; the large dose of heat creates sudden expansion of the cold anode. It is therefore advisable to practice tube *warm-up procedures,* as suggested by the manufacturer, before starting the day's examinations or after the tube has not been

Common Causes of X-ray Tube Failure

- Vaporized tungsten
- Pitted anode
- Cracked anode
- Gassy tube

used for several hours. Typical warm-up procedure consists of two exposures made by using 100 mA, 2-s exposure, and 70 kV. The long 2-s exposures distribute heat over the entire surface of the anode and promote uniform thermal expansion of the anode.

Gassy tube: If the tube vacuum begins to deteriorate, air molecules collide with and decelerate the high-speed electrons, thus decreasing the efficiency of x-ray production. The condition is called a "gassy tube" and eventually causes oxidation and burnout of the cathode filament.

Summary

- Filtration, expressed in millimeters of Al equivalent, removes low-energy x-rays from the primary beam, thereby
  - reducing patient skin dose
  - increasing the average energy of the beam
- Inherent + added filtration = total filtration.
- Inherent filtration includes the glass envelope, oil coolant/insulation.
- Added filtration consists of thin layers of Al and includes the collimator and its mirror.
- Equipment operated above 70 kV must have at least 2.5-mm Al equivalent.
- An adjustable collimator is used to define the size and shape of the x-ray and light fields; its light localizer includes a small light bulb and a 45° mirror.
- X-ray tube kW rating is usually between 20 and 80 kW.
- Excessive heat loading will cause accelerated tube aging and failure as a result of conditions such as pitted or cracked anode, gassy tube, or vaporized tungsten.
- Tube rating charts and anode cooling curves must be used to determine safe exposures and heat loading.

COMPREHENSION CHECK

1. List the three basic components of the x-ray tube (p. 421, 422).

2. Discuss the importance of the evacuated glass envelope (p. 422).

3. Identify the components of the cathode assembly (p. 422).

4. Describe thermionic emission (p. 422).

5. Describe how a double- or dual-focus tube differs from a single-focus tube (p. 422).

6. Explain why x-ray tube inherent filtration increases as the x-ray tube ages (p. 426).

7. Identify the current and voltage required by the filament circuit (p. 422).

8. Discuss why prolonged periods of rotor activation should be avoided (p. 422).

9. Describe the construction of the anode (p. 422).

10. Discuss the composition and function of the anode focal track (p. 422).

11. Discuss the value of anode rotation (vs. stationary anode) (p. 422).

12. Identify the device responsible for anode rotation and its two major parts (p. 422).

13. Identify two characteristics of tungsten that make it a desirable target material (p. 423).

14. Describe the line focus principle; distinguish between actual and effective focal spots (p. 424).

15. Describe the anode heel effect; relate it to focal track bevel (anode angle) (p. 425).

16. Discuss why heat removal mechanisms are important in x-ray tube construction; give examples of heat-reduction features (p. 425).

17. Determine heat units for 1φ, 3φ 6p, and 3φ 12p x-ray equipment (p. 425).

18. Determine safe exposure limits by using tube rating charts and anode cooling curves (p. 429).

19. Discuss at least three causes of x-ray tube failure (p. 422, 428, 430).

20. Differentiate between inherent and added filtration and identify the x-ray tube components that contribute to each (p. 426).

CHAPTER REVIEW QUESTIONS

1. Which of the following combinations will offer the greatest heat-loading capability?

   (A) 13° target angle, 1.2-mm actual focal spot

   (B) 7° target angle, 1.2-mm actual focal spot

   (C) 13° target angle, 1.0-mm actual focal spot

   (D) 7° target angle, 1.0-mm actual focal spot

2. The line focus principle expresses the relationship between

   (A) the actual and effective focal spots

   (B) exposure given to the IR and the resulting receptor exposure

   (C) SID used and resulting receptor exposure

   (D) grid ratio and lines per inch

3. Although the stated focal spot size is measured directly under the actual focal spot, focal spot size actually varies along the length of the x-ray beam. At which portion of the x-ray beam is the effective focal spot the smallest?

   (A) At its outer edge

   (B) Along the path of the central ray

   (C) At the cathode end

   (D) At the anode end

4. Design characteristics of x-ray tube targets that determine heat capacity include

   1. the rotation of the anode

   2. the diameter of the anode

   3. the size of the focal spot

   (A) 1 only

   (B) 1 and 2 only

   (C) 1 and 3 only

   (D) 1, 2, and 3

5. The electron cloud that forms on the cathode end of the x-ray tube is the product of a process called

   (A) electrolysis

   (B) thermionic emission

   (C) rectification

   (D) electromagnetic induction

6. Which of the following is/are characteristics of the x-ray tube?

   1. The target material should have a high atomic number and a high melting point

   2. The useful beam emerges from the port window

   3. The cathode assembly receives both low and high voltages

   (A) 1 only

   (B) 2 only

   (C) 1 and 2 only

   (D) 1, 2, and 3

7. Delivery of large exposures to a cold anode or the use of exposures exceeding tube limitation can result in

   1. increased tube output

   2. cracking of the anode

   3. rotor-bearing damage

   (A) 1 only

   (B) 1 and 2 only

   (C) 2 and 3 only

   (D) 1, 2, and 3

8. As electrons collide with the focal track of the anode disk, approximately 99% of their kinetic energy is changed to

   (A) x-rays

   (B) heat

   (C) tungsten vapor

   (D) recoil electrons

9. Conditions that contribute to x-ray tube damage include

   1. lengthy anode rotation

   2. exposures to a cold anode

   3. low-mAs/high-kV exposure factors

   (A) 1 only

   (B) 1 and 2 only

   (C) 1 and 3 only

   (D) 1, 2, and 3

10. Characteristics of the metallic element tungsten include

    1. ready dissipation of heat
    2. high melting point
    3. high atomic number

    (A) 1 only
    (B) 1 and 2 only
    (C) 2 and 3 only
    (D) 1, 2, and 3

11. Which of the following x-ray tube components is not located within the glass envelope?

    (A) Anode
    (B) Rotor
    (C) Cathode
    (D) Stator

12. Inherent filtration of the x-ray tube is composed of all the following components, *except*

    (A) glass envelope
    (B) aluminum sheets
    (C) oil coolant
    (D) tube window

Answers and Explanations

1. (B) The smaller the focal spot, the more limited the anode is with respect to the quantity of heat it can safely accept. As the target angle decreases, the actual focal spot can be increased while still maintaining a small effective focal spot. Therefore, group (B) offers the greatest heat-loading potential, with a steep target angle and a large actual focal spot. It must be remembered, however, *that a steep target angle increases the heel effect* and IR coverage may be compromised.

2. (A) The line focus principle is a geometric principle illustrating that the *actual focal spot is larger than the effective (projected) focal spot.* The actual focal spot (target) is larger, to accommodate heat over a larger area, and is angled so as to *project* a smaller focal spot, thus maintaining spatial resolution by reducing blur. The relationship between the exposure given to the IR and the resulting receptor exposure is expressed in the reciprocity law; the relationship between the SID and the resulting IR exposure is expressed by the inverse square law. Grid ratio and lines per inch are unrelated to the line focus principle.

3. (D) X-ray tube targets are constructed according to the *line focus principle*—the focal spot is angled (usually 12°–17°) to the vertical. As the actual focal spot is projected downward, it is foreshortened; thus, the effective focal spot is always smaller than the actual focal spot. As it is projected toward the *cathode* end of the x-ray beam, the effective focal spot becomes *larger* and approaches its actual size. As it is projected toward the anode end, and foreshortening becomes more pronounced, the effective focal spot becomes smaller.

4. (D) Each time an x-ray exposure is made, less than 1% of the total energy is converted to x-rays and the remainder (>99%) of the energy is converted to heat. Thus, it is important to use target material with a high atomic number and a high melting point. The larger the actual focal spot size, the larger is the area over which the generated heat is spread and the more tolerant the x-ray tube is. Heat is particularly damaging to the target if it is concentrated or limited to a small area. A target that rotates during the exposure is spreading the heat over a large area, the entire surface of the focal track. If the diameter of the anode is greater, the focal track will be longer and heat will be spread over an even larger area.

5. (B) The thoriated tungsten filament of the cathode is heated by its own filament circuit. The x-ray tube filament is made of thoriated tungsten and is part of the cathode assembly. Its circuit provides current and voltage to heat it to incandescence, at which time it undergoes *thermionic emission*—the liberation of valence electrons from the filament atoms. *Electrolysis* describes the chemical ionization effects of an electric current. *Rectification* is the process of changing AC to unidirectional current.

6. (D) Anode target material with a *high atomic number* produces higher energy x-rays more efficiently. Because a great deal of heat is produced at the target, the material should have a *high melting point* so as to avoid damage to the target surface. Most of the x-rays generated at the focal spot are directed downward and pass through the x-ray tube's *port window*. The cathode filament receives *low-voltage* current to heat it to the point of thermionic emission. Then, *high voltage* is applied to drive the electrons across to the focal track.

7. (C) A large quantity of heat applied to a cold anode can cause enough surface heat to crack the anode. Excessive heat to the target can cause pitting or localized melting of the focal track. Localized melts can result in vaporized tungsten deposits on the glass envelope, which can cause a filtering effect, decreasing tube output. Excessive heat also can be conducted to the rotor bearings, causing increased friction and tube failure.

8. (B) The vast majority of target interactions involve the incident electrons and outer shell tungsten electrons. No ionization occurs, and the energy loss is reflected in heat generation. The production of x-rays is an amazingly inefficient process: *More than 99% of the electron's kinetic energy is changed to heat energy and less than 1% into x-ray photon energy.* This presents a serious heat buildup problem in the anode because heat production is directly proportional to tube current.

9. (B) X-ray tube life may be extended by using exposure factors that produce a *minimum of heat,* that is, a lower milliampere seconds and higher kilovoltage combination, whenever possible. When the rotor is activated, the filament current is increased to produce the required electron source (thermionic emission). *Prolonged rotor time,* then, can lead to shortened filament life as a result of early vaporization. Large exposures to a cold anode will heat the anode surface, and the big temperature difference can cause cracking of the anode. This can be avoided by proper warming of the anode prior to use, thereby allowing sufficient dispersion of heat through the anode.

10. (D) The x-ray anode may be a molybdenum disk coated with a tungsten–rhenium alloy. Because tungsten has a *high atomic number* ($Z = 74$), it produces high-energy x-rays more efficiently. Because a great deal of heat is produced at the target, tungsten's *high melting point* (3410°C) helps avoid damage to the target surface. Heat produced at the target should be dissipated readily, and tungsten's *conductivity is similar to that of copper.* Therefore, as heat is applied to the focus, it can be conducted throughout the disk to equalize the temperature and thus avoid pitting, or localized melting, of the focal track.

11. (D) The stator is located outside of the glass envelope and consists of a series of electromagnets. Its purpose is to exert a drag on the rotor located within the envelope to produce a spinning motion on the anode stem. This will in turn rotate the anode disk for x-ray production. The anode, cathode, and rotor are all located within the glass envelope and under a vacuum environment.

12. (B) Inherent, or "built-in," filtration consists of equipment that can already be found in the x-ray tube as a part of its typical construction. The glass envelope provides the vacuum environment needed for efficient production of x-rays. The glass window provides an opening for the x-rays to exit the tube after their creation at the anode. The oil coolant is needed to help dissipate the overwhelming amount of heat produced with each exposure. All three of these components are inherently found in the x-ray tube as a part of its construction. To meet the necessary total thickness of aluminum filtration and to further reduce the amount of low-energy photons created during a radiographic exposure, additional sheets of aluminum are added. These sheets are, therefore, considered added filtration.

THE RADIOGRAPHIC CIRCUIT

The x-ray circuit can be divided into three portions:

1. The *low-voltage,* or *primary, circuit* contains most of the devices found on the control console.

2. The *filament circuit* varies the current sent to the filament to provide the required mA value.

3. The *high-voltage,* or *secondary, circuit* includes the high-voltage transformer, rectification system, and x-ray tube.

Primary Circuit Components

Primary or Low-Voltage Circuit Devices

Main switch and circuit breakers: These are usually located on a wall in or near the x-ray room (Fig. 13-37). Circuit breaker switches must be closed to energize the equipment.

Autotransformer: It is a variable transformer that operates on AC and enables the radiographer to select kilovoltage. The function and operation of autotransformers are discussed earlier in this section.

kV selector: It is used by the radiographer to choose the kilovoltage, often as kV major (in increments of 10) and kV minor (in increments of 2). In doing so, the appropriate number of coils (representing V) on the autotransformer is selected by the movable contact.

Types of X-ray Timers

- Mechanical
- Synchronous
- Impulse
- Electronic
- mAs
- Automatic exposure control (AEC) (ionization chamber/phototimer)

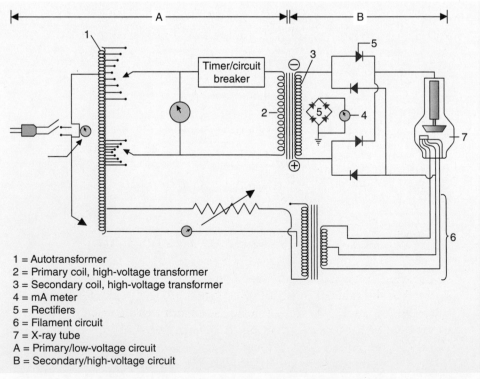

1 = Autotransformer
2 = Primary coil, high-voltage transformer
3 = Secondary coil, high-voltage transformer
4 = mA meter
5 = Rectifiers
6 = Filament circuit
7 = X-ray tube
A = Primary/low-voltage circuit
B = Secondary/high-voltage circuit

Figure 13-37. Simplified x-ray circuit. High-voltage current from the secondary transformer coil is rectified before it reaches the x-ray tube. (Reproduced with permission from Saia DA. *Lange Q&A Radiography Examination.* 7th ed. New York, NY: McGraw-Hill; 2009.)

Line voltage compensator: It functions to automatically adjust for any fluctuations in incoming voltage supply. A uniformly consistent and accurate voltage supply is required for predictable radiographic results. A small variation in voltage entering the primary transformer coil voltage represents a much larger variation as it leaves the secondary coil. The control consoles of some older x-ray units were equipped with line voltage compensators that were adjustable by the radiographer, but in equipment manufactured nowadays, the process takes place automatically within the machine.

Timer: It functions to regulate the length of x-ray exposure. Very simple timers such as the mechanical, synchronous, and impulse timers are rarely used in x-ray equipment manufactured nowadays because they do not permit very fast, accurate exposures. *Mechanical timers* are capable of exposures only as short as ¼ s; *synchronous timers* as short as $\frac{1}{60}$ s *Impulse timers* are more accurate and capable of exposures as short as $\frac{1}{120}$ s.

The *electronic timer* used in x-ray equipment manufactured nowadays is somewhat complex and based on a capacitor–resistor circuit. Electronic timers are very accurate and capable of rapid exposures as short as 1 ms (i.e., $\frac{1}{1000}$ or 0.001 s).

The *milliampere-second timer* (*mAs timer*) monitors the product of mA and time and terminates the exposure when the desired mAs has been reached. mAs timers are found on some mobile x-ray units. They are also found on some older, fixed x-ray units and display the mAs exposure value when exposure time is too short to permit the actual mA to register on the mA meter.

Another type of timer is the *AEC,* which functions to produce consistent radiographic results (Fig. 13-38). AECs have sensors that signal to terminate the exposure once a predetermined, known, and correct exposure has been reached.

AEC is used to automatically regulate the amount of ionizing radiation delivered through the anatomic part to the IR/radiation detector, regardless of the IR/radiation detector type, thereby serving to produce consistent and comparable radiographic results with minimum patient exposure. When AEC is installed in the x-ray circuit, it is calibrated to terminate the exposure once the predetermined desirable exposure has been made.

Exact positioning and centering are particularly critical when using AEC. The anatomic part of interest must be aligned (centered) accurately with respect to the AEC sensors; otherwise, the result can be over- or underexposure. The correct AEC sensors must be selected. If the value of interest (*VOI*) *is small,* AEC detectors not covered by anatomy are likely to cause premature termination of exposure, resulting in quantum noise. A large metal orthopedic prosthetic should not be positioned directly over an AEC sensor because an excessive exposure time can result, causing patient and image overexposure.

The type of AEC most often used, the *ionization chamber,* is located just beneath the tabletop, above the radiation detector. The part

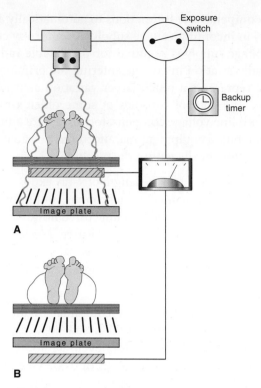

Figure 13-38. Two types of automatic exposure controls. AEC (A) consists of an *ionization chamber* located *under* the x-ray tabletop. The electrometer measures the number of ionizations and terminates the exposure once a predetermined quantity has been reached. AEC (B) is the *phototimer,* consisting of a PMT located *under the IP*. Note that a backup timer is in place to terminate the exposure should the AEC fail to do so. (Reproduced with permission from Saia DA. *Lange Q&A Radiography Examination.* 7th ed. New York, NY: McGraw-Hill; 2009.)

being imaged is centered to the sensor and exposed. When the predetermined quantity of air ionization has occurred within the chamber, as measured and determined by an electrometer, the exposure is automatically terminated.

Another type of AEC is the *phototimer,* located behind the radiation detector/IR. The phototimer consists of a special fluorescent screen that, when activated by x-ray, produces light and charges a PMT. When the correct charge has been reached, as determined by the electrometer, the exposure is automatically terminated.

A *backup timer* (the manual timer) is used to protect the patient from unnecessary exposure, and the x-ray tube from damage, should the AEC fail to operate properly. Additional discussion of AECs can be found in Chapter 12.

X-ray timer malfunction can cause undesirable fluctuation in receptor exposure. If the timer terminates the exposure prematurely, the image can be underexposed; if the exposure is delayed in terminating, the image can be overexposed. Electronic timers can be accurate to as low as 1 ms. The spinning-top test used to evaluate timer accuracy in single- and three-phase equipment cannot be used for three-phase or high-frequency equipment. The majority of exposure timers are now electronic and usually controlled by a microprocessor and accuracy evaluated with an oscilloscope.

Primary coil of the high-voltage transformer: It is the final component of the primary, or low-voltage, circuit. The low voltage entering the primary coil is stepped up to high kilovoltage in the secondary coil by means of mutual induction.

Exposure switch: It is a remote control switch that functions to start the x-ray exposure (the timer terminates the exposure).

Filament Circuit Components

The filament circuit is responsible for supplying low-voltage current (3–5 A, 10–12 V) to the filament of the x-ray tube. Because the incoming voltage (110–220 V) is greater than that required, a *step-down transformer* is placed in the filament circuit to make the required voltage adjustment. A *rheostat*, or other type of *variable resistor*, is placed in the filament circuit to adjust amperage and corresponds to the *mA selector* on the control console.

Secondary Circuit Components

Secondary or High-Voltage Circuit Devices

Secondary coil of high-voltage transformer: It carries the required high voltage for x-ray production (and proportionally smaller current value).

mA meter: It is located at the midpoint of the secondary transformer coil. Because it is grounded, it can be safely placed in the operator's console. The mA meter displays the tube current value.

Rectifiers: These comprise a system of diodes located between the secondary coil of the high-voltage transformer and the x-ray tube. Recall from earlier discussion that they allow current to flow in only one direction and function to change AC to unidirectional pulsating current. Current pulsations decrease with solid-state, 3φ rectification (3φ 6p rectification has a 13% ripple; 3φ 12p rectification has a 4% ripple).

X-ray tube: It is the final device in the secondary circuit. The filament of its negative electrode, the cathode, is heated by its own circuit to produce *thermionic emission*. As high voltage is applied, the thermionic electron cloud is driven to the anode target. The rapid deceleration of electrons, and their interaction with tungsten atoms of the target, results in an energy conversion to heat and x-rays (99.8% heat, 0.2% x-rays).

Circuitry Overview of a Single Exposure

1. X-ray machine is turned on. This activates the filament circuit and heats the x-ray tube filament (10–12 V, 3–5 A).

2. If the machine has been off overnight, warm-up exposures are made to warm the anode throughout (anode cracking can occur when surface heat is applied to a cold anode).

3. Appropriate technical factors are chosen on the control panel (machines having a line voltage compensator on the control panel should be adjusted to compensate for any incoming voltage fluctuation).

Primary/Low-Voltage Circuit Components

- Main switch/circuit breaker
- Autotransformer
- kV selector switch
- Line voltage compensator
- Timer
- Primary coil of high-voltage transformer
- Exposure switch

Secondary/High-Voltage Circuit Components

- Secondary coil of high-voltage transformer
- mA meter (grounded at midpoint of the secondary coil)
- Rectifiers
- X-ray tube

4. The rotor/exposure switch is often a two-stage exposure button that should be depressed completely in one motion; the first click heard after partial depression is the induction motor bringing anode rotation up to speed. At this time, the filament is heated to maximum (thermionic emission) and produces an electron cloud.

5. On complete depression of the rotor/exposure switch, the exposure is made. The moment the exposure button is depressed, the voltage selected by the autotransformer is sent to the step-up transformer where it is converted to the required high voltage (kV) and low amperage (mA). This high-voltage current then passes through the rectification system that changes AC to pulsating DC.

6. The applied high voltage (potential difference) propels the electron cloud to the anode where interactions between the high-speed electrons and tungsten target atoms convert electron kinetic energy to (99.8%) heat energy and (0.2%) x-ray photon energy.

Summary

- The three portions of the x-ray circuit are the low-voltage/primary circuit, the filament circuit, and the high-voltage/secondary circuit.

- Primary circuit devices include the main switch and circuit breaker, the autotransformer and kV selector, line voltage compensator, timer, primary coil of the high-voltage transformer, and exposure switch; most of the control console devices are in the primary circuit.

- The timer regulates the length of the x-ray exposure; types of timers include mechanical, impulse, synchronous, mAs timer, electronic timer, and AEC.

- There are two types of AECs: the ionization chamber, located above the IR and the phototimer, located behind the IR.

- A *backup timer* terminates the exposure should the AEC fail, thereby protecting the patient from excessive exposure and prolonging the life of the x-ray tube.

- A step-down transformer and a rheostat (or other variable resistor) are placed in the filament circuit to supply the x-ray tube with a low-voltage current.

- Secondary circuit devices include the secondary coil of the high-voltage transformer, mA meter, rectifiers, and x-ray tube; the grounded mA meter can display the tube current value on the control console.

- Rectifiers are located between the transformer's secondary coil and the x-ray tube; they change AC to unidirectional current.

COMPREHENSION CHECK

1. Identify the three portions of the x-ray circuit (p. 436).

2. Identify the components of the primary, or low-voltage, circuit (p. 436, 437).

3. Describe the various types of x-ray timers and identify their accuracy (p. 437).

4. Describe the two types of AECs and identify the location of each (p. 437, 438).

5. Discuss the importance of a backup timer (p. 438).

6. Describe the tests used to evaluate 3φ timers (p. 439).

7. Identify the function of the rheostat and transformer in the filament circuit (p. 439, 440).

8. Identify and describe the components of the secondary, or high-voltage, circuit (p. 439).

CHAPTER REVIEW QUESTIONS

1. An AEC device can operate on which of the following principles?
   1. A PMT charged by a fluorescent screen
   2. A parallel-plate ionization chamber charged by x-ray photons
   3. Motion of magnetic fields inducing current in a conductor
   (A) 1 only
   (B) 2 only
   (C) 1 and 2 only
   (D) 1, 2, and 3

2. Which of the following AEC devices is most commonly used in imaging equipment these days?
   (A) Phototimer
   (B) Ionization chamber
   (C) Sensor
   (D) Backup timer

3. The AEC backup timer functions to
   1. protect the patient from overexposure
   2. protect the x-ray tube from excessive heat
   3. increase or decrease programmed receptor exposure
   (A) 1 only
   (B) 1 and 2 only
   (C) 2 and 3 only
   (D) 1, 2, and 3

4. The voltage ripple associated with a three-phase, 12-pulse–rectified generator is about
   (A) 4%
   (B) 13%
   (C) 32%
   (D) 100%

5. Circuit devices that permit electrons to flow in only one direction are
   (A) solid-state diodes
   (B) resistors
   (C) transformers
   (D) autotransformers

6. Which of the following is/are component(s) of the secondary, or high-voltage, side of the x-ray circuit?
   1. Rectification system
   2. Autotransformer
   3. kV meter
   (A) 1 only
   (B) 1 and 2 only
   (C) 2 and 3 only
   (D) 1, 2, and 3

7. If the primary coil of a high-voltage transformer is supplied by 220 V and has 400 turns and the secondary coil has 100,000 turns, what is the voltage induced in the secondary coil?
   (A) 80 kV
   (B) 55 kV
   (C) 80 V
   (D) 55 V

8. A device used to ensure reproducible radiographs, regardless of tissue density variations, is the
   (A) automatic exposure control
   (B) penetrometer
   (C) autotransformer
   (D) anatomically programmed radiography

9. Accurate operation of the AEC device depends on
   1. tissue thickness and density
   2. positioning of the object with respect to the photocell
   3. beam restriction
   (A) 1 only
   (B) 1 and 2 only
   (C) 2 and 3 only
   (D) 1, 2, and 3

10. What is located between the secondary coil of the high-voltage transformer and the x-ray tube?
    (A) Timer
    (B) Rectifiers
    (C) Filament circuit
    (D) Autotransformer

11. In which part of the radiographic circuit can the x-ray tube be found?

    (A) Filament circuit

    (B) Secondary circuit

    (C) Exposure switch

    (D) Primary circuit

12. Where in the radiographic circuit can the step-down transformer be found?

    1. Filament circuit

    2. Primary, or low-voltage circuit

    3. Secondary, or high-voltage circuit

    (A) 1 only

    (B) 2 only

    (C) 3 only

    (D) 1 and 2 only

Answers and Explanations

1. (C) A parallel-plate *ionization chamber* is the most common type of AEC. A radiolucent chamber is located beneath the patient (between the patient and the IR). As photons emerge from the patient, they enter the chamber and ionize the air within it. Once a predetermined charge has been reached, the exposure is terminated automatically. The *phototimer* is another type of AEC that actually measures light. As x-ray photons penetrate and emerge from a part, a fluorescent screen beneath the IR glows and the fluorescent light charges a PMT. Once a predetermined charge has been reached, the exposure terminates automatically. Motion of magnetic fields inducing current in a conductor refers to the *principle of mutual induction.*

2. (B) AECs are used in equipment nowadays and serve to produce consistent and comparable results. The most commonly used type of AEC is the ionization chamber, located beneath the tabletop and above the IR. The part to be examined is centered to it (the sensor) and radiographed. When a predetermined quantity of ionization has occurred (equal to the correct receptor exposure), the exposure terminates automatically. The older type AEC, the phototimer, a small fluorescent screen, is positioned beneath the IR. Remnant radiation emerging from the patient, exposes the IR, exits, and the fluorescent screen emits light. Once a predetermined amount of fluorescence has been detected by the photocell sensor, the exposure is terminated automatically. In either case, the manual timer should be used as a backup timer; in case of AEC malfunction, the exposure would terminate, thus avoiding patient overexposure and tube overload.

3. (B) When an AEC is installed in an x-ray circuit, it is calibrated to produce radiographic densities as required by the radiologist. Once the part being radiographed has been exposed to produce the correct receptor exposure, the AEC automatically terminates the exposure. The manual timer should be used as a backup timer; in case the AEC fails to terminate the exposure, the backup timer would protect the patient from overexposure and the x-ray tube from excessive heat load. The master receptor exposure override generally is set on normal to produce the required receptor exposure. In special cases, when this produces excessive or insufficient receptor exposure, the master receptor exposure override may be adjusted to plus or minus position.

4. (A) *Voltage ripple* refers to the percentage drop from maximum voltage each pulse of current experiences. In single-phase rectified equipment, the entire pulse (half-cycle) is used; therefore, there is first an increase to the maximum (peak) voltage value and then a decrease to zero potential (90° past peak potential). The entire waveform is used; at 100 kV, the actual average kilovoltage output would be approximately 70 kV. Three-phase rectification produces almost constant potential, with small ripples (drops) in maximum potential between pulses. Approximately a 13% voltage ripple (drop from maximum value) characterizes the operation of three-phase, six-pulse generators. Three-phase, 12-pulse generators have about a 4% voltage ripple. HF current is most efficient and produces less than 1% voltage ripple. The HF generator is small in size and produces an almost constant potential waveform.

5. (A) *Rectifiers change AC into unidirectional current* by allowing current to flow through them in only one direction. Valve tubes are vacuum rectifier tubes found in older equipment. *Solid-state diodes* are the types of rectifiers used in x-ray equipment these days. Rectification systems are found between the secondary coil of the high-voltage transformer and the x-ray tube. *Resistors,* such as rheostats or choke coils, are circuit devices used to vary voltage or current. *Transformers,* operating on the principle of mutual induction, change the voltage (and current) to useful levels. *Autotransformers,* operating on the principle of self-induction, enable us to select the required kilovoltage.

6. (A) All circuit devices located *before* the primary coil of the high-voltage transformer are said to be on the *primary or low-voltage* side of the x-ray circuit. The timer, autotransformer, and (prereading) kilovoltage meter are all located in the *low*-voltage circuit.

The *secondary/high-voltage* side of the circuit begins with the *secondary coil* of the high-voltage transformer. The *mA meter* is connected at the midpoint of the secondary coil of the high-voltage transformer. Following the secondary coil is the *rectification system* and the *x-ray tube.*

Transformers are used to change the value of an AC. They operate on the principle of mutual induction. The secondary coil of the step-up transformer is located in the high-voltage (secondary) side of the x-ray circuit. The step-down transformer, or filament transformer, is located in the filament circuit and serves to regulate the voltage and current provided to heat the x-ray tube filament. The rectification system is also located on the high-voltage, or secondary, side of the x-ray circuit.

7. (B) The high-voltage, or step-up, transformer functions to *increase voltage* to the necessary kilovoltage. It *decreases the amperage* to milliamperage. The amount of increase or decrease *depends on the transformer ratio,* that is, the ratio of the number of turns in the primary coil to the number of turns in the secondary coil. The transformer law is as follows:

To Determine Secondary *V*	To Determine Secondary *I*
$\dfrac{V_s}{V_p} = \dfrac{N_s}{N_p}$	$\dfrac{N_s}{N_p} = \dfrac{I_p}{I_S}$

Substituting known values:

$$\frac{x}{220} = \frac{100{,}000}{400}$$

$$400x = 22{,}000{,}000$$

Thus, $x = 55{,}000$ V (55 kV).

8. (A) Radiographic reproducibility is an important concept in producing high-quality diagnostic images. Radiographic results should be consistent and predictable not only in terms of positioning accuracy but also with respect to exposure factors. AEC devices (phototimers and ionization chambers) automatically terminate the x-ray exposure once a predetermined quantity of x-rays has penetrated the patient, thus ensuring consistent results. A penetrometer can be used to demonstrate effects of kV on contrast. The autotransformer allows the radiographer to select kilovoltage at the console. Anatomically programmed radiography refers to the x-ray system's ability to provide predetermined technical exposure factors based on the anatomical part selected by the radiographer. APR will not automatically alter these suggested values based on the exposure received.

9. (C) The AEC automatically terminates the exposure when the proper receptor exposure has been reached. The important advantage of the phototimer, then, is that it can accurately duplicate receptor exposures. It is very useful in providing accurate comparison in follow-up examinations and in decreasing patient exposure dose by reducing the number of "retakes" needed because of improper exposure. The AEC automatically adjusts the exposure required for body parts with different thicknesses and densities. However, proper functioning of the phototimer depends on accurate positioning by the radiographer. The correct photocell(s) must be selected, and the anatomic part of interest must completely cover the photocell to achieve the desired receptor exposure. If collimation is inadequate and a field size larger than the part is used, excessive SR from the body or tabletop can cause the AEC to terminate the exposure prematurely, resulting in an underexposed image.

10. (B) The rectifiers are system of diodes located between the secondary coil of the high-voltage transformer and the x-ray tube. They allow current to flow in only one direction and function to change AC to unidirectional pulsating current. Current pulsations decrease with solid-state, three-phase rectification (3φ 6p rectification has a 13% ripple; 3φ 12p rectification has a 4% ripple).

11. (B) The x-ray tube, high-voltage transformer, and rectification system can all be found on the secondary, or high-voltage, circuit. Most of the control console devices can be found on the primary, or low-voltage, circuit. The filament circuit is responsible for supplying low-voltage current to the filament of the x-ray tube. The exposure switch is found on the primary circuit.

12. (A) The step-down transformer can be found in the filament circuit. Because the incoming voltage it receives is much greater than needed, a step-down transformer will reduce the voltage and increase the current as necessary. The primary coil of the high-voltage transformer is located on the primary circuit, whereas the secondary coil of the high-voltage transformer is located on the secondary circuit. The high-voltage transformer is a step-up transformer that increases voltage and decreases current as necessary.

COMPONENTS OF DIGITAL IMAGING

Anatomically Programmed Radiography

By using automatically programmed technique, or APR, the radiographer uses console graphics or a touch screen to *select the anatomic part, the desired position/procedure, and the relative size* (S, M, L) of the part to be imaged (Fig. 13-39). The unit's microprocessor chooses the appropriate preprogrammed mAs and kV algorithm for that particular part and size—from the "internal technique chart" predetermined and stored on installation. Both AEC and manual exposure factors are typically recommended so that under nonroutine conditions, the radiographer can modify the preset/programmed factors.

APR is used in conjunction with AEC and is therefore still highly dependent on the skillfulness of its user. Accurate positioning, photocell selection, and control of SR are essential to the production of quality images. See the "AEC" section(s) for review of these important factors.

Computer System Fundamentals. The computer system consists of the *hardware*, which is any physical component of the computer, and the *software*, which is a set of instructions or program to operate the computer.

The hardware consists of input and output devices. These devices allow information to be put into a computer and allow information to be directed outside the computer. The *central processing unit* is the primary control center for the computer consisting of a control unit, an arithmetic unit, and memory. The speed is measured in "millions of instructions per second." Most desktop computer speeds are given in megahertz (MHz). The *memory* is solid state. It is used by the computer during execution of a program. There are two types of memory. The first is *RAM*, or random access memory. This memory is volatile and will lose all information when the computer is turned off unless previously saved. Read-only memory, or *ROM*, is the memory that is hardwired into the computer, which means it stays in the computer even when the computer is turned off. ROM usually contains the booting instructions.

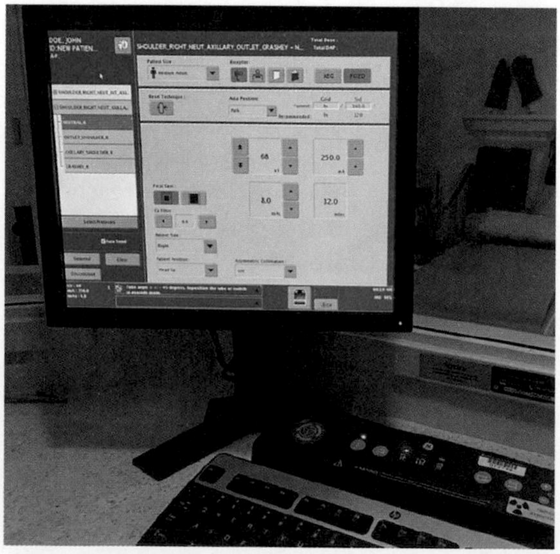

Figure 13-39. Acquisition workstation of APR unit. (Photo contributor: Richard Kovatch, RT(R).)

Pixel

- Two dimensional
- *Picture element*
- Measured in *XY* direction

Voxel

- The third dimension, depth
- *Volume element*
- Measured in *Z* direction

Bit

- *Binary digit*
- Smallest unit of computer data

Bit Depth

- Number of bits per pixel
- Determines gray scale

Matrix

- Number of pixels in *XY* direction making up a digital image

Field of View (FOV)

- How much of the part/patient is included in the matrix

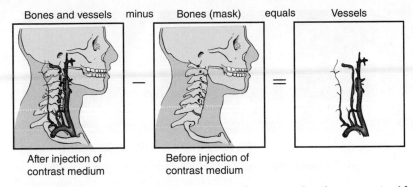

Bones and vessels   minus   Bones (mask)   equals   Vessels

After injection of
contrast medium

Before injection of
contrast medium

Figure 13-40. Digital subtraction angiography. Image details not required for diagnosis can be subtracted from an image. Only vessels containing contrast medium are visualized in the final image.

The *software* is a set of instructions the computer uses to function effectively, known as a *program*. Computer programming languages include, but are not limited to:

- Fortran: formula translation; used mainly in science and engineering applications.
- Basic: a beginner's all-purpose language with symbolic instructions and code.
- Cobol: common business-oriented language.
- Pascal: high-level mathematics.

Binary numbers: The computer hardware interprets all information as a simple "yes" or "no" decision. Current "on" implies "yes" and current "off" implies "no." This is symbolically represented with digits 1 and 0. A *bit* in computer terminology refers to an individual 1 or 0 and is a single bit of information. Bit *depth* refers to the number of *bits per pixel* and identifies the levels of gray/*gray scale*.

Image storage: Image storage is located in a *pixel* (Fig. 13-41A), which is a two-dimensional "picture element." Pixels are measured in the "*XY*" direction.

Typical Image Matrix Sizes Used in Medical Imaging Are

Nuclear medicine	128 × 128
Digital subtraction angiography (DSA) (Fig. 13-40)	1024 × 1024
CT	512 × 512
Chest radiography	2048 × 2048

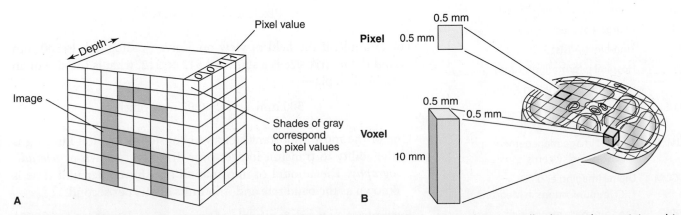

Figure 13-41. (A) A digital image may be likened to a three-dimensional object made up of many small cubes, each containing a binary digit or bit. The image is seen on one surface of the block, whose depth is the number of bits required to describe each pixel's gray level. **(B)** The third dimension in the matrix of pixels is the depth, which together with the pixel is called the voxel (volume element).

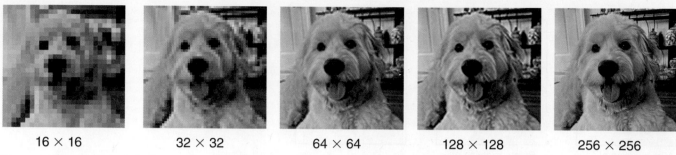

| 16 × 16 | 32 × 32 | 64 × 64 | 128 × 128 | 256 × 256 |

Figure 13-42. The matrix is the number of pixels in the *XY* direction. The larger the matrix size, the better the image resolution.

Digital Image Resolution Improves With

- Smaller pixel size
- Smaller pixel pitch
- Larger image matrix

Abbreviations

IP	Image plate
PSP	Photostimulable phosphor
PSL	Photostimulated luminescence
SPS	Storage phosphor screen
CR	Computed radiography
SNR	Signal-to-noise ratio
MTF	Modulation transfer function
PMT	Photomultiplier tube
PD	Photodiode
ADC	Analog-to-digital converter
APR	Anatomically programmed radiography
DQE	Detective quantum efficiency
CCD	Charge-coupled device
TFT	Thin-film transistor
HIS	Hospital information system
RIS	Radiology information system
PACS	Picture archiving and communication system
MIMPS	Medical image management and processing systems
DICOM	Digital Imaging and COmmunications in Medicine
EDR	Exposure data recognition
DEL	Detector element

The third dimension in the matrix of pixels is the depth that, together with the pixel, is called the *voxel* (Fig. 13-41B). The voxels are measured in the "Z" direction. The depth of the block is the number of bits required to describe the gray level that each pixel can take on. This is known as the *bit depth*.

The matrix is the number of pixels in the *XY* direction. The larger the matrix size, the better the image resolution (Fig. 13-42). The smaller the pixels and *pixel pitch* (i.e., distance between the center of one pixel to the center of adjacent pixel), the better the resolution.

A digital image is formed by a *matrix* of *pixels* in rows and columns. A matrix having 512 pixels in each row and column is a 512 × 512 matrix. The term *FOV* is used to describe how much of the part (e.g., 150-mm diameter) is included in the matrix. The matrix or FOV can be changed without affecting the other, but changes in either will change pixel size. As matrix size is increased, there are more and smaller pixels in the matrix, therefore, improved spatial resolution; *spatial resolution* is measured in line pairs per millimeter (lp/mm). Fewer and larger pixels result in a poor resolution "pixelly" image, that is, one in which you can actually see the individual pixel boxes (Fig. 13-42).

The size of a pixel can be calculated mathematically if the size of the FOV and the matrix are both known. To calculate the size of a pixel, one must divide the size of the FOV by the matrix.

$$\text{Pixel size} = \text{FOV/Matrix}$$

For example, if the field of view on a given radiograph is 500 mm and the matrix size is a standard 512 × 512, what is the size of an individual pixel?

$$500 \text{ mm} \div 512 = 0.97 \text{ mm/pixel}$$

One of the most important factors to consider in digital imaging is the ability to transmit images over distances, known as *teleradiography*. The amount of information transferred per unit time is known as the baud rate and is in units of bits per second.

Example: A network is capable of transmitting data at a rate of 9600 baud. If each pixel has a bit depth of 8 bits, how long will it take to transmit a 512 × 512 image?

Solution:

$$(512 \times 512 \text{ pixels})(8 \text{ bits}/\text{pixel})/9600 \text{ bits}/\text{s} = 128 \text{ s}.$$

There are three possible means of image transmission. *Telephone* wires offer low-transmission speed while using a modem. *Coaxial cable* will transmit at approximately 100 Mbaud. Finally, there are *fiber-optic cables* that are unaffected by electrical fields and therefore have less error than cables or wires with electrical signals.

Summary

- APR utilizes selection of anatomic part rather than selection of specific technical factors.
- There are two types of computer memory: RAM and ROM.
- A two-dimensional picture element is a pixel; a three-dimensional picture element is a voxel.
- Spatial resolution is measured in lp/mm.
- Spatial resolution improves with smaller pixel size, smaller pixel pitch, and larger image matrix.
- Images can be transmitted via telephone wires, coaxial cable, and fiber-optic cable.

The Image Plate

The IP used in CR has a *protective* function for the flexible PSP storage plate within; it can be conveniently placed in a Bucky tray or under the anatomic part and comes in a variety of sizes (Fig. 13-43A). The *PSP* within the IP is the *IR*.

IPs need not be light-tight because the PSP storage plate inside is *not light sensitive*. One corner of the IP's rear panel has a *memory chip* for patient information; the IP also has a thin *lead foil backing* to absorb any backscatter.

The Photostimulable Phosphor

Inside the IP is the all-important *PSP* storage plate, which is the actual IR.

The PSP has a layer of europium-activated barium fluorohalide ($BaFX:Eu^{2+}$; X = halogen) mixed with a binder substance. When the PSP receives x-ray photons, the x-ray energy interacts with the barium fluorohalide crystals to form the latent image.

The barium fluorohalide is usually *granular* or *turbid* phosphors. Other examples of turbid phosphors are Gd_2O_2S and rubidium chloride. *Needle*-shaped or *columnar* phosphors (usually CsI) have the advantage of *better x-ray absorption* and *less light diffusion* (Fig. 13-43B).

Just under the barium fluorohalide layer is a *reflective layer* that helps direct emitted light up toward the CR reader. Below the reflective layer is the *base,* behind that is an *antistatic layer,* and then the *lead foil* to absorb backscatter. There is a *protective layer* over the top of the barium fluorohalide.

PSP Storage Plate Layers

- Protective coat
- $BaFX:Eu^{2+}$ phosphors in binder material
- Reflective backing
- Polyester base support material
- Antistatic layer
- Lead foil backing

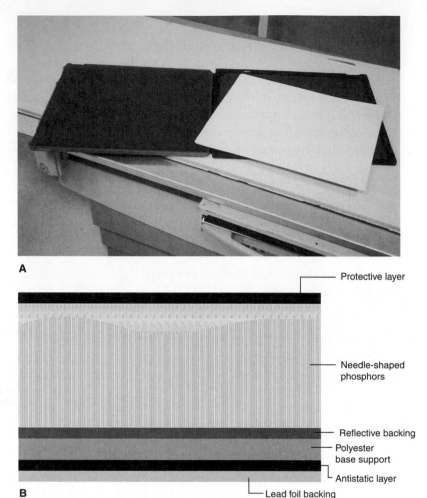

Figure 13-43. **(A)** The IP holds a PSP storage plate (the IR) between its front and rear panels. (Reproduced with permission from Shephard CT. *Radiographic Image Production and Manipulation.* New York, NY: McGraw-Hill; 2003.) **(B)** Barium fluorohalide is either granular or "needle-shaped." The "needlelike" phosphors have the advantage of *better x-ray absorption and less light diffusion.*

Some PSP storage plates are manufactured specifically for better resolution (e.g., for mammography). Some higher resolution PSP storage plates "read" the information from *both* sides of the PSP storage plates.

X-ray Absorption by PSP

When the barium fluorohalide absorbs x-ray energy, *electrons are released and they divide into two groups.* One electron group initiates *immediate luminescence* (primary excitation) during the excited state of Eu^{2+}. The other electron group *becomes trapped* within the phosphors halogen ions, forming a "color center" (also called "F center"). These are the phosphors that ultimately form the radiographic image because, when exposed to a *monochromatic* laser light source, these phosphors emit *polychromatic* light (secondary excitation), termed *PSL*.

The PSP layer can *store* its latent image for several hours; however, after approximately 8 h, noticeable image *fading* will occur. The europium activator is important for the *storage* characteristic of the PSPs; without europium, the latent image will not change to a manifest image.

Reading the PSP

After exposure, the IP is placed into the CR *scanner/reader* (Fig. 13-44A and B), where the PSP screen is automatically removed. The latent

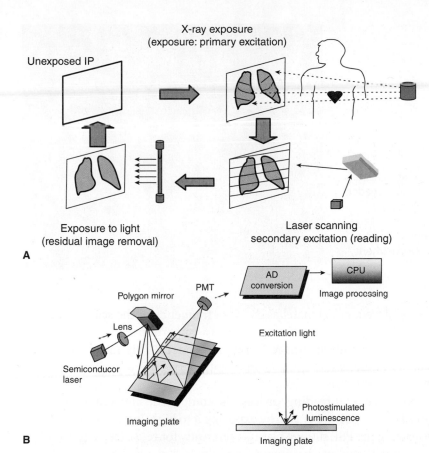

Figure 13-44. **(A)** The *recording, reading,* and *erasure cycle* of a CR PSP storage plate. The PSP is exposed to x-ray photons, scanned/read, and then erased for reuse. (Photo contributor: Courtesy of FUJIFILM Medical System USA.) **(B)** The latent image on the PSP screen is changed to a manifest image as it is moved at a constant speed and scanned by a narrow, high-intensity helium–neon laser or a solid-state laser to obtain the pixel data. (Photo contributor: Courtesy of FUJIFILM Medical System USA.)

image on the PSP is changed to a *manifest image* as it is moved at a *constant* speed and scanned by a narrow monochromatic *high-intensity helium–neon laser* or a *solid-state* laser to obtain the pixel data.

The longer wavelength light from the newer *solid-state lasers* has the advantage of being unlikely to interfere with the light being emitted by the PSPs. This appropriate (red, 430–550 nm) wavelength is absorbed by the "color center" and the electrons trapped there, causing PSL to occur during the excited state of Eu^{2+} (secondary excitation).

The phosphors are activated by a *monochromatic laser light*; however, PSL is a *different* color (bluish-purple, blue–green, etc.). These two lights (PSL and laser) must not interfere with each other. To improve the image SNR, the PSL (carrying the x-ray image) must be a different wavelength/color than, and physically separate from, the laser excitation light. An *optical filter* is used that permits *transmission* of the PSL but *attenuates* the laser light; this filter is mounted in front of a PMT (Fig. 13-44B).

The PMT or PD is used to detect the PSL and convert it to electrical signals. The electrical energy is sent to an *ADC*, where it becomes the *digital* image that is displayed, after a short delay, on a high-resolution monitor and/or printed out by a laser printer (hardcopy). The digitized images can also be manipulated in *postprocessing*, electronically *transmitted*, and stored/*archived*. Postprocessing manipulation can include *edge enhancement*; this technique can be used to improve the visibility of structures such as chest tubes by accentuating their edges.

An artifact associated with digital imaging and grids is "aliasing" (Fig. 13-45). If the direction of the lead strips and the grid lines per inch

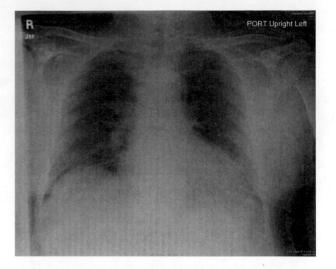

Figure 13-45. Aliasing artifact. If the direction of the lead strips and the grid frequency matches the scan frequency of the scanner/reader, this artifact can occur. Aliasing (sometimes called Moiré effect) appears as superimposed images slightly out of alignment, an image "wrapping" effect. This is most common in mobile radiography with stationary grids. (Photo contributor: Stamford Hospital, Department of Radiology.)

(i.e., grid frequency) matches the scan frequency of the scanner/reader, this artifact can occur. Aliasing appears as superimposed images slightly out of alignment, an image "wrapping" effect. This most commonly occurs in mobile radiography with stationary grids and can be a problem with DR FPDs.

Once the PSP-reading process is completed, any remaining data stored on the PSP are erased by exposing it to high-intensity light (called "erasure"); the PSP storage plate is then ready for reuse (see Fig. 13-44A).

As mentioned earlier, image *fading* will occur if there is a delay in reading the PSP. This is because after a time, trapped photoelectrons are released from the "color center" and are therefore unable to participate in PSL. PSL intensity *decreases* as the time interval between x-ray exposure and the image-reading process increases. If the exposed PSL is not delivered to the reader/processor for 8 h, PSL decreases by approximately 25%. Fading also increases as environmental temperature increases.

PSP Sensitivity

PSP storage plates are very sensitive (more than film emulsion) to not only x-rays but also ultraviolet, gamma, and particulate radiations. Environmental conditions are therefore an important consideration in the storage of PSP/storage screens and their IPs.

Building materials such as concrete, marble, and so on, constantly emit natural radiation; bedrock in some geographic areas contributes significantly to background radiation. If PSP storage plates are stored for extended periods of time, the possibility of artifacts must be considered. These artifacts typically appear as randomly placed small black spots. *If an IP and its PSP storage plate have been stored, unused, for an extended period of time (i.e., for 48 h), the PSP storage plate should be erased prior to use.*

The mechanical consistency and accuracy of the laser optics and transport systems of the CR scanner/reader are extremely important for image quality—inconsistent scanning motion can result in a wavy, or otherwise distorted, image. This is sometimes called *laser jitter* and should be evaluated monthly as part of the CR QA monitoring.

Steps in Reading the PSP Storage Plate

- IP into scanner/reader
- PSP automatically removed
- PSP moved at constant speed, scanned by a monochromatic laser to obtain pixel data
- PSL occurs during scanning
- Scanning laser and PSL must be different wavelengths and must not interact
- For better SNR, an optical filter attenuates the laser while transmitting the PSL
- PMT/PD detects the PSL and converts it to electrical signals
- Electrical signals sent to ADC and displayed on the monitor
- PSP erased by exposing it to high-intensity light; ready for reuse

Dynamic Range and Postprocessing

In CR, there is a *linear* relationship between the exposure, given the PSP storage plate and its resulting luminescence, as it is scanned by the laser. One of the biggest advantages of CR is the dynamic range of gray scale it offers—many, many more shades of gray are made available for viewing and diagnostic interpretation. Gray scale is variations in brightness resulting from intensity variations and made available for perception by the human eye by computer manipulation.

CR's wide dynamic range permits visualization of anatomic details having only slightly different absorption differentials and also permits the use of EDR, which automatically adjusts image brightness and contrast to meet diagnostic requirements.

Digital imaging affords much greater *dynamic range* and *exposure latitude;* technical inaccuracies can be effectively eliminated from the "raw" image through rescaling (normalizing). Overexposure of up to 500% and underexposure of up to 80% are reported as recoverable, thus eliminating most retakes (Fig. 13-46A–F). *This surely affords increased efficiency; however, this does not mean that images can be exposed arbitrarily.*

Postprocessing is the ability to manipulate the image after exposure (Fig. 13-47). Among other things, image manipulation postprocessing can be used for *grayscale/contrast* modification via *windowing.* The window *width* is related to the shades of gray; window *level* corresponds to the *brightness.*

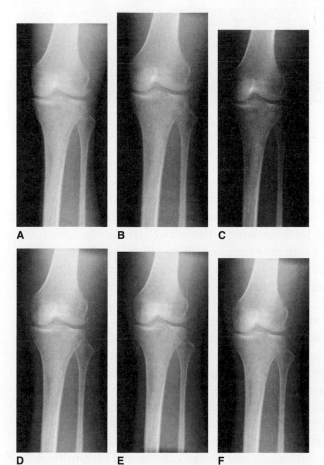

A   B   C

D   E   F

Figure 13-46. CR affords an almost infinite dynamic range/gray scale; technical inaccuracies can be effectively eliminated, but exposure dose must still be considered. In the images seen above, **(A)**, **(B)**, and **(C)** were made with conventional SF using at 65 kV and at 3.2, 6.3, and 12.5 mAs, respectively. Receptor exposure changes are easily identified. Images **(D)**, **(E)**, and **(F)** were made with CR using the same 3.2, 6.3, and 12.5 mAs, respectively. These images are identical—demonstrating how technical inaccuracies can be effectively eliminated with CR. Although the images are identical, the exposure dose is not! An approximation of the exposure dose can be determined from the exposure indicator: an "S" (sensitivity) number, "EI" (exposure index), or other "relative exposure index," depending on the manufacturer.

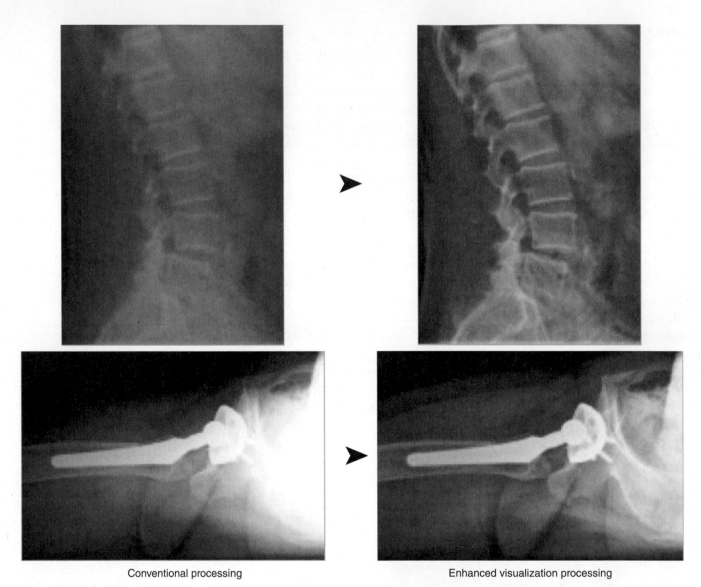

Conventional processing   Enhanced visualization processing

Figure 13-47. Lateral lumbar and lateral hip images on the left were processed with conventional processing technology. Images on the right are the result of enhanced visualization technology. (FUJIFILM Healthcare Americas Corp.)

Image *annotation* permits placement of labels, arrow indicators, markers and more on the digital image. These can be useful in pointing out important information to the viewer. Image inversion, or reversal, provides a different perspective by changing white to black and black to white. Image flip also provides another perspective by enabling *rotation* of the image over the horizontal and vertical axes. *Edge enhancement* creates images with higher resolution through less pixel averaging. This is useful for the visualization of small, complex, and high-contrast tissues. Image smoothing can be used to reduce the noise on an image but must not be used excessively for it could cause a loss of detail. Other postprocessing functions include highlighting, zoom, pan, and scroll.

Advancements in image processing have made significant improvements in visualization of anatomic details, practically eliminating the need for postprocessing. The advanced technology automatically recognizes tissue density differences and characteristics, and even orthopedic hardware. It automatically compensates for, and enhances, anatomic structures having widely different tissue densities and produces a uniformly diagnostic image.

Exposure Indication

CR offers *wide dynamic range and automatic optimization of the radiologic image.* When AEC is not used, CR can compensate for approximately 80% underexposure and 500% overexposure—this is termed EDR. This can be an important advantage, particularly in trauma and mobile radiography. The radiographer must still be vigilant in patient dose considerations—overexposure, although correctable via EDR, results in *increased patient dose;* underexposure results in decreased image quality because of increased image noise.

CR systems provide some type of *exposure indicator,* its name varies according to manufacturer: an *S* (sensitivity) number, *EI, REX* (reached EI), or other identifying EI depending on the manufacturer used. The manufacturer usually provides a chart identifying the acceptable *range* the exposure indicator numbers should be within for various examination types. Although in one manufacturer's system a high *S* number is related to *under*exposure, a high *EI* number in another manufacturer's system is related to *over*exposure—it is essential for radiographers to be knowledgeable about the various types of equipment they use.

> ### CR Resolution Increases As
>
> - PSP size decreases
> - Laser beam size decreases
> - Monitor matrix size increases

Summary

- The IP houses and protects the PSP; the PSP is not light sensitive.
- The PSP is usually barium fluorohalide and granular or turbid; when exposed to a laser light source, it emits PSL.
- A PMT or PD detects the PSL, converts it to electrical signals, and sends them to the ADC, where they become the digital image displayed on the monitor.
- The digitized images can also be manipulated in postprocessing, transmitted, and archived.
- Postprocessing manipulation can include edge enhancement; this technique can be used to improve the visibility of structures such as chest tubes by accentuating their edges.
- Windowing changes image contrast and/or brightness; window width controls the number of grays, whereas window level corresponds to the brightness.
- CR resolution is affected by size of PSP, laser beam, and monitor matrix.
- The terms *dynamic range* and *contrast resolution* are used to describe the range of grays a digital system is capable of resolving.
- Insufficient mAs can cause digital image noise (decreased SNR).
- The exposure indicator identifies the acceptable range of exposure for the part being imaged.

INDIRECT AND DIRECT DIGITAL IMAGING

CR/DR Differences

Although CR utilizes traditional x-ray tables and IPs to enclose and protect the flexible PSP, *DR* requires the use of somewhat different equipment. DR does not use IPs or a traditional x-ray table; it is a *direct-capture,* or *indirect-capture,* system of x-ray imaging (Fig. 13-48). DR eliminates IPs and their handling, DR affords the advantage of immediate display of the image (compared to the CR's slightly delayed image display), and DR exposures can be lower because of the detector's higher DQE (i.e., the ability to perceive and interact with x-ray photons). DR, like CR, also offers the advantage of image preview and postprocessing.

CR uses IPs that require an *identification process.* In DR, patient identification and demographics are selected from the RIS or HIS list.

Flat-Panel Detectors

As its name suggests, the digital detector is a flat, plate-like, panel—both x-ray *detection and digitization* take place in the flat panel. FPDs can be a *fixed* part of the x-ray unit and require no physical transportation of IPs, and no wear and tear on PSPs through a scanner/reader. There are also wired, and wireless, flat panels that send information directly to the computer. They were initially used almost exclusively in mobile imaging but are gaining use in general radiography. There are two types: *indirect* conversion (scintillation) systems and *direct* conversion (nonscintillation) systems. These digital imaging systems can differ in type of capture element, coupling element, and collection element (Fig. 13-49).

Indirect Systems. These use a two-step process that converts x-ray energy into light energy and then converts that light energy into electronic signals. In the *indirect* systems, remnant x-rays transmitted

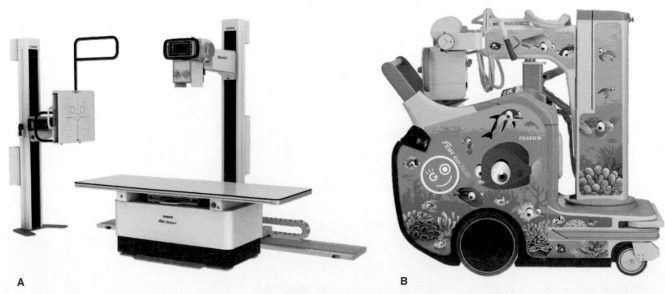

A   **B**

Figure 13-48. Direct-capture digital radiography units: **(A)** fixed and **(B)** mobile. (Photo contributor: FUJIFILM Healthcare Americas Corp.)

Digital Radiography					
Type	CR	Indirect DR	Indirect DR	Indirect DR	Direct DR
Capture element	Barium fluorohalide	CsI	CsI–cesium iodide/GdOD gadolinium oxysilfide	CsI- cesium Iodine	a-Se amorphous selenium
Coupling element		Lens or fiber optics	a-Si Amorphous silicon	Fiber optics or lens	a-Si
Collection element		CMOS	TFT	CCD	TFT

Figure 13-49. Indirect and direct digital radiography and their associated elements.

through the imaged part are *converted to light* through a columnar-needle scintillating phosphor such as CsI or the turbid formation phosphor Gd_2O_2S. The scintillation light is converted to electrons that are collected by photodetector coupling agents—TFTs or CCDs—where it is then changed to an electrical (analog) signal. The analog electrical signals are then digitized (by the ADC) and processed by the computer, producing an image.

The original *indirect flat-panel system* is the TFT system. Below its scintillation layer, the TFT system uses a highly transparent glass interface. Because glass is not a semiconductor like silicon, a thin film of *amorphous silicon* (a-Si) (i.e., in fluid form rather than crystalline) is deposited on both sides to function as *PD*. The top *scintillator layer* is usually CsI or Gd_2O_2S—also used in fluoroscopic systems. These phosphors absorb x-ray energy and change it into luminescent light energy. The a-Si functions to absorb the scintillation light energy and convert it into electrical charges (electrons). Immediately adjacent to the a-Si flat-panel layer is the *TFT array*, which functions to collect and readout electrical charges produced by the a-Si flat-panel layer.

The *CCD system* in DF is indirect because it requires a scintillator, but it is not an actual flat-panel system. The scintillation light is converted to an electrical charge at the CCD's silicon interface. The CCD collects the electrical charges and sends the signal to the ADC. Some advantages of CCDs are that they can respond to lower scintillation light levels, and they provide high-quality image data quickly. Systems *without* a scintillation/light conversion step have a *higher* DQE, with the exception of the new *CMOS* capture systems.

Direct Systems. *Direct* conversion FPDs utilize *no scintillation*; x-rays are *directly* converted to electric signals by the photoconductor a-Se—most commonly used because of its excellent x-ray absorption/conversion properties and spatial resolution. Below the a-Se layer is a *TFT array* that functions to collect and store the electrical charges. Electric charges are transmitted to the ADC for digitization.

Thus, the direct-capture system *eliminates the scintillator step* required in indirect DR. Because selenium has a relatively low Z number ($Z = 34$, compared with gadolinium [$Z = 64$] or cesium [$Z = 55$]), a-Se detectors are made thicker to improve detection, thus compensating for the low x-ray absorption of selenium. There is no diffusion of electrons, so spatial resolution is not affected in this manner.

The spatial resolution of direct digital systems is fixed and is related to the *detector element* (DEL) size of the TFT and its *fill factor*. The DEL is the sensing element of the TFT, and it is desirable that its largest portion is used for just that purpose. If 25% of the DEL is used for other functions, the DEL is said to have a *fill factor* of 75%. The greater the fill factor, the better the spatial resolution and SNR.

The larger the TFT DEL size, and the larger the fill factor, the better the spatial resolution. DEL size of 100 μm provides a spatial resolution of about 5 lp/mm (available only in some digital mammography systems). DEL size of 200 μm provides a spatial resolution of about 2.5 lp/mm (general radiography)—lower than that achieved with a 400-speed system in analog systems. A 100-speed system offers a spatial resolution of about 10 lp/mm—significantly greater than, and currently unachievable in, digital imaging.

Spatial resolution in digital imaging is fixed, but it is very important that radiographers are alert to the opportunities they have to utilize and control the remaining recorded detail factors (motion and geometric factors).

Portable detectors are available that can be used in conjunction with a mobile x-ray unit.

Monitor Display

Digital images are best viewed in areas with low ambient lighting levels that will avoid undesirable monitor screen glare (Fig. 13-50). Digital

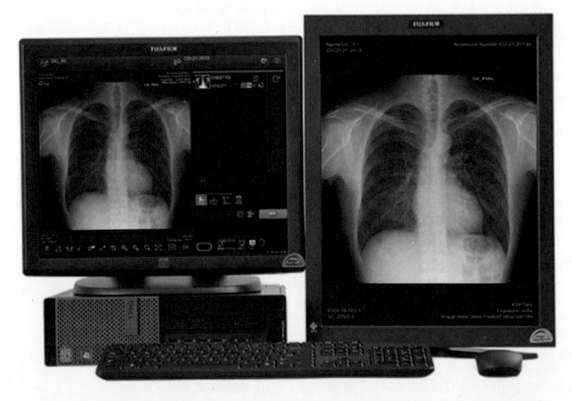

Figure 13-50. Low lighting levels provide optimal digital image visualization, avoiding monitor glare. (Photo contributor: FUJIFILM Healthcare Americas Corp.)

images usually have a black "mask" covering the white unexposed areas, further reducing objectionable ambient light and glare. If the radiographer views images in a brightly lit area, the image can appear excessively dark. The same image, when reviewed by the radiologist in the appropriate lighting, might look most adequate. As light level increases, the pupils of the eye contract and admit less light, causing images to appear dark. It is an effect similar to walking from a sunny day into a darkened theater.

Summary

- Indirect conversion detector: X-rays are converted to light scintillations, and light is converted to electric signals.
- a-Si in the indirect system absorbs scintillation energy, converting it to electric charges, which are then collected by the TFT array.
- Direct conversion detector: X-rays are converted directly to electric signals; there is no scintillation.
- The electric charges are transmitted to the ADC for digitization.
- Direct digital spatial resolution is related to DEL size and fill factor.
- Better resolution and SNR are achieved with larger DEL size and greater fill factor.
- Ideal digital image display areas strive to reduce ambient light and monitor glare.

COMPREHENSION CHECK

1. What is the primary control center for the computer consisting of a control unit, an arithmetic unit, and memory (p. 446)?

2. What are the two types of computer memory (p. 446)?

3. What term is used to describe how much of the part is included in the matrix (p. 446, 448)?

4. How do matrix size, pixel size, and FOV influence resolution (p. 448)?

5. What is the function of the CR PSP (p. 449)?

6. Describe how the image on the PSP is converted to the image seen on the monitor (p. 451).

7. What is the value of postprocessing (p. 451, 453, 454)?

8. Describe how windowing (width and level) affects the contrast and brightness of the diagnostic image (p. 453).

9. What term is commonly used to describe the range of grays a particular digital system is capable of resolving (p. 455)?

10. List three factors/features that determine CR resolution (p. 448, 449).

11. Define noise; explain how it might be encountered in CR (p. 455).

12. Describe the two types of indirect-capture digital images; identify which is the original flat-panel system (p. 457).

13. What portion of the indirect-capture system is absent in the direct-capture system (p. 457)?

14. What is a scintillator, and where is it used in digital imaging? Give examples of scintillators used (p. 457).

15. Describe the direct-capture digital imaging process (p. 457, 458).

CHAPTER REVIEW QUESTIONS

1. Image resolution improves as
   1. scintillation increases
   2. DEL size increases
   3. fill factor increases

   (A) 1 only
   (B) 1 and 2 only
   (C) 2 and 3 only
   (D) 1, 2, and 3

2. As digital image matrix size increases
   1. pixel size decreases
   2. resolution decreases
   3. pixel depth decreases

   (A) 1 only
   (B) 2 only
   (C) 1 and 2 only
   (D) 2 and 3 only

3. The luminescent light emitted by the PSP during the readout process is transformed into the image seen on the monitor by the
   (A) PSP
   (B) detector element (DEL)
   (C) ADC
   (D) helium–neon laser

4. Potential digital image postprocessing tasks include
   1. PACS/MIMPS
   2. annotation
   3. inversion/reversal

   (A) 1 only
   (B) 1 and 2 only
   (C) 2 and 3 only
   (D) 1, 2, and 3

5. Computed radiography resolution increases as
   1. laser beam size decreases
   2. monitor matrix size decreases
   3. PSP crystal size decreases

   (A) 1 only
   (B) 1 and 2 only
   (C) 1 and 3 only
   (D) 1, 2, and 3

6. Calculate the size of a pixel in an image with a 1024 × 1024 matrix and a 30-cm FOV.
   (A) 34.0 mm/pixel
   (B) 0.30 mm/pixel
   (C) 0.03 mm/pixel
   (D) 3.4 mm/pixel

7. Which of the following statements about the differences between CR and DR systems are true?
   1. CR uses imaging plates, whereas DR does not
   2. DR has a higher DQE and offers a lower patient dose
   3. CR images are displayed immediately after exposure

   (A) 1 only
   (B) 1 and 2 only
   (C) 2 and 3 only
   (D) 1, 2, and 3

8. As the size of the image matrix increases In digital imaging,
   1. FOV increases
   2. pixel size decreases
   3. spatial resolution increases

   (A) 1 only
   (B) 1 and 2 only
   (C) 2 and 3 only
   (D) 1, 2, and 3

9. In modern digital imaging systems, kV selection has a primary effect on
   1. photon energy
   2. photon penetration
   3. image contrast

   (A) 1 only
   (B) 1 and 2 only
   (C) 2 and 3 only
   (D) 1, 2, and 3

10. Digital radiographic imaging equipment provides a number of functions for optimization of image quality, including
    1. exposure data recognition
    2. automatic rescaling
    3. narrow latitude

    (A) 1 only
    (B) 1 and 2 only
    (C) 2 and 3 only
    (D) 1, 2, and 3

Answers and Explanations

1. (C) The spatial resolution of direct digital systems is fixed and is related to the DEL size of the TFT and its fill factor. The DEL is the sensing element of the TFT, and its largest portion should be used for its sensing function to maintain/improve resolution. For example, if 25% of the DEL is used for other functions, the DEL is said to have a fill factor of 75%.

The larger the TFT DEL size, and the larger the fill factor, the better the DQE/spatial resolution. DEL size of 100 μm provides a spatial resolution of about 5 lp/mm (available only in some digital mammography systems). DEL size of 200 μm provides a spatial resolution of about 2.5 lp/mm (general radiography)—lower than that achieved in 400-speed analog systems. A 100-speed analog system offers a spatial resolution of about 10 lp/mm—significantly greater than, and currently unachievable in, digital imaging.

2. (A) Pixel depth is directly related to shades of gray—called *dynamic range*—and is measured in *bits*. The greater the number of bits, the more shades of gray. For example, a 1-bit (2^1) pixel will demonstrate two shades of gray, whereas a 6-bit (2^6) pixel can display 64 shades, and a 7-bit (2^7) pixel will display 128 shades. However, pixel depth is unrelated to resolution.

A digital image is formed by a *matrix of pixels* (picture elements) in rows and columns. A matrix that has 512 pixels in each row and column is a 512×512 matrix. The term *FOV* is used to describe how much of the patient (e.g., 150-mm diameter) is included in the matrix. The matrix and the FOV can be changed independently without one affecting the other, but changes in either will change pixel size. As in analog radiography, *spatial resolution* is measured in lp/mm. As *matrix size is increased* (e.g., from 512×512 to 1024×1024), there are more and smaller pixels in the matrix and therefore *improved resolution*. Fewer and larger pixels result in poor resolution, a "pixelly" image, that is, one in which you can actually see the individual pixel boxes.

3. (C) The exposed IP is placed into the CR scanner/reader, where the PSP/SPS is removed automatically. The latent image appears as the PSP is scanned by a narrow, high-intensity *helium–neon laser* to obtain the pixel data. As the PSP plate is scanned in the CR reader, it releases a violet light—a process called *photostimulated luminescence (PSL)*. The luminescent light is converted to electrical energy, representing the *analog* image. The electrical energy is sent to an *ADC,* where it is digitized

and becomes the *digital* image that is displayed eventually (after a short delay) on a high-resolution monitor and/or printed out by a laser printer. The digitized images can also be manipulated in postprocessing, transmitted electronically, and stored/archived. A DEL, or detector element, is the sensing component of the TFT array in direct digital imaging systems. They are not found in PSP systems.

4. (C) Digital image postprocessing provides the opportunity for image optimization. Image annotation permits placement of labels, arrow indicators, and so on. Windowing allows adjustment of image contrast and/or brightness to diagnostic requirements. Contrast scale enhancement is the most valuable tool in digital imaging. Image minification, with larger matrix sizes, enables us to see tiny anatomic details and improve spatial resolution. Image inversion, or reversal, provides a different perspective by changing white to black and black to white. Image flip also provides another perspective by enabling us to rotate the image. Edge enhancement is useful for small and high-contrast tissues. Other postprocessing functions include highlighting, zoom, pan, and scroll. The pixel shift feature is important in DSA. Image subtraction is used to enhance contrast. If the part moves during acquisition of serial images, misregistration occurs, making the required exact superimposition impossible. Pixel shift is a function that can correct misregistration. Another emerging postprocessing task used in diagnostic functions is determining numeric pixel value for particular ROI. This feature has proved useful in bone densitometry, renal calculus recognition, and calcified lung nodule identification.

5. (C) Spatial resolution in CR is impacted by the size of the PSP, the size of the scanning laser beam, and monitor matrix size. *High-resolution monitors* (2–4 MP [megapixels]) are required for high-quality, high-resolution image display. *The larger the matrix size, the better is the image resolution.* Typical image matrix size (rows and columns) used in CR is 2048×2048. As in traditional radiography, *spatial resolution* is measured in lp/mm. As matrix size is increased, there are more and smaller pixels in the matrix and therefore improved spatial resolution. Other factors contributing to image resolution are the *size of the laser beam* and the *size of the PSP.* Smaller phosphor size improves resolution in ways similar to that of intensifying screens—anything that causes an increase in light diffusion will result in a decrease in resolution. Smaller phosphors in the PSP (SPS) plate allow less light diffusion. In addition, the scanning laser light must be of the correct intensity and size. A narrow laser beam is required for optimal resolution.

6. (B) Pixel size is determined by dividing the FOV by the matrix. In this case, the FOV is 30 cm; because the answer is expressed in millimeters, first change 30 cm to 300 mm. Then 300 divided by 1024 equals 0.29 mm:

$$30 \text{ cm} = 300 \text{ mm}$$

$$300 \div 1024 = 0.29 \text{ mm/pixel}$$

The FOV and the matrix size are independent of one another; that is, either can be changed, and the other will remain unaffected. However, pixel size is affected by changes in either the FOV or the matrix size. For example, if the matrix size is increased, pixel size decreases. If FOV is increased, pixel size increases. Pixel size is inversely related to resolution. As the pixel size increases, the resolution decreases.

7. (B) *CR* utilizes traditional x-ray tables and *IPs* to enclose and protect the flexible PSP screen, whereas *DR* requires the use of significantly different equipment. DR does not use IPs or a traditional x-ray table—it is a direct-capture/conversion, or indirect-capture/conversion, system of x-ray imaging. Many DR units eliminate IPs and their handling (some DRs use a wired or wireless detector); DR affords the advantage of *immediate display* of the image (compared to the CR's slightly delayed image display); and DR *exposures can be lower* because of the detector's *higher DQE* (i.e., ability to perceive and interact with x-ray photons of lower energies). DR, like CR, also offers the advantage of image preview and postprocessing.

8. (C) The FOV and matrix size are independent of one another; that is, either can be changed, and the other will remain unaffected. However, *pixel size is affected by changes in either the FOV or the matrix size*. For example, if matrix size is increased, pixel size decreases. If FOV increases, pixel size increases. Pixel size is inversely related to resolution. As the pixel size decreases, the resolution increases.

9. (B) In digital imaging, brightness and contrast are determined by computer software and monitor controls; however, the principal factor in good digital image visibility and patient dose is still the result of proper IR exposure. Selection of kV and mAs in digital imaging is similar to analog imaging, that is, kV still determines *penetration but not contrast*; mAs still determines *dose* but has *no impact on brightness*. The terms *density* and *brightness* do not mean the same thing and therefore are not used interchangeably.

10. (B) Digital imaging EDR and automatic rescaling offer *wide* latitude and automatic optimization of the VOI in the radiologic image. EDR, by using the selected processing algorithm and its LUT, enables compensation for approximately 80% underexposure and 500% overexposure. Although automatic/computerized optimization of the radiologic image is a wonderful tool, radiographers must be even more aware of their responsibility to keep patient dose to a minimum. Overexposure, although correctable via EDR, results in increased patient dose; underexposure results in decreased image quality because of increased image *noise*.

THE FLUOROSCOPIC SYSTEM

Equipment

Fluoroscopic x-ray examinations are performed to study the dynamics of various parts in *motion*. Fluoroscopy was performed almost exclusively in the very early days of radiology because of the lack of dependable x-ray tubes and image-recording systems (Fig. 13-51A). In the late 1940s and early 1950s, image intensification was developed and served to provide much brighter images at lower exposures. *Image intensifiers* (IIs) brighten (intensify) the conventional, or "dark," fluoroscopic image 5000–20,000 times. Fluoroscopic procedures used nowadays are much safer (lower exposure/mA) and brighter; the fluoroscopic image can be photographed still or moving or viewed with a television camera/CCD and projected onto a nearby or remote television monitor.

A fluoroscope has two principal components, an x-ray tube and a fluorescent screen, attached at opposite ends of a *C-shaped arm* (Fig. 13-52; see also Fig. 13-51B). The fluoroscopic *table* accommodates the patient and must be able to move to an upright position (90°) and to a Trendelenburg position (up to ~40°). Therefore, a 90/30 fluoroscopic table refers to one that will move upright (90°) and angle Trendelenburg up to 30°.

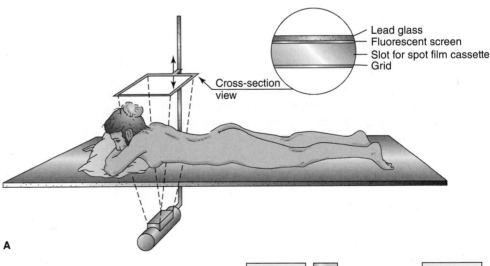

A

Figure 13-51. (A) Basic early fluoroscope. **(B)** Conceptualization of relationship and function of an image intensifier input screen, photocathode, and output screen. For every one x-ray photon interacting with the input screen, 5000 fluorescent light photons are emitted. Note the close (but not touching) relationship between the input screen and the photocathode for maintenance of resolution. The light photons interact with the photocathode, and approximately 150 electrons are emitted by the photoemissive metal. The photoelectrons then interact with the output screen, and 2000 fluorescent light photons are emitted for every electron.

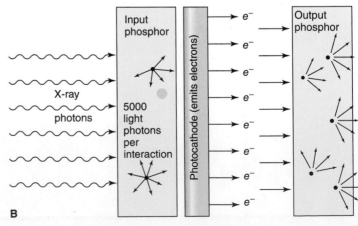

B

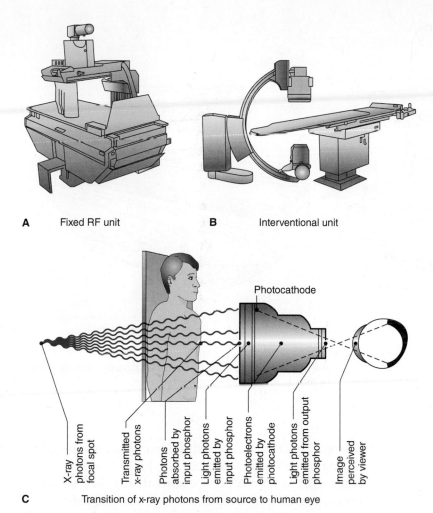

A Fixed RF unit **B** Interventional unit

Photocathode

X-ray photons from focal spot

Transmitted x-ray photons

Photons absorbed by input phosphor

Light photons emitted by input phosphor

Photoelectrons emitted by photocathode

Light photons emitted from output phosphor

Image perceived by viewer

C Transition of x-ray photons from source to human eye

Figure 13-52. A fluoroscope has two principal components; an x-ray tube and a fluorescent screen, attached at opposite ends of a C-shaped arm. **(A)** Traditional fixed RF unit and **(B)** *C-arm*. Especially useful in interventional procedures. **(C)** Transition of x-ray photons emerging from x-ray tube, through part under study, into image intensifier, to human eye.

Fluoroscopic x-ray tubes are standard rotating anode tubes, usually installed under the x-ray table but operated at much lower tube currents than radiographic tubes. Over-the-table fluoroscopic x-ray tubes result in higher radiation exposure to personnel than under-the-table x-ray tubes. Instead of the 50–1200 mA used in radiography, traditional image-intensified fluoroscopic tubes are operated at currents that range from 0.5 to 5.0 mA (averaging 1–3 mA). Higher mA is often used in pulsed and/or flat-panel fluoroscopy.

Patient dose is much higher in fluoroscopic than radiographic procedures because of the considerably shorter source-to-object distance used in fluoroscopy. Fluoroscopic *entrance exposure* is significantly greater than exit exposure as a result of attenuation processes within the patient. The typical entrance skin exposure (ESE) rate is 17.5 mGy/min (2 R/min); a *boost* mode is often available for special situations—using exposure rates of *up to 175 mGy (20 R/min)*. Use of the "boost" mode is permitted for only short periods of time and an *audible signal* is activated during its use.

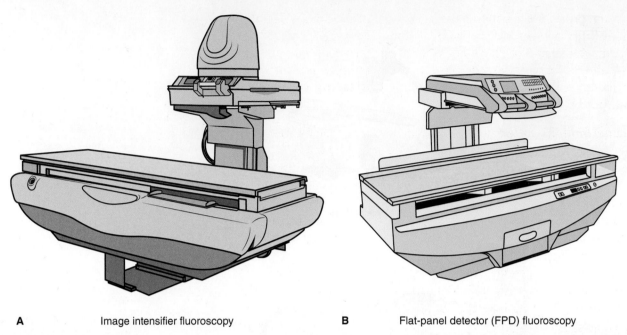

A   Image intensifier fluoroscopy   **B**   Flat-panel detector (FPD) fluoroscopy

Figure 13-53. (A and **B)** Digital fluoroscopy can be achieved with an image intensifier (II) system or with a flat-panel detector (FPD) system. Figure **A** illustrates image-intensified digital fluoroscopy. Note the location of the image intensifier atop the fluoroscopic tower. Figure **B** illustrates a flat-panel detector fluoroscopic system. Note the absence of an image intensifier.

Digital Fluoroscopy. In DF, the II output screen image is coupled via a CCD for viewing on a display monitor (Fig. 13-53A and B). A CCD converts visible light to an electrical charge that is then sent to the ADC for processing. When output screen light strikes the CCD cathode, a proportional number of electrons are released by the cathode and stored as digital values by the CCD. The CCD's rapid discharge time virtually eliminates image lag and is useful in high-speed imaging procedures such as cardiac catheterizations. CCDs have replaced the television camera associated with image intensification. They are more sensitive to the light emitted by the output phosphor; they are much more compact than a television camera and can efficiently capture the fluoroscopic image. In comparison to the television cameras, CCDs provide better resolution and contrast and have a higher DQE and SNR. CMOS efficiency in DF has improved greatly over the past decade. Advantages of CMOS over CCDs include significantly less cost, greater speed, and much more energy efficient (less power consumption). The CCD still provides somewhat better image quality.

DF also offers "road-mapping" capability. "Road-mapping" is a technique useful in procedures involving guidewire/catheter placement.

During the fluoroscopic examination, the most recent fluoroscopic image can be stored on the monitor (last image hold), thereby reducing the need for continuous x-ray exposure. This technique can offer significant reductions in patient and personnel radiation exposure.

Because DF images are obtained by using a pulsed (rather than continuous) x-ray beam, this significantly decreases patient dose—as long as the pulse rate is below 30 pps. Most DF static images can also be made with a lower mA because of the greater sensitivity of the CCD. Image acquisition rates are usually between 1 and 10 images per second. *Fewer frames per second result in lower patient dose.* Dose-reduction advantages can be nullified by taking superfluous digital spot images.

Flat-Panel Digital Fluoroscopy. In addition, instead of the fluoroscopic image being received by an II, it can be received by a *FPD* (Fig. 13-53B). The use of a fluoroscopic FPD can offer the benefit of further reduction in patient dose because of increased sensitivity to x-ray DQE. There is also increased temporal resolution, helping reduce motion unsharpness. There is improved contrast resolution, although spatial resolution is the same as, or not as good as, image intensification fluoroscopy.

In this system, *the x-ray tube must be able to turn on and off very quickly.* The term *interrogation time* refers to the time it takes the tube to reach the required technical factors. The term *extinction time* refers to the time it takes the tube to turn off. The required time is less than 1 ms.

Safety Features. For radiation protection purposes, the fluoroscopic tabletop exposure rate must not exceed 100 mGy$_a$/min and all fluoroscopic equipment must provide an SSD of *at least* 30 cm (for mobile) and 38 cm (for stationary) units between the x-ray source (focal spot) and the x-ray tabletop. Positioning the II *closer* to the patient *decreases the SID* and *decreases patient dose.* Patient dose decreases because as the SID is *decreased,* the number of x-ray photons at the input phosphor *increases;* this results in the automatic brightness control (ABC), *decreasing the mA* to compensate for the increase in x-ray photons.

A *5-min timer* is used to measure accumulated fluoroscopic examination time and make an audible sound or interrupt exposure after 5 min of fluoroscopy. X-ray production is usually activated by a foot switch (*dead man's switch*), thus leaving the fluoroscopist's hands free to handle the carriage and position and palpate the patient. The fluoroscopic tube is usually equipped with electrically driven collimating *shutters.* Leaded glass provides shielding from radiation passing through the intensifying screen, and the II is lead lined. A *Bucky slot cover* and a *protective curtain* also help reduce exposure to the fluoroscopist.

Some Radiation Safety Features of Fluoroscopic Equipment

- Maximum of 5 mA in traditional II fluoroscopy
- 30 cm minimum between the focal spot and the tabletop
- 100 mGy$_a$/min maximum tabletop exposure
- 5-min cumulative timer
- "Dead man's" switch
- Automatic collimation
- Bucky slot cover
- Protective curtain

Summary

- Fluoroscopes are used to examine moving parts and are occasionally equipped with a device to take cassette-loaded spot films.
- A fluoroscope has two major parts: an x-ray tube and a fluorescent screen, attached at opposite ends of a C-shaped arm.
- The fluoroscopic tube is usually located (at least 30 cm) under the x-ray table and usually operated at 1–3 mA (up to a maximum of 5 mA); mA automatically increases for fluoroscopic images.

- Fluoroscopic patient dose depends on exposure rate, tissue thickness or density, and length of exposure.
- Fluoroscopic patient dose decreases as the II is moved closer to the patient.
- Fluoroscopic "boost" mode can deliver up to 200 mGy$_a$/min.
- Many guidelines regulate the operation of fluoroscopic equipment because of the unavoidable high patient dose inherent in fluoroscopic procedures (because of the short focus-to-patient distance).
- IIs brighten the conventional, dark fluoroscopic image 5000–20,000 times.
- DF images are obtained by using a *pulsed* x-ray beam; this can significantly decrease patient dose.
- DF image acquisition rates are usually between 1 and 10 images per second; fewer frames per second result in lower patient dose.
- In DF, the fluoroscopic image can be received by an FPD; in this system, the x-ray tube must be able to turn on and off very quickly.

The Image Intensifier

The fluorescent layer of early conventional (or "dark") fluoroscopic screens was made of *zinc cadmium sulfide* (Patterson B-2 screen). The *input screen* of II tube is made nowadays of a thin layer of *CsI,* 12.7–30.5 cm (5–12 inches) in diameter and slightly convex in shape.

CsI is much more efficient than zinc cadmium sulfide because it absorbs, and converts to fluorescent light, a greater number of the x-ray photons striking it. For each absorbed x-ray photon, approximately 5000 light photons are emitted (see Fig. 13-51B). This fluorescent light strikes a *photocathode* made of a photoemissive metal. A number of electrons are subsequently released from the photocathode and focused toward the output side of the image tube. Although this step actually represents a *deamplification,* it has very little effect on the end result. A thin (0.2 mm) layer of glass or other transparent material is placed between the input screen and the photocathode to prevent chemical reaction between the two; otherwise, the two must be as close as possible to reduce light-spread and allow for maximum transfer of accurate information.

The electrons emitted from the photocathode are confined and focused toward the output end of the tube by negatively charged *electrostatic focusing lenses.* They then pass through the neck of the tube where they are accelerated through a potential difference of 25,000–35,000 V and strike the small 1.27–2.54 cm (½–1 inch) fluorescent *output phosphor* that is mounted on a flat-glass support (Fig. 13-54; see also Fig. 13-52).

The entire assembly is enclosed within a 2- to 4-mm thick vacuum glass envelope. The glass is then coated to prevent the entry of light. The glass tube is enclosed within a metal housing that functions to attenuate magnetic fields from outside the tube that would distort the electron paths within.

For undistorted focusing of electrons onto the output phosphor, each electron must travel the same distance, thus the slight curvature of the input phosphor.

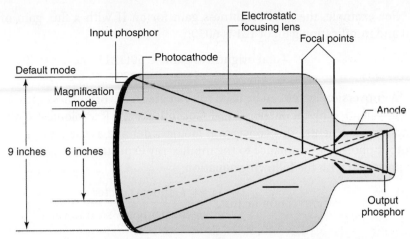

Figure 13-54. As field of view (patient area/normal vs. magnification mode) decreases, magnification of the output screen image increases and contrast and resolution improve. Note that the focal point on the 6-inch field, or mode, is further away from the output phosphor; therefore, the output image appears magnified. Because less minification takes place in this instance, the image is not as bright. Technical factors are automatically increased to compensate for the loss in brightness.

There are several occasions of information transfer within the II: from x-ray beam to input phosphor from input phosphor to photocathode, from photocathode to electron beam, from electron beam to output phosphor, and from output phosphor to the human eye (see Fig. 13-52). Thus, an electrical image is transformed to a light image, then back to an electron image, and finally back to a light image.

Electrons from the photocathode are accelerated as they travel toward the output phosphor. The gain in brightness achieved by the II is the result of this *electron acceleration (flux gain)* and *image minification. Flux gain* is defined as the ratio of light photons at the output phosphor to the number at the input phosphor. A typical II has a flux gain of approximately 50.

The image produced on the input phosphor of the II is reproduced as a minified image on the output screen. Because the output phosphor is much smaller than the input phosphor, the amount of fluorescent light emitted from it per unit area is significantly greater than the quantity of light emitted from the input phosphor. This process is called *minification gain* and is equal to the ratio of the diameters of the input and output phosphor squared:

$$\text{Minification gain} = \left(\frac{\text{Input phosphor diameter}}{\text{Output phosphor diameter}} \right)^2$$

For example, the minification gain for an II with an input phosphor of 11 inches and output phosphor of 1 inch is 121:

$$\text{Minification gain} = \left(\frac{11''}{1''} \right)^2$$

$$= 121$$

The total *brightness gain* of an II is the product of flux gain and minification gain:

$$\text{Total brightness gain} = \text{flux gain} \times \text{minification gain}$$

For example, the total brightness gain for an II with a flux gain of 50 and minification gain of 121 is 6050:

$$\text{Total brightness gain} = 50(121)$$
$$= 6050$$

A conversion factor can be used to evaluate an II's brightness gain, as recommended by the International Commission of Radiological Units and Measurements. This conversion factor is defined as the ratio of the output phosphor luminance to the input x-ray exposure rate. They have expressed it with the following equation:

$$\text{Conversion factor} = \frac{\text{Candela}/\text{meter}^2}{\text{Milliroentgen}/\text{second}}$$

The brightness, resolution, and contrast of an intensified image are greatest in the center of the image. Because the exposure rate is reduced at the periphery of the input phosphor and because there is less-than-exact peripheral electron focusing from the photocathode, brightness, resolution, and contrast are reduced (up to 25%) toward the periphery; this characteristic of IIs is called *vignetting*.

Input phosphor diameters of 5–12 inches are available. Although smaller diameter input phosphor improves resolution, it does not permit viewing of large patient areas.

A type of image distortion, called *pincushion distortion,* is common to intensified images and is caused by the curvature of the input phosphor and diminished electron-focusing precision at the image periphery. These types of distortion are not present in DR because there is no curvature.

There will always be some degree of magnification in image intensification (just as in radiography); the degree depends on the distance of the II from the patient.

Dual- and triple-field IIs are available that permit magnified viewing of fluoroscopic images. Magnified images are reduced in brightness unless the mA is automatically increased when the II is switched to the magnification mode (see Fig. 13-54). ESE can increase dramatically as the FOV decreases (i.e., as magnification increases).

Fluoroscopy units are frequently equipped with a last-view freeze-frame feature. This permits the fluoroscopist a longer view of on-screen anatomy without the need for continuous x-ray exposure.

With respect to patient dose, it should be recalled that positioning the II closer to the patient during fluoroscopy reduces the patient's dose. As the distance between the x-ray source/tube and the II/image receptor (i.e., the SID) is reduced (Fig. 13-55), the intensity of the x-ray photons at the II's input phosphor increases, stimulating the ABC to decrease the mA and thereby decreasing patient dose.

Summary

- The basic parts of the II are the input screen, photocathode, electrostatic focusing lenses, accelerating anode, and output screen, within a vacuum glass envelope.
- The process of energy conversion within the II is from electrical to light, to electrical, and back to light.

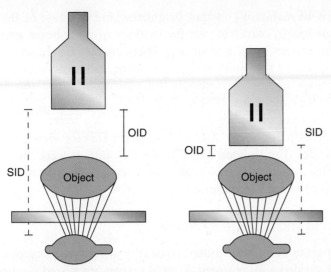

Figure 13-55. Positioning the image intensifier closer to the patient during fluoroscopy reduces patient dose. (Reproduced with permission from Saia DA. *Lange Q&A Radiography Examination*. 7th ed. New York, NY: McGraw-Hill; 2009.)

- CsI is the preferred phosphor for the II's input screen; for each x-ray photon it absorbs, it emits approximately 5000 light photons.
- Light photons strike the photocathode, which releases a number of electrons that are directed toward the neck of the II by the negatively charged focusing lenses.
- The input screen and the photocathode are slightly curved so that each electron travels the same distance to the output phosphor to prevent distortion.
- Electrons are accelerated by the anode's 25- to 30-kV potential, thus making the output image brighter (*flux* gain); the electrons strike the output screen and are converted to a much brighter, smaller (minification gain), and inverted fluorescent image.
- *Minification* gain is determined by dividing the input screen diameter by the output screen diameter and squaring the result; *total brightness* gain is equal to the product of flux gain and minification gain.
- Diminished resolution and contrast at the image periphery are called vignetting.
- Magnification results in some loss of brightness; mA is automatically increased to compensate (with a corresponding increase in dose).
- Last-view freeze-frame feature can significantly decrease patient dose.

Viewing Systems

The optical system of the II can transfer the output phosphor image to a mirror-viewing apparatus. Mirror viewing offers good resolution, but its disadvantages include limited viewing by one person at a time and limited fluoroscopist movement. In comparison, *closed-circuit television fluoroscopy* is far more convenient; it allows the fluoroscopist freedom of movement and permits simultaneous viewing by a number of people.

As body areas of different thicknesses and density are scanned with the II, image brightness and contrast require adjustment. The *ABC* functions to maintain constant brightness and contrast of the output phosphor image, correcting for fluctuations in x-ray beam attenuation with adjustments in kV and/or mA. There are also brightness and contrast controls on the monitor that the radiographer can regulate. Recall that positioning the II *closer* to the patient *increases the SSD and decreases the patient dose (ESE)*.

The II output phosphor image is *coupled* via a *television camera* (in analog fluoroscopy) or a CCD or CMOS (in DF) for viewing on a display monitor. The Vidicon and Plumbicon cameras were the most frequently used analog television cameras. They are approximately 6 inches in length and 1 inch in diameter.

Recording and Storage Systems

In addition to being transmitted to nearby or remote monitors, images can be recorded and/or stored. Digital images are stored electronically. They can also be put on a CD and used with the appropriate viewing program. The DF output phosphor image is coupled via a CCD for viewing on a display monitor (Fig. 13-56). CCDs have been used to replace the television camera associated with image intensification. They are much more compact than a television camera and can efficiently capture the fluoroscopic image. A CCD converts visible light to an electrical charge, which is then sent to the ADC for processing. When output phosphor light strikes the CCD cathode, a proportional number of electrons are released by the cathode and stored as digital values by the CCD. The CCD's rapid discharge time virtually eliminates image lag which makes it useful in high-speed imaging procedures such as cardiac catheterizations. In comparison to the television cameras, CCDs provide better resolution and contrast and have a higher DQE and SNR. In DF, CMOS efficiency has improved greatly over the past decade. Advantages of CMOS over CCDs include significantly less cost, greater speed, and much more energy efficient (less power consumption). The CCD still provides somewhat better image quality.

DF also offers "road-mapping" capability. During the fluoroscopic examination, the most recent fluoroscopic image can be stored on the

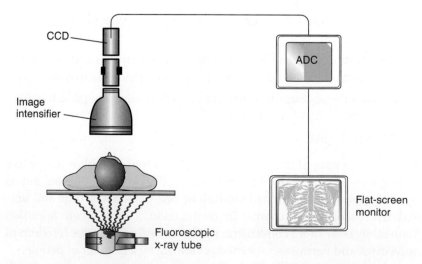

Figure 13-56. Image-intensified fluoroscopic unit with ancillary imaging devices.

monitor (image hold), thereby reducing the need for continuous x-ray exposure. This technique can offer a significant reduction in patient and personnel radiation exposure. DF offers lower patient dose because its x-ray beam is "pulsed" rather than continuous. The x-ray exposure turns on and off very quickly. The time it takes the x-ray tube to reach the required exposure is called the *interrogation time*. The term *extinction time* refers to the time required for the x-ray tube to switch off. Most DF static images can also be made with a lower mA because of the sensitivity of the CCD.

An *FPD* can be used to receive the fluoroscopic image. DF FPD images are also obtained by using a pulsed x-ray beam, decreasing patient dose, even though the exposures might be made at traditionally high mA—as long as the pulse rate is below 30 pps. Image acquisition rates are usually between 1 and 10 images per second. Fewer frames per second result in lower patient dose. FPDs have a higher DQE, higher temporal resolution, and higher contrast resolution. Flat-panel spatial resolution is not significantly better than image intensification fluoroscopic images.

Information Storage. The quantity of patient information and diagnostic image data stored by hospitals is ever increasing. It is essential that this information be stored, managed, and utilized efficiently. There is RIS that centrally processes and stores image data within a hospital, enabling image retrieval from the server by any department over the hospital network and displays image at the requesting department site. This eliminates the cumbersome task of sorting, conveying, and storing films. The HIS networks allow the archiving and distribution of vast amounts of image information from all modalities, managing it all with a single system. By using multiple connections over a network (e.g., PACS/MIMPS), image data can also be shared by multiple hospitals.

Advantages of Flat-Panel Fluoroscopy
• Pulsed x-ray beam
• Decrease patient dose
• Increased sensitivity to x-rays (DQE)
• Increased temporal resolution; decreased motion unsharpness
• Improved contrast resolution

Summary

- The optical system transfers the output screen image to either mirror viewing or television monitor (via Plumbicon or Vidicon camera).
- Television monitor viewing is more practical and convenient, although it involves some loss of image quality.
- ABC automatically adjusts kV or mA; brightness and contrast controls are also available for adjustment on the TV monitor.
- The output screen image is usually coupled to the television camera via a series of complex and precisely adjusted lenses and mirror.
- Videotape recordings, permitting immediate playback, may be made during the fluoroscopic procedure, although there is some loss of image resolution.
- In DF, the II output screen image is coupled via a CCD for viewing on a display monitor.
- Advantages of DF include higher SNR, less patient dose, postprocessing capability, and "road-mapping."

COMPREHENSION CHECK

1. Explain the purpose of fluoroscopy and the function of the fluoroscope (p. 464).

2. Identify the usual location of the fluoroscopy tube in relation to the patient table (p. 464).

3. Identify the fluoroscopic mA range of operation; what is "boost mode" (p. 465)?

4. List at least six fluoroscopic equipment features designed to reduce patient and personnel exposure (p. 467).

5. Explain why fluoroscopic exposure dose is greater than radiographic dose (p. 465).

6. Identify, with respect to the image intensifier (II) (p. 468, 469):

   A. composition of the input phosphor, and its characteristics and advantages

   B. action of the photocathode

   C. function of the electrostatic focusing lenses

   D. function and potential difference of the accelerating anode

   E. function and size of the output phosphor

   F. two components of total brightness gain

7. Determine minification gain (p. 469, 470).

8. Define vignetting (p. 470).

9. Discuss advantages and disadvantages of magnified images (p. 470).

10. Identify ways in which the fluoroscopic image can be recorded (p. 472).

11. Identify by what means the II compensates for varying body thicknesses (p. 471, 472).

12. Define what is meant by coupling (p. 472).

13. Identify the fluoroscopic monitor controls that can be regulated by the radiographer (p. 472).

14. Define/describe the terms *interrogation time* and *extinction time* (p. 467).

15. List comparisons between large and small fluoroscopic FOVs (p. 470).

16. What device couples the image intensifier and the TV monitor in digital fluoroscopy (p. 472)?

17. Describe the operation of CCDs (p. 472).

18. Compare the SNR of cameras such as Plumbicon and Vidicon to the SNR of CCDs (p. 472).

19. List four advantages of DF over analog fluoroscopy (p. 479).

20. Explain how and why DF can offer considerably less patient dose (p. 472, 473).

21. What is the advantage of "last image hold"? What is "road-mapping" technique (p. 472, 473)?

22. What are the advantages of FPD fluoroscopy (p. 473)?

CHAPTER REVIEW QUESTIONS

1. Which of the following systems functions to compensate for changing patient/part thicknesses during fluoroscopic procedures?

   (A) Automatic brightness control

   (B) Minification gain

   (C) Automatic resolution control

   (D) Flux gain

2. Patient dose during fluoroscopy is affected by the

   1. distance between the patient and the input phosphor

   2. amount of magnification

   3. tissue density

   (A) 1 only

   (B) 3 only

   (C) 2 and 3 only

   (D) 1, 2, and 3

3. In digital fluoroscopy systems, which of the following replaced the image intensifier's television camera tube?

   (A) Solid-state diode

   (B) Charge-coupled device

   (C) Photostimulable phosphor

   (D) Vidicon tube

4. ABC is used in fluoroscopy to adjust the

   1. kilovoltage (kV)

   2. milliamperage (mA)

   3. time (s)

   (A) 1 only

   (B) 1 and 2 only

   (C) 2 and 3 only

   (D) 1, 2 and 3

5. To maintain image clarity in an image-intensifier system, the path of electron flow from the photocathode to the output phosphor is controlled by the

   (A) accelerating anode

   (B) electrostatic lenses

   (C) vacuum glass envelope

   (D) input phosphor

6. Moving the image intensifier closer to the patient during fluoroscopy

   1. decreases the SID

   2. decreases patient dose

   3. improves image quality

   (A) 1 only

   (B) 1 and 2 only

   (C) 1 and 3 only

   (D) 1, 2, and 3

7. Which of the following is/are associated with magnification fluoroscopy?

   1. Higher patient dose than nonmagnification fluoroscopy

   2. Higher voltage to the focusing lenses

   3. Image intensifier focal point closer to the input phosphor

   (A) 1 only

   (B) 1 and 2 only

   (C) 2 and 3 only

   (D) 1, 2, and 3

8. Advantages of flat-panel fluoroscopy include

   1. decreased patient dose

   2. increased temporal resolution

   3. decreased DQE

   (A) 1 only

   (B) 1 and 2 only

   (C) 2 and 3 only

   (D) 1, 2, and 3

9. The total brightness gain of an image intensifier is the product of

   1. flux gain

   2. minification gain

   3. focusing gain

   (A) 1 only

   (B) 2 only

   (C) 1 and 2 only

   (D) 1 and 3 only

10. The term *interrogation time* refers to
    (A) the shortest possible exposure time permitted by a particular x-ray tube
    (B) the amount of time required for AM x-ray tube warm up
    (C) the time required for the x-ray tube to turn off
    (D) the time it takes the x-ray tube to reach the required technical factors

11. What calculates the ratio of light photons at the output phosphor to the number at the input phosphor?
    (A) Minification gain
    (B) Total brightness gain
    (C) Flux gain
    (D) Automatic brightness control

Answers and Explanations

1. (A) Parts being examined during fluoroscopic procedures change in thickness and density as the patient is required to change positions and as the fluoroscope is moved to examine different regions of the body that have varying thickness and tissue densities. The *ABC* functions to vary the required milliampere seconds and/or kilovoltage as necessary. With this method, patient dose varies and image quality is maintained. Minification and flux gain contribute to total brightness gain.

2. (D) Moving the II closer to the patient during fluoroscopy decreases the SID and patient dose (as SID is reduced, the intensity of the x-ray photons at the II's input phosphor increases; the ABC then automatically decreases the mA and therefore patient dose). Moving the II closer to the patient during fluoroscopy also decreases the OID and therefore magnification. As tissue density increases, a greater exposure dose is required.

3. (B) In DF, the II output phosphor image is coupled via a *CCD* for viewing on a display monitor. A CCD converts visible light to an electrical charge that is then sent to the ADC for processing. When output phosphor light strikes the CCD cathode, a proportional number of electrons are released by the cathode and stored as digital values by the CCD. The CCD's rapid discharge time virtually eliminates image lag and is particularly useful in high-speed imaging procedures such as cardiac catheterizations. CCD cameras have replaced analog cameras (such as the Vidicon and Plumbicon) in fluoroscopic equipment. CCDs are more sensitive to the light emitted by the output phosphor (than the analog cameras) and are associated with less "noise." DF photo-spot images are simply still-frame images that offer postprocessing capability. DF also offers "road-mapping" capability. "Road-mapping" is a technique useful in procedures involving guidewire/catheter placement. During the fluoroscopic examination, the most recent fluoroscopic image is stored on the monitor, thereby reducing the need for continuous x-ray exposure. This technique can offer significant reductions in patient and personnel radiation exposure.

4. (B) As body areas of different thicknesses and densities are scanned with the image intensifier, image brightness and contrast require adjustment. The ABC functions to maintain constant brightness and contrast of the output screen image, correcting for fluctuations in x-ray beam attenuation with adjustments in kilovoltage and/or milliamperage. There are also brightness and contrast controls on the monitor that the radiographer can regulate.

5. (B) The *input phosphor* of image intensifiers is usually made of CsI. The input phosphor receives remnant radiation emerging from the patient and converts it to a fluorescent light image. For each x-ray photon absorbed by CsI, approximately 5000 light photons are emitted. Directly adjacent to the input phosphor is the *photocathode,* which is made of a photoemissive alloy. As the light photons strike a photoemissive photocathode, a number of electrons are released (the electron image) from the photocathode and focused toward the output side of the image tube by voltage applied to the negatively charged *electrostatic focusing lenses*. The electrons are carefully focused by the lenses to maintain image resolution. The electrons are then accelerated through the *accelerating anode* in the neck of the tube and finally to the *output phosphor* for conversion back to light.

6. (D) Moving the image intensifier closer to the patient during fluoroscopy reduces the distance between the x-ray tube (source) and the image receptor, that is, the SID. It follows that the distance between the part being imaged (object) and the image receptor, that is, the OID, is also reduced. The shorter OID produces less magnification and better image quality. As the SID is reduced, the intensity of the x-ray photons at the image intensifier's input phosphor increases, stimulating the ABC to decrease the milliamperage and thereby *decreasing patient dose*.

7. (D) Image intensifier input phosphor diameters of 5–12 inches are available. Although smaller diameter input phosphors improve resolution, they do not permit a large FOV, that is, viewing of large patient areas.

Dual- and triple-field image intensifiers are available that permit *magnified* viewing of fluoroscopic images. To achieve magnification, the *voltage* to the focusing lenses is increased and a *smaller* portion of the input phosphor is used, thereby resulting in a smaller FOV. Because minification gain is now decreased, the image is not as bright. The mA is automatically increased to compensate for the loss in brightness when the image intensifier is switched to magnification mode. ESE can increase dramatically as the FOV decreases (i.e., as magnification increases).

As FOV decreases, *magnification* of the output phosphor image increases, there is less *noise* because increased mA provides a greater number of x-ray photons, and *contrast* and *resolution* improve. The *focal point* in the magnification mode is *further away from* the output phosphor (as a result of increased voltage applied to the focusing lenses) and therefore the output image is magnified.

8. (B) DF offers *lower patient dose* because its x-ray beam is "pulsed," rather than continuous. The x-ray exposure turns on and off very quickly, thereby *reducing motion unsharpness* (i.e., increasing temporal resolution). Image acquisition rates are usually between 1 and 10 images per second. Fewer frames per second result in lower patient dose. FPDs have a *higher DQE,* higher temporal resolution, and higher contrast resolution. DF also offers "road-mapping" capability. During the fluoroscopic examination, the most recent fluoroscopic image can be stored on the monitor (image hold), reducing the need for continuous x-ray exposure and offering a significant reduction in patient and personnel radiation exposure.

9. (C) The brightness gain of image intensifiers is 5000–20,000 times. This increase is accounted for in two ways. As the electron image is focused to the output phosphor, it is accelerated by high voltage (about 25 kV). The output phosphor is only a fraction of the size of the input phosphor, and this decrease in image size represents brightness gain, termed *minification gain.* The *ratio* of the number of x-ray photons at the input phosphor compared with the number light photons at the output

phosphor is termed *flux gain. Total brightness gain is equal to the product of minification gain and flux gain.*

10. (C) The use of a fluoroscopic FPD can offer the benefit of reduction in patient dose because of increased DQE and pulsed x-ray beam. The x-ray tube must be able to turn on and off very quickly. The term *interrogation time* refers to the time it takes the tube to reach the required technical factors. The term *extinction time* refers to the time it takes the tube to turn off. The required time is less than 1 ms.

11. (C) Flux gain is used to assess the ratio of light photons present at the output phosphor compared with the number that were initially at the input phosphor. Typical image intensifiers have a flux gain of approximately 50, meaning there are 50 times as many light photons at the output phosphor. This contributes to an increase in brightness for the image. Minification gain concerns the size difference in diameter of both phosphors. Because the output phosphor is much smaller than the input phosphor, light is concentrated over a smaller area. The product of flux gain and minification gain determines the overall brightness of the image, or the total brightness gain. Automatic brightness control is a method of maintaining image brightness by controlling kV and mA throughout a fluoroscopic procedure as various tissue densities are exposed.

COMPUTED TOMOGRAPHY

Computed tomography (CT) equipment (Fig. 13-57A) and images differ considerably from those produced by conventional *projection radiography* or by *CR/DR*. Both conventional radiography and CR/DR are based on the absorption of x-rays as they pass through the different tissues of a patient's body and the exiting x-rays interacting with a detection device (i.e., film emulsion, PSP, or other IR). This produces two-dimensional images that are made with reference to the *long axis of the body,* with anatomic structures superimposed on one another, and often degraded by SR fog. In CR/DR, analog images are changed to digital images with an ADC, although they are generally viewed as analog images for monitor display (see Fig. 13-44A and B).

Conventional tomography is called *axial tomography* because the image plane parallels the body's long axis, providing coronal and/or sagittal images. This procedure is infrequently performed nowadays.

CT images are *cross-sectional* (i.e., axial, perpendicular to the body's long axis), individual slices—called *transaxial* (or transverse) *images.* The

Terminology
Outdated: "CAT" scan
• Refers to computerized *axial* tomography
Correct: CT scan
• CT
• Axial images can be reconstructed and viewed in the sagittal and coronal planes

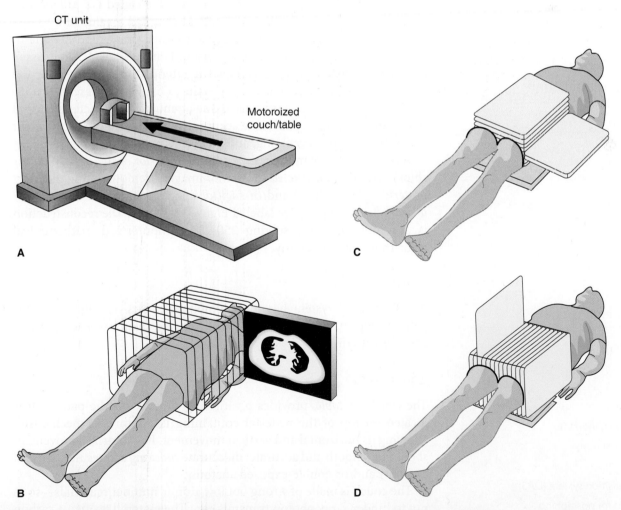

Figure 13-57. **(A)** A typical CT unit. **(B)** The helical/spiral CT x-ray tube, with detector arrays opposite it, rotates around the patient, obtaining axial "slices"/"sections" of information. These axial images **(B)** can be reconstructed into coronal **(C)** and/or sagittal **(D)** images. This is accomplished as the computer solves 250,000 mathematical algorithms simultaneously.

process of CT imaging allows very much improved perception of small tissue density differences; slice thickness is measured in millimeters.

The CT x-ray tube, and the rows of detectors opposite it, rotates around the patient (Fig. 13-57A–D). The CT images (two-dimensional or three-dimensional) are obtained by detecting and measuring the exit radiation from each slice, determining its attenuation and transmission characteristics, and converting to electrical signals, which are then changed to digital data. The digital data are transferred to a computer for reconstruction. The reconstructed images can then be displayed on a monitor, transmitted elsewhere, printed, and archived. The acquisition and reconstruction process in a seventh generation CT unit can normally be accomplished in under 20 s.

Sir Godfrey Newbold Hounsfield created the first CT unit, describing the reconstruction of data taken from multiple projection angles. Allan MacLeod Cormack worked with the complex mathematical algorithms required for image reconstruction. Their first commercial CT head scanner was available in 1971. In 1979, Hounsfield and Cormack shared the Nobel Prize in Medicine for their historic work with this new imaging science.

To express the beam attenuation characteristics of various tissues, the *Hounsfield Unit* (HU) is used. HUs can also be called *CT numbers* or tissue density values. Godfrey Hounsfield assigned a value of 0 to distilled water, a value of +1000 to dense osseous tissue, and a value of −1000 to air. There is a direct relationship between the HU and tissue attenuation coefficient. The greater the attenuation coefficient of the particular tissue, the higher the HU value. One HU represents a 0.1% difference between the particular tissue attenuation characteristics and that of distilled water. HU value accuracy can be affected by equipment calibration, volume averaging, and image artifacts.

Axial images (demonstrating *superior/inferior* structural relationships) can be *reconstructed* to *coronal* images (demonstrating *anterior/posterior* relationships) and/or *sagittal* images (demonstrating *medial/lateral* relationships)—see labeled Figure 13-58A–F. The reconstruction is accomplished by resolving 250,000 computerized mathematical algorithms simultaneously!

Component Parts

A CT imaging system has four component parts—a *couch/table* for patient support, a (doughnut-shaped) *gantry*, a *computer*, and *operating consoles* with display.

Couch/Table

The *couch*, or *table*, provides positioning support for the patient. It is located on top of the pedestal containing its motorized mechanism, allowing its horizontal and vertical movement. Its motorized movement should be smooth and accurate; inaccurate *indexing* can result in missed anatomy and/or double-exposed anatomy.

The couch is made of strong but low atomic number materials—so as not to hinder x-ray photon transmission. The material is often a carbon fiber, capable of weight limits up to 450 lb. Precise table motion is essential, and exceeding the weight limit can affect/damage the table's precise moving mechanism.

Common Hounsfield Units

+1000 = Bone

0 = Distilled water

−1000 = Air

CT Component Parts

- Couch/table
- Gantry
- X-ray tube
- Detector array
- High-voltage generator
- Collimator assembly
- Slip rings
- Digital acquisition system (DAS)
- Laser beams for positioning
- Computer
- Operating consoles

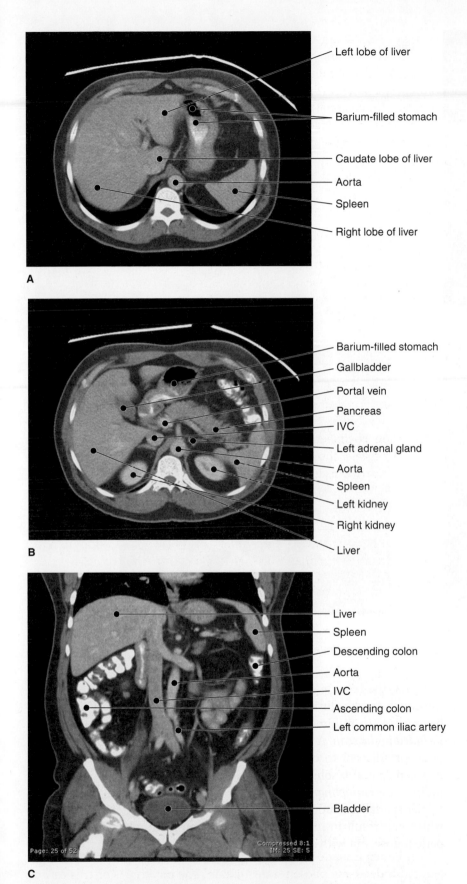

Left lobe of liver

Barium-filled stomach

Caudate lobe of liver

Aorta

Spleen

Right lobe of liver

A

Barium-filled stomach

Gallbladder

Portal vein

Pancreas

IVC

Left adrenal gland

Aorta

Spleen

Left kidney

Right kidney

Liver

B

Liver

Spleen

Descending colon

Aorta

IVC

Ascending colon

Left common iliac artery

Bladder

Page: 25 of 52

Compressed 8:1
IM: 25 SE: 5

C

Figure 13-58. **(A)** Superior and **(B)** inferior *axial* images; **(C)** anterior and **(D)** posterior *coronal* images; **(E)** medial and **(F)** lateral *sagittal* images. (*Continued*)

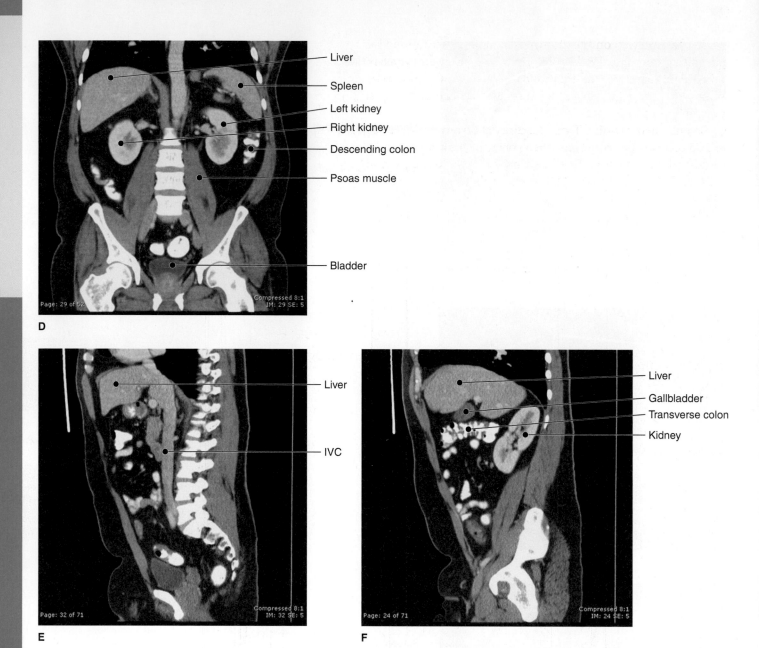

D

E

F

Figure 13-58. *(Continued)*

In CT, the term *pitch* refers to the relationship between the distance the couch travels during one x-ray tube rotation and the width of the beam/slice (in millimeters). *The pitch determines the amount of tissue included in the scan.* A pitch of 1.0 indicates that the slices will be contiguous, or adjacent to one another. This typically offers a good balance between spatial resolution and patient dose. Pitch values less than 1.0 indicate *oversampling* and can result in excessive exposure, but also a higher spatial resolution. Pitch values above 1.0 indicate *undersampling* which can result in missed data (i.e., anatomy/pathology) and a lower patient dose, but with a decrease in spatial resolution.

Gantry

The *gantry* component generally includes an x-ray tube, a detector array, a high-voltage generator, a collimator assembly, slip rings, DAS, and laser beams to assist positioning.

The patient/part on the motorized couch is surrounded by the circular gantry opening. Within the circular gantry assembly is the x-ray tube, facing an array of thousands of detectors (up to 60+ rows). In sixth-generation CT, the x-ray tube and detectors move around the patient within the gantry.

Seventh-generation CT can acquire data from multiple sections—up to 320 sections per rotation—the x-ray tube making many *pulsed exposures,* and the detector array receiving the transmitted photons.

In earlier generations of CT, the x-ray tube rotated 360° around the patient lying on a stationary couch to obtain a "slice" image. The couch would then advance a particular distance (called *indexing*), stop, and then the x-ray tube rotated 360° in the opposite direction for the next "slice" image, and so on.

The several generations of CT scanners have had various combinations of fixed and/or rotating x-ray tubes and detector arrays, and examination times have changed considerably during the evolution of CT.

Gantry Components
1. X-ray tube
2. Detector array
3. High-voltage generator
4. Collimator assembly
5. Slip rings
6. DAS
7. Laser beams for positioning

Computer

The CT computer must be capable of performing tens of thousands calculations, simultaneously, per slice—for considerably more than 100 slices per second.

A microprocessor or array processor is used for the all-important function of reconstruction. *Reconstruction* is defined as the time lapse between completion of imaging and the appearance of images.

Operating Consoles

The CT technologist uses one console to operate the CT machine, selecting the correct examination protocols, and entering patient demographics. Another console might be required for technologist postprocessing, archiving, and other administrative tasks. There may be a third display console available for the physician to view and manipulate images.

Generations of Computed Tomography

- First: *pencil* beam
  - Head scans only
  - Detectors opposite finely collimated beam
  - "Translation" time: time taken for the x-ray tube and two detectors to travel from one side of part to other side
  - After one translation, the x-ray tube/detector assembly rotated 1° (indexing)
  - Translation and indexing were repeated until examination completion, followed by computer reconstruction
  - Examination time more than 30 min; one to four sections acquired per rotation
- Second: divergent (but flat) *fan* beam (~10)
  - More data collected with about 30 detectors
  - 30° indexing
  - Reduced examination time (one-tenth of first-generation time!)
  - One to four sections acquired per rotation

- Third: *rotating tube and detector* array
  - This was recognized as the first multidetector CT
  - Had *thicker* fan beam (i.e., not flat) that now required different reconstruction algorithms
  - *Curved array* of approximately 250–900 detectors (covers at least 20 mm on the Z axis)
  - *Greater coverage* and *thinner slices* provide *higher resolution* images
  - Continuous tube operation—*no stop for translation*
  - 360° of data collected
  - *Pause* between each scan for table indexing
  - Reduced scan time; one to four sections acquired per rotation
- Fourth: *stationary detector ring* with rotating tube
  - Clockwise motion, followed by counterclockwise motion for next section
  - Greatly reduced examination time
  - One to four sections acquired per rotation
- Fifth: *electron beam;* ultrahigh-speed CT
  - 400–800 fixed detectors
  - For cardiac imaging specifically because of its speed
  - Four sections acquired per rotation
- Sixth: *helical or spiral CT*
- Similar to third generation because *x-ray tube and detectors rotate continuously* 360° around the patient (Fig. 13-59)

> ### Advantages of Helical Multislice CT
>
> - Reduced motion blur/artifacts
> - Greatly reduced scan time
> - Increase in tissue volume imaged
> - Lower volume contrast media needed
> - High-quality reconstruction

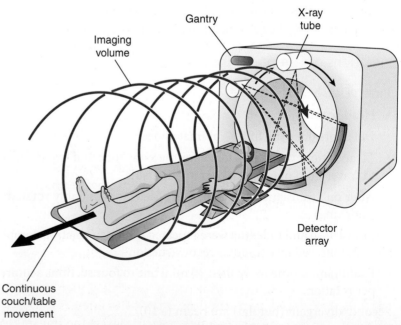

Figure 13-59. Achievement of *slip ring technology* allows *continuous* x-ray tube rotation and *simultaneous* couch movement, permitting acquisition of volume multislice scanning. The method of image acquisition lends itself to the term *helical* (or spiral) CT.

- Couch/table is *simultaneously* moving through gantry (no stop for indexing)
- *Made possible by slip ring technology,* which no longer made it necessary for the machine to stop and uncoil wires in the gantry between each rotation
- Complete volume of part (chest/abdomen) can be scanned in 30 s per one breath hold
- Slices of data can be adjusted by table speed—this is called *pitch,* that is, slices and their data can be right next to each other (called a pitch of 1); a pitch greater than 1 allows fast acquisition but can result in a thicker slice or a gap between slice data (information can be missed, image quality can decrease); a pitch less than 1 indicates overlap of slice data (can result in excessive patient exposure)
- Some helical/spiral CT units have a dual source (i.e., two x-ray tubes) for better resolution and for better balance
- Seventh: *multidetector/multisection CT*
  - Images *more than one section* (16–320) *per rotation*
  - *Multiple rows of detectors* collect the data, thereby decreasing patient dose and total scan time
  - Total scan time (e.g., for chest/abdomen) reduced to approximately 15 s

> ### Types of Three-Dimensional Multiplanar Reconstruction (MPR)
>
> - MIP (maximum intensity projection)
> - SSD (shaded surface display)
> - SVD (shaded volume display)

In the 1990s, the implementation of *slip ring technology* allowed *continuous* rotation of the x-ray tube (through elimination of cables) and simultaneous couch movement. Sixth-generation CT scanning is termed *helical* (or spiral) CT—permitting acquisition of volume multislice scanning. Nowadays, helical multislice scanners, using two or more rows of detectors, can obtain uninterrupted data acquisition of 128 "slices" per tube rotation and can perform *three-dimensional multiplanar reconstruction* (MPR). In MPR, two-dimensional transverse images are stacked on each other to form a three-dimensional compilation by using one of three types of MPR algorithms (MIP, SSD, SVD).

Although the *CT x-ray tube* is similar to direct projection x-ray tubes, the objective is a fan-shaped beam. The CT x-ray tube also has several particular requirements; it must have a very high short-exposure rating and must be capable of tolerating several million HUs while still having a small focal spot for optimal spatial resolution. To help tolerate the very high production of HUs, the anode must also be capable of high-speed rotation. The x-ray tube produces a pulsed x-ray beam (1–5 ms) using up to approximately 1000 mA and 140 kV.

The *scintillation detector array* is made of thousands of solid-state PDs. If the scintillation crystals are packed tightly together so that there is virtually no distance between them, x-ray absorption efficiency is increased, patient dose is decreased, SNR is increased, and imaging time is decreased. Detection efficiency is extremely high—approximately 90%. These solid-state scintillation crystal assemblies (cadmium tungstate or rare earth oxide ceramic crystals) convert the transmitted x-ray energy into light. The light is then converted into electrical energy (by a semiconductor PD) and finally converted into an electronic/digital signal by the DAS. From the DAS, binary data are sent to the array processor computer. The computer *reconstructs* the "raw" data into cross-sectional images. Here, additional processing operations and image manipulation can also be carried out. Digital image postprocessing provides the opportunity for image optimization. Image annotation permits placement of labels, arrow indicators, and so on. Windowing allows adjustment of image contrast and/or brightness to diagnostic requirements. Contrast scale enhancement is the most valuable tool in digital imaging. Image minification, with larger matrix sizes, enables us to see tiny anatomic details and improve spatial resolution. Image inversion, or reversal, provides a different perspective by changing white to black and black to white. Image flip also provides another perspective by enabling us to rotate the image. Edge enhancement is useful for small and high-contrast tissues. Other postprocessing functions include highlighting, zoom, pan, and scroll. The pixel shift feature is important in DSA. Image subtraction (see Fig. 13-40) is used to enhance contrast. If the part moves during acquisition of serial images, misregistration occurs, making the required exact superimposition impossible. Pixel shift is a function that can correct misregistration. Another emerging postprocessing task used in diagnostic functions is determining numeric pixel value for particular ROI. This feature has proved useful in bone densitometry, renal calculus recognition, and calcified lung nodule identification.

The *high-voltage generator* provides HF power to the CT x-ray tube, enabling the high-speed anode rotation and the production of high-energy pulsed x-ray photons. Similar to the HF x-ray tubes used in projection radiography, conventional 60-Hz full-wave rectified power is converted to a higher frequency of 500–25,000 Hz. The CT generator can be located in the CT room, outside the gantry. However, an *HF CT generator* is usually mounted within the gantry's rotating wheel, is solid state and small in size, and produces an almost constant potential waveform.

The *collimator assembly* has two parts: The *prepatient* collimator at the x-ray tube consists of multilevel beam restrictions so that the x-ray beam diverges very little. Collimation (and therefore scan volume) varies according to the procedure being performed. The prepatient collimator determines patient *dose*. The *predetector* collimator, or *postpatient* collimator, further confines the exit photons before they reach the detector array, reducing the scatter reaching the detectors and improving image *contrast*. The predetector collimator determines *slice thickness* (also called *sensitivity profile*).

Summary

- Correct terminology is "CT."
- Axial images can be reconstructed and viewed in the sagittal and coronal planes.
- The infrequently performed *conventional tomography* is called *axial tomography* because the image plane parallels the body's long axis, providing coronal and/or sagittal images.
- CT images are axial images that can be reconstructed into coronal and/or sagittal images.

CHAPTER 13   EQUIPMENT OPERATION AND QUALITY ASSURANCE   **487**

- In CT, the x-ray tube and detector arrays opposite it rotate around the patient, obtaining "slices"/"sections" of information.

- Exit radiation from each slice is measured; attenuation and transmission characteristics are determined and converted to electrical signals, changed to digital data, then and transferred to computer for reconstruction.

- In 1979, Hounsfield and Cormack shared the Nobel Prize in Medicine for their historic work with CT imaging.

- The HU is used in CT to express the beam attenuation characteristics of various tissues.

- A CT imaging system has four component parts—a *couch/table* for patient support, a (doughnut-shaped) *gantry,* a *computer,* and *operating consoles* with display.

- The CT gantry is composed of the x-ray tube, detector array, high-voltage generator, collimator assembly, slip rings, DAS, and laser beams for positioning.

- The term *pitch* refers to the relationship between the distance the couch travels during one x-ray tube rotation and the width of the beam/slice (in millimeters).

- The seven generations of CT scanners have had various combinations of fixed and/or rotating x-ray tubes and detector arrays, and examination times have changed considerably during the evolution of CT.

- *Slip ring technology* allows *continuous* rotation of the x-ray tube (by elimination of cables) and simultaneous couch movement.

- *Helical* (or spiral) CT permits acquisition of volume multislice scans; helical/spiral multislice scanners use two or more rows of detectors.

- Advantages of *helical multislice CT* include reduced motion blur/artifacts, decreased scan time, increased tissue volume imaged, need of lower volume contrast media, and high-quality reconstruction.

- CT x-ray tubes have high-speed anode rotation and produce a pulsed, fan-shaped beam that emerges from a small focal spot for optimal spatial resolution; they have a high short-exposure rating and can tolerate several million HUs.

- The scintillation detector array is made of thousands of very sensitive/efficient solid-state PDs.

- The scintillation assemblies convert the transmitted x-ray energy into light, which is next converted into electrical energy by PDs, and finally converted into a digital signal by the DAS.

- From the DAS, binary data are sent to the array processor computer, where "raw" data are reconstructed into cross-sectional images. This is where additional processing operations and image manipulation can be carried out as well (e.g., windowing, enhancement, measurements, three-dimensional postprocessing, volume rendering, and multiplanar reconstruction).

- The small-size, solid-state HF CT generator is usually mounted within the gantry's rotating wheel and produces an almost constant potential waveform.

- The *collimator assembly* has two parts. The x-ray tube *prepatient* collimator has multiple beam restrictions to minimize beam divergence; it determines patient dose. The *predetector/postpatient* collimator further confines the exit beam before it reaches the detector array, reducing exit scatter, improving image contrast, and determining slice thickness/sensitivity profile.

- The CT computer performs tens of thousands of calculations, simultaneously, per slice—for considerably more than 100 slices per second.

- *Reconstruction* is defined as the time lapse between completion of imaging and the appearance of images.

- The console is used by the CT technologist to operate the CT machine, select the examination protocols, and enter patient information; another console might be required for postprocessing, archiving, and other administrative tasks.

COMPREHENSION CHECK

1. Discuss why the term *CT scan* is correct and the term *CAT scan* outdated (p. 479).

2. Who were the two individuals most instrumental in the development of CT, and how were they recognized (p. 480)?

3. List the four component parts of a CT unit (p. 480, 481).

4. List the seven components of the CT gantry (p. 482, 483).

5. What kind of technology allows continuous rotation of the CT x-ray tube and simultaneous movement of the examination couch (p. 485)?

6. Describe what is meant by the CT term *pitch* and how it is related to *undersampling* and *oversampling. Discuss its effect on resolution* (p. 482).

7. What is meant by CT translation time (p. 483)?

8. What is the shape of the CT x-ray beam and how has it changed over the generations(p. 485)?

9. What rotates directly opposite the x-ray tube in the CT gantry (p. 483)?

10. What is the function of the CT prepatient collimator and the postpatient collimator (p. 486)?

11. What is meant by the CT term *reconstruction* (p. 483)?

12. What is meant by the term *indexing* when applied to the CT couch (p. 483)?

13. Differentiate between the seven generations of CT (p. 483, 484).

CHAPTER REVIEW QUESTIONS

1. The CT x-ray tube collimator having greatest impact on patient dose is the
   (A) prepatient collimator
   (B) predetector collimator
   (C) control collimator
   (D) gantry collimator

2. Axial CT images can be reconstructed to sagittal images that will demonstrate
   (A) superior/inferior structural relationships
   (B) anterior/posterior relationships
   (C) medial/lateral relationships
   (D) inferior/lateral relationships

3. The component parts of a CT imaging system include
   1. gantry
   2. computer
   3. table
   (A) 1 only
   (B) 1 and 2 only
   (C) 2 and 3 only
   (D) 1, 2, and 3

4. The CT term used to describe patient couch/table movement divided by x-ray beam width is
   (A) pitch
   (B) gantry
   (C) grid
   (D) array

5. The CT x-ray tube collimator having greatest impact on image contrast is the
   (A) prepatient collimator
   (B) predetector collimator
   (C) control collimator
   (D) gantry collimator

6. CT gantry components include
   1. x-ray tube
   2. detector array
   3. computer
   (A) 1 only
   (B) 1 and 2 only
   (C) 2 and 3 only
   (D) 1, 2, and 3

7. The time lapse between completion of CT imaging and the appearance of CT images is called
   (A) reformation
   (B) reconstruction
   (C) display time
   (D) reassembly

8. Requirements of CT x-ray tube include
   1. high-speed anode rotation for heat distribution
   2. high short-exposure rating for the pulsed beam
   3. large focal spot for less heat protection
   (A) 1 only
   (B) 1 and 2 only
   (C) 2 and 3 only
   (D) 1, 2, and 3

9. The CT x-ray tube collimator having greatest impact on sensitivity profile is the
   (A) prepatient collimator
   (B) predetector collimator
   (C) control collimator
   (D) gantry collimator

10. Transformation of two-dimensional CT images into three-dimensional images is accomplished by
    (A) multiplanar reformation
    (B) multiplanar reconstruction
    (C) interpolation
    (D) extrapolation

11. A pitch setting of less than one would provide
    1. 1. undersampling
    2. 2. higher resolution
    3. 3. oversampling
    (A) 1 only
    (B) 3 only
    (C) 1 and 2 only
    (D) 2 and 3 only

12. What generation of CT scanner did not have an x-ray tube and detector array that could rotate 360° around the patient?
    (A) Third generation
    (B) Fourth generation
    (C) Sixth generation
    (D) Seventh generation

Answers and Explanations

1. (A) The *collimator assembly* has two parts. The x-ray tube *prepatient* collimator has multiple beam restrictions to minimize beam divergence; it determines patient dose. The *predetector/postpatient* collimator further confines the exit beam before it reaches the detector array, reducing exit scatter, improving image contrast, and determining slice thickness/sensitivity profile.

2. (C) The CT x-ray tube, and the rows of detectors opposite it, rotates around the patient. The CT images are obtained by detecting and measuring the exit radiation from each slice, determining its attenuation and transmission characteristics, converting to electrical signals, which are then changed to digital data, and transferring the data to a computer for reconstruction. *Axial* images (demonstrating *superior/inferior* structural relationships) can be reconstructed to *coronal* images (demonstrating *anterior/posterior* relationships) and/or *sagittal* images (demonstrating *medial/lateral* relationships)—see labeled Figure 13-58A–E. The reconstruction is accomplished by resolving 250,000 computerized mathematical algorithms simultaneously!

3. (D) A CT imaging system has four component parts—a *couch/table* for patient support, a *gantry*, a *computer*, and *operating consoles* with display. The *couch*, or table, provides positioning support for the patient. The *gantry* component generally includes an x-ray tube, a detector array, a high-voltage generator, a collimator assembly, slip rings, DAS, and laser beams to assist positioning. The CT *computer* must be capable of performing tens of thousands calculations, simultaneously, per slice—for considerably more than 100 slices per second. The CT technologist uses one *console* to operate the CT machine, selecting the correct examination protocols, and entering patient demographics. Another console might be required for technologist postprocessing, archiving, and other administrative tasks. There may be a third display console available for the physician to view and manipulate images.

4. (A) In CT, the term *pitch* refers to the relationship between the distance the couch travels during one x-ray tube rotation and the width of the beam/slice (in millimeters). The pitch determines the amount of tissue included in the scan. Pitch values less than 1.0 indicate oversampling and can result in excessive exposure. Pitch values above 1.0 indicate undersampling and can result in missed data (i.e., anatomy/pathology).

5. (B) The *collimator assembly* has two parts. The x-ray tube *prepatient* collimator has multiple beam restrictions to minimize beam divergence; it determines patient dose. The *predetector/postpatient* collimator further confines the exit beam before it reaches the detector array, reducing exit scatter, improving image contrast, and determining slice thickness/sensitivity profile.

6. (B) A CT imaging system has four component parts—a couch/table for patient support, a gantry, a computer, and operating consoles with display. The *gantry* component generally includes an x-ray tube, a detector array, a high-voltage generator, a collimator assembly, slip rings, DAS, and laser beams to assist positioning.

7. (B) The CT computer must be capable of performing tens of thousands calculations, simultaneously, per slice—for considerably more than 100 slices per second. CT images are obtained by detecting and measuring the exit radiation from each slice, determining its attenuation and transmission characteristics, converting to electrical signals, which are then changed to digital data, and transferring the data to a computer for reconstruction. A microprocessor or array processor is used for the all-important function of reconstruction. *Reconstruction* is defined as the time lapse between completion of imaging and the appearance of images.

8. (B) Although the CT x-ray tube is similar to direct projection x-ray tubes, the objective is a fan-shaped beam. The CT x-ray tube also has several particular requirements; it must have a very *high short-exposure rating* and must be capable of tolerating several million HUs while still having a *small focal spot* for optimal spatial resolution. To help tolerate the very high production of HUs, the anode must also be capable of *high-speed rotation*. The x-ray tube produces a pulsed x-ray beam (1–5 ms) using up to approximately 1000 mA and 140 kV.

9. (B) The *collimator assembly* has two parts. The x-ray tube *prepatient* collimator has multiple beam restrictions to minimize beam divergence; it determines patient dose. The *predetector/postpatient* collimator further confines the exit beam before it reaches the detector array, reducing exit scatter, improving image contrast, and determining slice thickness/sensitivity profile.

10. (A) Implementation of slip ring technology allowed continuous rotation of the x-ray tube and simultaneous couch movement. Nowadays, helical multislice scanners, using two or more rows of detectors, can obtain uninterrupted data acquisition of 128 "slices" per tube rotation and can perform three-dimensional *MPR*. In MPR, two-dimensional transverse images are stacked on each other to form a three-dimensional compilation using one of three types of MPR algorithms (MIP, SSD, SVD).

Interpolation and extrapolation are algorithmic mathematical processes used in image reconstruction.

11. (D) A pitch less than one (<1) means that the patient will move slower through the CT gantry as the tube rotates around him or her. This causes sections of anatomy to be scanned more than once, resulting in oversampling. This in turn leads to a higher resolution on the CT image because more image data were acquired. Undersampling occurs with a pitch greater than one (>1).

12. (B) The concept of rotating both the x-ray tube and detector array around the patient was first introduced in the third generation of CT scanners. The fourth generation attempted something different, with a stationary detector ring and rotating x-ray tube. With the sixth generation, there was a return to the rotating of both tube and detector array, but without stopping to index the radiographic table. This was called spiral/helical scanning. Seventh-generation scanners have multiple rows of detectors that rotate around the patient along with the x-ray tube. This allows for many sections to be imaged in one rotation.

STANDARDS OF PERFORMANCE AND EQUIPMENT EVALUATION

Regulations and Rationale

NCRP Report No. 102 serves as a guide to good medical radiation practices by describing the federal regulations on equipment design, performance, and use. Manufacturers of x-ray equipment must follow guidelines that state maximum x-ray output at specific distances, total quantities of filtration, positive beam limitation (PBL), and other guidelines. Radiographers must practice safe *principles of operation; preventive maintenance* and *quality control* (QC) checks must be performed at specific intervals to ensure continued safe equipment performance. The term *quality assurance* refers to the *professionals* who operate the equipment. The Joint Commission (TJC) identifies some of these considerations as assigning responsibility, collecting and organizing data, delineating scopes of care, evaluation of care, action to improve care, and so on. The term *QC* involves regular evaluation of *equipment* to determine its safe and accurate operation. An associated term is *medical maintenance,* which refers to scheduled and unscheduled support services.

Radiologic QC involves monitoring and regulating the variables associated with image production and patient care. Every radiologic facility nowadays must establish QC guidelines and conduct QC programs to provide a consistent standard of care. A properly documented, ongoing, and effective QC program is required by hospital accrediting agencies and state departments of health.

The rationale behind QC is that a radiographic imaging system performing in an erratic and undependable manner results in repeat exposures, thus contributing to unnecessary patient dose and uneconomical use of time, equipment, and supplies. *Radiographic QC* is an organized and methodical evaluation of imaging components from the x-ray tube to the display monitor, with the purpose of decreasing repeat exposures, thereby decreasing patient radiation exposure and increasing cost-effectiveness. The *frequency of testing* ranges from daily scanner/reader checks to quarterly, semiannual, and annual equipment performance testing.

The position of QC technologist is an increasingly important one, requiring advanced knowledge and skills.

The QC program requires the combined efforts of the radiographer, the QC technologist, the service engineer, and the medical physicist. The radiographer must be alert to any equipment malfunctions or unusual occurrences and report them to the QC technologist without delay. The QC technologist, the service engineer, and the medical physicist are responsible for equipment testing, correlation of test results, any necessary corrections or modifications, and accurate documentation of their activities.

QC in digital/electronic imaging is expanding. There are some established parameters for consideration, but there is much more to be experienced and learned. Established maintenance procedures are discussed.

> **QA Versus QC**
>
> Quality assurance (QA): Comprehensive evaluation that aims to improve the quality of care being delivered to patients by analyzing the *human* elements of the process.
>
> Quality control (QC): Comprehensive evaluation of *equipment* to ensure its functionality and ability to produce high-quality images at the lowest radiation doses possible.

EQUIPMENT CALIBRATION

QC ensures the equipment safety and its accurate operation. Various components must be tested at specified intervals, and test results must be within specified parameters. Any deviation from those parameters

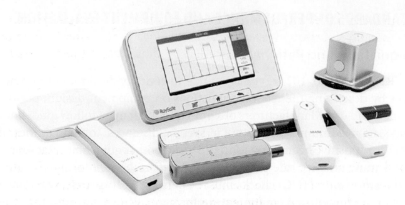

Figure 13-60. RaySafe X2 is a single diagnostic testing device for evaluation of many types of x-ray equipment and modalities: radiography, fluoroscopy, CT, mammography, and dental. It can simultaneously measure parameters such as kV, dose, dose rate, mAs, and HVL; no special settings needed. (Photo contributor: RaySafe, a division of Fluke Electronics Corporation.)

must be corrected. Examples of equipment components that are tested annually are the focal spot size, linearity, reproducibility, filtration, kV, and exposure time.

Fluke's 8000 Victoreen NERO mAx x-ray device (Fig. 13-60) is a single device capable of evaluating many types of x-ray imaging equipment available nowadays. It can simultaneously measure kV, exposure rate, and mA or mAs. It incorporates various filter cards to accurately measure kV and an ionization chamber to measure exposure rate. A device such as this can eliminate the need for several of the individual tests familiar to radiographers that are described.

Kilovoltage

Calibration of kV was formerly evaluated by using a Wisconsin test tool and cassette. The *digital kV test meters* are more convenient and simple to use. When various kVs are tested in the normal diagnostic range (40–150 kV), the selected kV and actual kV value should not differ by more than ±4 kV for *general diagnostic* equipment and by 5% of the nominal kV for *mammography* equipment.

Milliamperage

The accuracy of individual mA stations is related to *patient dose* and is essential for production of expected *receptor exposure* levels.

An *aluminum step-wedge* (penetrometer) can be used to evaluate each mA station. A series of exposures are made at a particular kV by *using the same mAs value at each mA station*, with exposure time adjusted to maintain a constant mAs. The resulting images should be identical. Performance of this test on properly calibrated equipment illustrates the *reciprocity law. Any variance should be within 10%.*

Linearity of mA can be evaluated by using a digital dosimeter (ionization chamber). Linearity tests the system's ability to produce expected changes in output intensity when the mAs is either increased or decreased. When the mAs is increased, the exposure intensity should also increase. When the mAs is decreased, the exposure intensity should decrease. *Linearity testing* is performed after generator modification or calibration and at least annually, and the acceptable variance is within 10%.

Timer

Timer accuracy is related to patient dose and the production of expected receptor exposure and should be tested at least on an annual basis. X-ray timer malfunction can cause undesirable fluctuation in receptor exposure. If the timer terminates the exposure prematurely, the image can be underexposed; if the exposure is delayed in terminating, the image can be overexposed. Electronic timers can be accurate to as low as 1 ms. The majority of exposure timers are now electronic and usually controlled by a microprocessor and accuracy evaluated with an oscilloscope. The use of a digital dosimeter, however, is a more simple and accurate measure of timer accuracy. The selected exposure time should be within 5% of the actual exposure time. Similar tests are used to evaluate the accuracy of automatic exposure devices.

Timer accuracy testing is performed after generator modification or calibration, when troubleshooting under- or overexposed images, and at least annually.

Beam Restriction

The collimator assembly (Fig. 13-61) includes a series of lead shutters, a mirror, and a light bulb. The mirror and the light bulb function to project the size, location, and center of the irradiated field. The bulb's emitted beam of light is deflected by a mirror placed at an angle of 45° in the path of the light beam. For the projected light beam to be the same size as the x-ray beam, the focal spot and the light bulb *must be exactly at the same distance* from the center of the mirror.

Congruence is a term used to describe the relationship between the collimator light field and the actual x-ray field—they must be congruent (i.e., match) to within 2% of the SID. *Centering* indication is required

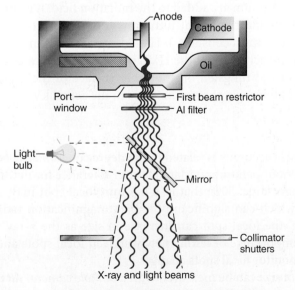

Figure 13-61. X-ray and light beams.

and must be within 1% of the central ray. PBL must not permit field size to exceed IR size. Collimators should be inspected and verified as accurate *semiannually,* that is, twice a year.

X-ray Tube Overload Protection

Warm-up procedures are performed at the beginning of the day to prevent excessive heat to a cold anode (which could crack the anode). Single-exposure overloads are avoided by programmed prevention of an exposure in excess of a particular predetermined amount. The *overload protection circuit testing* is performed after generator modification or calibration and at least annually.

Reproducibility

This test should be performed annually to evaluate *consistency* of x-ray tube output. A particular group of technical factors is selected, and a series of consecutive exposures (at least five) are made. The factors are changed between exposures and then changed back to the original technical factors. The digital radiation meter should register radiation output that does not vary more than 5%. If a radiographer notices an exposure fluctuation while using a particular group of technical factors, the *reproducibility* test is performed by using those factors but, alternately, changing to other technical factors between exposures.

Reproducibility testing is performed when troubleshooting a problem and at least annually.

Half-Value Layer

Half-value layer (HVL) testing provides beam quality information that is different from that obtained from kV testing. HVL is defined as the thickness of any absorber that will reduce x-ray beam intensity to one-half its original value. It is determined by measuring the beam intensity without an absorber and then recording the intensity as successive millimeters of aluminum are added to the radiation field. It is influenced by the type of rectification, total filtration, and kV. An x-ray tube HVL should remain almost constant. If HVL decreases, it is an indication of a decrease in the actual kV. If the HVL increases, it indicates the deposition of vaporized tungsten on the inner surface of the glass envelope (as a result of tube aging) or an increase in the actual kV.

Focal Spot Size

Focal spot size accuracy is related to the degree of *geometric blur,* that is, edge gradient or penumbra. Manufacturer tolerance for new focal spots is surprisingly large, 50%; that is, a 0.3-mm focal spot may actually be 0.45 mm (which can significantly impact magnification radiography). In addition, the focal spot can increase in size as the x-ray tube ages, hence the importance of *testing* newly arrived focal spots and periodic testing to monitor focal spots changes.

Focal spot size can be measured with a *pinhole camera, slit camera,* or *star pattern–type resolution device.* The *pinhole camera* is rather difficult to use accurately and requires the use of excessive tube (heat) loading. With a *slit camera,* two exposures are made: one measures the length of the focal spot and the other measures the width. The *star pattern–type,* or similar, resolution device can measure focal spot size *as a function of geometric blur* and is readily adaptable in a QC program to monitor focal spot changes over a period of time. It is recommended that focal spot size be checked on installation of a new x-ray tube and annually thereafter.

RADIOGRAPHIC AND FLUOROSCOPIC ACCESSORIES

Imaging Plates and Photostimulable Phosphors

Care and maintenance of IPs include monthly routine cleaning or as needed. The external surface must be kept clean, as a soiled surface can impair the IP's ability to travel through the scanner/reader; it can result in mechanical failure and system shutdown. If the IP can come in contact with any type of moisture such as body fluids or other contaminants, the IP should be appropriately bagged before use.

IPs and PSPs can collect dust and other particulate matter through normal use. The dust can be removed with a moisture-free air spray or by using a lint-free cloth. If the IP becomes soiled, it can be cleaned with anhydrous ethanol and thoroughly dried with a lint-free cloth.

Dust on PSPs has the effect of a clear pinhole artifact on the image. PSPs should be checked for physical damage too. Scratches appear as clear areas on the resulting image. If the PSP requires more than simple dusting, it can also be cleaned with anhydrous ethanol and dried thoroughly with a lint-free cloth or with a special PSP cleaner as recommended by the manufacturer. Using any other cleaner can cause breakdown of the PSP's protective coat. PSPs are flexible and have a sturdy protective coat but should be handled by their edges during cleaning. It is essential that the cleaner be completely dried because residual cleaner can cause the phosphors to swell, resulting in deterioration of the PSP.

Appropriate care ensures a maximum useful life. The life of the typical PSP is approximately 10,000 exposures.

Grids

Frequent, rigorous use or mishandling of clip-on/slip-on grids can result in damage and shifting of the lead strips. These unapparent structural changes result in artifacts that can hide or mimic pathology. Repeat exposures, with resultant patient dose increase, are often necessary. NCRP Report No. 99, Quality Assurance for Diagnostic Imaging, recommends that grid uniformity be evaluated periodically by imaging a homogeneous phantom with an exposure that will produce an optical density of approximately 1.2.

The report further states that moving grids in x-ray tables should be evaluated before installation and annually thereafter and that clip-on/slip-on grids and grid cassettes be evaluated every 6 months—or sooner if the grid is damaged or suspected of creating artifacts.

Fluoroscopic Exposure Rates

Maximum exposure rate in manual fluoroscopy should not exceed 21 mGy$_a$/min/mA or 100 mGy$_a$/min. If high-level "boost" mode is available, maximum allowable tabletop intensity is 200 mGy$_a$/min. Average size patients undergoing diagnostic fluoroscopic examinations commonly receive entrance exposures of up to 25 cGy (25 rad). In interventional procedures, entrance doses of 100 cGy can be delivered. In consideration of these potentially high doses, it is imperative that the exposure rates are checked regularly. *Generator output testing* is performed whenever the fluoroscopic system is serviced and at least every 6 months.

Lead Aprons and Gloves

Personnel fluoroscopic shielding apparel such as lead aprons, gloves, and thyroid shields should be *fluoroscoped annually* to detect any cracks that may have developed in the leaded vinyl.

Proper care is required to help prolong the useful life of lead apparel. If soiled, it can be cleaned with a damp cloth. Lead aprons should not be folded or carelessly dropped to the floor, for that facilitates development of cracks in the leaded vinyl. Lead aprons and gloves should be hung on appropriate racks when not in use. Lead apparel that is cracked will not protect the wearer as intended. Radiation is able to penetrate these areas more easily, leading to additional exposure of the wearer.

ADDITIONAL DIGITAL IMAGING CONSIDERATIONS

A good QC program is essential to consistent, effective operation of digital imaging equipment. There are some established parameters for consideration, but there is much more to be experienced and learned. Established maintenance procedures are covered here.

Established maintenance procedures include a *daily check* on the printer/processor according to the manufacturer's recommendations. The air intakes on the *reader* should be cleaned weekly or according to the manufacturer's recommendations.

The *laser* in the CR reader should be checked monthly for evidence of "jitter." Regular *contrast evaluation* is recommended; this confirms the consistency of the x-ray exposure, CR reader, workstation display, and hardcopy printer. A *sharpness* test is performed to evaluate the x-ray tube performance, CR reader optics, monitor display, and hardcopy printer.

The assessment of the EI/sensitivity checks the calibration and consistency of the actual x-ray exposures as well as the PMT of the CR reader.

Other tests include assessment of image *noise, artifacts, erasure* thoroughness, and *linearity* testing. A special phantom is provided to evaluate all system components/characteristics (Fig. 13-62).

Digital display devices require regular evaluation. Monitor *luminance* is assessed via photometric evaluation by using a luminance meter.

Ambient light can impact image contrast, and best viewing of the monitor's digital image is usually straight on (rather than from an

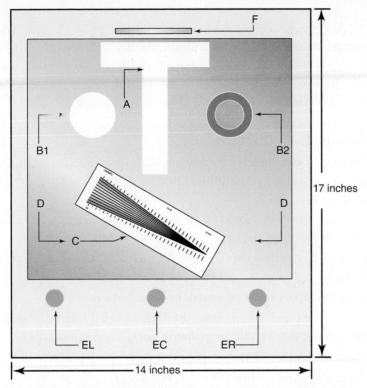

Figure 13-62. CR requires a regular QA program, just as other imaging systems and system components. The figure shows a typical CR test phantom; it is used to evaluate the accuracy of several system components/characteristics. (Photo contributor: FUJIFILM Healthcare Americas Corp.)

angle). Consequently, increased importance is placed on the ergonomic design of image viewing areas.

The grayscale and spatial resolution of the monitors must also be tested regularly by using one of the SMPTE (Society of Media Professionals, Technologists and Engineers) or AAPTM (American Association of Physicists in Medicine) TG18 test grid patterns. This ensures that the monitor can adequately depict the radiographic image free of monitor distortion or limited contrast and detail.

Liquid crystal display (LCD) monitors are being rapidly replaced by light-emitting display (LED) monitors. LEDs provide backlight for LCDs. In addition to improved lighting, the display device is more energy efficient, has a longer life, has a larger viewable area, and is thinner.

Summary

- The function of QC is to provide consistent, high-quality radiographs, thus reducing patient dose and increasing cost-effectiveness.
- QC programs involve evaluation and documentation of all imaging components from the x-ray tube to the display monitor.
- Kilovoltage accuracy can be determined by using a Wisconsin test cassette or digital meter and must be accurate to within 5 kV (±10%).

- Milliamperage accuracy is determined by using an aluminum step-wedge or digital dosimeter and must be accurate to within 10%.
- Timer accuracy is evaluated and must be accurate to within 5%. Reproducibility refers to tube output consistency and must not vary more than 5%.
- HVL is tested periodically to evaluate x-ray beam quality; HVL should remain almost constant.
- Focal spot size is tested by using a pinhole camera, slit camera, or star pattern–type resolution device on installation and every year thereafter.
- IPs and their PSPs should be visually checked and correctly cleaned on a regular basis.
- Dust and scratches on CR PSPs create artifacts on the processed images.
- Grid cassettes should be tested for damaged lead strips.
- Lead gloves and aprons must be fluoroscoped annually to detect any cracks; they should be properly hung when not in use.
- CR printer/processors should have a daily check performed.
- Reader air intakes should be checked weekly.

COMPREHENSION CHECK

1. Describe the value of a QC program (p. 493).

2. Identify the method used for kV calibration and the required degree of accuracy (p. 494).

3. Describe how mA linearity can be evaluated, and identify the required degree of accuracy (p. 494, 495).

4. Explain what is meant by reproducibility, and identify the degree of accuracy required (p. 496).

5. Define HVL, and list the three factors that influence it (p. 496).

6. Explain how tube aging can result in increased HVL (p. 496).

7. Identify when the focal spot size should be checked and the three devices that can be used to determine focal spot size (p. 496, 497).

8. Describe the important relationship between the focal spot, mirror, and collimator light bulb (p. 495).

9. Explain when/how to check the condition of a grid (p. 497).

10. Explain the necessity of QA checks on monitor luminance (p. 498).

11. Describe the proper care, storage, and checking of lead apparel (p. 498).

12. How often should checks be made on CR printer/processors? How often the air intakes be checked (p. 498)?

13. How should CR IPs and PSPs be checked and cleaned (p. 497)?

14. If a CR PSP has particles of dust on it, how will that appear on the digital image (p. 497)?

15. If a CR PSP is scratched, how will that appear on the digital image (p. 497)?

16. Explain exposure reciprocity, and identify the degree of accuracy required (p. 494).

17. Identify the two test patterns commonly used for QC on a monitor (p. 499).

CHAPTER REVIEW QUESTIONS

1. What devices are used to measure the focal spot size?
   1. Slit camera
   2. Pinhole camera
   3. Aluminum step-wedge
   (A) 1 only
   (B) 1 and 2 only
   (C) 2 and 3 only
   (D) 1, 2, and 3

2. HVL is affected by
   1. kV
   2. filtration
   3. focal spot
   (A) 1 only
   (B) 1 and 2 only
   (C) 2 and 3 only
   (D) 1, 2, and 3

3. The term that refers to the consistency of x-ray tube output over a series of exposures is
   (A) reproducibility
   (B) linearity
   (C) half-value layer
   (D) reconstruction

4. With what frequency should the protective apparel, such as aprons and gloves, be checked for defects?
   (A) Daily
   (B) Monthly
   (C) Bimonthly
   (D) Annually

5. The focal spot size should be evaluated on installation and then
   (A) annually
   (B) monthly
   (C) biweekly
   (D) semiannually

6. The x-ray system's ability to produce expected changes in output intensity when the mAs is either increased or decreased is
   (A) exposure reproducibility
   (B) exposure linearity
   (C) half-value layer
   (D) reconstruction

7. HVL can increase as a result of
   1. an increase in kV
   2. vaporized tungsten on the inner surface of the glass envelope
   3. a decrease in kV
   (A) 1 only
   (B) 1 and 2 only
   (C) 2 and 3 only
   (D) 1, 2, and 3

8. Equipment used to evaluate the accuracy of individual mA stations includes the
   1. aluminum step-wedge
   2. pinhole camera
   3. slit camera
   (A) 1 only
   (B) 1 and 2 only
   (C) 2 and 3 only
   (D) 1, 2, and 3

9. Advantages of LED display over LCD display include
   1. less power consumption
   2. improved lighting
   3. thinner design
   (A) 1 only
   (B) 1 and 2 only
   (C) 2 and 3 only
   (D) 1, 2, and 3

10. If the distance from the focal spot to the center of the collimator's mirror is 12 inches, what distance should the illuminator's light bulb be from the center of the mirror?
    (A) 3 inches
    (B) 6 inches
    (C) 9 inches
    (D) 12 inches

Answers and Explanations

1. (B) Focal spot size can be measured with a *pinhole camera, slit camera,* or *star pattern–type resolution device.* The *pinhole camera* is rather difficult to use accurately and requires the use of excessive tube (heat) loading. With a *slit camera,* two exposures are made: one measures the length of the focal spot and the other measures the width. The *star pattern–type,* or similar, resolution device can measure focal spot size as a function of geometric blur and is readily adaptable in a QC program to monitor focal spot changes over a period of time. It is recommended that focal spot size be checked on *installation* of a new x-ray tube and *annually* thereafter. An aluminum step-wedge can be used to demonstrate the effect of kV on contrast in analog imaging.

2. (B) HVL is defined as the thickness of any absorber that will reduce x-ray beam intensity (kerma) to one-half its original value. It is determined by measuring the beam intensity (kerma) without an absorber and then recording the intensity as successive millimeters of Al are added. It is influenced by the type of *rectification,* total *filtration,* and *kV.* X-ray tube HVL should remain almost constant. If HVL decreases, it is an indication of a decrease in the actual kV. If the HVL increases, it indicates the deposition of vaporized tungsten on the inner surface of the glass envelope (as a result of tube aging) or an increase in the actual kV.

3. (A) The term *reproducibility* refers to *consistency* of x-ray tube output. A particular group of technical factors is selected, and a series of consecutive exposures (at least five) is made. The factors are changed between exposures and then changed back to the original technical factors. The digital radiation meter should register radiation output that does not vary more than 5%. *Reproducibility testing* is performed when troubleshooting a problem and at least annually.

4. (D) Personnel fluoroscopic shielding apparel such as lead aprons, gloves, and thyroid shields should be *fluoroscoped annually* to detect any cracks that may have developed in the leaded vinyl.

Proper care is required to help prolong the useful life of lead apparel. If soiled, it can be cleaned with a damp cloth. Lead aprons should not be folded or carelessly dropped to the floor, for that facilitates the development of cracks in the leaded vinyl. Lead aprons and gloves should be hung on appropriate racks when not in use.

5. (A) Focal spot size accuracy is related to the degree of *geometric blur.* Manufacturer tolerance for new focal spots is quite large. In addition, the focal spot can increase in size as the x-ray tube ages, hence the importance of testing *newly arrived* focal spots and *annual* testing to monitor focal spots changes.

6. (B) Linearity of mA can be evaluated by using a digital dosimeter (ionization chamber). Linearity tests the system's ability to produce expected changes in output intensity when the mAs is either increased or decreased. When the mAs is increased, the exposure intensity should also increase. When the mAs is decreased, the exposure intensity should decrease. Linearity testing is performed after generator modification or calibration and at least annually, and the acceptable variance is within 10%.

7. (B) HVL testing provides beam quality information that is different from that obtained from kV testing. HVL is defined as the thickness of any absorber that will reduce x-ray beam intensity (kerma rate) to one-half its original value. It is determined by measuring the beam intensity/kerma without an absorber and then recording the intensity as successive millimeters of Al are added. It is influenced by the type of rectification, total filtration, and kV. The x-ray tube HVL should remain almost constant. If HVL decreases, it is an indication of a decrease in the actual kV. If the HVL increases, it indicates the deposition of vaporized tungsten on the inner surface of the glass envelope (as a result of tube aging) or an increase in the actual kV.

8. (A) Focal spot size can be measured with a *pinhole camera, slit camera,* or *star pattern–type resolution device.* The aluminum step-wedge, or penetrometer, can be used to evaluate each mA station. The accuracy of each mA station is related to patient dose and is important for production of expected receptor exposure levels.

9. (D) LCD monitors are being rapidly replaced by LED monitors. LEDs provide backlight for LCDs. In addition to improved lighting, the display device is more energy efficient, has a longer life, has a larger viewable area, and is thinner.

10. (D) The collimator assembly includes a series of lead shutters, a mirror, and a light bulb. The mirror and the light bulb function to project the size, location, and center of the irradiated field. The bulb's emitted beam of light is deflected by a mirror placed at an angle of 45° in the path of the light beam. *For the projected light beam to be the same size as the x-ray beam, the focal spot and the light bulb must be exactly at the same distance from the center of the mirror.*

PART V

Practice Test

Practice Test

This practice test is intended to simulate the actual certification examination. Set aside special time for this test after your preparations for the actual examination are complete. Try to *simulate the actual examination environment* as much as possible. Choose a quiet place free from distractions and interruptions, gather the necessary materials, and arrange to be uninterrupted for *up to 3 h*.

Each of the numbered items or incomplete statements in this section is followed by answers or completions of the statement. Select the lettered answer or completion that is *best* in each case.

1. The percentage of incoming x-ray photons that are detected and absorbed by the receptor describes
   (A) DEL
   (B) FOV
   (C) DQE
   (D) TFT

2. Which of the following is/are used to account for relative radiosensitivity of various tissues and organs?
   1. Radiation weighting factors (W_r)
   2. Tissue weighting factors (W_t)
   3. Absorbed dose
   (A) 1 only
   (B) 2 only
   (C) 2 and 3 only
   (D) 1, 2, and 3

3. Which of the following statements regarding Figure 14-1A is/are true?
   1. The first and second metatarsal bases are superimposed on the medial and intermediate cuneiforms
   2. Articulations around the sinus tarsi and cuboid are well demonstrated
   3. The plantar surface and the IR form a 30° angle
   (A) 1 only
   (B) 2 only
   (C) 2 and 3 only
   (D) 1, 2, and 3

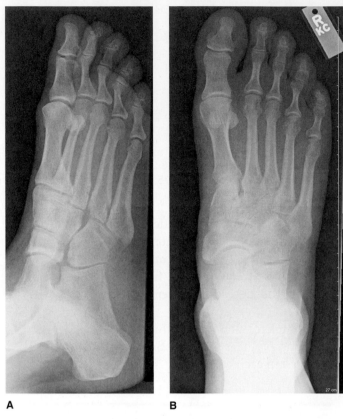

A　　　　　　　　**B**

Figure 14-1. **(A)** and **(B)**. (Photo contributor: Conrad P Ehrlich, MD.)

4. Photostimulable luminescence (PSL) occurs when the photostimulable phosphor (PSP) is exposed to

 (A) monochromatic laser light

 (B) barium fluorohalide

 (C) high-energy x-ray photons

 (D) low-energy x-ray photons

5. What is the relationship between source-to-image-receptor distance (SID), x-ray beam intensity, and receptor exposure?

 (A) As SID increases, beam intensity increases and receptor exposure increases

 (B) As SID increases, beam intensity increases and receptor exposure decreases

 (C) As SID increases, beam intensity decreases and receptor exposure increases

 (D) As SID increases, beam intensity decreases and patient dose decreases

6. A patient experiencing syncope should be placed in which of the following positions?

 (A) Dorsal recumbent with head elevated

 (B) Dorsal recumbent with feet elevated

 (C) Lateral recumbent

 (D) Seated with feet supported

7. Symptoms of imminent anaphylactic shock include

 1. dysphasia

 2. urticaria

 3. constriction of the throat

 (A) 1 only

 (B) 2 only

 (C) 2 and 3 only

 (D) 1, 2, and 3

8. Which of the following is/are well demonstrated in the oblique position/projection of the lumbar spine?

1. Zygapophyseal joints

2. Intervertebral foramina

3. Intervertebral joints

(A) 1 only

(B) 1 and 2 only

(C) 2 and 3 only

(D) 1, 2, and 3

9. Which of the following digital postprocessing actions removes high-frequency noise from the digital image?

(A) Windowing

(B) Smoothing

(C) Aliasing

(D) Edge enhancement

10. Which of the following ethical principles is most closely related to *avoidance of deception*?

(A) Autonomy

(B) Beneficence

(C) Fidelity

(D) Veracity

11. *Somatic effects* of radiation refer to effects that are manifested

(A) in the descendants of the exposed individual

(B) during the life of the exposed individual

(C) in the exposed individual and his or her descendants

(D) in the reproductive cells of the exposed individual

12. The left colic flexure is formed by the junction of the

(A) transverse and ascending colon

(B) descending and transverse colon

(C) descending and sigmoid colon

(D) cecum and ascending colon

13. The term *interrogation time* refers to

(A) the shortest possible exposure time permitted by a particular x-ray tube

(B) the amount of time required for x-ray tube AM warming

(C) the time required for the x-ray tube to turn off

(D) the time it takes the x-ray tube to reach the required technical factors

14. An increase in added filtration will result in

1. an increase in maximum energy of the x-ray beam

2. a decrease in x-ray intensity

3. an increase in effective energy of the x-ray beam

(A) 1 only

(B) 1 and 2 only

(C) 2 and 3 only

(D) 1, 2, and 3

15. What does the letter I represent in Figure 14-2?

(A) Lunate

(B) Pisiform

(C) Trapezoid

(D) Hamate

16. Symptoms of shock include

1. pallor and weakness

2. increased pulse rate

3. fever

(A) 1 only

(B) 1 and 2 only

(C) 1 and 3 only

(D) 1, 2, and 3

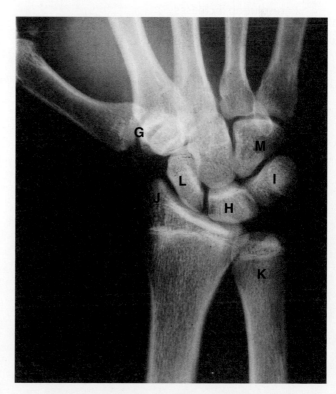

Figure 14-2. (Photo contributor: Bob Wong, RT.)

17. The term *health care–associated infection* (HAI) often replaces which of the following terms?

    (A) Upper respiratory infection

    (B) Urinary tract infection (UTI)

    (C) Suppressed infection

    (D) Nosocomial infection

18. The term *effective dose* refers to

    (A) whole-body dose

    (B) localized organ dose

    (C) absorbed dose

    (D) radiation weighting factor

19. With the body in the erect position, the diaphragm moves

    (A) 2–4 inches higher than when in the recumbent position

    (B) 2–4 inches lower than when in the recumbent position

    (C) 2–4 inches superiorly

    (D) very slightly

20. With all other factors constant, as a digital image's matrix size increases

    1. pixel size decreases

    2. resolution increases

    3. pixel size increases

    (A) 1 only

    (B) 2 only

    (C) 1 and 2 only

    (D) 2 and 3 only

21. The AP recumbent projection of an average sthenic stomach during a GI examination will usually demonstrate

    1. barium-filled fundus

    2. double contrast of distal stomach portions

    3. barium-filled duodenum and pylorus

    (A) 1 only

    (B) 1 and 2 only

    (C) 1 and 3 only

    (D) 1, 2, and 3

22. The American Hospital Association's (AHA's) Patient Care Partnership reviews what patients can/should expect during a hospital stay, including

    1. protection of patient privacy

    2. help with billing claims

    3. help when leaving the hospital

    (A) 1 only

    (B) 1 and 2 only

    (C) 2 and 3 only

    (D) 1, 2, and 3

23. Figure 14-3 is representative of which of the following?

    (A) Bremsstrahlung radiation

    (B) Characteristic radiation

    (C) Photoelectric Effect

    (D) Compton Scatter

24. Advantages of moving the image intensifier closer to the patient during traditional fluoroscopy include

    1. increased object-to-image-receptor distance (OID)

    2. decreased patient dose

    3. improved image quality

    (A) 1 only

    (B) 1 and 2 only

    (C) 2 and 3 only

    (D) 1, 2, and 3

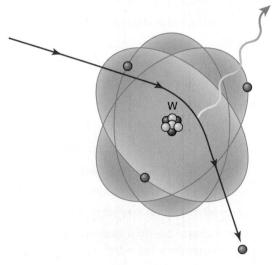

Figure 14-3.

25. Manual exposure control was used and the exposure factors selected for a particular nongrid x-ray image were 400 mA, 20 ms, and 90 kV. Another image using a 6:1 grid is requested. Which of the following groups of factors is *most* appropriate?

    (A) 400 mA, 20 ms, 110 kV

    (B) 200 mA, 80 ms, 100 kV

    (C) 300 mA, 80 ms, 90 kV

    (D) 400 mA, 90 ms, 90 kV

26. Which of the subparts of Figure 14-4 most likely demonstrates the wave form produced by single-phase rectified equipment?

    (A) Figure A

    (B) Figure B

    (C) Figure C

    (D) Figure D

27. Which of the following factor(s) is/are important in determining thickness of protective barriers?

    1. Distance between the x-ray source and the barrier

    2. Occupancy factor time

    3. Workload (mA-min/week)

    (A) 1 only

    (B) 1 and 2 only

    (C) 2 and 3 only

    (D) 1, 2, and 3

28. An autoclave is used for

    (A) dry heat sterilization

    (B) chemical sterilization

    (C) gas sterilization

    (D) steam sterilization

29. Which aspect of the forearm should be closest to the IR when examining the fourth and fifth fingers in the lateral position?

    (A) Anterior

    (B) Posterior

    (C) Medial

    (D) Lateral

30. Which of the following imaging procedures does *not* require use of ionizing radiation to produce an image?

    1. Diagnostic sonography

    2. Computed tomography (CT)

    3. Magnetic resonance imaging

    (A) 1 and 2 only

    (B) 1 and 3 only

    (C) 2 and 3 only

    (D) 1, 2, and 3

31. Which of the following digital artifacts can result if the direction of the grid's lead strips and the grid frequency match the scan frequency of the scanner/reader?

    (A) Phantom image

    (B) Skipped scan lines

    (C) Aliasing

    (D) Grid lines

32. Examples of primary radiation barriers include

    1. x-ray room walls

    2. control booth

    3. lead aprons

    (A) 1 only

    (B) 1 and 2 only

    (C) 2 and 3 only

    (D) 1, 2, and 3

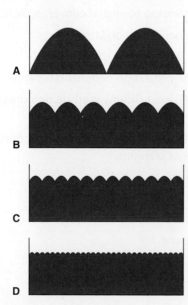

Figure 14-4.

33. Which formula would the radiographer use to determine the total number of heat units produced with a given exposure using three-phase, 12-pulse equipment?

    (A) mA × time × kV
    (B) mA × time kV × 3.0
    (C) mA × time kV × 1.4
    (D) mA × time kV × 1.8

34. Diseases whose mode of transmission is air include

    1. tuberculosis
    2. mumps
    3. rubella

    (A) 1 only
    (B) 1 and 2 only
    (C) 1 and 3 only
    (D) 1, 2, and 3

35. Which of the following image matrix sizes will provide the best spatial resolution?

    (A) 256 × 256
    (B) 512 × 512
    (C) 1024 × 1024
    (D) 2048 × 2048

36. The image seen in Figure 14-5 was made in which of the following positions?

    (A) AP erect
    (B) PA recumbent
    (C) Right lateral decubitus
    (D) Dorsal decubitus

37. Advantages of light-emitting display (LED) over liquid crystal display (LCD) include

    1. less power consumption
    2. improved lighting
    3. thinner design

    (A) 1 only
    (B) 1 and 2 only
    (C) 2 and 3 only
    (D) 1, 2, and 3

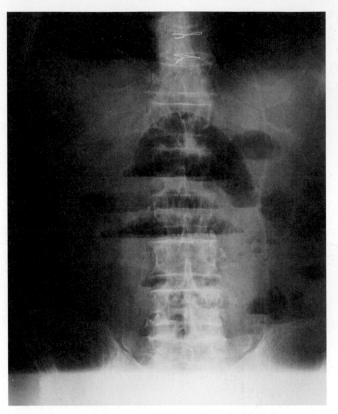

Figure 14-5. (Photo contributor: Stamford Hospital, Department of Radiology.)

38. What transforms the violet light emitted by the PSP into the image seen on the monitor?

    (A) The photostimulable phosphor
    (B) The scanner/reader
    (C) The analog-to-digital converter (ADC)
    (D) The helium–neon laser

39. In trauma imaging of the skull

    1. the AP projection demonstrates anterior cranium
    2. the AP axial /Towne method demonstrates posterior cranium
    3. the AP axial/reverse Caldwell demonstrates anterior cranium

    (A) 1 only
    (B) 1 and 2 only
    (C) 2 and 3 only
    (D) 1, 2, and 3

40. A profile view of the glenoid fossa can be obtained with the CR directed perpendicular to the glenoid fossa and the patient rotated

    (A) 20°, affected side down
    (B) 20°, affected side up
    (C) 45°, affected side down
    (D) 45°, affected side up

41. Characteristics of nonstochastic/early tissue effects of radiation include that

    1. they have predictability
    2. they have a threshold
    3. severity is directly related to dose

    (A) 1 only
    (B) 1 and 2 only
    (C) 2 and 3 only
    (D) 1, 2, and 3

42. Chemical substances that are used to kill pathogenic bacteria are called

    1. antiseptics
    2. germicides
    3. disinfectants

    (A) 1 only
    (B) 1 and 2 only
    (C) 2 and 3 only
    (D) 1, 2, and 3

43. Potential educational Honor Code violations include

    1. falsification of clinical competency documents
    2. cheating and/or plagiarism
    3. violating patient confidentiality

    (A) 1 only
    (B) 1 and 2 only
    (C) 2 and 3 only
    (D) 1, 2, and 3

44. In which of the following locations can the pulse be detected only with the use of a stethoscope?

    (A) Wrist
    (B) Apex of the heart
    (C) Groin
    (D) Neck

45. Patient dose during fluoroscopic examinations varies with

    1. magnification
    2. patient size
    3. length of examination

    (A) 1 only
    (B) 1 and 2 only
    (C) 2 and 3 only
    (D) 1, 2, and 3

46. The image seen in Figure 14-6B was obtained in which of the following positions?

    (A) AP erect
    (B) AP recumbent
    (C) PA erect
    (D) PA recumbent

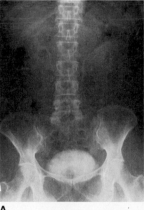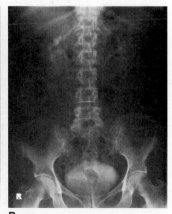

A   B

Figure 14-6. **(A)** and **(B)**. (Photo contributor: Stamford Hospital, Department of Radiology.)

47. What portion of a computed radiography system records the radiologic image?

    (A) The photostimulable phosphor

    (B) The scanner/reader

    (C) The emulsion

    (D) The image plate (IP)

48. Which of the following bones participate(s) in the formation of the knee?

    1. Femur

    2. Tibia

    3. Patella

    (A) 1 and 2 only

    (B) 1 and 3 only

    (C) 2 and 3 only

    (D) 1, 2, and 3

49. Adult tissues that are relatively insensitive to radiation exposure include

    1. muscle tissue

    2. nerve tissue

    3. epithelial tissue

    (A) 1 only

    (B) 1 and 2 only

    (C) 2 and 3 only

    (D) 1, 2, and 3

50. To better demonstrate ribs below the diaphragm

    1. suspend respiration at the end of full exhalation

    2. suspend respiration at the end of deep inhalation

    3. perform the examination in the recumbent position

    (A) 1 only

    (B) 2 only

    (C) 1 and 3 only

    (D) 2 and 3 only

51. The term used to describe a wall toward which the x-ray beam may be directed is

    (A) secondary barrier

    (B) primary barrier

    (C) leakage barrier

    (D) scattered barrier

52. When reviewing patients' blood chemistry levels, what is considered the normal creatinine range?

    (A) 0.6–1.5 mg/100 mL

    (B) 4.5–6.0 mg/100 mL

    (C) 8–25 mg/100 mL

    (D) Up to 50 mg/100 mL

53. The phenomenon that can occur between the time a PSP is exposed to x-rays and the time it is read by the scanner/reader is termed

    (A) excitation

    (B) photostimulable luminescence

    (C) scatter

    (D) fading

54. Arrange the following tissues in the order of decreasing radiosensitivity.

    1. Liver cells

    2. Intestinal crypt cells

    3. Muscle cells

    (A) 1, 3, 2

    (B) 2, 3, 1

    (C) 2, 1, 3

    (D) 3, 1, 2

55. The histogram demonstration of pixel value distribution can be changed/affected by which of the following?

    1. Selection of processing algorithm

    2. Processing delay

    3. Centering

    (A) 1 only

    (B) 1 and 2 only

    (C) 2 and 3 only

    (D) 1, 2, and 3

56. Glenohumeral joint dislocation can be evaluated with which of the following?
    1. Inferosuperior axial
    2. Transthoracic lateral
    3. Scapular Y projection
    (A) 1 only
    (B) 1 and 2 only
    (C) 2 and 3 only
    (D) 1, 2, and 3

57. A patient is usually required to drink barium sulfate suspension to demonstrate which of the following structure(s)?
    1. Pylorus
    2. Sigmoid
    3. Duodenum
    (A) 1 and 2 only
    (B) 1 and 3 only
    (C) 2 and 3 only
    (D) 3 only

58. By which of the following dose–response curves are late or long-term effects of radiation exposure generally represented?
    (A) Linear threshold
    (B) Linear nonthreshold
    (C) Nonlinear threshold
    (D) Nonlinear nonthreshold

59. Which of the following pathologic conditions will most likely offer greatest resistance to the passage of x-ray photons?
    (A) Fibrosarcoma
    (B) Osteomalacia
    (C) Paralytic ileus
    (D) Ascites

60. The image intensifier's input phosphor is generally composed of
    (A) cesium iodide
    (B) zinc cadmium sulfide
    (C) gadolinium oxysulfide
    (D) calcium tungstate

61. The position seen in Figure 14-7, used to demonstrate the intercondyloid fossa, requires that the CR be directed
    (A) vertically to the joint space
    (B) parallel to the long axis of the femur
    (C) perpendicular to the long axis of the tibia
    (D) parallel to the long axis of the tibia

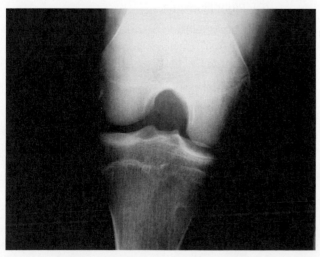

A

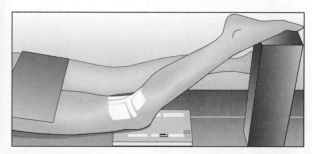

B

Figure 14-7. **(A)** and **(B)**.

62. Factors impacting spatial resolution in indirect digital imaging include
    1. pixel pitch
    2. sampling frequency
    3. DEL size of the TFT
    (A) 1 only
    (B) 1 and 2 only
    (C) 2 and 3 only
    (D) 1, 2, and 3

63. Double-contrast examinations of the stomach or large bowel are performed for better visualization of
    (A) position of the organ
    (B) size and shape of the organ
    (C) diverticula
    (D) gastric or bowel mucosa

64. If the exposure rate at 3 feet from the fluoroscopic table is 15 mGy$_a$/min, what will be the exposure rate for 4 min at a distance of 5 feet from the table?
    (A) 2.7 mGy$_a$
    (B) 5.4 mGy$_a$
    (C) 10.8 mGy$_a$
    (D) 16.2 mGy$_a$

65. The medical suffix *plasia* refers to
    (A) embryonic
    (B) condition
    (C) movement
    (D) development

66. What projection of the calcaneus is obtained with the leg extended, plantar surface vertical and perpendicular to the IR, and CR directed 40° caudad?
    (A) Axial plantodorsal projection
    (B) Axial dorsoplantar projection
    (C) Lateral projection
    (D) Weight-bearing lateral

67. Structures found within the mediastinum include all of the following, *except* the
    (A) esophagus
    (B) thymus
    (C) heart
    (D) terminal bronchiole

68. A student radiographer who is younger than 18 years must not receive an annual occupational dose greater than
    (A) 1 mSv (0.1 rem)
    (B) 5 mSv (0.5 rem)
    (C) 50 mSv (5 rem)
    (D) 100 mSv (10 rem)

69. Proper body ergonomics includes a wide base of support. The base of support is the portion of the body
    (A) in contact with the floor or other horizontal surface
    (B) in the midportion of the pelvis or lower abdomen
    (C) passing through the center of gravity
    (D) none of the above

70. Which of the following is demonstrated in a 25° LPO position with the CR entering 1 inch medial to the elevated anterior superior iliac spine?
    (A) Left sacroiliac joint
    (B) Right sacroiliac joint
    (C) Left ilium
    (D) Right ilium

71. Accurate operation of the automatic exposure control (AEC) device is dependent on
    1. thickness and density of the object
    2. positioning of the object with respect to the ionization chamber
    3. beam restriction
    (A) 1 only
    (B) 1 and 2 only
    (C) 2 and 3 only
    (D) 1, 2, and 3

72. Major effect(s) of deoxyribonucleic acid (DNA) irradiation includes
    1. malignant disease
    2. chromosome aberration
    3. cell death
    (A) 1 only
    (B) 1 and 2 only
    (C) 2 and 3 only
    (D) 1, 2, and 3

73. The voltage ripple associated with a three-phase, 12-pulse rectified generator is approximately
    (A) 100%
    (B) 32%
    (C) 13%
    (D) 3%

74. Which of the following is a condition in which an occluded blood vessel stops blood flow to a portion of the lungs?
    (A) Pneumothorax
    (B) Atelectasis
    (C) Pulmonary embolism
    (D) Hypoxia

75. The PSP is exposed to a narrow laser beam
    (A) on the display monitor
    (B) in the scanner/reader
    (C) in the cassette
    (D) on the x-ray table

76. What is the best way to reduce magnification distortion?
    (A) Use a small focal spot
    (B) Increase the SID
    (C) Decrease the OID
    (D) Use a shorter exposure time

77. The enteral route of drug administration includes
    1. intravenous
    2. oral
    3. nasogastric (NG) tube
    (A) 1 only
    (B) 1 and 2 only
    (C) 2 and 3 only
    (D) 1, 2, and 3

78. The energy of x-ray photons has an inverse relationship with
    1. photon wavelength
    2. applied mA
    3. applied kV
    (A) 1 only
    (B) 1 and 2 only
    (C) 1 and 3 only
    (D) 1, 2, and 3

79. Cervical spine positions performed to demonstrate the intervertebral foramina closest to the IR are
    (A) RAO and LAO
    (B) RPO and LPO
    (C) AP
    (D) lateral

80. A patient was positioned for a radiographic projection with the x-ray tube, grid, and IR properly aligned but with the body part angled. Which of the following will result?
    (A) Grid cutoff at the periphery of the image
    (B) Grid cutoff along the center of the image
    (C) Increased receptor exposure at the periphery
    (D) Image distortion

81. The product of absorbed dose (D) and radiation a weighting factor (W_r) is
    (A) EqD
    (B) EfD
    (C) TEDE
    (D) W_t

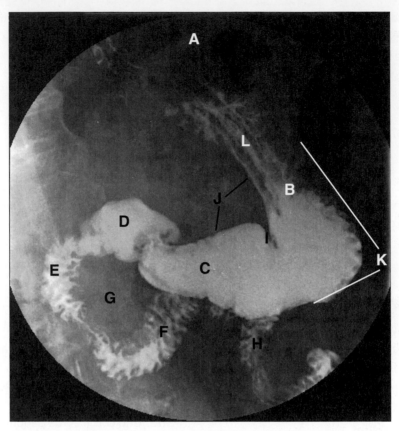

Figure 14-8. (Photo contributor: Stamford Hospital, Department of Radiology.)

82. What does the letter D represent in Figure 14-8?

    (A) Mucosal folds

    (B) Fundus

    (C) Duodenum

    (D) Jejunum

83. What does the letter F represent in Figure 14-8?

    (A) Jejunum

    (B) Ascending duodenum

    (C) Descending duodenum

    (D) Bulb of duodenum

84. What structure occupies the area represented by the letter G in Figure 14-8?

    (A) Gallbladder

    (B) Right lobe of the liver

    (C) Head of the pancreas

    (D) Hepatic flexure of the colon

85. In what position was the radiograph seen in Figure 14-8 made?

    (A) AP

    (B) LPO

    (C) RAO

    (D) Lateral

86. The purposes of an advanced health care directive, or living will, include all of the following, *except*

    (A) preserving a person's right to make decisions regarding his or her own health care

    (B) naming the individual authorized to make health care decisions for him or her

    (C) ensuring that only the patient's personal physician can make health care decisions for him or her

    (D) including specifics regarding do not resuscitate (DNR), do not intubate (DNI), and other end-of-life decisions

87. As a result of the anode heel effect, x-ray beam intensity is greatest along the
    (A) path of the central ray (CR)
    (B) anode end of the beam
    (C) cathode end of the beam
    (D) transverse axis of the IR

88. The function of *shuttering* is to
    (A) remove bright, unexposed areas outside the collimated field
    (B) prevent overexposure
    (C) prevent underexposure
    (D) substitute for, or supplement, collimation

89. Which of the following medical equipment is used to determine blood pressure?
    1. Pulse oximeter
    2. Stethoscope
    3. Sphygmomanometer
    (A) 1 and 2 only
    (B) 1 and 3 only
    (C) 2 and 3 only
    (D) 1, 2, and 3

90. Which of the following statements regarding human gonadal cells is/are accurate?
    1. The female oogonia reproduce only during fetal life
    2. The male spermatogonia reproduce continuously
    3. Both male and female stem cells reproduce only during fetal life
    (A) 1 only
    (B) 2 only
    (C) 1 and 2 only
    (D) 3 only

91. Circuit devices that permit electrons to flow in only one direction are
    (A) solid-state diodes
    (B) resistors
    (C) transformers
    (D) autotransformers

92. Exposure rate increases with an increase in
    1. mA
    2. kV
    3. SID
    (A) 1 only
    (B) 1 and 2 only
    (C) 2 and 3 only
    (D) 1, 2, and 3

93. Characteristics of anemia include
    1. decreased number of circulating red blood cells
    2. decreased hemoglobin
    3. hematuria
    (A) 1 only
    (B) 1 and 2 only
    (C) 1 and 3 only
    (D) 1, 2, and 3

94. Grid interspace material can be made of
    1. carbon fiber
    2. aluminum
    3. plastic fiber
    (A) 1 only
    (B) 1 and 2 only
    (C) 2 and 3 only
    (D) 1, 2, and 3

95. Which of these radiation exposure situations is likely to be the most harmful?
    (A) A large dose to a specific area all at once
    (B) A small dose to the whole body over a period of time
    (C) A large dose to the whole body all at one time
    (D) A small dose to a specific area over a period of time

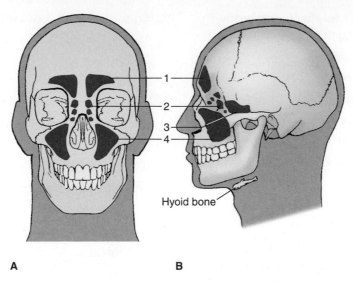

Hyoid bone

A   B

Figure 14-9. **(A)** and **(B)**.

96. What structure is indicated by the *number 3* in Figure 14-9?

(A) Maxillary sinuses

(B) Mastoid sinuses

(C) Sphenoid sinuses

(D) Ethmoid sinuses

97. Which of the following positions would best demonstrate the proximal tibiofibular articulation?

(A) AP

(B) 90° Mediolateral

(C) 45° Internal rotation

(D) 45° External rotation

98. Chemical substances that inhibit the growth of pathogenic microorganisms without necessarily killing them are called

1. antiseptics

2. germicides

3. disinfectants

(A) 1 only

(B) 1 and 2 only

(C) 2 and 3 only

(D) 1, 2, and 3

99. Which of the following is a vasopressor and may be used for an anaphylactic reaction or cardiac arrest?

(A) Nitroglycerin

(B) Epinephrine

(C) Hydrocortisone

(D) Digitoxin

100. Excessive absorption of useful x-ray photons by a grid is called

(A) grid selectivity

(B) contrast improvement factor

(C) grid cutoff

(D) latitude

101. Examples of destructive pathologic conditions include

1. emphysema

2. pneumoperitoneum

3. osteoporosis

(A) 1 only

(B) 2 only

(C) 2 and 3 only

(D) 1, 2, and 3

102. In which aspect of the orbital wall a "blowout fracture" usually occurs?

(A) Superior

(B) Inferior

(C) Medial

(D) Lateral

103. Required components of a digital fluoroscopy (DF) system include
    1. computer
    2. video monitor
    3. image manipulation console
    (A) 1 only
    (B) 1 and 2 only
    (C) 2 and 3 only
    (D) 1, 2, and 3

104. Which activator is required for barium fluorohalide to retain its luminous properties?
    (A) Cesium
    (B) Iodine
    (C) Europium
    (D) Gadolinium

105. Under which of the following conditions is biologic material most sensitive to radiation exposure?
    (A) Anoxic
    (B) Hypoxic
    (C) Oxygenated
    (D) Deoxygenated

106. Radiographic *subject unsharpness* is a result of
    1. object plane is not parallel with the CR
    2. object plane is not parallel with the IR
    3. anatomic details of interest are not in the path of the CR
    (A) 1 only
    (B) 1 and 2 only
    (C) 2 and 3 only
    (D) 1, 2, and 3

107. Order the following cell types in terms of radiosensitivity, from greatest to least.
    1. Osteoblasts
    2. Spermatogonia
    3. Myocytes
    (A) 1, 2, 3
    (B) 1, 3, 2
    (C) 2, 1, 3
    (D) 3, 1, 2

108. Special beam-shaping optics are used in the CR reader to keep the infrared laser scanning light finely focused to
    1. collect analog data
    2. improve signal-to-noise ratio (SNR)
    3. maintain good spatial resolution
    (A) 1 only
    (B) 1 and 2 only
    (C) 2 and 3 only
    (D) 1, 2, and 3

109. Which of the following is a fast-acting vasodilator used to lower blood pressure and relieve the pain of angina pectoris?
    (A) Digitalis
    (B) Dilantin
    (C) Nitroglycerin
    (D) Cimetidine (Tagamet)

110. Typical characteristics of the android pelvis, in comparison with the gynecoid pelvis, include
    1. smaller pubic arch/angle
    2. more narrow, vertical
    3. pelvic inlet larger and more round
    (A) 1 only
    (B) 1 and 2 only
    (C) 2 and 3 only
    (D) 1, 2, and 3

111. A radiographic image exhibiting few shades of gray between black and white is said to possess
    (A) no contrast
    (B) high contrast
    (C) low contrast
    (D) little contrast

112. A small bottle containing a single dose of medication is termed
    (A) an ampule
    (B) a vial
    (C) a bolus
    (D) a carafe

113. An increase in kV will have which of the following effects?

1. More scattered radiation will be produced

2. The exposure rate will increase

3. Radiographic contrast will increase

    (A) 1 only

    (B) 1 and 2 only

    (C) 2 and 3 only

    (D) 1, 2, and 3

114. Which of the following is the most proximal structure on the adult ulna?

    (A) Capitulum

    (B) Styloid process

    (C) Coronoid process

    (D) Olecranon process

115. In Figure 14-10, the letter E represents the

    (A) trochlea

    (B) capitulum

    (C) lateral epicondyle

    (D) medial epicondyle

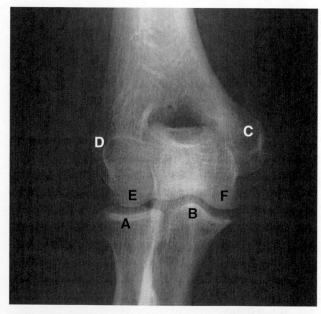

Figure 14-10. (Photo contributor: Stamford Hospital, Department of Radiology.)

116. In Figure 14-10, the letter D represents the

    (A) trochlea

    (B) capitulum

    (C) lateral epicondyle

    (D) medial epicondyle

117. What is the intensity of scattered radiation perpendicular to and 1 m from the patient compared with the useful beam at the patient's surface?

    (A) 0.01%

    (B) 0.1%

    (C) 1.0%

    (D) 10.0%

118. In which of the following projections or positions will subacromial or subcoracoid dislocation be best demonstrated?

    (A) Tangential

    (B) AP axial

    (C) Transthoracic lateral

    (D) PA oblique scapular Y

119. A 3-inch object to be radiographed at 36-inch SID lies 4 inches from the IR. What will be the image width?

    (A) 2.6 inches

    (B) 3.3 inches

    (C) 26.0 inches

    (D) 33.0 inches

120. The sternoclavicular joints are best demonstrated with the patient PA and

    (A) in a slight oblique, affected side adjacent to the IR

    (B) in a slight oblique, affected side away from the IR

    (C) erect, weight bearing

    (D) erect, with and without weights

121. Which of the following criteria is/are required for accurate visualization of the greater tubercle in profile?

1. Epicondyles parallel to the IR

2. Arm in external rotation

3. Humerus in the AP position

    (A) 1 only

    (B) 1 and 3 only

    (C) 2 and 3 only

    (D) 1, 2, and 3

122. All of the following positions are likely to be used for both single- and double-contrast examinations of the large bowel, *except*

(A) lateral rectum

(B) AP axial rectosigmoid

(C) right and left lateral decubitus abdomen

(D) RAO and LAO abdomen

123. In which of the following conditions is protective or "reverse" isolation required?

1. Tuberculosis

2. Burns

3. Leukemia

(A) 1 only

(B) 1 and 2 only

(C) 2 and 3 only

(D) 1, 2, and 3

124. Which of the following devices functions to produce "hard copies" of digital images?

(A) Digitizer

(B) Laser printer

(C) Histogram

(D) CRT

125. Image resolution improves as

1. scintillation increases

2. DEL size decreases

3. fill factor increases

(A) 1 only

(B) 1 and 2 only

(C) 2 and 3 only

(D) 1, 2, and 3

126. The *best* way to control voluntary motion is

(A) immobilization of the part

(B) careful explanation of the procedure

(C) short exposure time

(D) physical restraint

127. The manubrial notch, a bony landmark used in radiography of the sternoclavicular joints, is located at the same level as the

(A) vertebra prominens

(B) first thoracic vertebra

(C) third thoracic vertebra

(D) ninth thoracic vertebra

128. Which of the following functions to protect the x-ray tube and the patient from overexposure in the event the AEC device fails to terminate an exposure?

(A) Circuit breaker

(B) Backup timer

(C) Rheostat

(D) Fuse

129. Potential digital image postprocessing tasks include

1. PACS/MIMPS

2. annotation

3. inversion/reversal

(A) 1 only

(B) 1 and 2 only

(C) 2 and 3 only

(D) 1, 2, and 3

130. In order to be considered as legitimate legal evidence, each x-ray image must contain certain essential and specific patient information, including

1. date of examination

2. side marker

3. referring physician

(A) 1 only

(B) 1 and 2 only

(C) 2 and 3 only

(D) 1, 2, and 3

131. In the lateral projection of the foot, the

1. plantar surface should be perpendicular to the IR

2. metatarsals should be superimposed

3. talofibular joint should be visualized

(A) 1 only

(B) 1 and 2 only

(C) 2 and 3 only

(D) 1, 2, and 3

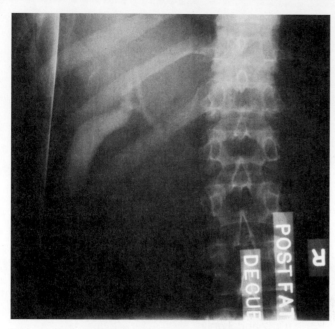

Figure 14-11. (Photo contributor: Stamford Hospital, Department of Radiology.)

132. The image artifact seen in Figure 14-11 is representative of
    (A) a processor artifact
    (B) an exposure artifact
    (C) a handling artifact
    (D) mechanical artifact

133. The technical factor that is used to regulate x-ray beam intensity is
    1. milliamperage
    2. exposure time
    3. kilovoltage
    (A) 1 only
    (B) 2 only
    (C) 1 and 2 only
    (D) 1, 2, and 3

134. Types of cell repair mechanisms following irradiation include
    1. DNA repair
    2. cell cycle arrest
    3. apoptosis
    (A) 1 only
    (B) 1 and 2 only
    (C) 2 and 3 only
    (D) 1, 2, and 3

135. The mechanical device used to correct an ineffectual cardiac rhythm is a
    (A) defibrillator
    (B) cardiac monitor
    (C) crash cart
    (D) resuscitation bag

136. The term that refers to parts closer to the source or beginning is
    (A) cephalad
    (B) caudad
    (C) proximal
    (D) medial

137. The blue-green PSL that corresponds to the visible x-ray image occurs
    1. immediately upon the initial prompt emission of light
    2. sometime after the initial prompt emission of light
    3. upon stimulation by finely focused infrared light
    (A) 1 only
    (B) 1 and 2 only
    (C) 2 and 3 only
    (D) 1, 2, and 3

138. An abnormal passage between organs is a/an
    (A) fistula
    (B) polyp
    (C) diverticulum
    (D) abscess

139. During GI radiography, the position of the stomach often varies depending on
    1. respiratory phase
    2. body habitus
    3. patient position
    (A) 1 and 2 only
    (B) 1 and 3 only
    (C) 2 and 3 only
    (D) 1, 2, and 3

140. The type of shock associated with pooling of blood in the peripheral vessels is classified as
    (A) neurogenic
    (B) cardiogenic
    (C) hypovolemic
    (D) septic

141. The AP axial projection (Towne method) of the skull *best* demonstrates the
    (A) occipital bone
    (B) frontal bone
    (C) facial bones
    (D) sphenoid bone

142. The uppermost portion of the iliac crest is approximately at the same level as that of the
    (A) costal margin
    (B) umbilicus
    (C) xiphoid tip
    (D) fourth lumbar vertebra

143. Devices that serve to collect PSL and transmit it to an ADC include
    1. photomultiplier tube
    2. photodiode
    3. charge-coupled device (CCD)
    (A) 1 only
    (B) 1 and 2 only
    (C) 2 and 3 only
    (D) 1, 2, and 3

144. An algorithm, as used in x-ray imaging, is a
    (A) geometric formula
    (B) series of specific exposure factors
    (C) series of variable instructions
    (D) series of predetermined exposure factors

145. The type(s) of radiation produced at the tungsten target is/are
    1. photoelectric
    2. characteristic
    3. bremsstrahlung
    (A) 1 only
    (B) 1 and 2 only
    (C) 2 and 3 only
    (D) 1, 2, and 3

146. Which of the following statements is/are true regarding swallowing dysfunction, or modified barium swallow, studies?
    1. Fluoroscopic images are made in the AP position
    2. The speech therapist prepares the contrast media
    3. Contrast filled images of the mouth, pharynx, and cervical esophagus are recorded
    (A) 1 only
    (B) 1 and 2 only
    (C) 2 and 3 only
    (D) 1 and 3 only

147. Characteristics of the typical diagnostic x-ray tube and its construction include that
    1. the target material should have a high atomic number and melting point
    2. the useful beam emerges from the port window
    3. the cathode assembly receives both low and high voltages
    (A) 1 only
    (B) 2 only
    (C) 1 and 2 only
    (D) 1, 2, and 3

148. During respiratory motion, the act of
    1. expiration raises the diaphragm
    2. inspiration elevates the ribs
    3. inspiration depresses the abdominal viscera
    (A) 1 only
    (B) 1 and 2 only
    (C) 2 and 3 only
    (D) 1, 2, and 3

149. The stomach of an asthenic patient is *most* likely to be located
    (A) high, transverse, and lateral
    (B) low, transverse, and lateral
    (C) high, vertical, and toward the midline
    (D) low, vertical, and toward the midline

150. The term *voxel* is associated with all of the following, *except*
   - (A) bit depth
   - (B) volume element
   - (C) measured in *Z* direction
   - (D) FOV

151. In which body position would a patient suffering from orthopnea experience the *least* discomfort?
   - (A) Fowler
   - (B) Trendelenburg
   - (C) Recumbent
   - (D) Erect

152. The position illustrated in Figure 14-12 can be improved by
   - (A) bringing the chin up more
   - (B) bringing the chin down more
   - (C) angling the CR caudad
   - (D) opening the mouth more

153. Inspiration and expiration projections of the chest may be performed to demonstrate
   1. pneumothorax
   2. foreign body
   3. atelectasis
   - (A) 1 only
   - (B) 1 and 2 only
   - (C) 1 and 3 only
   - (D) 1, 2, and 3

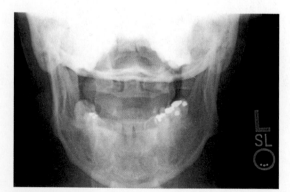

Figure 14-12.

154. Types of positive contrast agents include
   1. barium sulfate suspension
   2. water-based iodinated media
   3. carbon dioxide
   - (A) 1 only
   - (B) 2 only
   - (C) 1 and 2 only
   - (D) 1 and 3 only

155. Which of the following best describes correct hand hygiene?
   - (A) The radiographer's hands should be thoroughly washed with soap and warm running water, for at least 15 s after each patient
   - (B) The radiographer's hands should be thoroughly washed with soap and warm running water, for at least 15 s before each patient
   - (C) The radiographer's hands should be thoroughly washed with soap and warm running water, for at least 15 s before and after each patient
   - (D) The radiographer's hands and forearms should always be kept higher than the elbows during cleansing

156. Radiation exposure to the developing fetus can cause
   1. intellectual disability
   2. growth retardation
   3. organ damage
   - (A) 1 only
   - (B) 1 and 2 only
   - (C) 2 and 3 only
   - (D) 1, 2, and 3

157. Which of the following is/are characteristics of a 16:1 grid?
   1. It absorbs more useful radiation than an 8:1 grid
   2. It has greater centering latitude than an 8:1 grid
   3. It is used with higher kV exposures than an 8:1 grid
   - (A) 1 only
   - (B) 1 and 3 only
   - (C) 2 and 3 only
   - (D) 1, 2, and 3

158. The automatic exposure device that is located immediately under the x-ray table is the
    (A) ionization chamber
    (B) scintillation camera
    (C) photomultiplier
    (D) photocathode

159. What pixel size has a 512 × 512 matrix with a 20-cm FOV?
    (A) 0.07 mm/pixel
    (B) 0.40 mm/pixel
    (C) 0.04 mm/pixel
    (D) 4.0 mm/pixel

160. kV selection in digital imaging has an effect on
    1. photon energy
    2. penetration
    3. image contrast
    (A) 1 only
    (B) 1 and 2 only
    (C) 2 and 3 only
    (D) 1, 2, and 3

161. Figure 14-13A and B is most often used to evaluate which of the following conditions?
    (A) Subluxation
    (B) Spondylolisthesis
    (C) Whiplash injury
    (D) Cervical rib

162. Digital radiographic imaging equipment provides a number of functions for optimization of image quality, including
    1. exposure data recognition (EDR)
    2. automatic rescaling
    3. narrow latitude
    (A) 1 only
    (B) 1 and 2 only
    (C) 2 and 3 only
    (D) 1, 2, and 3

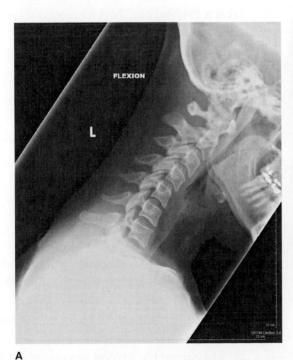
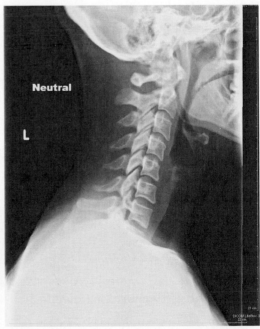

A   B

Figure 14-13. (A) and **(B)**. (Photo contributor: Conrad P. Ehrlich, MD.)

163. Advantages of flat panel fluoroscopy include
    1. decreased patient dose
    2. increased temporal resolution
    3. decreased DQE
    (A) 1 only
    (B) 1 and 2 only
    (C) 2 and 3 only
    (D) 1, 2, and 3

164. The number of gray shades that an imaging system can reproduce is termed
    (A) postprocessing
    (B) resolution
    (C) dynamic range
    (D) modulation transfer function (MTF)

165. The energy of ionizing electromagnetic radiations is measured in
    (A) mA
    (B) mAs
    (C) keV
    (D) kV

166. What is the function of a slit camera?
    1. To measure focal spot size
    2. To determine laser beam accuracy
    3. To regulate SID resolution
    (A) 1 only
    (B) 1 and 2 only
    (C) 1 and 3 only
    (D) 1, 2, and 3

167. Which of the following systems functions to compensate for changing patient/part thicknesses during fluoroscopic procedures?
    (A) Automatic brightness control (ABC)
    (B) Minification gain
    (C) Automatic resolution control
    (D) Flux gain

168. The structure labeled number 2 in Figure 14-14 is the
    (A) left subclavian artery
    (B) brachiocephalic artery
    (C) left common carotid artery
    (D) left vertebral artery

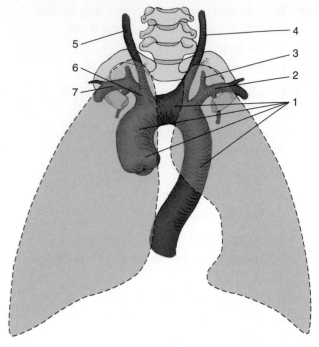

Figure 14-14. (Adapted from Dohetry GM, ed. *Current Surgical Diagnosis and Treatment,* 12th ed. New York: McGraw Hill; 2006: 824.)

169. What is the fetal dose limit for pregnant radiographers for the entire gestation period?
    (A) 1.0 mSv (0.1 rem)
    (B) 5.0 mSv (0.5 rem)
    (C) 50 mSv (5.0 rem)
    (D) 100 mSv (10 rem)

170. What type of precaution prevents the spread of infectious agents in aerosol form?
    (A) Strict isolation
    (B) Protective isolation
    (C) Airborne precautions
    (D) Contact precautions

171. When a radiographer is obtaining patient history, both subjective and objective data should be obtained. An example of *subjective* data is
    (A) the patient appears to have a productive cough
    (B) the patient has a blood pressure of 130/95
    (C) the patient complains of RUQ pain
    (D) the patient has a palpable mass in the left breast

172. An accurately positioned oblique projection of the first through fourth lumbar vertebrae will demonstrate the classic "Scotty dog." What bony structure does the Scotty dog's "ear" represent?

(A) Superior articular process

(B) Pedicle

(C) Transverse process

(D) Pars interarticularis

173. Figure 14-15 was made in which of the following positions?

(A) Right lateral decubitus

(B) Left lateral decubitus

(C) PA recumbent

(D) AP erect

174. What minimum total amount of filtration (inherent plus added) is required in an x-ray equipment operated above 70 kV?

(A) 2.5-mm Al equivalent

(B) 3.5-mm Al equivalent

(C) 2.5-mm Cu equivalent

(D) 3.5-mm Cu equivalent

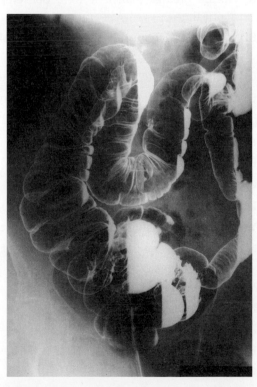

Figure 14-15. (Photo contributor: Stamford Hospital, Department of Radiology.)

175. A CR histogram is a graphic representation of

(A) grayscale values of the imaged part

(B) a characteristic curve of the imaged part

(C) *D*max

(D) *D*min

176. Proper care of leaded apparel includes

1. periodic check for cracks

2. careful folding following each use

3. routine laundering with soap and water

(A) 1 only

(B) 1 and 2 only

(C) 2 and 3 only

(D) 1, 2, and 3

177. The sum of effective dose equivalent from external and internal radiation sources is expressed as

(A) EqD

(B) EfD

(C) TEDE

(D) W_t

178. A radiograph obtained with a parallel grid demonstrates decreased receptor exposure on its lateral edges. This is most likely caused by

(A) static electrical discharge

(B) the grid off-centered

(C) improper tube angle

(D) decreased SID

179. What is meant by the term *controlled area*?

1. One that is occupied by people trained in radiation safety

2. One that is occupied by people who wear radiation monitors

3. One whose occupancy factor is 1

(A) 1 and 2 only

(B) 2 only

(C) 1 and 3 only

(D) 1, 2, and 3

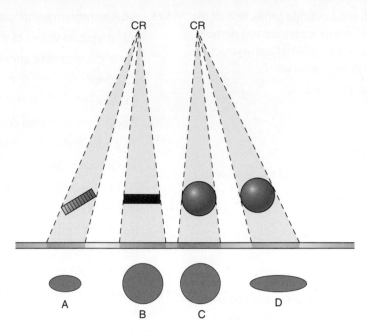

Figure 14-16.

180. Image A, seen in Figure 14-16, is representative of
    1. magnification
    2. distortion
    3. elongation
    4. foreshortening
    (A) 2 only
    (B) 1 and 2 only
    (C) 2 and 3 only
    (D) 2 and 4 only

181. All of the following statements concerning respiratory structures are true, *except*
    (A) the right lung has two lobes
    (B) the uppermost portion of the lung is the apex
    (C) each lung is enclosed in pleura
    (D) the trachea bifurcates into mainstem bronchi

182. To demonstrate the pulmonary apices with the patient in the AP erect position, the
    (A) CR is directed 15°–20° cephalad
    (B) CR is directed 15°–20° caudad
    (C) exposure is made on full exhalation
    (D) patient's shoulders are rolled forward

183. The effects of radiation on biologic material are dependent on several factors. If a quantity of radiation is delivered to a body over a long period of time, the effect
    (A) will be greater than if it were delivered all at one time
    (B) will be less than if it were delivered all at one time
    (C) has no relation to how it is delivered in time
    (D) is solely dependent on the radiation quality

184. In which quadrant is the sigmoid colon located?
    (A) LLQ
    (B) LUQ
    (C) RLQ
    (D) RUQ

185. Patient dose during fluoroscopy is affected by the
    1. distance between the patient and the input phosphor
    2. amount of magnification
    3. tissue density
    (A) 1 only
    (B) 3 only
    (C) 2 and 3 only
    (D) 1, 2, and 3

186. The four major arteries supplying the brain include the

   1. brachiocephalic artery

   2. common carotid arteries

   3. vertebral arteries

   (A) 1 and 2 only

   (B) 1 and 3 only

   (C) 2 and 3 only

   (D) 1, 2, and 3

187. The total brightness gain of an image intensifier is a result of

   1. flux gain

   2. minification gain

   3. focusing gain

   (A) 1 only

   (B) 2 only

   (C) 1 and 2 only

   (D) 1 and 3 only

188. Radiographers use monitoring devices to record their monthly exposure to radiation. The types of devices suited for this purpose include

   1. pocket dosimeter

   2. thermoluminescent dosimeter (TLD)

   3. optically stimulated luminescence (OSL)

   (A) 1 only

   (B) 1 and 2 only

   (C) 2 and 3 only

   (D) 1, 2, and 3

189. The AP projection of the scapula requires that the

   1. patient's arm be abducted at right angles to the body

   2. patient's elbow be flexed with hand supinated

   3. exposure be made during quiet breathing

   (A) 1 and 2 only

   (B) 1 and 3 only

   (C) 3 only

   (D) 1, 2, and 3

190. The radiograph seen in Figure 14-17 illustrates the joint space obscured by the

   (A) medial femoral condyle

   (B) lateral femoral condyle

   (C) intercondylar eminences

   (D) tibial tuberosity

191. The processes of the temporal include the

   1. mastoid

   2. zygomatic

   3. styloid

   (A) 1 only

   (B) 1 and 2 only

   (C) 2 and 3 only

   (D) 1, 2, and 3

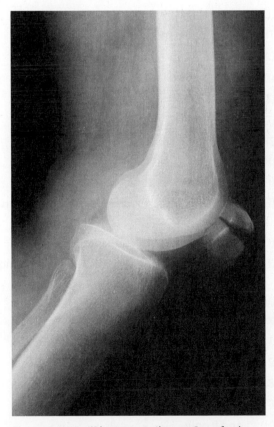

Figure 14-17. (Photo contributor: Stamford Hospital, Department of Radiology.)

192. When a patient is received in the radiology department with a urinary Foley catheter bag, it is important to
    (A) place the drainage bag above the level of the bladder
    (B) place the drainage bag at the same level as the bladder
    (C) place the drainage bag below the level of the bladder
    (D) clamp the Foley catheter

193. The total number of x-ray photons produced at the target is contingent on
    1. tube current
    2. target material
    3. square of the kilovoltage
    (A) 1 only
    (B) 1 and 2 only
    (C) 2 and 3 only
    (D) 1, 2, and 3

194. The *most* effective method of sterilization is
    (A) dry heat
    (B) moist heat
    (C) pasteurization
    (D) freezing

195. The radiographer's main objective regarding personal radiation safety is
    (A) not to exceed his or her dose limit
    (B) to keep personal exposure as far below the dose limit as possible
    (C) to avoid whole-body exposure
    (D) to wear protective apparel when "holding" patients for exposures

196. Which of the following conditions generally require(s) an increase in technical factors?
    1. Congestive heart failure
    2. Pleural effusion
    3. Emphysema
    (A) 1 only
    (B) 1 and 2 only
    (C) 1 and 3 only
    (D) 1, 2, and 3

197. The artifacts seen in Figure 14-18 are representative of
    (A) grid lines
    (B) Moiré artifact
    (C) surgical clips
    (D) hair braids

198. Which of the following generator types has the advantages of having compact size, producing nearly constant potential voltage, and decreasing patient dose?
    (A) Single-phase, full-wave
    (B) Three-phase, six-pulse
    (C) Three-phase, 12-pulse
    (D) High frequency

199. The dose of radiation that will cause a noticeable skin reaction is called the
    (A) linear energy transfer (LET)
    (B) source skin distance
    (C) skin erythema dose
    (D) SID

200. Correct treatment of epistaxis includes
    1. tilt head back
    2. breath through mouth
    3. refrain from speaking
    (A) 1 only
    (B) 1 and 2 only
    (C) 2 and 3 only
    (D) 1, 2, and 3

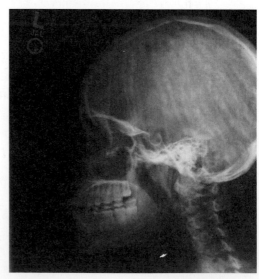

Figure 14-18. (Photo contributor: Stamford Hospital, Department of Radiology.)

Answers and Explanations

1. (C) DQE describes the percentage of incoming x-ray photons that are detected and absorbed by the receptor for transformation to the x-ray image. Receptor systems having higher DQEs have the ability to produce high-quality images at lower doses. In CR, the receptor is the PSP. Digital receptors include TFTs and CCDs. DR can be either direct or indirect conversion. Systems without a scintillation/light conversion step generally have a higher DQE.

2. (B) The *tissue weighting factor* (W_t) represents the relative tissue radiosensitivity of irradiated material (e.g., muscle vs. intestinal epithelium vs. bone). The *radiation weighting factor* (W_r) is a number assigned to different types of ionizing radiations to better determine their effect on tissue (e.g., x-ray vs. alpha particles). The W_r of different ionizing radiations is dependent on the LET of that particular radiation. The following formula is used to determine *effective dose* (E): E = Radiation weighting factor (W_r) × Tissue weighting factor (W_t) × Absorbed dose.

3. (D) Figure 14-1A is a medial oblique projection of the foot. The foot is rotated medially so that the *plantar surface* and the *IR* form a 30° angle—the *CR* and the *plantar surface* form a 60° angle. This position should demonstrate the third through fifth metatarsals completely free of superimposition when positioned correctly. Articulations around the cuboid and sinus tarsi should be well demonstrated, as well as the tuberosity of the base of the fifth metatarsal. The basis of the first and second metatarsals are superimposed on the medial and intermediate cuneiforms.

Figure 14-1B is the dorsoplantar projection of the foot; the CR is perpendicular to the plantar surface.

4. (A) The PSP screen within the IP has a layer of europium-activated barium fluorohalide ($BaFX:Eu^{2+}$; X = halogen) mixed with a binder substance. This layer serves as the *IR* when exposed to x-rays. Just under the barium fluorohalide layer is a *reflective layer,* then the *base,* then an *antistatic layer,* and finally a layer of *lead foil* to absorb backscatter. Over the top of the barium fluorohalide is a *protective layer.* When the barium fluorohalide absorbs x-ray energy, *electrons are released and they divide into two groups.* One electron group initiates *immediate luminescence* during the excited state of Eu^{2+}. The other electron group *becomes trapped* within the phosphor's halogen ions, forming a "color center." These are the phosphors that ultimately form the radiographic image because when exposed to a *monochromatic* (often infrared) laser light

source, these phosphors emit *polychromatic* light, termed *photostimulated luminescence.*

5. (D) According to the inverse square law of radiation, the intensity (exposure rate) of radiation from its source is inversely proportional to the distance squared. Therefore, as distance from the source of radiation is increased, exposure rate decreases. If x-ray photon exposure rate decreases, proportionally fewer photons will be received by the IR.

6. (B) Syncope, or fainting, is a result of a drop in blood pressure caused by insufficient blood (oxygen) to the brain. The patient should be helped into a dorsal recumbent position with feet elevated to facilitate blood flow to the brain.

7. (C) Adverse reactions to the intravascular administration of iodinated contrast are not uncommon, and although the risk of a life-threatening reaction is relatively rare, the radiographer must be alert to recognize and deal effectively should a serious reaction occur. Minor reaction is characterized by flushed appearance and nausea and a few hives (urticaria). *Early* symptoms of a possible anaphylactic reaction include *constriction of the throat,* possibly caused by laryngeal edema, *dysphagia* (difficulty swallowing), increased urticaria, itching of the palms and soles, hypotension, and a change in heart rate. The radiographer must maintain the patient's airway, summon the radiologist, and call a "code." *Dysphasia* refers to difficulty speaking and is not a typical allergic reaction.

8. (A) The first through fourth lumbar articular facets (forming *zygapophyseal joints*) are 45° to the midsagittal plane and therefore are well demonstrated in the *oblique* projection. The zygapophyseal joints of L5–S1 are best demonstrated in a 35° oblique. The lumbar *intervertebral foramina* lie 90° to the midsagittal plane and are therefore demonstrated in the *lateral* position. *Intervertebral joints* are well visualized in the *lateral* projection of all the vertebral groups.

9. (B) Image *smoothing* (or low-pass filtering) is a type of spatial frequency filtering performed in digital image postprocessing by averaging each pixel frequency with surrounding pixel values to remove high frequency noise. This results in a reduction of noise and contrast, and is useful for viewing small structural details. *Windowing* is a postprocessing adjustment of digital image brightness and contrast. *Aliasing* is an artifact that can occur in digital imaging with insufficient sampling frequency. *Edge enhancement* is also a postprocessing function that can be used to emphasize small high contrast tissues.

10. (D) *Veracity* is not only telling the truth but also not practicing deception. *Autonomy* is the ethical principle related to the theory that patients have the right to decide what will or will not be done to them. *Beneficence* is related to the idea of doing good and being kind. *Fidelity* is faithfulness and loyalty.

11. (B) *Somatic effects* of radiation refer to the effects experienced directly by the exposed individual such as erythema, epilation, and cataracts. *Genetic effects* of radiation exposure are caused by irradiation of the reproductive cells of the exposed individual and transmitted from one generation to the next.

12. (B) The approximately 5-foot-long large intestine (colon) functions in the formation, transport, and evacuation of feces. The colon commences at the terminus of the small intestine; its first portion is the saclike *cecum* in the RLQ, located inferior to the ileocecal valve. The ascending colon is continuous with the cecum and is located along the right side of the abdominal cavity. It bends medially and anteriorly, forming the *right colic* (hepatic) flexure. The colon traverses the abdomen as the transverse colon and bends posteriorly and inferiorly to form the *left colic* (splenic) flexure. The descending colon continues down the left side of the abdominal cavity, and at about the level of the pelvic brim, in the LLQ, the colon moves medially to form the S-shaped *sigmoid* colon. The rectum, approximately 5 inches in length, lies between the sigmoid and the anal canal.

13. (C) The use of a fluoroscopic flat panel detector can offer the benefit of reduction in patient dose because of increased DQE and pulsed x-ray beam. *The x-ray tube must be able to turn on and off very quickly.* The term *interrogation time* refers to the time it takes the tube to reach the required technical factors. The term *extinction time* refers to the time it takes the tube to turn off. The required time is less than 1 ms.

14. (C) Added aluminum filtration removes more low-energy photons; therefore, there is a decrease in the *number* of photons in the x-ray beam—that is, beam *intensity*. Because low-energy photons are removed, the overall average energy of the x-ray beam is increased. This process can also be called beam *hardening* because its average energy is increased. The maximum energy of the beam is unchanged as long as the kV remains unchanged.

15. (B) The wrist is composed of eight carpal bones arranged in two rows (proximal and distal). The proximal row consists of (from lateral to medial) the scaphoid, lunate, triquetrum, and pisiform. The distal row (from lateral to medial) includes the trapezium, trapezoid, capitate, and hamate. The radiograph seen in Figure 14-2 is a *PA projection of the wrist*. The letter L represents the *scaphoid*, which is the most *lateral* carpal of the *proximal* row. Just medial to the scaphoid is the lunate (H). The letter I indicates the pisiform, which is seen superimposed on the triquetrum. The letter M points out the most *medial* carpal of the *distal* row, the *hamate*. The joints of the wrist include the *intercarpal joints* and the *radiocarpal joint*.

16. (B) A patient going into shock may exhibit *pallor* and *weakness,* a significant *drop in blood pressure,* and an *increase in pulse rate*. The patient may also experience *apprehension* and *restlessness* and have *cool, clammy skin*. A radiographer recognizing these symptoms should call the patient to the physician's attention immediately. Fever is not associated with shock.

17. (D) The control and prevention of infection are a hospital-wide effort. Each department has its own infection control protocol, designed according to the risks unique to its services.

The most susceptible to infection include the sick, infirm, immunocompromised, very young, poorly nourished, weak, or fatigued—all who have a diminished natural resistance to infection. HAIs, formerly called *nosocomial infections,* are infections acquired by *patients* (susceptible hosts) while they are in the hospital, unrelated to the condition for which the patients were hospitalized.

18. (A) Tissue weighting factor (W_t) represents the relative *tissue* radiosensitivity of irradiated material. Radiation weighting factor (W_r) is a number assigned to different types of ionizing *radiations* to better determine their effect on tissue. The W_r of different ionizing radiations is dependent on the LET of that particular radiation. The following formula is used to determine *effective dose* (*E*): E = Radiation weighting factor (W_r) × Tissue weighting factor (W_t). The *effective dose* describes whole-body dose. Whole-body dose is always less than the exposure dose received by the irradiated part. For example, the entrance skin exposure of a PA chest is approximately 70 mrem, whereas the effective dose is 10 mrem. The effective (whole body) dose is much less because much of the body is not included in the primary beam. Occupational dose limits are expressed as effective dose.

19. (B) When the body is erect, the diaphragm is more easily moved to a lower position during inspiration. For this reason, chest radiography is performed erect to allow maximum lung expansion. With the body in the supine position, the abdominal viscera exert greater pressure on the diaphragm and it usually assumes a position 2–4 inches higher than that when erect.

20. (C) A digital image is formed by a *matrix* of *pixels* (picture elements) in rows and columns. A matrix having 512 pixels in each row and column is a 512 × 512 matrix. The term *field of view* is used to describe how much of the patient (e.g., 150 mm diameter) is included in the matrix. The matrix and/or FOV can be changed without affecting the other, but changes in either will change pixel size. As in traditional radiography, *spatial resolution* is measured in line pairs per millimeter (*lp/mm*). As matrix size is increased, there are more and smaller pixels in the matrix and therefore improved resolution. Fewer and larger pixels result in a poor resolution "pixelly" image, that is, one in which you can actually see the individual pixel boxes.

21. (B) With the body in the AP recumbent position, barium easily flows into the fundus of the stomach, displacing it somewhat superiorly. The fundus, then, is filled with barium, whereas the air that had been in the fundus is displaced into the gastric body, pylorus, and duodenum, illustrating them in double-contrast fashion. Air contrast delineation of these structures allows us to see through the stomach to retrogastric areas and structures. Barium-filled duodenum and pylorus are best demonstrated in the RAO position.

22. (D) The AHA replaced the patient's Bill of Rights with the *Patient Care Partnership—Understanding Expectations, Rights, and Responsibilities*. Their plain-language brochure includes the essentials of the Bill of Rights and reviews what patients can/should expect during a hospital stay.

The Patient Care Partnership statement addresses *high-quality hospital care*, combining skill, compassion, and respect and the right to know the identity of caregivers. It includes a *clean* and *safe environment*, free from neglect and abuse, and information about anything unexpected that occurred during the hospital stay. The Patient Care Partnership identifies *involvement in your care*: It elaborates on patient discussion/understanding of their condition and treatment choices with their physician, patients' responsibility to provide complete and correct information to the caregiver, understanding who should make decisions for patients if they cannot make those decisions (including "living will" or "advance directive").

The Patient Care Partnership statement identifies *protection of your privacy*, describing the ways in which patient information is safeguarded. It also describes *help when leaving the hospital*—availability of and/or instruction regarding follow-up care. Finally, the Patient Care Partnership statement addresses *help with your billing claims,* including filing claims with insurance companies and assisting those without health coverage.

These patient rights can be exercised on the patient's behalf by a *designated surrogate* or *proxy* decision maker.

23. (A) Figure 14-3 illustrates the production of bremsstrahlung (brems) radiation (A)—an interaction between a high-speed electron and a tungsten (W) nucleus. A high-speed electron is accelerated from the x-ray tube filament toward a tungsten atom within the anode focal track. The negative electron is attracted by the positive tungsten nucleus. The electron is "braked"/slowed down as it changes direction. The energy it loses when it is "braked" is given up in the form of an x-ray photon, that is, brems (or braking) radiation. Characteristic radiation (B) is produced at the target when a high-speed electron ejects a K shell electron, creating a vacancy. The vacancy is filled when an L shell electron drops down to the K shell. The energy lost in the transition is given up in the form of characteristic radiation. The photoelectric effect (C) and Compton scatter (D) are interactions between ionizing radiation and tissue.

24. (C) Moving the image intensifier *closer to the patient* during fluoroscopy *reduces* the distance between the x-ray tube (source) and the image intensifier (IR); that is, the *SID* is reduced. It follows that the distance between the part being imaged (object) and the image intensifier (IR) is also reduced; that is, the *OID* is reduced (Fig. 14-19). The shorter OID produces *less magnification* and *better image quality*. As SID is reduced, the intensity of the x-ray photons at the image intensifier's input phosphor increases, stimulating the ABC to decrease the mA (milliamperage), thereby *decreasing the patient dose*.

25. (C) The addition of a grid will help clean up the scattered radiation produced by higher kV, but it requires mAs adjustment. The original mAs is 8 (400 mA x 20 ms [0.02 s]). The new mAs should be 24 because, according to the grid conversion factors listed below, the addition of a 6:1 grid requires that the original mAs be multiplied by a factor of 3:

No grid	= 1 × original mAs
5:1 grid	= 2 × original mAs
6:1 grid	= 3 × original mAs
8:1 grid	= 4 × original mAs
12:1 grid	= 5 × original mAs
16:1 grid	= 6 × original mAs

8 mAs × 3 = 24 mAs. The adjustment therefore requires 24 mAs at 90 kV.

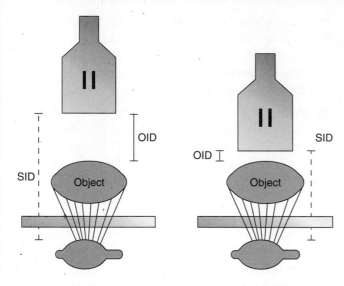

26. (A) Voltage ripple refers to the percentage drop from maximum voltage each pulse of current experiences. In single-phase rectified equipment, the entire pulse (half-cycle) is used (A); therefore, there is first an increase to maximum (peak) voltage value and a subsequent decrease to zero potential (90° past peak potential). The entire waveform is used; if 100 kV were selected, the actual average kilovoltage output would be approximately 70. Three-phase rectification produces (B) almost constant potential with small ripples (drops) in maximum potential between pulses. Approximately, a 13% voltage ripple (drop from maximum value) characterizes the operation of three-phase, six-pulse generators (C). Three-phase, 12-pulse generators have approximately a 4% voltage ripple (D).

27. (D) The closer the x-ray source is to the barrier (wall), the greater the thickness necessary. Occupancy factor refers to the degree of occupancy of the department adjacent to the barrier; a stairway would require less shielding than a busy work area. Workload is important in determining barrier thickness and refers to the number of examinations performed in the x-ray room measured in mA-min/week; the greater the number of examinations per week, the greater the barrier thickness required. Use factor is also important in determining barrier thickness and refers to the amount of time x-rays are directed to a particular wall; the greater the amount of time, the greater the thickness required.

28. (D) Sterilization is the complete elimination of all living microorganisms and can be accomplished by several methods. *Pressurized steam,* in an *autoclave,* is probably the most familiar means of sterilization; the pressure allows higher temperatures to be achieved. *Gas or chemical* sterilization is used for items unable to withstand moisture and/or high temperatures. Other methods of sterilization include *dry heat,* ionizing *radiation,* and microwaves (*non*ionizing radiation).

29. (C) When examining the third through fifth fingers in the lateral position, the *medial* side of the forearm (*ulnar side*) should be closest to the IR. This *minimizes magnification* by achieving the shortest possible OID. The terms *medial* and *lateral* are identified while viewing the part in the anatomic position.

30. (B) Neither diagnostic sonography nor magnetic resonance imaging requires the use of ionizing radiation to produce an image. CT does require ionizing radiation to produce an image. Sonography requires the use of high-frequency sound waves (ultrasound) to produce images of soft-tissue structures and certain blood vessels within the body. Magnetic resonance imaging relies on the use of a very powerful magnet and specially designed coils that send and receive radiowave signals to produce the image.

31. (C) An artifact associated with digital imaging and grids is *aliasing* or the *Moiré effect.* If the direction of the lead strips and the grid lines per inch (i.e., grid frequency) matches the scan frequency of the scanner/reader, this artifact can occur. Aliasing appears as superimposed images slightly out of alignment, an image "wrapping" effect. This most commonly occurs in mobile radiography with stationary grids and can be a problem with digital radiography (DR) flat panel detectors. Phantom images are usually associated with incomplete erasure.

32. (A) *Primary radiation barriers* protect against direct exposure from the primary (useful) x-ray beam and have much greater attenuation capability than *secondary barriers,* which protect only from leakage and scattered radiation. Examples of primary barriers are the lead *walls* and *doors* of a radiographic room, that is, any surface that could be struck by the useful beam. Primary protective barriers of typical installations generally consist of walls with $\frac{1}{16}$-inch (1.5-mm) lead thickness and 7 feet height.

Secondary radiation includes *leakage* and *scattered* radiation. The control booth wall is a secondary barrier; therefore, the primary beam must never be directed toward it. The x-ray tube housing must reduce leakage radiation to less than 100 mR/h at a distance of 1 m from the housing. Lead aprons, lead gloves, portable x-ray barriers, and the like are also designed to protect the user from exposure to *scattered* radiation and will not protect from the primary beam.

33. (C) The number of *heat units* produced during a given exposure with single-phase equipment is determined by multiplying mA × s × kV. A correction factor is required with three-phase equipment. Unless the equipment manufacturer specifies otherwise, three-phase and high-frequency equipment heat units are determined by multiplying mA × s × kV × 1.4.

34. (D) *Indirect contact* involves transmission of microorganisms via *airborne* contamination, *fomites,* and *vectors.* *Airborne* precaution is required for pathogenic organisms that are capable of persistent suspension in air, such as varicella, rubeola, and tuberculosis. They *require that the patient wear a mask* to avoid the spread of acid-fast bacilli (in bronchial secretions of patients with tuberculosis) or other pathogens during coughing. If the patient is unable or unwilling to wear a mask, the radiographer must wear one. The radiographer should wear gloves, but a gown is required only if flagrant contamination is likely. Patients infected with *airborne precaution* require a *private, specially ventilated (negative pressure) room.* A private room is indicated for all patients on *droplet precaution,* that is, diseases transmitted via large droplets expelled from the patient while speaking, sneezing, or coughing. The pathogenic droplets can infect others when they come in contact with mouth or nasal mucosa or conjunctiva.

Rubella (German measles), *mumps,* and *influenza* are among the diseases spread by *droplet* contact; a *private room is required* for the patient, and health care practitioners must use *gown* and *gloves.*

35. (D) Image storage is located in a *pixel,* which is a two-dimensional "picture element" measured in the *XY* direction. The third dimension in the matrix of pixels is the *depth* that together with the pixel is called the *voxel,* measured in the *Z* direction.

A digital image is formed by a *matrix* of *pixels* in rows and columns. The *matrix* is the number of pixels in the *XY* direction. *The larger the matrix size, the better the image resolution.*

A matrix having 512 pixels in each row and column is a 512 × 512 matrix. The term *field of view* is used to describe how much of the patient (e.g., 150-mm diameter) is included in the matrix. The matrix and/or FOV can be changed without one affecting the other, but changes in either will change the pixel size. *As in traditional radiography, spatial resolution is measured in line pairs per millimeter (lp/mm). As matrix size is increased, there are more and smaller pixels in the matrix and therefore improved*

resolution. Fewer and larger pixels result in a poor-resolution "pixelly" image, that is, one in which you can actually see the individual pixel boxes.

Typical image matrix sizes used in radiography are as follows:

Nuclear medicine	128 × 128
Digital subtraction angiography	512 × 512
Computed tomography	512 × 512
Chest radiography	2048 × 2048

36. (A) The AP projection provides a general survey of the abdomen, showing the size and shape of the liver, spleen, and kidneys. When performed in the *erect* position, it should demonstrate both hemidiaphragms. The *erect* position is used to demonstrate air/fluid levels (as seen in the radiograph; Fig. 14-5). Air or fluid levels will be clearly demonstrated only if the CR is directed *parallel* to them. The manner (direction) in which the levels are seen indicates the position in which the image was obtained.

37. (D) LCD monitors are being rapidly replaced by LED monitors. LEDs provide backlight for LCDs. In addition to improved lighting, the display device is more energy efficient, has a longer life, has a larger viewable area, and is thinner.

38. (C) The exposed IP is placed into the CR scanner/reader, where the PSP plate is automatically removed. The latent image appears as the PSP is scanned by a narrow high-intensity *helium–neon laser* to obtain the pixel data. As the PSP is scanned in the CR reader, it releases a violet light—a process called *photostimulated luminescence.*

The luminescent light is converted to electrical energy representing the *analog* image. The electrical energy is sent to an ADC where it is digitized and becomes the *digital* image that is eventually displayed (after a short delay) on a high-resolution monitor and/or printed out by a laser printer. The digitized images can also be manipulated in postprocessing, electronically transmitted, and stored/archived.

39. (D) Imaging a patient with traumatic injury, especially to the skull, requires careful attention to patient condition throughout the procedure. Cervical spine injury must be ruled out before any attempt to position the skull. Images usually obtained include AP, AP axial/reverse Caldwell, and AP axial/Towne method. The AP and reverse Caldwell are used to evaluate the anterior cranium. The AP axial projection (Towne method) is used to evaluate posterior cranium/occipital bone. The OML and MSP should be perpendicular to the image receptor. The CR enters at the nasion and perpendicular to the MSP in the AP projection. In the AP axial/reverse Caldwell, the CR is directed to the nasion at a cephalad angle of 15°. In the AP axial/Towne method the CR is directed 30° caudad to the OML, passing through the EAM and exiting the foramen magnum.

40. (C) A profile view of the glenoid fossa can be obtained in the AP oblique projection (*LPO* or *RPO*, Grashey method). In the anatomic position, the bony glenoid fossa is seen to project *posteriorly* and *laterally* approximately 40°. Therefore, if the shoulder is positioned with the body rotated 35°–45° *toward the affected side,* the glenoid fossa will be placed parallel with the CR (*perpendicular to the IR*) and a profile view of the fossa is obtained.

41. (D) *Nonstochastic* effects are early tissue reactions. They are somatic effects having predictable threshold responses; that is, a certain quantity of radiation must be received before the effect occurs, and the greater the dose, the more severe the effect. Examples of nonstochastic effects/early tissue reactions are erythema, blood changes, cataract formation, and epilation. *Stochastic* effects of radiation are nonthreshold and randomly occurring. Examples of stochastic effects include carcinogenesis and genetic effects. The chance of occurrence of stochastic effects is directly related to the radiation dose; that is, as radiation dose increases, there is a greater likelihood of genetic alterations or development of cancer.

42. (C) Some chemical agents used in health care facilities function to kill pathogenic microorganisms, whereas others function to inhibit the growth/spread of pathogenic microorganisms. Germicides and disinfectants are used to kill pathogenic microorganisms, and antiseptics (such as alcohol) are used to stop their growth/spread. *Sterilization* is another associated term and refers to killing of all microorganisms and their spores.

43. (D) A question every primary pathway candidate for certification must answer on his or her ARRT® application, in addition to reading and signing the "Written Consent under FERPA," is "Have you ever been suspended, dismissed, or expelled from an educational program that you have attended to meet ARRT certification requirements?"

The ARRT can obtain specific parts of a graduate's educational records concerning violations to an honor code.

Some examples of reportable infractions are listed as follows:

- Cheating and/or plagiarism
- Falsification of eligibility requirements (e.g., clinical competency information)
- Forgery or alteration of any document related to qualifications or patient care
- Abuse, neglect, or abandonment of patients
- Sexual contact without consent or harassment to any member of the community, including patients
- Conduct that is seriously obscene or offensive
- Practicing in an unsafe manner or outside the scope of professional training
- Violating patient confidentiality (HIPAA)
- Attempted or actual theft of any item not belonging to the student (including patients' property)
- Attending class or clinical setting while under the influence of alcohol, drugs, or other substances

(Adapted from The American Registry of Radiologic Technologists Standards of Ethics. "ARRT Standards of Ethics", 2022. https://www.arrt.org/pages/earn-arrt-credentials/initial-requirements/ethics/ethics-requirements)

44. (B) As blood pulsates through the arteries, a throb can be detected. This throb or *pulse* can be readily palpated where the arteries are superficial. (Examples are *wrist, groin, neck,* and posterior surface of the *knee.*) The apical pulse can be detected with a stethoscope.

45. (D) Patient dose during fluoroscopy can be significant. Many guidelines are in place to keep patient dose, and radiation worker dose, to a minimum. Fluoroscopic magnification technique requires increased exposure and increased patient dose. The greater the patient size and the greater the length of the fluoroscopic examination, the greater the patient dose.

46. (B) Radiograph A was performed *PA* and radiograph B was performed *AP*, as evidenced by the bony pelvis anatomy. The PA projection (image A) shows the ilia more foreshortened, giving the pelvis a "closed" appearance, whereas the AP projection shows the ilia and bladder area more "open." Technical factors were selected appropriately, for the required anatomic structures are well visualized: renal shadows, psoas muscle, lumbar transverse processes, and inferior margin of the liver. There is no evidence of the radiographs having been obtained in an erect position, as the hemidiaphragms are not included, and the gas patterns appear without leveling.

47. (A) The CR IP houses the PSP. This PSP with its layer of europium-activated barium fluorohalide serves as the *IR* as it is exposed in the traditional manner and receives the latent image. The PSP can *store* the latent image for several hours; after approximately 8 h, noticeable image fading will occur. Once the IP is placed into the CR processor (*scanner* or *reader*), the PSP is automatically removed. The latent image on the PSP is changed to a manifest image as it is scanned by a narrow, high-intensity *helium–neon laser* to obtain the pixel data. As the PSP is scanned in the "reader," it releases a violet light—a process called *photostimulated luminescence.*

48. (D) The knee is the largest and one of the most complex joints of the body. It is formed by three bones—the proximal tibia, the patella, and the distal femur—which articulate to form two joints, the *femorotibial* (hinge joint) and *femoropatellar* (gliding joint).

However, the knee actually consists of three articulations: (i) the patellofemoral joint, (ii) the lateral, and (iii) the femorotibial joint. The femorotibial joint can be further described as the lateral femorotibial joint (lateral femoral condyle with tibial plateau) and the medial femorotibial joint (medial femoral condyle with tibial plateau).

The knee is a diarthrotic articulation classified as a bicondylar, or modified hinge joint. The patellofemoral joint is actually a gliding joint. The knee's principal motion is in one direction; it has limited rotation motion.

49. (B) Because *muscle* and *nerve* tissues perform specific functions and do not divide, they are relatively *insensitive* to radiation exposure. *Epithelial* cells cover the outer surface of the body and line body cavities as well as tubes and passageways leading to the exterior. They contain very little intercellular substance and are devoid of blood vessels. Because *epithelial* cells constantly regenerate through mitosis, they are very *radiosensitive.*

50. (C) Ribs below the diaphragm are best demonstrated with the diaphragm elevated. This is accomplished by placing the patient in a recumbent position and taking the exposure at the end of exhalation. Conversely, the ribs above the diaphragm are best demonstrated with the diaphragm depressed. Placing the patient in the erect position and taking the exposure at the end of deep inspiration accomplish this.

51. (B) Protective barriers are classified as either primary or secondary. Primary barriers protect from the useful, or primary, x-ray beam and consist of a certain thickness of lead. They are located anywhere the primary beam can possibly be directed, for example, the walls of the x-ray room. The walls of the x-ray room usually require $\frac{1}{16}$ inch (1.5 mm) thickness of 7 foot high lead. Secondary barriers protect from secondary (scattered and leakage) radiation. Secondary barriers are control booths, lead aprons and gloves, and the wall of the x-ray room above 7 feet. Secondary barriers require much less lead than do primary barriers.

52. (A) *Creatinine* is a normal alkaline constituent of urine and blood, but increased quantities of creatinine are present in advanced stages of renal disease. Creatinine and *BUN* (blood urea nitrogen) blood chemistry levels should be checked before beginning an examination requiring the use of an iodinated contrast agent. Increased levels may forecast increased possibility of contrast media–induced renal effects and poor visualization of the renal collecting systems. Normal creatinine range is 0.6–1.5 mg/100 mL (100 mg = 1 dL). Normal BUN range is 8–25 mg/100 mL.

53. (D) The phenomenon in which the radiographic information recorded on the PSP upon exposure to x-rays *decreases* with the elapsed time until it is read by the scanner/reader is termed *fading.* This occurs because the photoelectrons generated by x-ray excitation upon exposure of the PSP are thermally released over time and are therefore unable to contribute to photostimulated luminescence upon scanning/reading. Luminescence decreases by approximately 25% within 8 h of exposure. The greater the elapsed time and the greater the environmental temperature, the greater will be the degree of fading.

54. (C) According to Bergonié and Tribondeau, the most radiosensitive cells are undifferentiated, rapidly dividing cells such as lymphocytes, intestinal crypt (of Lieberkühn) cells, and spermatogonia. Liver cells are among the types of cells that are somewhat differentiated and capable of mitosis. These characteristics render them somewhat radiosensitive. Muscle cells, as well as nerve cells and red blood cells, are highly differentiated and do not divide. Therefore, in the order of *decreasing* sensitivity (from least to greatest sensitivity), the cells are intestinal crypt cells, liver cells, and muscle cells.

55. (D) Histogram appearance can be affected by a number of things. *Positioning and centering accuracy* can have a significant effect on histogram appearance. Other factors affecting histogram appearance include selection of the *correct processing algorithm* (e.g., chest vs. femur), changes in *scatter, SID, OID,* and *collimation*—in short, anything that affects scatter and/or dose. Another factor affecting histogram appearance in CR is *delay in processing* from the time of exposure, which can result in *fading* of the image.

56. (C) Although the *inferosuperior axial* projection can be used to evaluate the glenohumeral joint, the required abduction of the arm would be contraindicated when evaluating a shoulder for possible dislocation. The *transthoracic* lateral projection is used to evaluate the glenohumeral joint and the upper humerus when the patient is unable to abduct the arm (as in dislocation). The *scapular Y* projection is an oblique projection of the shoulder and is used in demonstrating anterior or posterior dislocation.

57. (B) *Oral* administration of barium sulfate is used to demonstrate the upper digestive system, esophagus, fundus, body, and pylorus of the stomach and barium progression through the small bowel. The large bowel, including sigmoid colon, is usually demonstrated via *rectal* administration of barium.

58. (C) Tissue is most sensitive to radiation exposure when in an *oxygenated* condition. Anoxic refers to a general lack of oxygen in tissue; hypoxic refers to tissue with little oxygen. Anoxic and hypoxic tumors are typically avascular (with little or no blood supply) and are therefore more radioresistant.

59. (D) The ability of x-ray photons to penetrate a body part has a great deal to do with the composition of that part (e.g., bone vs. soft tissue vs. air) and the presence of any pathologic condition. Pathologic conditions can alter the normal nature of the anatomic part. Some conditions such as osteomalacia, fibrosarcoma, and paralytic ileus (obstruction) result in a decrease in body tissue density. When body tissue density decreases, x-rays will penetrate the tissues more readily, that is, more x-ray penetrability. In conditions such as ascites, where body tissue density increases as a result of accumulation of fluid, x-rays will not readily penetrate the body tissues, that is, less x-ray penetrability.

60. (A) The image intensifier's input phosphor receives the remnant beam from the patient and converts it to a fluorescent light image. To maintain resolution, the input phosphor is made of cesium iodide crystals. *Cesium iodide* is much more efficient in this conversion process than the phosphor previously used, zinc cadmium sulfide. Calcium tungstate was the phosphor used in cassette-intensifying screens for many years prior to the development of rare earth phosphors such as gadolinium oxysulfide.

61. (D) The knee is formed by the proximal tibia, patella, and distal femur, which articulate to form the *femorotibial* and *patellofemoral* joints. The distal posterior femur presents two large *medial* and *lateral condyles* separated by the deep *intercondyloid fossa*. Two small prominences, the medial and lateral epicondyles, are just superior to the condyles. The femoral and tibial condyles articulate to form the femorotibial joint. Figure 14-7 illustrates positioning for the *intercondyloid fossa* (Camp–Coventry method). The patient is PA recumbent with the knee flexed so that the tibia forms 40° angle with the tabletop, with foot rested on support. The CR is directed 40° caudad (perpendicular to the long axis of the tibia) to the knee joint. This results in a *PA axial* (superoinferior) projection of the intercondyloid fossa, tibial plateau, and eminences. It is called the *tunnel view*.

62. (B) Spatial resolution in *indirect* digital imaging improves with increased *sampling frequency* (pixels/mm or pixel density), smaller *pixel pitch,* smaller *pixel size,* and larger image matrix. The smaller the pixels and *pixel pitch* (i.e., distance between the center of one pixel to the center of adjacent pixel), the better the resolution.

DEL size of the TFT is related to *direct* digital imaging.

63. (D) Double-contrast studies of the stomach or large intestine involve coating the organ with a thin layer of barium sulfate and then introducing air. This permits seeing through the organ to structures behind it and especially allows visualization of the mucosal lining of the organ. A barium-filled stomach or large bowel demonstrates position, size, and shape of the organ and any lesion that projects out from its walls such as diverticula. Polypoid lesions, which project inward from the wall of an organ, may go unnoticed unless a double-contrast examination is performed.

64. (D) The intensity or exposure rate of radiation at a given distance from a point source is inversely proportional to the square of the distance. This is the inverse square law of radiation and is expressed in the following equation:

$$\frac{I_1}{I_2} = \frac{D_2^2}{D_1^2}$$

Substituting known values:

$$\frac{15 \text{ mGy}_a}{x \text{ mGy}_a} = \frac{25}{9}$$

$$25x = 135$$

$$x = 5.4 \text{ mGy}_a/\text{min; therefore, } 21.6 \text{ mGy}_a \text{ in 4 min.}$$

65. (D) The medical suffix *plasia* refers to development, formation, growth, or proliferation. The suffix denoting embryonic is *blast*. Condition is indicated by the suffix *osis*. The suffix *kinesia* is used to refer to motion or movement.

66. (B) An axial *dorsoplantar* projection is described; the CR enters the dorsal surface of the foot and exits the plantar surface. The *plantodorsal* projection is done in the *supine* position and requires cephalad angulation. The CR enters the plantar surface and exits the dorsal surface.

67. (D) The mediastinum is the space between the lungs that contains the heart, great vessels, trachea, esophagus, and thymus gland. It is bound anteriorly by the sternum and posteriorly by the vertebral column and extends from the upper thorax to the diaphragm.

68. (A) Because the established dose-limit formula guideline is used for occupationally exposed persons 18 years and older, guidelines had to be established In the event a student entered the clinical component of a radiography educational program prior to the age of 18 years. The guideline states that the occupational dose limit for students *younger than 18 years* is 1 mSv (0.1 rem/100 mrem*)* in any given year.

69. (A) Proper body ergonomics/mechanics includes a wide base of support. The *base of support* is the part of the body in touch with the floor or other horizontal plane. The *center of gravity* is the midpoint of the pelvis or lower abdomen, depending on body build. The *line of gravity* is the abstract line passing through the center of gravity, vertically. Proper body ergonomics can help prevent painful back injuries by making proficient use of the muscles in the arms and legs.

70. (B) The sacroiliac joints angle posteriorly and medially 25° to the median sagittal plane. Therefore, to demonstrate the sacroiliac joints with the patient in the *AP* position, the *affected* side must be elevated 25°. This places the joint space perpendicular to the IR and parallel to the CR. Therefore, the *LPO* position will demonstrate the *right sacroiliac joint* and *RPO* position will demonstrate the left. When performed with the patient in the *PA* position, the *unaffected* side will be elevated 25°.

71. (C) The AEC automatically terminates the exposure when the proper density has been recorded on the IR. The important advantage of the phototimer, then, is that it can accurately duplicate radiographic densities. It is useful in providing accurate comparison in follow-up

examinations and in decreasing patient exposure dose by decreasing the number of "retakes" because of improper exposure. The AEC automatically adjusts the exposure required for body parts having different *thicknesses* and *densities*. Remember that proper functioning of the AEC depends on accurate positioning by the radiographer. The correct *ionization chamber*(s) must be selected, and the anatomic part of interest must completely cover the ionization chamber to achieve the desired density. If *collimation* is inadequate, and a field size larger than the part is used, excessive scattered radiation from the body or tabletop can cause the AEC to terminate the exposure prematurely, resulting in an underexposed radiograph.

72. (D) *Chromosome aberration, cell death,* and *malignant disease* are major effects of DNA irradiation, often as a result of abnormal metabolic activity. If the damage happens to the DNA of a germ cell, the radiation response may not occur until one or more generations later.

73. (D) Voltage ripple refers to the percentage drop from maximum voltage each pulse of current experiences. In single-phase rectified equipment, the entire pulse (half-cycle) is used; therefore, there is first an increase to maximum (peak) voltage value and a subsequent decrease to zero potential (90° past peak potential). The entire waveform is used; if 100 kV were selected, the actual average kilovoltage output would be approximately 70. Three-phase rectification produces almost constant potential with just small ripples (drops) in maximum potential between pulses. Approximately, a 13% voltage ripple (drop from maximum value) characterizes the operation of three-phase, six-pulse generators. Three-phase, 12-pulse generators have approximately a 4% voltage ripple.

74. (C) Blood pressure in pulmonary circulation is relatively low and therefore pulmonary vessels can easily become blocked by blood clots, air bubbles, or fatty masses, resulting in a *pulmonary embolism*. If the blockage stays in place, it results in an extra strain on the right ventricle, which is now unable to pump blood. This occurrence can result in congestive heart failure. *Pneumothorax* is air in the pleural cavity. *Atelectasis* is a collapsed lung or part of a lung. *Hypoxia* is a condition of low tissue oxygen.

75. (B) CR uses special phosphor plates inside IPs to record the radiologic image. Upon exposure, a latent image is produced on the PSP, which is located inside the IP. The IP is placed in the CR reader, and the PSP is automatically removed. The PSP is scanned with a narrow laser beam to obtain the pixel data, which can then be displayed on a monitor as the radiographic image.

76. (C) There are two types of distortion: size and shape. *Shape distortion* relates to the alignment of the x-ray tube, the part to be radiographed, and the IR. There are two kinds of shape distortion: *elongation* and *foreshortening*. *Size distortion* is *magnification* and is related to the OID and SID. Magnification can be reduced by either increasing the SID or decreasing the OID. However, an increase in SID must be accompanied by an increase in mAs (milliampere seconds) to maintain density. It is therefore preferable, in the interest of exposure time, to reduce OID whenever possible. Use of short exposure time is beneficial for reducing motion unsharpness.

77. (C) The term *enteral* refers to the digestive tract. Therefore, enteral routes are any route of administration that involves administration through the digestive tract. That includes oral or rectal administration or by way of an NG tube.

78. (A) As kV is increased, more *high-energy* photons are produced and the overall energy of the primary beam is increased. *Photon energy is inversely related to wavelength;* that is, as photon energy increases, wavelength decreases. An increase in milliamperage serves to increase the number of photons produced at the target but is unrelated to their energy.

79. (A) The cervical intervertebral foramina lie 45° to the midsagittal plane and 15°–20° to a transverse plane. When the *posterior oblique* position (LPO and RPO) is used, the cervical intervertebral foramina demonstrated are those *further* from the IR. There is therefore some magnification of the foramina. In the *anterior oblique* position (LAO and RAO), the foramina disclosed are those *closer* to the IR.

80. (D) Proper *alignment* of the x-ray tube, body part, and IR is required to avoid image *distortion* in the form of *foreshortening* or *elongation*. *Foreshortening* will usually result when the *part* is out of alignment. *Elongation* is often a result of *angulation of the x-ray tube*. Grid lines or grid cutoff will occur when the *grid* itself is off center or is not in alignment with the x-ray tube.

81. (A) Important dosimetry considerations include not only the amount of radiation received but also the *type* of ionizing radiation and the degree of sensitivity of the irradiated *tissues*. Equivalent dose (*EqD*) is the product of absorbed dose (*D*) and radiation weighting factor (*W*$_r$). The weighting factor of x-rays and gamma radiation is 1;

the *W*$_r$ of beta particles is 10 and that of alpha particles is 20. The *EqD* unit of measure in biological material is the Sievert. Effective dose (EfD) describes the dose to specific *tissues* (*W*$_t$), as well as exposure from particular type(s) of radiation. Reproductive cells are highly radiosensitive and have a weighting factor of 0.2. Stomach, colon, and lung tissues have a weighting factor of 0.12. The weighting factor of liver, esophagus, thyroid, bladder, and breast tissues is 0.05. Skin is relatively radiation insensitive; its weighting factor is 0.01. EfD is the product of absorbed dose (*D*), radiation weighting factor (*W*$_r$), and tissue weighting factor (*W*$_t$). Its unit of measure is the Sievert. EfD can be used to express the amount of radiation received in a particular x-ray examination. TEDE, total effective dose equivalent, is the sum of effective dose equivalent from external and internal radiation sources. It is useful for occupational exposure, particularly to those in higher radiation areas such as interventional procedures and nuclear medicine. The TEDE limit to the occupationally exposed is 0.05 Sievert (50 mSv) and 0.001 Sievert (1.0 mSv) for the general public.

82–84. (82, A; 83, B; 84, C) The *stomach* is the dilated, saclike portion of the GI tract. When the stomach (or a portion of it) is empty, its mucosal lining forms soft folds called *rugae* (L). Exteriorly, the stomach presents a *greater curvature* (K) on its lateral surface and a *lesser curvature* (J) on its medial surface. The proximal opening of the stomach is the cardiac sphincter; the pyloric sphincter is located at its distal end. The portion of the stomach around the distal esophagus is called the *cardia;* that portion superior to the esophageal juncture is the *fundus* (A). The major portion of the stomach is the *body* (B); the distal portion is the *pylorus* (C). The *incisura angularis* (I) is located on the lesser curvature and marks the beginning of the pylorus (C). The distal opening of the pylorus is the pyloric sphincter. The small intestine is composed of the duodenum, jejunum, and ileum. The duodenum is the shortest portion (~12 inches). It begins just beyond the pyloric sphincter and is divided into four portions: the *duodenal cap* or *bulb* (D), *descending duodenum* (E), transverse duodenum, and *ascending duodenum* (F). These portions form the C-shaped *duodenal loop* that is occupied by the *head of the pancreas* (G). The ascending duodenum terminates at the duodenojejunal flexure that marks the beginning of the 9-foot *jejunum* (H). It should be noted that the lengths of intestine usually quoted are those present at autopsy and can be up to 50% longer than actual (living) size because of loss of muscle tone following death.

85. (C) Because the fundus is the most *posterior* portion of the stomach, it readily fills with barium when the patient is in the *AP* or *LPO* position. With the patient in the *PA* or *RAO* position, the barium moves to the more distal portions of the stomach. Figure 14-8 illustrates the RAO position. It is in this position that peristalsis is most active and the stomach's emptying mechanism can be evaluated. To evaluate the stomach adequately, preliminary patient preparation is required. The upper GI tract must be empty; patients should be questioned about their preparation and a preliminary "scout image" taken to check abdominal contents.

86. (C) Many people believe that potential legal and ethical issues can be avoided by creating an *advance health care directive* or *living will*. Because all persons have the right to make decisions regarding their own health care, this legal document preserves that right in the event an individual is unable to make those decisions. The directive names the individual authorized to make all health care decisions and can include specifics regarding *DNR, DNI,* and/or other end-of-life decisions.

87. (C) Because the anode's focal track is beveled (angled, facing the cathode), x-ray photons can freely diverge toward the cathode end of the x-ray tube. However, the "heel" of the focal track prevents x-ray photons from diverging toward the anode end of the tube. This results in varying intensity from the anode to the cathode, fewer photons at the anode end, and more photons at the cathode end. *The anode heel effect is most noticeable using large IR sizes, short SIDs, and steep target angles.*

88. (A) *Shuttering* is used to remove the bright unexposed areas outside of the collimated field that contribute to *veil glare*. Glare interferes with accurate perception of details. Shuttering is *never* a substitute for adequate collimation.

89. (C) A *pulse oximeter* is used to measure a patient's pulse rate and oxygen saturation level. A *stethoscope* and a *sphygmomanometer* are used together to measure blood pressure. The first sound heard is the systolic pressure and the normal range is 110–140 mm Hg. When no more sound is heard, the diastolic pressure is recorded. The normal diastolic range is 60–90 mm Hg. Elevated blood pressure is called *hypertension. Hypotension,* low blood pressure, is not of concern unless it is caused by injury or disease; in that case, it results in shock.

90. (C) The development of male and female reproductive stem cells has important radiation protection implications. Male reproductive stem cells reproduce continuously. However, the female reproductive stem cells develop only during fetal life; women are born with all the reproductive cells they will ever have. Children have their reproductive futures ahead of them.

91. (A) Some x-ray circuit devices, such as transformers and autotransformers, will operate only on AC. The efficient operation of the x-ray tube, however, requires the use of unidirectional current, so current must be *rectified* before it gets to the x-ray tube. The process of full-wave rectification changes the negative half-cycle to a useful positive half-cycle. An x-ray circuit rectification system is located between the secondary coil of the high-voltage transformer and the x-ray tube. Rectifiers are solid-state diodes made of *semiconductive materials* such as silicon, selenium, or germanium that conduct electricity *in only one direction.* Thus, a series of rectifiers placed between the transformer and the x-ray tube function to change AC to a more useful unidirectional current.

92. (B) The *quantity* of x-ray photons produced at the target is the function of mAs. The *quality* (wavelength, penetration, and energy) of x-ray photons produced at the target is the function of kV. The kV also has an effect on exposure rate, because an increase in kV increases the number of high-energy x-ray photons produced at the target. Exposure rate *decreases* with an increase in SID.

93. (B) Anemia is a blood condition characterized by a decreased number of circulating red blood cells and decreased hemoglobin levels and has many causes. Adequate hemoglobin is required to provide oxygen to the body. Anemia is treated according to its cause. *Hematuria* is the term used to describe blood in the urine and is unrelated to anemia.

94. (C) Grids are composed of alternating strips of lead and radiolucent interspace material. The interspace material is either aluminum or plastic fiber. Aluminum resists moisture, is sturdier, and provides a "smoother" appearance with less visible grid lines—but requires a higher mAs and therefore increases patient dose. Plastic fiber interspace material can be affected by moisture, resulting in warping. Carbon fiber is often used as IP-front material because of its durability and homogeneity.

95. (C) The greatest effect of, and response to, irradiation is brought about by a *large dose of radiation, to the whole body, delivered all at one time*. Whole-body radiation can depress many body functions. With a fractionated dose, the effects would be less severe because the body would have an opportunity to repair between doses.

96. (C) There are four sets of paranasal sinuses: (i) *frontal*, (ii) *ethmoidal*, (iii) *maxillary*, and (iv) *sphenoidal* (Fig. 14-9). The left and right *frontal* sinuses (*number 1*) are usually asymmetrical and are located behind the glabella and superciliary arches of the frontal bone. The *ethmoidal* sinuses (*number 2*) are composed of 6–18 thin-walled air cells occupying the bony labyrinth of the ethmoid bone. The *frontal* and *ethmoidal sinuses* are demonstrated in the PA axial projection (Caldwell position). The *maxillary* sinuses (antra of Highmore; *number 4*) are the largest of the paranasal sinuses and are located in the body of the maxillae. They are particularly prone to infection and collections of stagnant mucus. The maxillary sinuses are well demonstrated in the *parietoacanthial* projection (Waters position). The *sphenoidal* sinuses (*number 3*) are located in the body of the sphenoid bone and are usually asymmetrical. They are well demonstrated in the *submentovertical (SMV)* projection. All paranasal sinuses are demonstrated in the *lateral* projection, although the left and right of each group are superimposed. Radiography of the paranasal sinuses must be performed in the erect position so that any *fluid levels* may be demonstrated and to distinguish between fluid and other pathology such as *polyps*.

97. (C) In the *AP* projection, the proximal fibula is at least partially superimposed on the lateral tibial condyle. *Medial rotation* of 45° will "open" the proximal tibiofibular articulation. *Lateral rotation* will obscure the articulation even more.

98. (A) Some chemical agents used in health care facilities function to *kill* pathogenic microorganisms, whereas others function to *inhibit the growth/spread* of pathogenic microorganisms. Germicides and disinfectants are used to kill pathogenic microorganisms, and antiseptics (such as alcohol) are used to stop their growth/spread. *Sterilization* is another associated term and refers to killing of all microorganisms and their spores.

99. (B) Epinephrine (Adrenalin) is the vasopressor used to treat an anaphylactic reaction or cardiac arrest. *Nitroglycerin* is a vasodilator. *Hydrocortisone* is a steroid that may be used to treat bronchial asthma, allergic reactions, and inflammatory reactions. *Digitoxin* is used to treat cardiac fibrillation.

100. (C) Grids are used in radiography to *absorb scattered radiation* before it reaches the IR, thus improving radiographic contrast. Contrast obtained with a grid compared with contrast without a grid is termed *contrast improvement factor*. The greater the percentage of scattered radiation absorbed than absorbed nonscattered radiation, the greater the "selectivity" of the grid. If a grid absorbs an abnormally large amount of useful/primary radiation because of improper centering, tube angle, or tube distance, *grid cutoff* occurs.

101. (D) Normal tissue variants and pathologic processes that alter tissue thickness and composition can have a significant effect on image density. The radiographer must be aware of these variants and processes to make an appropriate and accurate selection of technical factors. Normal variants of muscle development result from different lifestyles, occupations, and age and will affect image density. Other than normal variants that influence image density/brightness and, consequently, the selection of technical factors are age, gender, and pathology. Various abnormal pathologic conditions, disease processes, and trauma can affect tissue density and hence density.

Some pathologic conditions are called *destructive*, such as osteoporosis, osteomalacia, pneumoperitoneum, emphysema, and conditions involving necrosis or atrophy. These conditions can cause an undesirable increase in image density unless they are recognized and appropriate changes made in exposure factors. Other conditions such as ascites, rheumatoid arthritis, and Paget's disease are *additive*, and an increase in exposure factors is required to maintain adequate density/brightness.

102. (B) The bony walls of the orbit are thin, fragile, and subject to fracture. A direct blow to the eye results in a pressure that can cause fracture. That fracture is usually to the *orbital floor* (inferior aspect of the bony orbit). Because the fracture results from increased pressure within the eye, it is called a "blowout" fracture.

103. (D) The advantages of DF over conventional fluoroscopy include higher speed acquisition and availability of postprocessing for image/contrast enhancement. Although DF fundamentally appears the same as conventional fluoroscopy, DF has special requirements: a computer, two video monitors, and an operating console that is far more complex than the conventional console. A computer is located between the TV camera (or CCD) and the TV monitor and serves to convert the analog image to a digital image. The operating console has many special function keys for patient data entry, data acquisition, image display, and image postprocessing manipulation. Two video monitors are required; the second monitor is for display of the subtracted image.

104. (C) When the barium fluorohalide absorbs x-ray energy, electrons are released and they divide into two groups: One electron group initiates *immediate lumines-cence* during the excited state of Eu^{2+}; the other electron group becomes trapped within the phosphor's halogen ions, forming a "color center." These are the phosphors that ultimately form the radiographic image because when exposed to a *monochromatic* laser light source, these phosphors emit *polychromatic* light, termed *photo-stimulated luminescence*.

The PSP layer (or SPS) can *store* its latent image for several hours; however, after approximately 8 h, notice-able image *fading* will occur. The europium activator is important for the *storage* characteristic of the PSPs; it also has functions similar to the sensitization specks within film emulsion. Without europium, the image will not become manifest.

105. (B) Late, long-term effects of radiation can occur in tissues that have survived a previous irradiation months or years earlier. These late effects, such as carcinogenesis and genetic effects, are "all-or-nothing" effects—either the organism develops cancer or it does not. Most late effects *do not have a threshold dose;* that is, *any* dose, however small, theoretically can induce an effect. Increasing that dose increases the likelihood of the occurrence but does not affect its severity; these effects are termed *stochastic. Nonstochastic effects* are those that do not occur below a particular threshold dose and that increase in severity as the dose increases.

106. (C) A certain amount of object unsharpness is an inherent part of every radiographic image because of the position and shape of anatomic structures within the body.

For the shape of anatomic structures to be accurately recorded, the structures must be *parallel* to the *x-ray tube* (*perpendicular* to the CR) and the *IR* and *aligned* with the *CR.*

Image details away from the path of the CR will be exposed by more divergent rays, resulting in *rotation distortion*. This is why the CR must be directed to the part of greatest interest.

The shape of anatomic structures lying at an angle within the body or placed away from the CR will be mis-represented on the IR. There are two types of shape distor-tion. If a linear structure is not parallel to the long axis of the part/body and not parallel to the IR, that anatomic structure will appear *smaller*—it will be *foreshortened*. On the other hand, *elongation* occurs when the x-ray tube is angled.

107. (C) Tissue cell radiosensitivity is influenced by their degree of maturity, their degree of mitotic activity, and

their particular function. Immature (undifferentiated or precursor) cells are more radiosensitive. Spermatogonia are primitive male sex cells and the most radiosensitive of the three. Osteoblasts have intermediate radiosensi-tivity, whereas myocytes (muscle cells) have less mitotic activity and are the least radiosensitive of the three listed.

108. (C) When the IP is accepted by the scanner/reader, the PSP is automatically removed. The PSP's latent image is converted to a *visible PSL image* as it is moved and scanned by a narrow monochromatic *high-intensity helium–neon laser* or *solid-state* laser to obtain the pixel data.

To improve the image SNR and maintain spatial resolution, the image-carrying PSL must be a different wavelength (color) from, and physically separate from, that of the laser excitation light. An *optical filter* is used that permits *transmission* of the PSL but *attenuates* the laser light; this filter is mounted in front of a photo-multiplier tube (PMT).

The PMT or photodiode (PD) is used to detect and collect the PSL's analog data and convert it to electrical signals. The electrical energy is sent to an *ADC* where it becomes the *digital* image that can be displayed and/or printed out by a laser printer. The digitized images can also be manipulated in *postprocessing*, electronically *transmitted*, and stored/*archived*.

109. (C) Angina pectoris is a spasmodic chest pain fre-quently caused by oxygen deficiency in the myocardium. The pain often radiates down the left arm and up to the left jaw. Angina pectoris attacks are frequently associ-ated with exertion or emotional stress in individuals with coronary artery disease. Pain may be relieved with a vasodilator such as *nitroglycerin* given sublingually or transdermally. *Digitalis* is used to treat congestive heart failure. *Dilantin* is used in the control of seizure disorders, and *Tagamet* is used to treat duodenal ulcers.

110. (B) The average *female* (*gynecoid*) *pelvis* differs from the average *male* (*android*) *pelvis* in that it is shallower, and its bones are generally more delicate. The pelvic outlet is wider and more circular in the female; the ischial tuberosi-ties and acetabula are further apart; and the angle formed by the pubic arch is also greater in the female. All these bony characteristics facilitate the birth process.

Following are the male (android) pelvis characteristics:

- Narrower, more vertical
- Deeper from anterior to posterior
- Pubic angle smaller
- Pelvic inlet narrower and heart-shaped/round

111. (B) Radiographic contrast is described as the difference between densities in the radiographic image. It is the function of radiographic contrast to make details visible. Radiographs exhibiting many shades of gray are said to possess *long-scale,* or *low,* radiographic contrast; that is, there are *many grays,* and there is only *little difference between the various shades of gray.* Conversely, radiographs exhibiting *few shades of gray* are said to possess *short-scale,* or *high,* radiographic contrast. These images have a very *noticeable difference between radiographic densities.*

112. (A) Injectable medications are available in two different kinds of containers. An *ampule* usually holds a single dose of medication. A *vial* is a small bottle that holds several doses of the medication. The term *bolus* is used to describe an amount of fluid to be injected. A *carafe* is a narrow-mouthed container not likely to be used for medical purposes.

113. (B) An increase in kilovoltage (photon energy) will result in a *greater number* (i.e., exposure rate) of scattered photons (Compton interaction). These scattered photons carry no useful information and contribute to radiation *fog.* Using manual technique, or in analog imaging, an increase in kV produces a *decrease* in (i.e., *lower*) image contrast.

114. (D) The distal humerus articulates with the proximal radius and ulna to form the elbow joint. At its proximal end, the ulna presents the *olecranon process,* found at the proximal and posterior end of the *semilunar (trochlear) notch.* The *coronoid process* is seen at the distal and anterior end of the semilunar notch. Specifically, the semilunar notch of the ulna articulates with the trochlea of the distal medial humerus. The *capitulum* is lateral to the trochlea and articulates with the radial head.

115. (B); 116. (C) Figure 14-10 shows an AP projection of the elbow joint. The distal humerus articulates with the radius and ulna to form the elbow joint. The lateral aspect of the distal humerus presents a raised, smooth, rounded surface—the *capitulum* (E)—that articulates with the superior surface of the *radial head* (A). The *trochlea* (F) is on the medial aspect of the distal humerus and articulates with the semilunar notch of the ulna. Just proximal to the capitulum and trochlea are the *lateral* (D) and *medial* (C) *epicondyles*; the medial is more prominent and palpable. The coronoid fossa is found on the anterior distal humerus and functions to accommodate the *coronoid process* (B) with the elbow in flexion.

117. (B) The patient is the most important radiation scatterer during both radiography and fluoroscopy. In general, at 1 m from the patient, *the intensity is reduced by a factor of 1000* to approximately 0.1% of the original intensity. Successive scatterings can render the intensity to unimportant levels.

118. (D) The "scapular Y" refers to the characteristic *Y* formed by the body of the scapula, acromion, and coracoid processes. The patient is positioned in a PA oblique position—an RAO or LAO, depending on which is the affected side. The midcoronal plane is adjusted approximately 60° to the IR, and the affected arm is left relaxed at the patient's side. The scapular Y position is used to *demonstrate anterior* (subcoracoid) or *posterior* (subacromial) *humeral dislocation.* The humerus is normally superimposed on the scapula in this position; any deviation from this may indicate dislocation.

119. (B) Magnification is part of every radiographic image. Anatomic parts within the body are at various distances from the IR and therefore have various degrees of magnification. The formula used to determine amount of image magnification is

$$\frac{\text{Image size}}{\text{Object size}} = \frac{\text{SID}}{\text{SOD}}$$

Substituting known values:

$$\frac{x}{3''} = \frac{36'' \text{ SID}}{32'' \text{ SOD}} = (\text{SOD} = \text{SID} - \text{OID})$$
$$32x = 108$$
$$x = 3.37 \text{ image width}$$

120. (A) Sternoclavicular joints should be performed in a PA position whenever possible to keep OID to a minimum. The *oblique* position (15°) opens the joint *closest* to the IR. The erect position may be used but is not required. Weight-bearing images are not recommended.

121. (D) The greater and lesser tubercles are prominences on the proximal humerus separated by the intertubercular (bicipital) groove. The AP projection of the humerus/shoulder places the *epicondyles parallel to the IR* and the shoulder in *external rotation* and demonstrates the *greater tubercle in profile.* The lateral projection of the humerus places the shoulder in extreme internal rotation with the epicondyles perpendicular to the IR and demonstrates the lesser tubercle in profile.

122. (C) Radiographic examinations of the large bowel generally include the AP or PA axial position to "open" the S-shaped sigmoid colon, the lateral position especially for the rectum, and the LAO and RAO (or LPO and RPO) to "open" the colic flexures. Left and right decubitus positions are usually used only in double-contrast BEs to better demonstrate double contrast of the medial and lateral walls of the ascending and descending colon.

123. (C) Protective or "reverse" isolation is used to keep the susceptible patient from becoming infected. Patients who have suffered burns have lost a very important means of protection, their skin, and therefore have increased susceptibility to bacterial invasion. Patients whose immune systems are depressed lose the ability to combat infection and hence are more susceptible to infection. Active tuberculosis requires airborne precautions.

124. (B) Film images can be scanned and digitized by a special machine called an image digitizer. Interpretation of digital images is made from the *LED* display monitor; this is called "soft copy display." "Hard copies" can be made with a *laser printer*. A *laser camera* records the displayed image by exposing a film with laser light; it can also record several images on one film. The *laser printer* is connected for processing of the images.

125. (C) The spatial resolution of direct digital systems is fixed and is related to the *DEL* size of the TFT and its *fill factor*. The DEL is the sensing element of the TFT and its largest portion should be used for its sensing function to maintain/improve resolution. For example, if 25% of the DEL is used for other functions, the DEL is said to have a *fill factor* of 75%.

The larger the TFT DEL size, and the larger the fill factor, the better the spatial resolution. DEL size of 100 μm provides a spatial resolution of about 5 lp/mm (available only in some digital mammography systems). DEL size of 200 μm provides a spatial resolution of about 2.5 lp/mm (general radiography)—lower than that achieved with a 400-speed-intensifying screen in analog systems. A 100-speed-intensifying screen system offers a spatial resolution of about 10 lp/mm—significantly greater than, and currently unachievable in, digital imaging.

126. (B) Patients who are able to cooperate are usually able to control *voluntary* motion if they are provided with an adequate explanation of the procedure. Once patients understand what is needed, most will cooperate to the best of their ability (by suspending respiration and holding still for the exposure). Certain body functions and responses, such as heart action, peristalsis, pain, and muscle spasm, cause *involuntary* motion uncontrollable by the patient. The best way to control involuntary and voluntary motion is by always selecting the shortest possible exposure time. Voluntary motion may also be minimized by careful explanation, immobilization, and (as a last resort and only in certain cases) restraint.

127. (C) The *manubrial* or *jugular notch* Is the depression on the superior border of the manubrium and is located at the level of the *third thoracic* vertebra. The *vertebra prominens* is at the level of the *seventh cervical* vertebra.

128. (B) An AEC is calibrated to produce radiographic densities as required by the radiologist for interpretation purposes. Once the part being radiographed has been exposed to produce the required optical density, the AEC automatically terminates the exposure. The manual timer should be used as a *backup timer* should the AEC fail to terminate the exposure, thus protecting the patient from overexposure and the x-ray tube from excessive *heat* load. *Circuit breakers* and *fuses* are circuit devices used to protect circuit elements from overload. In case of current surge, the circuit is broken (opened), thus preventing equipment damage. A *rheostat* is a type of variable resistor.

129. (C) Digital image postprocessing provides the opportunity for image optimization. Image annotation permits placement of labels, arrow indicators, and so on. Windowing allows adjustment of image contrast and/or brightness to diagnostic requirements. Contrast scale enhancement is the most valuable tool in digital imaging. Image minification, with larger matrix sizes, enables us to see tiny anatomic details and improve spatial resolution. Image inversion, or reversal, provides a different perspective by changing white to black and black to white. Image flip also provides another perspective by enabling us to rotate the image. Edge enhancement is useful for small and high-contrast tissues. Other postprocessing functions include highlighting, zoom, pan, and scroll. The pixel shift feature is important in digital subtraction angiography. Image subtraction is used to enhance contrast. If the part moves during acquisition of serial images, misregistration occurs, making the required exact superimposition impossible. Pixel shift is a function that can correct misregistration. Another emerging postprocessing task used in diagnostic functions is determining numeric pixel value for particular ROI (region of interest). This feature has proved useful in bone densitometry, renal calculus recognition, and calcified lung nodule identification.

130. (B) X-ray images are often subpoenaed as court evidence in cases of medical litigation. In order to be considered as legitimate legal evidence, each x-ray image must contain certain essential and specific patient information. Essential information that *must* be included on each image is patient identification, the identity of the facility where the x-ray study was performed, the date on which the study was performed, and a right- or left-side marker.

Other useful information that *may* be included, but that is not considered essential, is additional patient demographics such as their date of birth, identity of the referring physician, time of day when the study was performed, and identity/initials of the radiographer performing the examination.

131. (B) When the foot is positioned for a lateral projection, the plantar surface should be perpendicular to the IR so as to superimpose the metatarsals. This may be accomplished with the patient lying on either the affected or unaffected side (usually affected), that is, mediolateral or lateromedial. The talofibular articulation is best demonstrated in the medial oblique projection of the ankle.

132. (B) Exposure-type artifacts are those that appear on the radiograph as a result of image formation processes and are probably the most common type of image artifact. A *foreign body* in the IP or within the body part will cast its image on the radiographic image. Similarly, artifacts commonly occur from closing, dentures, jewelry, and imaging accessories. These are *exposure-type artifacts*. In Figure 14-11, a right lateral decubitus projection of the gallbladder, a foam pad, and the sheet have been imaged to produce the exposure artifact. *Processing artifacts* occur during PSP processing as a result of equipment malfunction/error.

133. (C) Technical factors that are used to regulate the *number* (intensity) of x-ray photons produced at the target are milliamperage and exposure time (mAs). Beam intensity and exposure dose are directly proportional to mAs; if the mAs is cut in half, the number of x-ray photons will decrease by one-half. Although kV is used primarily to regulate beam quality it does have an impact on been intensity, although the relationship is not proportional.

134. (D) The majority of cell damage occurring after irradiation is repairable. The three types of potential damage to *DNA* are base damage, single-strand break, and double-strand break. Of these, base damage and single-strand break are more readily repairable whereas double-strand DNA break can be more problematic. In cell cycle arrest, the cell can temporarily stop trying to repair itself. *Cell cycle arrest* can occur between the G1 and S stages, during S, or between G2 and M. The human body works to take care of its whole unit. If a cell and/or its genetic content are damaged enough so that its progeny could lead to production of malignant neoplasm or death of the whole unit, it is far better that the cell be sacrificed for the well-being of the whole unit (entire body). That is termed *apoptosis*, "cell suicide," for the benefit of the whole unit.

135. (A) The mechanical device used to correct an ineffectual cardiac rhythm is a *defibrillator*. The two paddles attached to the unit are placed on a patient's chest and used to introduce an electric current in an effort to correct the dysrhythmia. A *cardiac monitor* is used to display, and sometimes record, electrocardiogram (ECG) readings and some pressure readings. The *crash cart* is a supply cart with various medications and equipment necessary for treating a patient who is suffering from a myocardial infarction or other serious medical emergencies. It is periodically checked and restocked, usually by nursing staff, although radiographers may be responsible for a daily check of the plastic throwaway locks. These locks are used to ensure that the cart has not been tampered with or supplies inadvertently used in nonemergency situations. A resuscitation bag is used for ventilation, for example, during cardiopulmonary resuscitation.

136. (C) There are many terms (with which the radiographer must be familiar) that are used to describe radiographic positioning techniques. *Cephalad* refers to that which is toward the head, and *caudad* to that which is toward the feet. Structures close to the source or beginning are said to be *proximal*, whereas those lying close to the midline are said to be *medial*.

137. (C) When barium fluorohalide absorbs x-ray energy, *electrons are released and they divide into two groups*: One electron group initiates *immediate* luminescence during the excited state of Eu^{2+}; the other electron group becomes *trapped* within the phosphor's halogen ions, forming a "color center." These trapped phosphors are the phosphors that ultimately form the radiographic image because when exposed to a *monochromatic* laser light source, these phosphors emit *polychromatic* light, termed *photostimulated luminescence*. The PSP layer *stores* its latent image for several hours; however, after approximately 8 h, noticeable image *fading* will occur. The europium activator is important for the *storage* characteristic of the PSPs; it also has functions similar to the sensitization specks within film emulsion; without europium, the image will not become manifest.

138. (A) A *fistula* is an abnormal tubelike passageway between organs or an organ and the surface. Fistulas can result from abscesses, injuries, malignancies, inflammation of neighboring tissues, and ionizing radiation exposure. A *polyp* is a tumor with either a pedicle (pedunculated, or having a stalk) or a broad base (sessile), commonly found in vascular organs projecting inward from its mucosal wall. They are usually removed surgically because, although usually benign, they can become malignant. A *diverticulum* is an *outpouching* from the wall of an organ, such as the colon. An *abscess* is a localized collection of pus as a result of inflammation.

139. (D) When performing GI radiography, the position of the stomach may vary depending on the respiratory phase, body habitus, and patient position. *Inspiration* causes the lungs to fill with air and the diaphragm to descend, thereby pushing the abdominal contents downward. On *expiration*, the diaphragm will rise, allowing the abdominal organs to ascend. The *body habitus* is an important factor in determining the size and shape of the stomach. An asthenic patient may have a long, J-shaped stomach, whereas the stomach may be transverse in a hypersthenic patient. The body habitus is an important consideration in determining the positioning and placement of the IR. The *patient position* can also alter the position of the stomach. If a patient turns from the RAO position into the AP position, the stomach will move into a more horizontal position. Although the cardiac sphincter and the pyloric sphincter are relatively fixed, the fundus is quite mobile and will vary in position.

140. (A) The type of shock associated with pooling of blood in the peripheral vessels is classified as *neurogenic shock*. This occurs in cases of trauma to the central nervous system, resulting in decreased arterial resistance and pooling of blood in peripheral vessels. *Cardiogenic shock* is related to cardiac failure, as a result of interference with heart function. It can occur in cases of cardiac tamponade, pulmonary embolus, or myocardial infarction. *Hypovolemic shock* is related to loss of large amounts of blood, from either internal bleeding or hemorrhage associated with trauma. *Septic shock* is a result of massive infection; *anaphylactic shock* results from contact with substances to which the individual has become sensitized, for example, a medication or bee sting.

141. (A) The *AP axial* projection (Towne method) of the skull is used to demonstrate the *occipital* bone. The skull is positioned AP and the CR is directed caudally. This serves to project the anterior structures inferiorly and away from superimposition on the occipital bone. The frontal bone is best demonstrated in the PA projection and the facial bones in the parietoacanthial (Waters) position. The sphenoid bone can be seen in the lateral and basal projections.

142. (D) Surface landmarks, prominences, and depressions are useful to the radiographer in locating anatomic structures not visible externally. The *costal margin* is at about the same level as L3. The *umbilicus* is approximately at the same level as the L3–L4 interspace. The *xiphoid* tip is at about the same level as T10. The fourth lumbar vertebra is approximately at the same level as the *iliac crest*.

143. (D) In the CR reader, a PMT or PD is used to detect PSL and convert it to electrical signals. The electrical energy is sent to an ADC where it becomes the *digital image* that is displayed, after a short delay, on a high-resolution monitor.

In indirect-capture DR, a flat panel detector uses cesium iodide or gadolinium oxysulfide as the scintillator, that is, which captures x-ray photons and emits light. That light is then transferred directly to the ADC via a photodetector coupling agent—a CCD or TFT.

144. (C) An algorithm is a series of computerized step-by-step instructions used to solve a problem. The instructions are flexible, that is, variable, and various options are checked to produce the best possible results from the range of available options.

Radiographically speaking, the algorithm will test a range of variations to produce the best possible group of exposure factors for the anatomic particular part and circumstances.

145. (C) X-ray photons are produced in two ways as high-speed electrons interact with target atoms. First, if the high-speed electron is attracted by the nucleus of a tungsten atom and changes its course, the energy given up as the electron is "braked" in the form of an x-ray photon. This is called *bremsstrahlung* (braking) radiation and is responsible for the majority of x-ray photons produced at the conventional tungsten target. Second, a high-speed electron may eject a tungsten K-shell electron, leaving a vacancy in the shell. An electron from a higher energy level, for example, the L shell, drops down to fill the vacancy, emitting the difference in energy as a K-characteristic ray. *Characteristic radiation* comprises only approximately 15% of the primary beam.

146. (C) Swallowing dysfunction, or modified barium swallow, studies are performed to observe the swallowing mechanism. The radiographer prepares the patient and assists with the procedure. Thin and thick barium is prepared by the speech therapist for comparisons of swallowing mechanism. A very thick barium and/or a solid such as a cracker is also often used. The radiologist performs fluoroscopy and records images in the standing or seated lateral position.

147. (D) Anode target material of *high atomic number* produces higher energy x-rays more efficiently. Because a great deal of heat is produced at the target, the material should have a *high melting point* so as to avoid damage to the target surface. Most of the x-rays generated at the focal spot are directed downward and pass through the x-ray tube's *port window*. The cathode filament receives *low-voltage* current to heat it to the point of thermionic emission. Then *high voltage* is applied to drive the electrons across to the focal track.

148. (D) With inspiration, the diaphragm is depressed, that is, moved into a lower position. The ribs and sternum are elevated. As the ribs are elevated, their angle is decreased. Radiographic density can vary considerably in appearance depending on which phase of respiration the exposure is made.

149. (D) The four body types (from largest to smallest) are hypersthenic, sthenic, hyposthenic, and asthenic. The abdominal viscera of the *asthenic* person are generally located quite low, vertical, and toward the midline. The opposite is true of the *hypersthenic* person: Organs are located high, transverse, and laterally.

150. (D) Digital image storage is located in a *pixel*, which is a *two-dimensional* "*pi*cture *el*ement," measured in the *XY direction*. The third dimension, *Z* direction, in the matrix of pixels is the *depth* that is called the *voxel* (*vo*lume *el*ement). The *depth* of the block is the number of bits required to describe the gray level that each pixel can take on—known as the bit depth.

Bit depth in CT is approximately 2^{12} with a dynamic range of almost 5000 gray shades, approximately 2^{14} in CR/DR with a dynamic range of more than 16,000 gray shades, and approximately 2^{16} in digital mammography with a dynamic range of more than 65,500 gray shades. The matrix is the number of pixels in the *XY* direction. As matrix size increases, for a fixed FOV, pixel size is smaller and better spatial resolution results. An electronic/digital image is formed by a matrix of pixels in rows and columns. A matrix having 512 pixels in each row and column is a 512 × 512 matrix (a typical CT image).

The term *FOV* is used to describe how much of the patient is included in the matrix. Either the matrix or the FOV can be changed without one affecting the other, but changes in either will change pixel size. As FOV increases, for a fixed matrix size, the size of each pixel increases and spatial resolution decreases. Fewer and larger pixels result in a poor-resolution "pixelly" or "mosaicked" image, that is, one in which you can actually see the individual pixel boxes.

151. (D) Orthopnea is a respiratory condition in which the patient has difficulty breathing (*dyspnea*) in any position other than erect. The patient is usually comfortable in the erect, standing, or seated position. The *Trendelenburg position* places the patient's head lower than the rest of the body. The *Fowler position* is a semierect position, and the *recumbent position* is lying down.

152. (B) The radiograph in Figure 14-12 shows the odontoid process superimposed on the base of the skull. The maxillary teeth can be seen very superior to the base of the skull. *Bringing the chin down* will move the base of the skull up and permit visualization of the C1–C2 structures. A diagnostic image of C1–C2 depends on adjusting the flexion of the neck *so that the maxillary occlusal plane and the base of the skull are superimposed*. Accurate adjustment of these structures will usually allow good visualization of the odontoid process and the atlantoaxial articulation. Too much flexion superimposes teeth on the odontoid process; too much extension superimposes the base of the skull on the odontoid process.

153. (D) Phase of respiration is exceedingly important in thoracic radiography; lung expansion and the position of the diaphragm strongly influence the appearance of the finished radiograph. Inspiration and expiration radiographs of the chest are taken to demonstrate air in the pleural cavity (*pneumothorax*), to demonstrate *atelectasis* (partial or complete collapse of one or more pulmonary lobes) degree of *diaphragm excursion*, or to detect the presence of a *foreign body*. The expiration image will require a somewhat greater exposure to compensate for the diminished quantity of air in the lungs.

154. (C) Contrast media may be described as either positive (radiopaque) or negative (radiolucent). *Positive, or radiopaque, contrast agents* have a higher atomic number than the surrounding soft tissue, resulting in a greater attenuation or absorption of x-ray photons, thereby producing a higher radiographic contrast.

Examples of positive contrast media are iodinated (both water- and oil-based) agents and barium sulfate suspensions. *Negative,* or *radiolucent, contrast agents* used are air and various gases. Because the atomic number of air is also quite different from that of soft tissue, an artificially high subject contrast can be produced. The advantage of carbon dioxide over air is that it is absorbed more rapidly by the body.

155. (C) The most important precaution in the practice of aseptic technique is proper hand hygiene. The radiographer's hands should be thoroughly washed with soap and warm running water, for at least 15 s before and after each patient examination, or by using an alcohol sanitizer. If the faucet cannot be operated with the knee, it should be opened and closed using paper towels. The hands and forearms should always be kept lower than the elbows; care should be taken to wash all surfaces and between fingers. The radiographer's uniform should not touch the sink. Hand lotions should be used to prevent hands from chapping; broken skin permits the entry of microorganisms. Disinfectants, antiseptics, and germicides are substances used to kill pathogenic bacteria; they are frequently used in handwashing substances. Alcohol-based hand sanitizers have been recommended as an alternative to handwashing with soap and water, except when there is visible soiling or after caring for a patient with *Clostridium difficile* infection.

156. (D) The *developing fetus* is particularly sensitive to radiation exposure. The law of Bergonié and Tribondeau states that *stem cells,* which give rise to a specific type of cell, as in hematopoiesis, are particularly radiosensitive, as are *young cells* and tissues. It also states that *cells with a high rate of proliferation* (mitosis) are more sensitive to radiation. Radiation exposure, especially between the 2nd and 6th weeks following conception (the period of major organogenesis), can cause *organ damage, intellectual disability, growth retardation, microcephaly,* and *genital deformities.*

157. (B) High kilovoltage exposures produce large amounts of scattered radiation, and high ratio grids are often used with high kilovoltage techniques in an effort to absorb more of this scattered radiation. However, as more scattered radiation is absorbed, *more primary radiation is absorbed* as well. This accounts for the *increase in mAs required* when changing from 8:1 to 16:1 grid. In addition, precise *centering* and *positioning* become more critical; a small degree of inaccuracy is *more likely to cause grid cutoff* in a high ratio grid.

158. (A) AEC devices function to produce consistent and comparable image results. In one type of AEC, there is an *ionization chamber* just beneath the tabletop above the IR. The part to be examined is centered to the sensor(s) and radiographed. When a predetermined quantity of ionization has occurred (equal to the correct receptor exposure), the x-ray exposure terminates automatically. In the *phototimer* type of AEC, a small fluorescent screen is positioned beneath the IR. When remnant radiation emerging from the patient exposes the PSP (or film) and exits, the fluorescent screen emits light. Once a predetermined amount of fluorescent light is "seen" by the photocell sensor, the exposure is terminated.

A scintillation camera is used in nuclear medicine. A photocathode is an integral part of the image intensification system.

159. (B) Pixel size is determined by dividing the FOV by the matrix. In this case, the FOV is 20 cm; because the answer is expressed in millimeters, first change 20 cm to 200 mm. Then 200 divided by 512 equals 0.39 mm:

$$20\ cm = 200\ mm$$
$$200 \div 512 = 0.39\ mm/pixel$$

FOV and matrix size are independent of one another; that is, either can be changed, and the other will remain unaffected. However, pixel size is affected by changes in either FOV or matrix size. For example, if matrix size is increased, pixel size decreases. If FOV is increased, pixel size increases. Pixel size is inversely related to resolution. As pixel size increases, resolution decreases.

160. (B) In *digital* imaging, brightness and contrast are determined by computer software and monitor controls. *However, the principal factor in good digital image visibility and patient dose is still the result of proper IR exposure.* Selection of kV and mAs in digital imaging is similar to analog imaging, that is, kV still determines *penetration but not contrast*; mAs still determines *dose* but has *no impact on brightness.* The terms *density* and *brightness* do not mean the same thing and therefore are not used interchangeably.

161. (C) Fractures and/or dislocations of the cervical spine are usually caused by acute *hyperflexion* or *hyperextension* as a result of indirect trauma. *Whiplash* injury is caused by a sudden, forced movement in one direction and then the opposite direction (as in rear-end automobile impacts). Whiplash symptoms frequently include neck pain and stiffness, headache, and pain and numbness of the upper extremities. Whiplash is often evidenced radiographically by straightening or reversal of the normal lordotic curve and demonstrated in lateral projections performed in flexion and extension.

162. (B) Digital imaging EDR and *automatic rescaling* offer *wide* latitude and automatic optimization of the values of interest in the radiologic image. EDR, using the selected processing algorithm and its lookup table (LUT), enables compensation for approximately 80% underexposure and 500% overexposure. Although automatic/computerized optimization of the radiologic image is a wonderful tool, radiographers must be even more aware of their responsibility to keep patient dose to a minimum. Overexposure, although correctable via EDR, results in *increased patient dose;* underexposure results in decreased image quality because of increased image *noise.*

163. (B) DF offers *lower patient dose* because its x-ray beam is "pulsed," rather than continuous. The x-ray exposure turns on and off very quickly, thereby *reducing motion unsharpness* (i.e., increasing temporal resolution). Image acquisition rates are usually between 1 and 10 images per second. Fewer frames per second result in lower patient dose. Flat panel detectors have a *higher DQE*, higher temporal resolution, and higher contrast resolution. DF also offers "road-mapping" capability. During the fluoroscopic examination, the most recent fluoroscopic image can be stored on the monitor (image hold), reducing the need for continuous x-ray exposure and offering a significant reduction in patient and personnel radiation exposure.

164. (C) The term *dynamic range* refers to the number of shades of gray an imaging system can reproduce. Although the human eye can perceive about 30 shades of gray, and analog imaging can demonstrate about 1000 shades of gray, digital imaging can demonstrate more than 16,000 gray shades. The postprocessing function of *windowing* enables perception of many gray shades. This can also be called *contrast resolution.* The term *resolution* refers to the ability to see adjacent separate objects as separate and is measured in lp/mm. *MTF* expresses the mathematical process for *measuring* resolution.

165. (C) The components of the electromagnetic spectrum are identified in different ways. *Wavelength* is used to identify visible light. *Frequency* is used to identify radiowaves. Units of *energy* are used to identify ionizing electromagnetic radiations. The unit *keV* (kiloelectron volt) is used to identify the x-ray photon energies produced by diagnostic x-ray equipment. The unit *kV*

(kilovolts) describes the voltage required to produce the x-rays within the x-ray tube. The units mA and mAs are quantitative units identifying the number or quantity of x-rays available.

166. (A) A quality control program requires the use of a number of devices to test the efficiency of various parts of the imaging system. A *slit camera,* as well as a star-pattern or pinhole camera, is used to test focal spot size. A parallel-line resolution test pattern is used to test the resolution capability of intensifying screens.

167. (A) Parts being examined during fluoroscopic procedures change in thickness and density as the patient is required to change positions and as the fluoroscope is moved to examine different regions of the body that have varying thickness and tissue densities. The *ABC* functions to vary the required milliampere seconds and/or kilovoltage as necessary. With this method, patient dose varies, and image quality is maintained. Minification and flux gain contribute to total brightness gain.

168. (A) Figure 14-14 illustrates the aortic arch (number 1) and its three main branches—the brachiocephalic artery (number 6), the left common carotid artery (number 4), and the left subclavian artery (number 2). The right common carotid artery (number 5) and the right subclavian artery (number 7) are branches of the brachiocephalic artery. The vertebral arteries are the first main branches of the subclavian arteries. The left vertebral artery is labeled number 3.

169. (B) The pregnant radiographer poses a special radiation protection consideration, as the safety of the unborn individual must be considered. It must be remembered that the developing fetus is particularly sensitive to radiation exposure. Established guidelines state that the occupational radiation exposure to the *fetus* must not exceed 0.5 rem (500 mrem or 5 mSv) during the entire gestation period—not to exceed 50 mrem in 1 month.

170. (C) Category-specific isolations have been replaced by *transmission-based precautions: airborne, droplet,* and *contact.* Under these guidelines, some conditions or diseases can fall into more than one category. *Airborne precaution* is implemented with patients suspected or known to be infected with the *tubercle bacillus* (TB), *chickenpox* (varicella), and *measles* (rubeola). Airborne precaution *requires that the patient wear a mask* to avoid the spread of bronchial secretions or other pathogens during coughing. Aerosols can remain airborne for extended periods of time and may be inhaled. If the patient is unable or unwilling to wear a mask, the radiographer must wear one. The radiographer should wear gloves, but a gown is required only if flagrant contamination is likely. Patients under airborne precaution require a *private, specially ventilated (negative-pressure) room.*

A private room is also indicated for all patients on *droplet precaution,* that is, diseases transmitted via *large droplets* expelled from the patient while speaking, sneezing, or coughing. The pathogenic droplets can infect others when they come in contact with mouth or nasal mucosa or conjunctiva. *Rubella* (German measles), *mumps,* and *influenza* are among the diseases spread by droplet contact; *a private room is required* for the patient, and health care practitioners should use *gown* and *gloves.* Any diseases spread by direct or close *contact,* such as *MRSA* (methicillin-resistant *Staphylococcus aureus*), *conjunctivitis,* and *hepatitis A,* require *contact precaution. Contact precaution* procedures require a *private patient room* and the use of *gloves, mask,* and *gown* for anyone coming in direct contact with the infected individual or his or her environment.

171. (C) Obtaining a complete and accurate history from the patient for the radiologist is an important aspect of a radiographer's job. Both subjective and objective data should be collected. *Objective* data include signs and symptoms that can be observed such as a cough, a lump, or elevated blood pressure. *Subjective* data relate to what the patient feels and to what extent. A patient may experience pain, but is it mild or severe? Is it localized or general? Does the pain increase or decrease under different circumstances? A radiographer should explore this with the patient and document additional information on the requisition for the radiologist.

172. (A) The 45° oblique position of the lumbar spine is generally performed for demonstration of the zyg*apophyseal joints.* In a correctly positioned oblique lumbar spine, *Scotty dog* images are demonstrated. The Scotty dog's *ear* corresponds to the superior articular process, *nose* to the transverse process, *eye* to the pedicle, *neck* to the pars interarticularis, *body* to the lamina, and *front foot* to the inferior articular process.

173. (B) The pictured radiograph was made in the *left lateral decubitus* position. It is part of a series of radiographs made during an air-contrast (double-contrast) barium enema (BE) examination. A *double-contrast examination* of the large bowel is performed to see *through* the bowel to its posterior wall and to visualize any *intraluminal* (e.g., polypoid) *lesions* or *masses.* Various body positions are used to redistribute the barium and air. To demonstrate

the medial and lateral walls of the bowel, decubitus positions are performed. The radiograph presents a left lateral decubitus position because the *barium has gravitated* to the left side (the side of the splenic flexure). The *air rises* and delineates the medial side of the descending colon and the lateral side of the ascending colon.

174. (A) The x-ray tube's glass envelope and oil coolant are considered inherent (built-in) filtration. Thin sheets of aluminum are added to make *a total of at least 2.5-mm Al equivalent filtration in equipment operated above 70 kV.* This is done to remove the low-energy photons that serve to contribute only to patient skin dose.

175. (A) The CR scanner/reader recognizes numerous tissue density values of the part and constructs a *grayscale histogram* of these values represented in the imaged part. A histogram is a *graphic representation* defining all these values. The radiographer selects a *processing algorithm* by selecting the anatomic part and particular projection on the computer. The CR unit then matches that information with a particular LUT. Hence, *histogram analysis* and use of the appropriate LUT together function to produce predictable image quality in CR.

176. (A) Protective aprons and gloves are made of lead-impregnated vinyl or leather. They should be checked annually for cracks via radiographic or fluoroscopic means. Otherwise, minimal care is required. Lead aprons and gloves should always be hung on appropriate hangers. Glove supports permit air to circulate within the glove. Apron hangers provide convenient storage without folding. If lead aprons are folded, or left in a careless heap, cracks are more likely to form. If lead aprons or gloves become soiled, cleaning with a damp cloth and appropriate solution is all that is required. Excessive moisture should be avoided.

177. (C) Important dosimetry considerations include not only the amount of radiation received but also the *type* of ionizing radiation and the degree of sensitivity of the irradiated *tissues.* Equivalent dose (EqD) is the product of absorbed dose (D) and radiation weighting factor (W_r). The weighting factor of x-rays and gamma radiation is 1; the W_r of beta particles is 10, and that of alpha particles is 20. The EqD unit of measure in biological material is the Sievert. Effective dose (EfD) describes the dose to specific *tissues* (W_t), as well as exposure from particular type(s) of radiation. Reproductive cells are highly radiosensitive and have a weighting factor of 0.2. Stomach, colon, and lung tissues have weighting factor of 0.12. The weighting factor of liver, esophagus, thyroid, bladder, and breast tissues is 0.05. Skin is relatively radiation insensitive; its weighting factor is 0.01. EfD is the product of absorbed dose (D), radiation weighting factor (W_r), and tissue weighting factor (W_t). Its unit of measure is the Sievert. EfD can be used to express the amount of radiation received in a particular x-ray examination. *TEDE, total effective dose equivalent*, is the sum of effective dose equivalent from external and internal radiation sources. It is useful for occupational exposure, particularly to those in higher radiation areas such as interventional procedures and nuclear medicine. The TEDE limit to the occupationally exposed is 0.05 Sievert (50 mSv) and 0.001 Sievert (1.0 mSv) for the general public.

178. (D) The lead strips in a parallel grid are *parallel to each other* and therefore *not to the x-ray beam*. The more divergent the x-ray beam, the more likely there will be cutoff/*decreased* receptor exposure at the lateral edges of the radiograph. This problem becomes more pronounced at short SIDs. If there were a centering or tube angle problem, there would more likely be a noticeable receptor exposure *loss* on one side *or* the other.

179. (D) A controlled area is one that is occupied by radiation workers trained in radiation safety and who wear radiation monitors. The exposure rate in a *controlled area* must not exceed 100 mR/week; its occupancy factor is considered to be 1, indicating that the area may always be occupied and therefore requiring maximum shielding. An *uncontrolled area* is one occupied by the general population; the exposure rate there must not exceed 10 mR/week. Shielding requirements vary according to several factors, one being *occupancy factor*.

180. (D) Anatomical structures can be misrepresented because of their distance from the image receptor, because of their position with respect to the image receptor, and/or because of the direction/angulation of the central ray. This misrepresentation is termed distortion. The two types of distortion are size (magnification) and shape. Shape distortion is either foreshortening or elongation. Foreshortening occurs when the anatomic part is not parallel with the image receptor (A). Elongation occurs when the x-ray tube is angled (D). Positioning of the anatomic part and/or tube angulation can be used to advantage to remove superimposed structures so that others can be better visualized. Size distortion/magnification occurs when there is distance between the object being imaged and the image receptor (B and C). There are varying degrees of unavoidable size distortion/magnification in every x-ray image.

181. (A) The trachea (windpipe) bifurcates into left and right *mainstem bronchi,* each entering its respective lung hilum. The *left* bronchus divides into *two* portions, one for each lobe of the left lung. The *right* bronchus divides into *three* portions, one for each lobe of the right lung. The lungs are conical in shape, consisting of upper pointed portions, termed the *apices* (plural for apex), and the broad lower portions (or *bases*). The lungs are enclosed in a double-walled serous membrane called the *pleura*.

182. (A) When the shoulders are relaxed, the clavicles are usually carried below the pulmonary apices. To examine the portions of the lungs lying behind the clavicles, the CR is directed cephalad 15°–20° to project the clavicles above the apices when the patient is examined in the AP position.

183. (B) The effects of a quantity of radiation delivered to a body are dependent on the amount of radiation received, size of the irradiated area, and how the radiation is delivered in time. If the radiation is delivered in portions over a period of time, it is said to be *fractionated* and has a less harmful effect than if the radiation was delivered all at once. Therefore, cells have an opportunity to repair and some recovery occurs between doses.

184. (A) The approximately 5-foot long large intestine (colon) functions in the formation, transport, and evacuation of feces. The colon commences at the terminus of the small intestine; its first portion is the saclike *cecum* in the RLQ, located inferior to the ileocecal valve. The *ascending colon* is continuous with the cecum and is located along the right side of the abdominal cavity. It bends medially and anteriorly forming the right colic (*hepatic*) flexure. The colon traverses the abdomen as the *transverse colon* and bends posteriorly and inferiorly to form the left colic (*splenic*) flexure. The *descending colon* continues down the left side of the abdominal cavity and at about the level of the pelvic brim, in the LLQ, the colon moves medially to form the S-shaped *sigmoid* colon. The rectum, approximately 5 inches in length, lies between the sigmoid and the anal canal.

185. (D) Moving the image intensifier closer to the patient during fluoroscopy decreases the SID and patient dose (as SID is reduced, the intensity of the x-ray photons at the image intensifier's input phosphor increases; the ABC then automatically decreases the mA and therefore patient dose). Moving the image intensifier closer to the patient during fluoroscopy also decreases the OID and therefore magnification. As tissue density increases, a greater exposure dose is required.

186. (C) Major branches of the common carotid arteries (internal carotids) function to supply the anterior brain, whereas the posterior brain is supplied by the vertebral arteries (branches of the subclavian). The brachiocephalic (innominate) artery is unpaired and is one of the three branches of the aortic arch from which the right common carotid artery is derived. The left common carotid artery comes directly off the aortic arch.

187. (C) The brightness gain of image intensifiers is 5000–20,000. This increase is accomplished in two ways. First, as the electron image is focused on the output phosphor, it is accelerated by high voltage. (This is *flux gain*.) Second, the output phosphor is only a fraction of the size of the input phosphor, and this image size decrease represents another brightness gain, termed *minification gain*. *Total brightness gain is equal to the product of minification gain and flux gain.*

188. (C) The OSL is rapidly becoming the most commonly used personnel monitor nowadays. Film badges and TLDs have been successfully used for years. A pocket dosimeter is used primarily when working with large amounts of radiation and when a daily reading is desired.

189. (D) With the patient in the AP position, the scapula and the upper thorax are normally superimposed. With the arm abducted, elbow flexed, and hand supinated, much of the scapula is drawn away from the ribs. The patient should not be rotated toward the affected side, as this causes superimposition of ribs on the scapula. The exposure is made during quiet breathing to obliterate pulmonary vascular markings.

190. (A) The knee is formed by the proximal tibia, patella, and distal femur, which articulate to form the femorotibial and patellofemoral joints. The distal posterior femur presents two large medial and lateral condyles separated by the deep intercondyloid fossa. Two small prominences, the medial and lateral epicondyles, are just superior to the condyles. The femoral and tibial condyles articulate to form the femorotibial joint. In the lateral position, the *medial femoral condyle, being farther from the IR, is magnified.* Its magnified image obscures the knee joint space unless correction is made. Angulation of 5° cephalad will *superimpose the magnified medial femoral condyle on the lateral condyle* and permit a *better view of the joint space.*

191. (D) The eight cranial bones include the paired temporal bones. The temporal bones have a squamous portion, a mastoid portion, a petrous portion, and styloid portion. The three *processes* associated with each temporal bone are mastoid process, the zygomatic process, and the temporal styloid process.

192. (C) When caring for a patient with an indwelling Foley catheter, place the drainage bag and tubing *below the level of the bladder* to maintain the gravity flow of urine. Placement of the tubing or bag above or at level with the bladder will allow backflow of urine into the bladder. This reflux of urine can increase the chance of UTI.

193. (D) The greater the *number of electrons* comprising the electron stream and bombarding the target, the greater the number of x-ray photons produced. Although kV is usually associated with the energy of the x-ray photons, because *a greater number of more energetic electrons* will produce more x-ray photons, an increase in kV will also increase the *number* of photons produced. Specifically, the quantity of radiation produced increases as the *square* of the kV. The material composition of the tube target also plays an important role in the number of x-ray photons produced. The higher the *atomic number,* the denser and more closely packed the atoms comprising the material, therefore the greater the chance of an interaction between a high-speed electron and target material.

194. (B) The most effective method of sterilization is *moist heat,* using steam under pressure. This is known as autoclaving. Sterilization by dry heat requires higher temperatures for longer periods of time than moist heat. Pasteurization is moderate heating with rapid cooling and is frequently used in commercial preparation of milk and alcoholic beverages such as wine and beer. It is not a form of sterilization. Freezing can also kill some microbes but is not a form of sterilization.

195. (B) Even the smallest exposure to radiation can be harmful. It must, therefore, be every radiographer's objective to keep his or her occupational exposure as far below the dose limit as possible. Radiology personnel should never hold patients during an x-ray examination.

196. (B) *Emphysema* is abnormal distention of alveoli (or tissue spaces) with air. The presence of abnormal amounts of air makes it necessary to decrease from normal exposure factors. *Congestive heart failure* and *pleural effusion* involve abnormal amounts of fluid in the chest and thus require an *increase* in exposure factors.

197. (D) Before the radiologic examination begins, patients often need to change their clothing and/or remove radiopaque objects (e.g., jewelry, dentures, and braided hair) from superimposition on structures of interest. Figure 14-18 illustrates multiple *braids* of hair superimposed on skull structures. Whereas loose hair is radiolucent, hair that is braided becomes more dense and is often imaged radiographically. The ensuing artifacts can interfere with accurate diagnosis.

198. (D) Conventional 60-Hz full-wave rectified power is converted to a higher frequency of 500–25,000 Hz in the most recent generator design—the *high-frequency generator*. The high-frequency generator is small in size, in addition to producing a nearly constant potential waveform. High-frequency generators first appeared in mobile x-ray units and were then adopted by mammography and CT equipment. Nowadays, more and more radiographic equipment use high-frequency generators. Their compact size makes them popular, and the fact that they produce nearly constant potential voltage helps improve image quality and decrease patient dose (fewer low-energy photons to contribute to skin dose).

199. (C) Erythema is the reddening of skin as a result of exposure to large quantities of ionizing radiation. It was one of the first somatic responses to irradiation demonstrated to the early radiology pioneers. The effects of radiation exposure to the skin follow a *nonlinear, threshold dose–response relationship*. An individual's response to skin irradiation depends on the dose received, period of time over which it was received, size of the area irradiated, and individual's sensitivity. The dose that it takes to bring about a noticeable erythema is called the *skin erythema dose*.

200. (C) *Epistaxis* is the medical term for nosebleed. It is a fairly common, and not usually serious, event. Epistaxis is often caused by prolonged exposure to dry air, causing the nasal membranes to dry out. In this condition, the membranes are much more susceptible to bleeding and infection. The patient should be instructed to keep their head level, to breathe through their mouth, and to pinch the midportion of the nose for approximately 8–10 min or until the event has subsided.

Subspecialty List

1. Image production/image acquisition and technical evaluation
2. Safety/radiation physics and radiobiology
3. Procedures
4. Image production/equipment operation and quality assurance
5. Image production/image acquisition and technical evaluation
6. Patient care
7. Patient care
8. Procedures
9. Safety/radiation physics and radiobiology
10. Patient care
11. Safety/radiation physics and radiobiology
12. Procedures
13. Image production/equipment operation and quality assurance
14. Image production/image acquisition and technical evaluation
15. Procedures
16. Patient care
17. Patient care
18. Safety/radiation protection
19. Procedures
20. Image production/image acquisition and technical evaluation
21. Procedures
22. Patient care
23. Image production/image acquisition and technical evaluation
24. Safety/radiation protection
25. Image production/image acquisition and technical evaluation
26. Image production/equipment operation and quality assurance
27. Safety/radiation protection
28. Patient care
29. Procedures
30. Image production/equipment operation and quality assurance
31. Image production/image acquisition and technical evaluation
32. Safety/radiation protection
33. Image production/equipment operation and quality assurance
34. Patient care
35. Image production/image acquisition and technical evaluation
36. Procedures
37. Image production/equipment operation and quality assurance
38. Image production/equipment operation and quality assurance
39. Procedures
40. Procedures
41. Safety/radiation protection
42. Patient care
43. Patient care
44. Patient care
45. Safety/radiation protection
46. Procedures
47. Image production/equipment operation and quality assurance
48. Procedures
49. Safety/radiation physics and radiobiology
50. Procedures
51. Safety/radiation protection
52. Patient care
53. Image production/equipment operation and quality assurance
54. Safety/radiation physics and radiobiology
55. Image production/image acquisition and technical evaluation
56. Procedures
57. Procedures
58. Safety/radiation physics and radiobiology
59. Procedures
60. Image production/equipment operation and quality assurance
61. Procedures
62. Image production/image acquisition and technical evaluation

63. Procedures
64. Safety/radiation protection
65. Procedures
66. Procedures
67. Procedures
68. Safety/radiation protection
69. Patient care
70. Procedures
71. Image production/image acquisition and technical evaluation
72. Safety/radiation physics and radiobiology
73. Image production/equipment operation and quality assurance
74. Patient care
75. Image production/image acquisition and technical evaluation
76. Image production/image acquisition and technical evaluation
77. Patient care
78. Image production/radiation physics and radiobiology
79. Procedures
80. Image production/image acquisition and technical evaluation
81. Safety/radiation physics and radiobiology
82. Procedures
83. Procedures
84. Procedures
85. Procedures
86. Patient care
87. Safety/radiation physics and radiobiology
88. Image production/image acquisition and technical evaluation
89. Patient care
90. Safety/radiation physics and radiobiology
91. Image production/equipment operation and quality assurance
92. Image production/image acquisition and technical evaluation
93. Patient care
94. Image production/equipment operation and quality assurance
95. Safety/radiation protection
96. Procedures
97. Procedures
98. Patient care
99. Patient care
100. Image production/image acquisition and technical evaluation
101. Procedures
102. Procedures
103. Image production/equipment operation and quality assurance
104. Image production/image acquisition and technical evaluation
105. Safety/radiation physics and radiobiology
106. Image production/image acquisition and technical evaluation
107. Safety/radiation physics and radiobiology
108. Image production/image acquisition a technical evaluation
109. Patient care
110. Procedures
111. Image production/image acquisition and technical evaluation
112. Patient care
113. Image production/image acquisition and technical evaluation
114. Procedures
115. Procedures
116. Procedures
117. Safety/radiation protection
118. Procedures
119. Image production/image acquisition and technical evaluation
120. Procedures
121. Procedures
122. Procedures
123. Patient care
124. Image production/equipment operation and quality assurance
125. Image production/image acquisition and technical evaluation
126. Procedures

127. Procedures
128. Image production/equipment operation and quality assurance
129. Image production/equipment operation and quallty assurance
130. Patient care
131. Procedures
132. Image production/image acquisition and technical evaluation
133. Image production/image acquisition and technical evaluation
134. Safety/radiation physics and radiobiology
135. Patient care
136. Procedures
137. Image production/image acquisition and technical evaluation
138. Patient care
139. Procedures
140. Patient care
141. Procedures
142. Procedures
143. Image production/image acquisition and technical evaluation
144. Image production/image acquisition and technical evaluation
145. Safety/radiation physics and radiobiology
146. Procedures
147. Image production/equipment operation and quality assurance
148. Procedures
149. Procedures
150. Image production/image acquisition and technical evaluation
151. Procedures
152. Procedures
153. Patient care
154. Procedures
155. Patient care
156. Safety/radiation physics and radiobiology
157. Image production/image acquisition and technical evaluation

158. Image production/image acquisition and technical evaluation
159. Image production/equipment operation and quality assurance
160. Image production/image acquisition and technical evaluation
161. Procedures
162. Image production/image acquisition and technical evaluation
163. Image production/equipment operation and quality assurance
164. Image production/image acquisition and technical evaluation
165. Image production/equipment operation and quality assurance
166. Image production/equipment operation and quality assurance
167. Image production/equipment operation and quality assurance
168. Procedures
169. Safety/radiation protection
170. Patient care
171. Patient care
172. Procedures
173. Procedures
174. Safety/radiation protection
175. Image production/image acquisition and technical evaluation
176. Safety/radiation protection
177. Safety/radiation physics and radiobiology
178. Image production/image acquisition and technical evaluation
179. Safety/radiation protection
180. Image production/image acquisition and technical evaluation
181. Procedures
182. Procedures
183. Safety/radiation physics and radiobiology
184. Procedures
185. Safety/radiation protection
186. Procedures

187. Image production/equipment operation and quality assurance

188. Safety/radiation protection

189. Procedures

190. Procedures

191. Procedures

192. Patient care

193. Image production/equipment operation and quality assurance

194. Patient care

195. Safety/radiation protection

196. Procedures

197. Image production/image acquisition and technical evaluation

198. Image production/equipment operation and quality assurance

199. Safety/radiation physics and radiobiology

200. Patient care

Index

Note: Page numbers followed by *b*, *f*, and *t* indicates text in box, figure, and table respectively.

A

Abdomen
    acute, 45
    plain image of, 324
    quadrants and regions of, 94*f*
    radiographic examination of, 191
Abdominal pain, 205, 206f
Abduction, 97*b*
Acceptance, 21
Acetabulum, 135
Acromioclavicular joints, 127t
Acromioclavicular separation, 128*f*
Actual focal spot (AFS), 369
Acute radiation syndrome (ARS), 266–267
    central nervous system, 266
    gastrointestinal, 266
    hematopoietic, 266
    stages, 267, 267*b*
Acute abdomen, 45
Adam's apple. *See* Laryngeal prominence
Added filtration, 278
Adduction, 97*b*
AEC. *See* Automatic exposure control (AEC)
Airborne transmission of infectious microorganisms, 56
Air Kerma, 307*b*
Air-gap technique, 286–287, 340*f*
ALARA (as low as reasonably achievable) principle, 274
Alcohol-based hand sanitizers, 57
Allergen, 40, 78
Allergic reactions, 40–41
    anaphylactic responses, 42
    latex products and, 41–42
Allergy, 40, 78
Alternating current (AC), 409–411, 4410*b*
Aluminum filtration, 278
American Registry of Radiologic Technologists (ARRT), 9–10

Ethics Committee, 9
Rules of Ethics, 9
Standards of Ethics, 9–10
Amphiarthrotic joints, 106, 154
Anaphylaxis, 78
Anatomically programmed technique, 352–353
Anatomic snuff box, 111
Anger, 21
Angina pectoris, 229
Angstrom, 250, 404
Ankle
    AP projection of, 143*f*
    medial oblique projection of, 143*f*
    mortise, 130
    positions/projections of, 142*t*
Annual occupational dose-equivalent limit, 293
Annulus fibrosus, 131
Anode heel effect, 344
    conditions, 344*b*
    radiographic illustration of, 345*f*
Antecubital vein, 71, 72*f*
Antisepsis, 54
Aperture diaphragms, 274
Apophysis, 108
Appendicitis, 203
ARRT. *See* American Registry of Radiologic Technologists (ARRT)
ARS. *See* Acute radiation syndrome (ARS)
Arthritis, 108
Arthrography, 142
Arthrology, 106
Articulation, 114
    amphiarthrotic, 154
    classification, 107, 108*b*
    diarthrotic, 106
    synarthrotic, 108b
Assessment, patient's, 69
Assault, 7
Asthenic habitus, 95
Asthenic stomach, 94*f*
Atelectasis, 191
Atherosclerosis of coronary arteries, 229
Atlantoaxial joint, 156
Atlanto-occipital joint, 156
Atlas, 156
Atrophic and necrotic conditions, 343*b*
Attenuating sterile gloves, 300

Attenuation, 253
Automatic exposure control (AEC), 350–352
    backup timer, 285
    ionization chamber, 284–285, 284*f*
    minimum response time, 285
    phototimer, 285,
    positioning, 351
    technique charts, 351–352
Automatic rescaling, 349
Autotransformers, 412–413
    fixed-ratio transformer, 412
    iron core, 410
Avascular necrosis of femoral head, 135

B

Ball and socket joint, 107
Bargaining behavior, 21
Barium enema (BE) examination, 208
Bartholin duct, 199
Battery, 7, 409
Beam filtration, 9
Beam restriction, 274, 274b
    accuracy, 276
    types of, 274
        aperture diaphragms, 274
        collimators, 275
        cones and cylinders, 274–275, 274*f*
Beta-adrenergic blockers, 80
Bicondylar joint, 107
Biliary system, 196–197
    common bile duct, 196
    cystic duct, 196
    gallbladder, 196
    hepatic ducts, 196
    radiographic examinations of, 197
Binary digit, 346*b*
Biologic Effects of Ionizing Radiation (BEIR) VII report, 251
Biomedical waste 59, 62
Bipartite patella, 133
Bladder trigone, 214, 215*f*
Blood-borne pathogens, 54
Body habitus, 91–95
    hypersthenic, 93, 93*f*, 95
    hyposthenic, 93, 93*f*, 95
    sthenic, 93, 93*f*, 95
Body mechanics
    concepts, correct use of, 29–30
    physical ergonomics, 29–30

Body planes, 91, 91f
  coronal plane, 91
  median sagittal plane, 91
  midcoronal plane, 91
  sagittal plane, 91
  transverse/horizontal plane, 91
Body surface landmarks and localization
    points, 95, 95f
Body systems, 189–196
Bone malignancies, 265
Bone marrow, 108
Bone(s), 108104
  articulation, 105
  cavities (depressions), 105
  long, 106
    anatomy of, 106f
  prominences, 105
  tissue, 106
    cancellous (spongy), 106
    compact, 106
Boxer's fracture, 111
Brachycephalic skull, 170
Brain, 224
Breast shields, 280
"Breathing technique," 373, 374f
Bremsstrahlung (Brems) radiation,
    252
Bronchi, 190
Bunion, 130

C

Calcaneus, 141, 141t
Calcific tendonitis, 117
Calcium channel blockers, 80
Camp–Coventry method, 145f
Capillaries, 227
Carcinogenesis, 265
Cardiac notch, 202
Cardiac sphincter, 199, 202
Cardiopulmonary arrest, 46
Cardiopulmonary circulation, 228f
Cardiopulmonary resuscitation
    (CPR), 46
Carpal bones, 107
Carpal tunnel syndrome, 111–112
Carpometacarpal joints, 111
Carriers, 56
Cataractogenesis, 265
Cauda equina, 224
Cecum, 203, 204b
Cell cycle, cell radiosensitivity during,
    260, 260f

Centers for Disease Control and
    Prevention (CDC), 58–63
Central nervous system (CNS), 224–226,
    224f
  brain, 224
  meninges, 224
  myelography, 225, 225f
  radiographic examination, 224
  spinal cord, 224, 224f
  terminology and pathology related to,
    226
Central venous catheters (CVCs), 35
Cerebral artery hemorrhage, 224
Cerebrospinal fluid (CSF), 224
Cerebrovascular accident (CVA), 46
Cervical spine, 156–160, 157f, 158t, 159f
  fractures/dislocations of, 157
  osteoarthritis in, 158
  positions/projections of, 158t, 159f
Cervix, 222
Characteristic radiation, 252–253
Chest drainage system, 34
Chest radiography, 98
  axial and decubitus, 195t
  dextrocardia, 196f
  emphysema, 46
  PA and lateral, 193t, 194f
Choanae, 189
Cholecystitis, 196
Cholecystokinin, 196
Circulatory system, 227–232
  abdominal aorta, 229–230
  angiographic procedures, 230
  aorta, 229, 229f
  aortic arch, 227f, 229
  arteries of lower limb, 227f
  ascending aorta, 227f
  digital subtraction angiography, 363
  terminology and pathology related to,
    232
  thoracic aorta, 227f, 229
  venography, 232, 232f
  vessels, 231
Circumduction, 97b
Clavicle, 116
  fractured, AP projection of, 123f
  positions/projections of, 139
Clavicular fractures, 116
Closed-circuit television fluoroscopy, 471
Closed-core transformer, 412, 412f
Clostridium difficile (C. difficile)
    infection, 55, 61

Coccyx, 165t, 166
Code of Federal Regulations (CFR), 309
Colles fracture, 113, 113f
Collimators, 275, 275f
Colon, 203
Common law, 7
Communication
  challenges
    cultural differences, 21–22
    elderly patients, 22–23
    impediments, 21–22
    infants and children, 22–23
    medical terminology, 22
    misunderstandings of gestures, 22
    non–English-speaking patients, 23
  facial expression, 17
  with patients
    examination instructions, 20
    patient education, 19–20
    patient identification, 18
    verbal and nonverbal, 18–19
  strategies to improve, 22–24
  unspoken/nonverbal, 17–18
Compressions, 46, 216
Compton scatter, 253–254
Computed tomography (CT) equipment,
    479–480
Computerized radiography (CR),
    285
Condylar joint, 107f
Constipation, 76
Constitution, 7
Contact precautions, 61b
Contrast enema, 76
Contrast enhancement, 348
Contrast media
  contraindications and patient
    education, 76–77
  multiple examinations, scheduling of,
    75–76
  negative, 75
  patient history and use of, 69–70
  patient preparation, 74
  positive, 75
  purpose of, 75
  reactions and complications, 77–79
  for urographic procedures, 216
Contrast resolution, 324, 341
Control booth, 297, 298f
Controlled area, 297
Convulsion, 44
Coronoid process, 112, 177

Court decisions, 7
Cranial bones, 172, 172*b*
    ethmoid bone, 173
    frontal bone, 172
    occipital bone, 175–176
    parietal bones, 172
    sphenoid bone, 173–175
    temporal bones, 176
Cricoid (hyaline) cartilage, 190
Crossed grid, 336
Cultural groups, 21
Cuneiform bones, 119
Current, 407
Cylinder cones, 274–275, 274*f*
Cystic duct, 196

D

10-day rule, 263
Degenerative arthritis, 108, 343*b*, 351*b*.
    See also osteoarthritis
Deglutition, 189
Deliberate motion, 373
Deltoid tuberosity, 114
Denial, 21
Deoxyribonucleic acid (DNA), 259
Depression, 21
Destructive Pathologic Conditions, 341*b*,
    351
Detective quantum efficiency (DQE),
    362
Detector element, 458
Diabetic patients, 77
Diagnostic x-rays. *See* X-rays
Diarthrotic joints, 106
    types of, 107
        ball-and-socket, 107
        bicondylar, 107
        condyloid, 107
        gliding (plane), 107
        hinge, 107
        pivot, 107
        saddle, 107
Diastole, 228
Digestive system, 199–213
    accessory organs, 199
    esophagus, 199–201
    GI tract, 199
    large intestine (colon), 199
    layer of GI tract, 199
    peritoneum, 201
    salivary glands, 199

small intestine, 203
stomach, 210
terminology and pathology related to,
    213
Digital fluoroscopy (DF), 466, 467
Digital imaging, 498–499
Digital imaging exposure data/field
    recognition (EDR/EFR), 34
Digital radiography (DR), 395
Digital subtraction angiography (DSA),
    447, 447*f*
Direct contact, diseases transmission by,
    56
Direct current (DC), 409
Direct ion storage dosimeter (DIS), 313
Disinfectants, 54–55
Disinfection, 54
Dislocations
    of elbow, 114
    of shoulder, 114
Distal radioulnar joint, 112
Distal tibiofibular joint, 131
Diverticula, 204
Documentation, 39, 80
Dolichocephalic skull, 170
Dose-area product (DAP) meter,
    257
Dosimeter
    direct ion storage, 313
    film badge, 310
    optically stimulated luminescence,
        310–311, 310*f*
    thermoluminescent, 311–312
Double-contrast studies, 75
    of stomach and large intestine, 204
Droplet contact, 61, 68
Droplet precaution, 61
Duodenum, 203
Dynamic range, 348

E

Edge gradient/penumbra, 369
Effective dose (EfD), 258
Effective dose equivalent, 258
Effective (or projected) focal spot (EFS),
    369
Elbow
    AP projection of, 115*f*
    fat pads, 114
    lateral projection of, 124*f*
    medial (internal) oblique view of, 124*f*
    positions/projections of, 119*t*

Electricity
    alternating current, 409–410, 409*f*
        electromagnet, 410
        helix, 410
        mutual induction, 410
Electromagnetic radiation, 249–252
    frequency, 249
    wavelength, 249
Electromagnetic spectrum, 403, 403*f*
Embryonic resorption, 262
Emergencies
    acute abdomen, 45
    cardiopulmonary arrest, 46
    convulsions, 44
    epistaxis, 43–44
    fractures, 43
    postural hypotension, 44
    respiratory failure, 45–46
    seizure, 45
    shock, 45
    spinal injuries, 43
    stroke, 46
    syncope, 44
    unconsciousness, 45
    vertigo, 44
    vomiting, 43
Emphysema, 32, 191*f*, 343*b*
Endoscopic retrograde
    cholangiopancreatography
    (ERCP), 197, 197*t*
Enteroclysis, 76, 208
Epiglottis, 190
Epilation, 266
Epistaxis, 43–44
Epiphyseal line, 108
Epiphysis, 108
Epithelial tissue, 260
Equipment
    dedicated, 408
    fixed, 407
    mobile, 408–409
    motion, 373
Ergonomic transfer devices, 30
Esophageal varices, 201
Esophagus, 201
    RAO of barium-filled, 203*f*
Ethmoidal sinuses, 181
Ethical conduct, 3
Ethics, 3
    ARRT standards, 9–10
    honor/integrity, 10
    standards of, 9–10

Ethnocentrism, 22
Eversion, 97*b*
Exposure data recognition (EDR), 392
Exposure index (EI), 382
Exposure indicator (EI) values, 8
Exposure switch, 297, 439
Extension, 97*b*
Extravasation, 77

F

Face mask, 33
Facial bones, 176, 176*b*, , 182*t*
   inferior nasal conchae, 170
   lacrimal, 176
   mandible, 177
   maxillae, 176–177
   nasal, 176
   palatine, 177
   vomer, 177
   zygomatic/malar, 176
Facial expression, 17
Fallopian tubes, 221, 223*f*
False imprisonment, 7
Fat pads, elbow, 114
Febrile patient, 37
Female reproductive system, 221–224
   hysterosalpingography, 222–224, 222*t*
   ovaries, 221, 223*f*
   oviducts, 221
   terminology and pathology related to, 224
   uterus, 221
Femorotibial joint, 132–133
Femur, 134–135, 134*f*, 135*f*
   positions/projections of, 139*t*
Fertilization, 221
Fetal irradiation, 262
Fibula, 132
Film badge dosimeter, 311
Filtration, 277–278, 278*b*, 341
   added, 277
   collimators, 426
   inherent, 277
   NCRP guidelines, 278, 309
   purpose of, 277
Fingers, positions/projections of, 119*t*
Fixed kV technique chart, 351, 352b
Flat contact shields, 279, 280
Flexion, 97*b*
Floating ribs, 169
Fluoroscopic system, 464
Fluoroscopy, 287
   occupational exposure and, 293

Focal spot blooming phenomenon, 425
Focal spot blur, 369
Focal spot size, 369–372
Focused grid, 335, 335*b*
Foot
   lateral projection of, 140*f*
   medial oblique view of, 140*f*
   positions/projections of, 139*t*
Forearm
   AP projection of, 112*f*
   lateral projection of, 112*f*
Fractionation and protraction, 261
Fractures, 43. *See also* specific type
Frequency, 249, 250*f*
Frontal sinuses, 172185*f*

G

Gait belts, 30
Gallbladder, 196
   PA projection of, 198*f*
   sonographic imaging, 197*f*
Gallbladder attack, 196
Gallstones, 196
Gastritis, 202
Gastrointestinal (GI) tubes, 34
Generators, 344–346
Genetic effects, radiation-induced, 262, 265
Genetically significant dose, 264–265
Geometric distortion
   distance, 365
   factors, 363
   OID, 365
   SID, 365
Germ cells, 252
Germicides, 55
Gonadal shields
   types of, 281, 282*f*
      contour contact shields, 283
      flat contact shields, 280
      shadow shields, 280
   use of, 280
Graininess, 349, 363
   causes of, 349*b*
Grayscale, 349
Greater trochanter, 134
Greater tubercle, fractures of, 114
Grid errors
   angulation, 336
   off-center, 336
   off-focus, 336

off-level errors, 336
   upside-down grid, 336
Grids, 286, 286*f*
   characteristics, 336–340
   defined, 333
   errors, 336
   factor, 338, 338*b*
   formula, 339
   high-ratio, 286
   low-ratio, 286
   types of, 335
   use of, 333

H

HAIs. *See* Health care-associated infections (HAIs)
Hallux valgus, 130
Haversian (osteon) system, 106
Heart, 2228
   chambers, 2228
   wall, 228
Hand hygiene, 54–55
HBV infections, 58
Health care–associated infections (HAIs), 55
Heartburn, 199
Heel bone, 119
Heimlich maneuver, 33, 46
Heimlich maneuver, 33
Hematoma, 77, 81
Hematopoiesis, 108
Heparin lock, 71
Hepatic ducts, 196
Hepatitis B, 58
Hepatitis B, 58
Hepatopancreatic ampulla, 196
Hepatopancreatic sphincter (of Oddi), 196
Herniated nucleus pulposus (HNP), 156
Hiatal hernia, 201, 202
High-frequency generator, 414–415
High-Voltage Transformers, 411–412
Hinge joint, 107, 132
Hip, 149
   AP oblique (modified Cleaves) view of, 148*f*
Histogram, 347
Honor Code, 10
Horizontal (cross-table) lateral projection, 43
Hospital Infection Control Practices Advisory Committee (HICPAC), 58

Hospital personnel, 57
Hoyer patient lift, 30
Humeral fractures, 114
Humerus, 114
Hyaline cartilage, 109
Hydronephrosis, 214
Hypersthenic habitus, 95
Hypersthenic stomach, 94
Hyposthenic habitus, 95
Hysterosalpingography, 222, 224

I

Ileocecal valve, 203
Ileum, 203, 203*b*
Iliac crest, 137
Iliopectineal line, 137
Ilium, 137
Image plates (IPs), 61
Image processing
  digital display, 390
    exposure field recognition, 390
    histograms and LUTs, 391–392
    partition pattern recognition, 390, 390*f*
    postprocessing/image manipulation, 393–394
  image identification, 382
  IPs and PSPs, 497
Image quality, 323
  contrast resolution, 324
  detective quantum efficiency (DQE), 362
  spatial resolution, 324–325
Image receptors, 285
Immobilization devices, 98
Incisura angularis, 202
Indirect contact, diseases transmission by, 56
Infection
  chain of, 55–57
    mode of transmission, 56–57
    portals of entry, 57
    portals of exit, 56
    susceptible hosts, 57
  Clostridium difficile (C. difficile), 55, 61
  HBV, 58
  health care–associated infections (HAIs), 55
  hepatitis B, 58
  HIV/AIDS, 58
  nosocomial, 57

prevention and control, basic guidelines, 58–59
reservoir of, 55–56
transmission-based precautions, 60t
  airborne, 60
  contact, 61–62
  contaminated material disposal, 62–63
  droplet, 61
  by health care practitioners, 59
  patients in contact isolation, 61
  patient with compromised immune system, 62
  radiographic table and other equipment, 61
  use of PPE, 59
Infiltration, 31, 77
Inflammatory response, 40
Influenza, 56
Informed consent, 4
Infusion injection, 71
Inherent filtration, 277–278
Innominate bone, 135, 136*f*
Inspissation, 76
Intercarpal joints, 111
Intercondylar eminence (tibial spine), 131
Intercondylar fossa, 132, 132*f*
International Commission on Radiological Protection (ICRP), 316
Interphalangeal joints (IPJs), 111
Interpreter, use of, 23
Intervertebral disks, 162
Intravenous pyelography (IVP), 216
Intravenous urogram (IVU), 75, 216, 216*f*
Inverse square law, 296–297
Inversion, 97*b*
Iodinated contrast agents, 77, 79
Ionic contrast media, 77
Ionization chamber, 284–285
Ionizing radiations, 249–252. *See also* X-ray photons
  attenuation, 253
  biologic effects of, 258–262
  dose–response curves, 255, 255*f*
    linear, 255*f*, 255
    nonlinear, 255*f*, 255
  early/short-term effects, 256, 256*b*
  genetic effects, –262
    children, 264

    females, 263–264
    genetically significant dose, 264–265
    males, 264
    pregnancy, 2
  long-term/delayed effects, 256, 256*b*
  low-LET radiation, 255
  man-made, 251
  molecular effects of, 259–260
    direct effect, 259
    indirect effect, 259–260
  natural background radiation, 250–251
  risk, types of, 257
    nonstochastic/deterministic, 257
    stochastic/probabilistic, 257
  somatic effects, 265–266
Irritant contact dermatitis, 41
Ischial tuberosity, 137
Ischium, 135
IVU. *See* Intravenous urogram (IVU)

J

Jejunum, 203
Jewelry artifact, 98*f*
Joint, 106. *See also* specific joint arthritis, 108

K

Kidney, ureter, and bladder (KUB) images, 216
Kidneys, 214, 214*f*
Kilovoltage (kV), 276
Knee
  bony anatomy of, 145
  horizontal beam lateral projection of, 90*f*
  ligaments, 132, 133*ff*
Kyphosis, 154

L

Labrum, 135
Large intestine (colon), 208–209
  radiographic examination of, 197,197t 204197
Laryngeal cartilages, 190
Laryngeal prominence, 192
Laryngopharynx, 189
Larynx, 189
Last menstrual period (LMP), 263
Lateral condyle, 131
Lateral epicondyle, 132
Lateral epicondylitis (tennis elbow), 114
Law of Bergonié and Tribondeau, 258

Lead aprons, 283, 287, 298b, 299f
    attenuation characteristics of, 298b
Lead gloves, 295, 299
Lead shutters, 275
Leakage radiation, 294–295
LET. See Linear energy transfer (LET)
Libel, 8
Litigation, 7
Litigation in radiology
    errors or delays in diagnosis, 8
    guilty of assault or battery, 7
    intentional (misconduct) torts, 7
    patient falls and positioning injuries, 8
    pregnancy, 8
Light localization apparatus, 275
Linear energy transfer (LET), 259–262
Linear-no-threshold (LNT) risk model,
    255
Long bone measurement, 142, 147t
Lordosis, 154
Lower leg, positions/projections of, 131
Low-LET radiation, 255, 259
Lumbar puncture, 224, 226
Lumbar spine, 162–166
Lumbarization, 162
Lungs, 189
Lymphocytes, 260

M

Magnetic field, 410
Malpractice, 8
Mammography, 278
Mandible, 183t
Man-made ionizing radiation, 251, 316
Material Safety Data Sheets (MSDSs), 63
Maxillary sinuses, 188, 242
Mechanical ventilators, 33–34
Mechanical ventilators, 33
Medial condyle, 134
Medial epicondyle, 114, 114f
Medial malleolus, 131
Median nerve, 112
Medical asepsis, 54
Medical malpractice lawsuits, 8
Medical radiation, 251, 251b
Medical terminology of radiologic
    procedures, 22
Medications
    administration of, 70
        IV fluids and for, 71
        routes of, 68
        venipuncture, 71–72, 72f

and applications, 79t
    equipment, 70–71
    laboratory values and, 78–79
    reactions and complications, 77
Menisci, knee, 133
Mesocephalic skull, 170
Metacarpals, 110f, 111
Metacarpophalangeal (MCPs) joints, 111
Metaphysis, 108
Metatarsal bones, 119
Metformin (Glucophage), 79
Microorganisms, 53, 57
Micturition, 214
Miller–Abbott tube, 35
Milliampere seconds (mAs), 276, 276b
Mills, R. Walter, 91
Mitral valve, 246
Mobile lead barrier, 300, 300f
Mobile radiography, 61
    occupational exposure in, 293
Modulation Transfer Function, 361
Monitoring devices, 309
Motion, reducing of, 97
    deliberate, 373
    equipment, 373
    intentional, 374f
    involuntary, 97, 373
    voluntary, 97, 373
Motor control, 37
Motors, 408
Moving grid, 286, 335, 497
Multidrug-resistant organisms
    (MDROs), 56
Multipartite patella, 133
Mumps, 61
Muscle spasm, 43
Mutual induction, 410
Myelography, 225, 225f, 226f
Myocardial infarction, 229

N

Nares, 189
Nasal bones, 176, 182t, 183f
Nasal cannula, 33
Nasal prongs, 33
Nasoenteric (NE) tubes, 34–35
Nasogastric (NG) tubes, 34–35
Nasointestinal (NI) tubes, 34–35
Nasopharynx, 189
National Council on Radiation
    Protection and Measurements
    (NCRP)

on collimators, 275
    dose limits, 315b
    on filtration, 291
    patient protection, recommendations
        for, 291
    on personal monitoring, 293
    reports, 301
Natural background radiation, 251
NCRP. See National Council on
    Radiation Protection and
    Measurements (NCRP)
Needle for injection, 72, 73f
Negligence theory of liability, 8
Negligent/unintentional torts, 8
Neural/vertebral arch, 154b, 155
Neutropenic isolation, 64
N95 respirators, 60
Noise, 363
Nonionic contrast media, 82
Nonrebreathing mask, 33
Nonverbal communication, 18–19
Nosocomial infections, 57
Nosebleed. See Epistaxis
Nosocomial infections. See Health care-
    associated infections (HAIs)
NPO (nothing by mouth), 76, 78
Nucleus pulposus, 156

O

Objective signs, 37
Object-to-image-receptor distance
    (OID), 286
Obturator foramen, 137
Occupational exposure, 293–294
Occupational radiation sources
    leakage radiation, 294–295
    and NCRP guidelines, 295
    scattered radiation, 294
Occupationally acquired infection, 59
Official written report, 315, 315f
Oil-base contrast myelography, 226f
Oil-based contrast media, 5
Olecranon fossa, 112, 114
Olecranon process, 112
On a New Kind of Rays, 307
Operative cholangiography, 197, 197t
Optically stimulated luminescence (OSL)
    dosimeters, 310–311
Orbit, 171f, 172
Orbital fractures, 181
Oropharynx, 190
Os calcis. See Calcaneus

Osgood–Schlatter disease, 132
Osseous tissue, 106
Osteoarthritis, 108
Osteocytes, 106
Osteology, 105
Osteomalacia, 343*b*
Osteoporosis, 108, 160, 343*b*
  risk factors for, 108
Ovaries, 222, 223*f*
Oxygen enhancement ratio (OER), 261
Oxygen masks, 33
Oxygen therapy, 32–34
  methods of delivery, 33–34
  symptoms of inadequate oxygen
    supply, 33

P

Paget disease, 151*f*
Paleness, 37
Paranasal sinuses, 181–188
Parenteral administration, 72
Parietal pleura, 191
Parotid gland, 199
Particulate radiation, 309
Patella, 132
  tangential sunrise projection of, 146*f*
Patellar fractures, 133, 133*f*
Pathogenic microorganisms, 54
Pathogens, 54
Pelvic fractures, 43
Patient
  assistance and transfer, 29–32
    ambulatory inpatients, 29
    body mechanics rules, use of, 29–30
    elderly or thin patients, 31
    ergonomic transfer devices, using, 30
    form wheelchair or stretcher, 31
    of patients with IV infusions, 31
    of patients with tracheostomy tube,
      31
    safety/comfort guidelines, 30–32
    of sedated, senile, and in shock
      patients, 31
  confidentiality, 3–4
  consent, 4
  rights of, 3–5
  confidentiality, 3–4
  consent, 4
  rights of, 3–5
  structure position, 367
  structure shape, 367
  variables, 324

Patient's Bill of Rights, 4–5
Patient Care Partnership, 4–5
Patient dose
  beam restriction for reducing of, 274–276
  filtration, impact of, 277–278
  technical factors on, impact of
    generator type, 277
    mAs and kV, 277
Patient education, 19–20
Patient identification, 18
Patient monitoring
  assessment, 36
  blood pressure measurements, 38–39
  body temperature, 37–38
  physical signs, 37
  pulse rate, 38, 38*t*
  respiratory rate, 38
  symptoms of inadequate oxygen
    supply, 38
  vital signs, 37–39
Patient protection, 273–274
  beam restriction, 274–276
  filtration, 277–278
  grids and air-gap technique, 286–287
  image receptors, 285
  NCRP recommendations for, 287
  patient exposure, reducing, 284–285
  shielding, 279–283
  technical factors and, 276–277
Patient support equipment
  oxygen, 32–34
  suction, 34
  tubes and catheters, 34–36
Pelvic fractures, 137
Pelvic girdle, 135, 136*f*
Pelvic inlet, 137
Pelvis
  AP projection of, 130*f*, 141*f*
  bony anatomy of, 128–131, 129*f*, 130*f*,
    131*f*
  female and male, 131, 131*b*, 131*f*
  positions/projections of, 140*t*
Pericardium, 228
Perichondrium, 109
Peritoneal folds, 202
Peritoneum, 343b
Peritonitis, 76
Personnel protection
  ALARA principle, use of, 294
  methods of
    cardinal principles, 296
    inverse square law, 96–297

occupational exposure and, 293–294
primary and secondary barriers
  NCRP guidelines, 295
  protective accessories, 300
  protective apparel and care, 298–300
radiation sources and, 294–295
  leakage radiation, 294–295
  NCRP guidelines, 297, 309
  scattered radiation, 294
special considerations
  fluoroscopic units and procedures,
    301
  mobile units, 301
  pregnancy, 300–301
Phalangeal fractures, 111
Phalanges, 130
Pharynx, 190*b*
Phlebitis, 77
Peripherally inserted central catheter
  (PICC), 35
Personal care, 55
Personal protection equipment (PPE), 59
Photoelectric effect, 253, 253*f*, 247
Photon interactions, 406*b*
  coherent (classical) scatter, 406
  Compton scatter, 253–405
  photoelectric effect, 405
  tissue attenuation, 406
Phototimer, 284, 284*f*
Pivot joint, 107
Plane joint, 107
Pleural cavity, 191
Pneumothorax, 191
Pocket dosimeter, 310*b*, 312, 313*f*
Portals of entry, 57
Portals of exit, 56
Positioning and general terminology, 92*b*
  anteroposterior projection, 92*f*
  left anterior oblique position, 92*f*
  left lateral position, 92*f*
  left posterior oblique position, 92*f*
  posteroanterior projection, 92*f*
  right anterior oblique position, 92*f*
  right lateral position, 92*f*
  right posterior oblique position, 92*f*
Positive beam limitation (PBL), 276
Postural hypotension, 44
Powered air-purifying respirator
  (PAPR), 60
Pregnancy, irradiation during, 262
Primary radiation barriers, 297
Private law, 7

Prominences, 105,
Pronation, 97*b*
Proximal radioulnar joint, 113
Proximal tibiofibular joint, 132
Pubic symphysis, 137
Pubic tubercles, 137
Public law, 7
Pulmonary artery, 228f
Pulmonary veins, 229
Pulse, 228
Pyloric sphincter, 202

Q

Quality assurance, 261, 274, 274
Quantum mottle, 363

R

Radial head and neck, fractures of,
    113
Radial notch, 113
Radiation
    monitors, 310*b*
    protection rules, 296*b*
    quality factor for, 309*t*
    weighting factor, 258
Radiation exposure and monitoring
    evaluation and maintenance of records,
        313
    monitoring devices for, 309–315
        direct ion storage dosimeter, 313
        film badge, 311, 311f
        NCRP guidelines for use of, 295
        optically stimulated luminescence,
            310–311, 310f
        pocket dosimeter, 312, 313f
        thermoluminescent dosimeter, 311,
            312f
    units of measurement, 307–309
Radiobiology, 258
Radiocarpal joints, 107f, 111
Radiographer
    assessment of duty, 7–8
    burden to disprove negligence, 8
    communication skills (*See*
        Communication)
    defamation against, 8
    listening skills, 20
    patient identification and verification, 7
    pregnant, 300–301
    radiographic examinations, 34
    voice and rate of speech, 19

Radiographic circuit, 436
    digital imaging, anatomically
        programmed radiography, 446–449
    dynamic range and postprocessing,
        453–455
    exposure indication, 455
    filament circuit components, 439
    indirect and direct digital imaging, 456
        CR/DR differences, 456
        flat panel detectors, 456–458, 457f
    monitor display 458–459
    overview, 439
    photostimulable phosphor, 449
    primary/low-voltage circuit devices,
        436
    PSP sensitivity, 452
    secondary circuit components, 439
    X-ray absorption by PSP, 450
Radiographic illustration, anode heel
    effect of, 345f
Radiologic examinations, 20
Radioresistant tissue, 260
Radiosensitive tissues, 258
Radius, 107
Rebreathing mask, 33
Recoil electron, 259
Recording and Storage Systems, 472–473
Rectification system, 414
Rectum, 204
Relative biologic effectiveness (RBE),
    259,
Rem (radiation equivalent man),
    309
Renal pyramid, 214, 215f
Renal sinus, 214
Reservoir of infection, 55–56
Resolution, 324–325, 349
    defined, 349
    noise in, 349
    spatial, 361
Respiratory failure, 45–46
Respiratory system, 189–196, 189f
    bronchi, 191
    functions of, 190
    lower, 190
    lungs, 191
    nose, 190
    radiographic examinations, 191
        mobile chest radiography, 192
        positioning and selection of technical
            factors, 191–192, 181f
    trachea, 190

Rib(s), 169–170, 156f, 170t
    false, 169
    floating, 169
    fracture, 43, 169
    intercostal spaces, 169
Right to privacy, 7
Roentgen, 307, 307*b*, 308
Rotation, 97*b*
Rotator cuff, 116b, 117*b*
    injuries to, 117
Rubella, 61
Rugae, 201

S

Sacralization, 163
Sacrococcygeal joint, 163
Sacroiliac joints, 136f
    positions/projections of, 165*t*,
Sacrum, 163, , 165*t*, 166f
Saddle joint, 107f
Sail sign, 114
Salivary glands, 199, 200f, 201*b*,
Salpingitis, 221
Scapula, 107f, 114
    AP projection of, 112f
    lateral projection of, 112f
    positions/projections of, 121*t*
Scapular fractures, 117
Scattered radiation, 294, 331–333, 331f,
    331*b*
    beam restriction, 331, 331*b*
    factors, 331*b*
Scoliosis, 154
Scoliosis series, 167f, 167t, 264,
Secondary radiation, 297
    barriers, 297, 298f
Seizure, 45
Semilunar notch, 112
Sengstaken–Blakemore tube, 35
Sesamoid bones, 130
Shadow shields, 279
Shielding, 279–283, 282f
    patient position, 283
    rationale for use, 279
    types and placement of shields, 279–
        283
Shock, 45
Shoulder
    arthrography, 142
    in external rotation, 126f
    PA oblique projection, 126f
    positions/projections of, 119*t*

Sialography, 199
Sigmoid colon, 204
Sinus tarsi syndrome (STS), 119
Sinus tarsus, 119
Skeletal system, 105–108. *See also*
    Appendicular skeleton; Axial
    skeleton
  functions of, 105, 106*b*
Skin cancers, 265
Skin erythema, 266
Skull, 170, 171*f*, 172*f*
  anterior view, 171*f*
  AP axial (Towne method) projection
    of, 172*f*
  basal view, 174*f*
  baselines used in radiography, 175*f*
  cranial bones, 172–176, 172*b*,
    ethmoid bone, 173
    frontal bone, 172
    occipital bone, 175–176
    parietal bones, 172
    sphenoid bone, 173
    temporal bones, 176
  facial bones, 176, 176*b*
    inferior nasal conchae, 170
    lacrimal, 170
    mandible, 176
    maxillae, 176–177
    nasal, 177
    palatine, 177
    vomer, 177
    zygomatic/malar, 176
  fossae and principal foramina, 173*f*
  lateral projection of, 180*f*
  lateral view, 166*f*
  orbits, 181, 181*t*
  PA skull, 179*f*
  posterior view, 172*f*
  SMV skull, 174*f*, 180*f*
  sutures, 170
SLAP tears, 117
Small intestine, 204–204, 203*b*
  radiographic examination of, 197, 197*t*
Software processing algorithms, 349
Somatic effects, of radiation, 265–267
  blood cell effects, 266–267
  carcinogenesis, 265
  cataractogenesis, 265
  early, 265
  embryologic/fetal effects, 266
  late, 265
  life span shortening, 265–266

occupationally exposed personnel, 265
  reproductive risks, 266
  skin effects, 266
Source-to-skin distance, 287
Spatial resolution
  defined, 325
  factors, 325*b*
Sphenoidal sinuses, 188
Sphygmomanometer, 39, 228
Spinal cord, 224, 224*f*
Spinal injuries, 43
Spinnaker sail sign, 114
Splint, 43
Spontaneous abortion, 262
Spur formation, 130
Standard precautions, 58–63
Standards of Ethics, 9–10
  ARRT, 9–10
  Honor Code, 10
Stationary grids, 335
Statutory law, 7
Step-up transformers, 411, 413*b*
Sterile technique, 55
Sterile corridor, 55
Sterilization. *See* Surgical asepsis
Sternal angle, 169
Sternal fractures, 169
Sternoclavicular joints, 166, 168*t*
Sthenic habitus, 93*b*, 93*f*, 95
Stochastic effects, 255, 257
Stomach, 201*f*, 202, 202*b*, 202*f*
  lateral projection, 189*f*
  LPO of, 149*f*
  PA projection of, 198*f*
Stress fractures, 130
Stroke, 46
Subjective signs, 37
Sublingual gland, 199
Submandibular glands, 199
Submandibular sialography, 199, 201*f*
Subtalar joint, 119
Suction, 34
Supination, 97*b*
Surgical asepsis, 54
Susceptible hosts, 57
Sustentaculum tali, 199
Sutures, 170
Swallowing/deglutition dysfunction
    study, 201*t*
Synarthrotic joints, 106
Syncope, 44
Systole, 228

T

Talus, 131
Target theory, 259
Tarsal bones, 119*b*
Temporomandibular joint (TMJ), 107f,
    184*t*
TFT array, 462
Thermoluminescent dosimeter (TLD),
    311, 312*f*
Thoracentesis, 191
Thoracic spine, 160, 160*f*, 161*t*, 161*f*
Threshold, 255
Thumb, 109
  positions/projections of, 119*t*
Thyroid cancers, 265
Thyroid cartilage, 190
Tibia and fibula, 130
  AP projection of, 137*f*
  lateral projection of, 140*f*
  positions/projections of, 139*t*
Tibial plateau, 131
Tibial tuberosity, 132
Tissue radiosensitivity, 260
Tissue weighting factor, 258, 309
Toes, positions/projections of, 140*t*
Tonsils, 189
Trabeculae, 106
Trachea (windpipe), 190*f*, 190
Transformer, 412
Transformer losses, 412*b*
Transient ischemic attack (TIA), 46
Transitional vertebrae, 162
Trochlea, 115
T-tube cholangiography, 197
Tubes and catheters, 34–36
Tungsten (W), 423

U

Ulna, 112, 112*f*
Ulnar notch, 113
Ulnar styloid, fractures of,
    113
Unconsciousness, 45
Unsplinted fracture, 43
Urinary catheterization, 35
Urinary tract infections (UTIs), 35
Unconsciousness, 45
Units of measurement, 307–309
  gray, 308
  sievert, 308–309
Unsplinted fracture, 43
Ureter, 214

Urethra, 214
Urinary bladder, 214
Urinary catheterization, 35
Urinary tract infections (UTIs), 35
Urinary system, 214–218, 215*f*
  bladder, 214, 214*f*
  functions of, 214
  kidneys, 214, 215*f*
  patient preparation and procedure,
    215–216
  terminology and pathology related to,
    218
  types of examinations, 216
    bladder positioning for IVU, 219*t*
    intravenous urography (IVU), 216
    kidney, ureter, and bladder (KUB), 216,
      217*f*, 219*t*
    retrograde urograms, 218, 218*f*
    RPO projection, 218*f*
    voiding cystourethrogram, 220*f*
  ureters, 214
Uterus, 221, 223*f*

V

Valsalva maneuver, 192
Variable kV technique chart, 351
Vector-borne transmission of infectious
  microorganisms, 57
Vehicle transmission of infectious
  microorganisms, 56
Veins, 207
Venipuncture, 71–72, 72*f*
Venography, 232, 232*f*
Venturi mask, 33
Verbal communication, 18–19

Vermiform appendix, 203
Vertebral column, 154–156, 155*f*
  cervical spine, 156–160, 157*f*, 158*t*,
    159*f*
  coccyx, 163, , 165*t*, *166f*
  lumbar, 162, 162*f*, 163, 163*t*, 164*f*, 165*f*
  sacrum, 163, 165*t*, 166*f*
  scoliosis series, 167*f*, 167*t*
  thoracic spine, 160, 160*f*, 161*t*,
Vertebral foramen, 154
Vertigo, 40, 44
Virtual grid technology, 339, 388–389
Visceral pleura, 191
Visibility, 326–327, 326*b*, 349
Vital signs, 37–39
Vomiting, 43
Volvulus, 203

W

Wafer grid, 335
Water-based contrast media, 77
Wavelength, 249, 250*f*, 403
Wharton duct, 199, 201*b*
Whiplash injury, 157
Wrist
  bony anatomy of, 110*f*, 111
  fractures of, 111
  lateral projection of, 122*f*
  PA projection of, 122*f*
  positions/projections of, 119*t*
  radial flexion/deviation maneuver of,
    122*f*
  semipronation oblique projection of,
    122*f*
Written communication, 18–19

X

X-ray circuit devices
  autotransformer, 413–414
  transformer, 413–414
X-ray examination requests, 6
X-ray photons, 404
  interactions, 406*b*
X-ray transformers, 409
X-ray tube, 421
  "braking" radiation, 421
  characteristic radiation, 421
  component parts, 421–423
    glass envelope, 422
    filament circuit, 422
  radiographic tube rating charts, 429*f*
  safe operation and care, 427–428
    rating, 427*b*
    tube failure, 428–429
    tube limits, 428*b*
X-ray tube failure
  cracked anode, 429–430
  gassy tube, 430
  pitted anode, 428–429
  vaporized tungsten, 428
X-rays, 252, 421. *See also* Ionizing
    radiations
  production of, 252–253

Z

Zero-gravity protection systems, 299,
    299*f*
Zygapophyseal joints, 156
Zygomatic arches, 179*t*